Springer
Milano
Berlin
Heidelberg
New York
Hong Kong
London
Paris
Tokyo

A. Gullo (Ed.)

Anaesthesia, Pain, Intensive Care and Emergency Medicine - A.P.I.C.E.

Proceedings of the

18th Postgraduate Course in Critical Care Medicine

Trieste, Italy - November 14-17, 2003

Volume II

Springer

Prof. ANTONINO GULLO, M.D.
Head, Department of Perioperative Medicine
Intensive Care and Emergency
Trieste University School of Medicine
Trieste, Italy

Springer-Verlag Italia
A member of Springer Science+Business Media
http://springeronline.com

ISBN 978-88-470-0235-7 ISBN 978-88-470-2189-1 (eBook)
DOI 10.1007/978-88-470-2189-1

SPIN 10960011

Table of Contents

PERIOPERATIVE MEDICINE

Authors Index

Abbott B.G.
Section of Cardiovascular Medicine, Yale University School of Medicine, New Haven, CT (USA)

Alexander R.
Department of Anaesthesia, Worcestershire Royal Hospital, Worcester (U.K.)

Aliberti G.
Nuclear Medicine Unit, National Institute for Cancer Research, Milan (Italy)

Allaria B.
Department of Intensive Care, National Institute for Cancer Research, Milan (Italy)

Albrecht R.
Department of Anaesthesia, Kantonsspital / University Clinics, Basel (Switzerland)

Almeida de Oliveira S.
Division of Thoracic and Cardiovascular Surgery, University of Sao Paulo Medical School, Sao Paulo (Brazil)

Antolini F.
Department of Anaesthesia and Intensive Care, Faenza Hospital, Faenza (Italy)

Atlee J.L.
Department of Anesthesiology, Medical College of Wisconsin, Froedtert Memorial Lutheran Hospital, Milwaukee, Wisconsin (U.S.A.)

Attanasio A.
Department of Anaesthesia and Intensive Care, Sondrio General Hospital, Sondrio (Italy)

Auler Jr J.O.C.
Anaesthesia and ICU Department, Heart Institute (InCor), University of Sao Paulo Medical School, Sao Paulo (Brazil)

Aya Otsuki D.
Veterinary School, Heart Institute (InCor), University of Sao Paulo Medical School, Sao Paulo (Brazil)

Bandeira Margarido C.
Anaesthesia and ICU Department, Heart Institute (InCor), University of Sao Paulo Medical School, Sao Paulo (Brazil)

Baue A.E.
Former Chairman, Department of Surgery, and Donald Guthrie Professor of Surgery, Yale University School of Medicine, New Haven, CT (USA)

Berlot G.
Department of Perioperative Medicine, Intensive Care and Emergency, Trieste University School of Medicine, Trieste (Italy)

Bertin-Maghit M.
Centre for Skin Burns, Edouard Herriot Hospital, Lyon (France)

Besso J.
Intensive Care Unit, Caracas Medical Centre, Caracas (Venezuela)

Bhagwanjee S.
Department of Anaesthesiology, University of the Witwatersrand, Johannesburg (South Africa)

Boerma E.C.
Department of Intensive Care, Medisch Centrum Leeuwarden, Leeuwarden (The Netherlands)

Bossaert L.
Department of Intensive Care and Emergency Medicine, University Hospital, Antwerp (Belgium)

Busoni P.
Department of Anaesthesia and Intensive Care, "A. Meyer" Paediatric Hospital, Florence (Italy)

Butera J.M.
Department of Intensive Care, Hospital Italiano, Buenos Aires (Argentina)

Camussi G.
Centre for Experimental Research and Medical Sciences (CERMS), S. Giovanni Battista Hospital, Turin (Italy)

Candiani A.
Department of Anaesthesiology and Intensive Care, Brescia University Hospital, Brescia (Italy)

Caramez M.P.
Departments of Anesthesiology and Critical Care and Respiratory Care, Harvard Medical School, Massachusetts General Hospital, Boston, Massachusetts (U.S.A.)

Carollo T.
Department of Intensive Care, Erasme Hospital, Free University of Brussels (Belgium), and Department of Perioperative Medicine, Intensive Care and Emergency, Trieste University School of Medicine, Trieste (Italy)

Castaratato C.
Intensive Care Unit, Hospital Italiano, Buenos Aires (Argentina)

Cecchini V.
Anaesthesia and Intensive Care Clinic, University of Udine School of Medicine, Udine (Italy)

Cerchiari E.
Department of Anaesthesia and Intensive Care, Maggiore Hospital, Bologna (Italy)

Chierego M.L.
Department of Intensive Care, Erasme Hospital, Free University of Brussels (Belgium), and Department of Perioperative Medicine, Intensive Care and Emergency, Trieste University School of Medicine, Trieste (Italy)

Cooper P.J.
Cardiac Mechano-Electric Feedback Lab, University Laboratory of Physiology, Oxford (U.K.)

Corti A.
Second Department of Anaesthesia, Intensive Care and Abdominal Transplantation, Niguarda Ca' Granda Hospital, Milan (Italy)

Corwin H.L.
Section Critical Care Medicine, Departments of Medicine and Anesthesiology, Dartmouth Hitchcock Medical Center, Dartmouth Medical School, Lebanon, NH (U.S.A.)

Costa M.G.
Anaesthesia and Intensive Care Clinic, University of Udine School of Medicine, Udine (Italy)

Crimi E.
Departments of Anaesthesia and Critical Care Medicine, Division of Respirology, St. Michael's Hospital, University of Toronto (Canada)

Dalsasso M.
Department of Pharmacology and Anaesthesiology, Padua University Medical School, Padua (Italy)

Das U.N.
EFA Sciences LLC, Norwood, MA (U.S.A.)

De Angelis V.
Transfusion Medicine Department, Maggiore Hospital, Trieste (Italy)

De Gasperi A.
Second Department of Anaesthesia, Intensive Care and Abdominal Transplantation, Niguarda Ca' Granda Hospital, Milan (Italy)

de Latorre F.J.
Department of Intensive Care, University Hospital Vall d'Hebron, Barcelona (Spain)

Del Curto S.
Department of Anaesthesia and Intensive Care, Sondrio General Hospital, Sondrio (Italy)

Del Sorbo L.
Departments of Anaesthesia and Critical Care Medicine, Division of Respirology, St. Michael's Hospital, University of Toronto (Canada)

Dell'Oste C.
Department Anaesthesia and Intensive Care, IRRCS Burlo Garofolo Children's Hospital, Trieste (Italy)

Della Rocca G.
Anaesthesia and Intensive Care Clinic, University of Udine School of Medicine, Udine (Italy)

DeVita M.A.
Department of Internal Medicine, Section of Palliative Care and Medical Ethics, University of Pittsburgh School of Medicine, Pittsburgh, PA (U.S.A.)

Downey G.P.
The Toronto General Hospital Research Institute of University Health Network, Toronto (Canada)

Faybik P.
Department of Anaesthesiology and General Intensive Care, University Hospital, Vienna (Austria)

Favaro M.
Department of Intensive Care, National Institute for Cancer Research, Milan (Italy)

Feihl F.
Division of Clinical Pathophysiology, Department of Internal Medicine, Vaudois University Hospital, Lausanne (Switzerland)

Freo U.
Department of Pharmacology and Anaesthesiology, Padua University Medical School, Padua (Italy)

Galimberti G.
Department of Perioperative Medicine, Intensive Care and Emergency, Trieste University School of Medicine, Trieste (Italy)

Gallesio A.O.
Adult Intensive Care Service, Hospital Italiano, Buenos Aires (Argentina)

Gazmuri R.J.
Department of Medicine, Division of Critical Care, and Department of Physiology & Biophysics, Finch University of Health Sciences/The Chicago Medical School North Chicago, Illinois (U.S.A.)

Greher M.
Department of Anaesthesiology and General Intensive Care, University of Vienna General Hospital, Vienna (Austria)

Guarneri B.
Department of Clinical Neurophysiology, Brescia General Hospital, Brescia (Italy)

Gueugniaud P.-Y.
Department of Anaesthesia and Intensive Care, CHU Lyon South, Pierre Benite (France)

Gullo A.
Department of Perioperative Medicine, Intensive Care and Emergency, Trieste University School of Medicine, Trieste (Italy)

Haitsma J.J.
Department of Anaesthesiology, University Hospital Rotterdam, Rotterdam (The Netherlands)

Hedenstierna G.
Department of Medical Sciences, Clinical Physiology, University Hospital, Uppsala (Sweden)

Hetz H.
Department of Anaesthesiology and General Intensive Care, University Hospital, Vienna (Austria)

Hillman K.
Department of Intensive Care, University of New South Wales, Sydney (Australia)

Himmelseher S.
Department of Anaesthesiology, Munich Technical University Clinic, Munich (Germany)

Holzer A.
Department of Anaesthesiology and General Intensive Care, University of Vienna, Vienna (Austria)

Iapichino G.
Department of Anaesthesiology and Intensive Care, San Paolo University Hospital, Milan (Italy)

Illievich U.M.
Department of Anaesthesiology and General Intensive Care, University of Vienna, Vienna (Austria)

Ince C.
Department of Physiology, Academic Medical Centre, University of Amsterdam, Amsterdam (The Netherlands)

Iscra F.
Department of Perioperative Medicine, Intensive Care and Emergency, Trieste University School of Medicine, Trieste (Italy)

Ivani G.
Department of Anaesthesiology and Intensive Care, Regina Margherita Children's Hospital, Turin (Italy)

Jevtovic-Todorovic V.
Department of Anesthesiology, University of Virginia Health System, Charlottesville, VA (U.S.A.)

Kacmarek R.M.
Department of Anesthesiology, Harvard Medical School, and Department of Respiratory Care, Massachusetts General Hospital, Boston, Massachusetts (U.S.A.)

Kaestle S.
Institute of Physiology, Charité - Campus Benjamin Franklin, Berlin (Germany)

Klimek M.
Sub-department "Central Location", Department of Anaesthesiology, Erasmus MC, University Medical Centre, Rotterdam (The Netherlands)

Kochs E.
Department of Anaesthesiology, Munich Technical University Clinic, Munich (Germany)

Kohl P.
Cardiac Mechano-Electric Feedback Lab, University Laboratory of Physiology, Oxford (U.K.)

Krismer A.C.
Department of Anaesthesiology and Critical Care Medicine, Leopold-Franzens-University, Innsbruck (Austria)

Kruger A.
Department of Anaesthesiology, University of the Witwatersrand, Johannesburg (South Africa)

Kuebler W.M.
Institute of Physiology, Charité - Campus Benjamin Franklin, Berlin (Germany)

Kuppe H.
Institute of Anaesthesiology, Berlin Heart Centre, Berlin (Germany)

La Cara M.F.
Department of Anaesthesia and Intensive Care, Maggiore Hospital, Bologna (Italy)

Lachmann B.
Department of Anaesthesiology, Erasmus Medical Centre, Rotterdam (The Netherlands)

Lachmann R.A.
Department of Anaesthesiology, Erasmus Medical Centre, Rotterdam (The Netherlands)

Latronico N.
Department of Anaesthesiology and Intensive Care, Brescia University Hospital, Brescia (Italy)

Leendertse-Verloop K.
Department of Anaesthesiology, University Hospital Rotterdam, Rotterdam (The Netherlands)

Leykin Y.
Second Department of Anaesthesia and Intensive Care, "S. Maria degli Angeli" Hospital, Pordenone (Italy)

Lindner K.H.
Department of Anaesthesiology and Critical Care Medicine, Leopold-Franzens-University, Innsbruck (Austria)

Linklater G.T.
Roxburghe House, Department of Palliative Medicine, Grampian Universities Hospitals Trust, Milltimber, Aberdeen (U.K.)

López J.
Intensive Care Unit, Caracas Medical Centre, Caracas (Venezuela)

Lupia E.
Section of Clinical Pathophysiology, Department of Internal Medicine, University of Turin, Turin (Italy)

Lyons G.
Department of Obstetric Anaesthesia, St James' University Hospital, Leeds (U.K.)

Manzi R.
Department of Intensive Care, National Institute for Cancer Research, Milan (Italy)

Mariano F.
Nephrology and Dialysis Unit, Department of Medicine, CTO Hospital, Turin (Italy)

Martins S.
Institute for Health Policy Studies, University of California, San Francisco (U.S.A.)

Mazza E.
Second Department of Anaesthesia, Intensive Care and Abdominal Transplantation, Niguarda Ca' Granda Hospital, Milan (Italy)

Melloni C.
Department of Anaesthesia and Intensive Care, Faenza Hospital, Faenza (Italy)

Mercurio G.
Departments of Anaesthesia and Critical care Medicine, Division of Respirology, St. Michael's Hospital, University of Toronto (Canada)

Metzler H.
Department of Anaesthesiology and Intensive Care Medicine, University Hospital of Graz, Graz (Austria)

Milesi S.
Second Department of Anaesthesia and Intensive Care, "S. Maria degli Angeli" Hospital, Pordenone (Italy)

Montrucchio G.
Nephrology and Dialysis Unit, Department of Medicine, CTO Hospital, Turin (Italy)

Moraes T.J.
Department of Medicine, Division of Respirology, The University of Toronto, Toronto, Ontario (Canada)

Mossetti V.
Department of Anaesthesiology and Intensive Care, Regina Margherita Children's Hospital, Turin (Italy)

Muchada R.
Department of Anaesthesia and Intensive Care, "Eugène André" Hospital, Lyon (France)

Nap R.
University Hospital Groningen (The Netherlands)

Negri E.M.
Faculty of Medicine, Sao Paulo University, Thoracic Department, AC Camargo Cancer Hospital, Sao Paulo (Brazil)

Negrini D.
Department of Experimental and Clinic Biomedical Sciences, Insubria University, Varese (Italy)

Ori C.
Department of Pharmacology and Anaesthesiology, University of Padua, Padua (Italy)

Papadakos P.J.
Department of Critical Care Medicine, University of Rochester, Rochester (U.S.A.)

Parrinello M.
Anaesthesia and Critical Care Medicine, Heart Institute (InCor), Medical Faculty, Sao Paulo University, Sao Paulo (Brazil), and Department of Perioperative Medicine, Intensive Care and Emergency, Trieste University School of Medicine, Trieste (Italy)

Paruk F.
Department of Anaesthesiology, University of the Witwatersrand, Johannesburg (South Africa)

Pellis T.
Department of Perioperative Medicine, Intensive Care and Emergency, Trieste University School of Medicine, Trieste (Italy)

Petit P.
Centre for Skin Burns, Edouard Herriot Hospital, Lyon (France)

Pezzi A.
Department of Anaesthesiology and Intensive Care, San Paolo University Hospital, Milan (Italy)

Piller F.
Department of Perioperative Medicine, Intensive Care and Emergency, Trieste University School of Medicine, Trieste (Italy)

Pitzorno C.
Department of Cardiology, Cattinara Hospital, Trieste (Italy)

Piva M.
Department of Perioperative Medicine, Intensive Care and Emergency, Trieste University School of Medicine, Trieste (Italy)

Požar Lukanović N.
Clinical Department of Anaesthesiology and Intensive Care, Medical Centre, Ljubljana (Slovenia)

Prosperi M.
Department of Anaesthesia and Intensive Care, Sondrio General Hospital, Sondrio (Italy)

Pru C.
Dialysis Unit, Caracas Medical Centre, Caracas (Venezuela)

Radrizzani D.
Department of Anaesthesiology and Intensive Care, San Paolo Unviersity Hospital, Milan (Italy)

Randino A.
Department of Perioperative Medicine, Intensive Care and Emergency, Trieste University School of Medicine, Trieste (Italy)

Reis Miranda D.
Department of Anaesthesiology, Erasmus-MC, Rotterdam (The Netherlands)

Reis Miranda D.
Critical Care Medicine, Faculty of Medical Sciences, University of Groningen (The Netherlands)

Resta M.
Department of Intensive Care, National Institute for Cancer Research, Milan (Italy)

Rizzi S.
Department of Anaesthesiology and Intensive Care, Padua University, Padua (Italy)

Rocco P.R.M.
Laboratory of Pulmonary Investigation, Carlos Chagas Filho Biophysics Institute, Federal University of Rio de Janeiro, Rio de Janeiro (Brazil)

Roncarati A.
Department of Anaesthesiology and Intensive Care, Padua University, Padua (Italy)

Rossi R.
Laboratory Medicine Unit, National Institute for Cancer Research, Milan (Italy)

Rupreht J.
Department of Anaesthesiology, University Hospital Rotterdam, Rotterdam (The Netherlands)

Rupreht R.
Department of Anaesthesiology, University Hospital Rotterdam, Rotterdam (The Netherlands)

Sá Malbouisson L.M.
Anaesthesia and ICU Department, Heart Institute (InCor), University of Sao Paulo Medical School, Sao Paulo (Brazil)

Sarti A.
Department of Anaesthesiology and Intensive Care, IRCCS Burlo Garofolo Children's Hospital, Trieste (Italy)

Scheidegger D.
Department of Anaesthesia, Kantonsspital / University Clinics, Basel (Switzerland)

Schellinger P.D.
Department of Neurology, University Heidelberg, Heidelberg (Germany)

Scott Wilner L.
Department of Critical Care Medicine, University of Pittsburgh School of Medicine, Pittsburgh, PA (U.S.A.)

Semeraro F.
Department of Anaesthesia and Intensive Care, Maggiore Hospital, Bologna (Italy)

Seymour J.
School of Nursing and Midwifery, University of Sheffield, Sheffield (U.K.)

Sfogliaferri F.
Department of Anaesthesia and Intensive Care, Faenza Hospital, Faenza (Italy)

Sinagra G.F.
Department of Cardiology, Cattinara Hospital, Trieste (Italy)

Spiss C.K.
Department of Anaesthesiology and General Intensive Care, University of Vienna, Vienna (Austria)

Steltzer H.
Department of Anaesthesiology and General Intensive Care, University Hospital, Vienna (Austria)

Sutcliffe A.J.
Department of Anaesthesia and Critical Care, Queen Elizabeth Hospital, Birmingham (U.K.)

Suzuki T.
Division of Respiratory Medicine, Department of Pediatrics, the Hospital for Sick Children, Toronto, Ontario (Canada)

Taglieri D.
Department of Anaesthesiology, Erasmus Medical Center Rotterdam, Rotterdam (The Netherlands), and Department of Perioperative Medicine, Intensive Care and Emergency, Trieste University School of Medicine, Trieste (Italy)

Takezawa J.
Department of Emergency and Intensive Care Medicine, Nagoya University School of Medicine, Nagoya (Japan)

Toller W.
Department of Anaesthesiology and Intensive Care Medicine, University Hospital of Graz, Graz (Austria)

Tomasini A.
Department of Perioperative Medicine, Intensive Care and Emergency, Trieste University School of Medicine, Trieste (Italy)

Tschernich H.
Department of Anaesthesiology and General Intensive Care, University of Vienna, General Hospital, Vienna (Austria)

Ummenhofer W.
Department of Anaesthesia, Kantonsspital / University Clinics, Basel (Switzerland)

Vidyarthi V.
Medical Service, Section of Critical Care Medicine, North Chicago VA Medical Center, North Chicago, Illinois (U.S.A.)

Vincent J.-L.
Department of Intensive Care, Erasme University Hospital, Free University of Brussels (Belgium)

Vitali Serdoz L.
Department of Cardiology, Cattinara Hospital, Trieste (Italy)

Viviani M.
Department of Perioperative Medicine, Intensive Care and Emergency, Trieste University School of Medicine, Trieste (Italy)

Wenzel V.
Department of Anaesthesiology and Critical Care Medicine, Leopold-Franzens-University, Innsbruck (Austria)

Whitfield R.
Pre-hospital Emergency Research Unit (PERU), Welsh Ambulance Services NHS Trust / University of Wales College of Medicine, Lansdowne Hospital, Cardiff (U.K.)

Woodhead K.M.
Independent Operating Theatre Consultant, President International Federation of Perioperative Nurses (U.K.)

Woollard M.
Pre-hospital Emergency Research Unit (PERU), Welsh Ambulance Services NHS Trust / University of Wales College of Medicine, Lansdowne Hospital, Cardiff (U.K.)

Zecchin M.
Department of Cardiology, Cattinara Hospital, Trieste (Italy)

Zhang H.
Departments of Anaesthesia and Critical Care Medicine, Division of Respirology, St. Michael's Hospital, University of Toronto (Canada)

Zimpfer M.
Department of Anaesthesiology and General Intensive Care, University of Vienna, General Hospital, Vienna (Austria)

Zin A.
Fernandes Figueira Institute, FIOCRUZ, Rio de Janeiro (Brazil)

Zin W.A.
Federal University of Rio de Janeiro, Carlos Chagas Filho Institute of Biophysics, Rio de Janeiro (Brazil)

Zobel G.
Paediatric Intensive Care Unit, Department of Paediatrics, University of Graz, Graz (Austria)

Abbreviations

$(dZ/dt)_{max}$, maximum rate of impedance change
15-HETE, 15-hydroxyeicosa-tetraenoic acid
A-aDO$_2$, arterial-alveolar oxygen difference
ABFi, indexed aortic blood flow
ABSI, abbreviated burn severity index
Acc, intr aortic blood acceleration
ACCP, American College of Chest Physicians
ACE, angiotensin converting enzyme
ACI, acceleration index
ACS, acute coronary syndrome
AECC, American-European Consensus Conference
AED, automatic external defibrillator
AFB, atrial fibrillation
AFT, atrial flutter
ALF, acute liver failure
ALI, acute lung injury
ALS, advanced life support
AM, actual mortality
AM, alveolar macrophages
AMI, acute myocardial infarction
ANH, acute normovolaemic haemodilution
ANP, atrial natriuretic peptide
ANTU, α-naphtylthoiurea
AP, action potential
AP, arterial pressure
APC, antigen presenting cells
APRV, airway pressure release ventilation
ARDS, acute respiratory distress syndrome
ARF, acute renal failure
ARF, acute respiratory failure
ASA, American Society of Anaesthesiologists
ATLS, advanced trauma life support™
ATP, adenosine triphosphate
AV, atrioventricular
AVDO$_2$, arteriovenous oxygen difference
AVJR, AV junctional rhythm
AVJT, AV junctional tachycardia
AVS, advanced vital support
BAL, bioartificial liver
BAL, bronchoalveolar lavage
BALF, bronchoalveolar lavage fluid
BB, ß-blockers
BIS, bispectral index
BLA, bronchoalveolar lavage
BNP, B natriuretic peptide
BP, blood pressure
BSI, blood system infection
CABG, coronary artery bypass grafting
CAD, coronary artery disease
cAMP, cyclic adenosine monophosphate
CAP, community acquired pneumonia
CBF, central blood flow
CBV, central blood volume
CCM, critical care medicine
CCO, continuous cardiac output
CHD, coronary heart disease
CHF, congestive heart failure
CI, cardiac index
CIM, critical illness myopathy
CIP, critical illness polyneuropathy
CMR, cerebral metabolic rate

$CMRO_2$, cerebral metabolic rate for oxygen
CO, cardiac output
COP, colloid oncotic pressure
COPD, chronic obstructive pulmonary disease
COX-2, cyclo-oxygenase-2
CPAP, continuous positive airway pressure
CPB, cardiopulmonary bypass
CPC, Chest Pain Centers
$cPLA_2$, cytosolic phospholipase A_2
CPP, cerebral perfusion pressure
CPR, cardiopulmonary resuscitation
CRT, cardiac resynchronisation therapy
CS, chondroitin sulphate
CSE, combined spinal epidural
CSF, cerebral spinal fluid
CTD, continuous thermodilution
CTG, cardiotachograph
CTGF, connective tissue growth factor
CVC, central venous catheter
CVP, central venous pressure
CVVHD, continuous veno-venous haemodialysis
DAD, diffuse alveolar damage
DAP, diastolic arterial pressure
DC, direct current
DCCT, Diabetes Control and Complications Trial
DDR, diastolic depolarisation rate
DES, desflurane
DIC, disseminated intravascular coagulation
DKA, diabetic ketoacidosis
DNAR, do-not-attempt-resuscitation
DNR, do-not-resuscitate
DTICH, delayed traumatic intracerebral haemorrhage
DVT, deep vein thrombosis
DWI, diffusion-weighted imaging
E, elastance
EAT, ectopic atrial tachycardia
EBM, evidence-based medicine
ECG, electrocardiogram
ECM, extracellular matrix
ED, emergency department
EDHF, endothelium-derived hyperpolarising factor
EDV, end-diastolic volume
EELV, end-expiratory lung volume
EIT, electric impedance tomography
ELAD, extracorporeal liver assist device
EM, expected mortality
EMD, electromechanical dissociation
EMS, emergency medical system
EPEC, Education for Physicians on End-of-life Care
EPO, erythropoietin
ER, emergency room
ESICM, European Society of Intensive Care Medicine
ET, ejection time
EVLW, extravascular lung water
FDA, Food and Drug Administration
FDG, ^{18}F-fluorodeoxyglucose
FFA, free fatty acids
fMRI, functional magnetic resonance imaging
FRC, functional residual capacity
FT, flow time
GABA, γ-amino-butyric acid
GAG, glycosaminoglycan
GCS, Glasgow Coma Scale
GFR, glomerular filtration rate

GIC, gastrointestinal complications
GIK, glucose-insulin-potassium
GIT, gastrointestinal tract
GP, general practitioner
HAECs, human aortic endothelial cells
HD, haemodialysis
HDF, haemodiafiltration
HDLs, high-density lipoproteins
HELLP, *h*aemolysis, *e*levated *l*iver enzymes, *l*ow *p*latelet count
HELP, Hospitalized Elderly Longitudinal Project
HES, hydroxyethyl starch
HF, heart failure
HFO, high frequency oscillation
HGF, hepatocyte growth factor
HMCAS, hyperdense middle cerebral artery sign
HNP, human neutrophil peptides
HOC, hypertrophic cardiomyopathy
HR, heart rate
HRP, heart rate period
HS, heparan sulphate
hs-CRP, high-sensitivity C-reactive protein
HSP, heat shock proteins
HSR, heat stress response
HT, highly intensive/complex treatment
HTN, hypertensive
IC, index of contractility
ICAM-1, intracellular adhesion molecule-1
ICD, implanted cardioverter-defibrillators
ICG, indocyanine green
ICH, intracerebral haemorrhage
ICO, intermittent cardiac output
ICP, intracranial pressure
ICU, intensive care unit
IFN, interferon
IFNγ, interferon-γ
IGF, insulin-like growth factor
IGT, impaired glucose tolerance
IHD, ischaemic heart disease
IL, interleukin
IL-1ra, IL-1 receptor antagonist
IL-6, interleukins-6
ILCOR, International Liaison Committee on Resuscitation
iNOS, inducible nitric oxide synthase
IPPV, intermittent positive pressure ventilation
IPS, infection probability score
ISS, interstitial space
ITBV, intrathoracic blood volume
ITP, immune thrombocytopoenia
ITP, intrathoracic pressure
IUR, intra-uterine resuscitation
IVS, intravascular space
LAD, left anterior descending coronary artery
LBBB, left bundle branch block
LCX, left circumflex coronary artery
LDH, lactate dehydrogenase
LE, labelled erythrocytes
LIDO-Trial, Levosimendan infusion versus Dobutamine in severe low Output heart failure
LIS, lung injury score
LPS, lipopolysaccharide
LT, less intensive treatment
LTB_4, leukotriene B_4
LV, left ventricle
LVEDA, left ventricular end diastolic area
LVEDV, left ventricular end diastolic volume

LVET, left ventricular ejection time
LVOT, left ventricular outflow tract obstruction
LVSV, left-ventricular stroke volume
LVSWI, left ventricular systolic work index
MAC, minimum alveolar concentration
MAP, mean arterial pressure
MAP, monophasic action potential
MAPK, mitogen-activated protein kinase
MARS, molecular adsorbent recirculating system
MBL, mannose-binding lecitin
MCP, monocyte chemoattractant protein
MDP, maximum diastolic potential
MEF, meccano-electric feedback
MI, myocardial infarction
MIBI, technetium-99m-labelled sestamibi
MIF, migration inhibitory factor
MIGET, multiple inert gas elimination technique
MIP-2, macrophage inflammatory protein-2
MMP, matrix metalloproteinases
MODS, multiple organ dysfunction
MOF, multiple organ failure
mPaw, mean airway pressure
MPI, myocardial perfusion imaging
MPM, Mortality Prediction Model
MR, mitral regurgitation
MSP, maximum systolic potential
MTT, mean transit time
NABIS:H, National Acute Brain Injury Study: Hypothermia
NAD$^+$/NADH, nicotinamide adenine dinucleotide
NE, neutrophil elastase
NEFA, nonesterified fatty acid
NF-?B, nuclear factor ?B
NHS, National Health Service
NIHSS, National Institutes of Health Stroke Scale
NMDA, N-methyl-D-aspartate
NNIS, National Nosocomial Infection Survey
NO, nitric oxide
NPO, neurogenic pulmonary oedema
NPPV, noninvasive positive pressure ventilation
NPV, negative predictive value
NSCSA, National Sentinel Caesarean Section Audit
NTG, nitroglycerin
NYHA, New York Heart Association
OHCA, out-of-hospital cardiac arrest
OLC, open lung concept
OLT, orthotopic liver transplantation
OPS, orthogonal polarisation spectral imaging
PAB, premature atrial beat
PAC, pulmonary artery catheter
PAD, public access defibrillation
PADSS, Post Anaesthesia Discharge Scoring System
PAED, public access emergency defibrillation
PAF, platelet activating factor
PAMPs, pathogen-associated molecular patterns
PAOP, pulmonary artery occluded pressure
PAP, pulmonary artery pressure
PAR 1, protease activated receptor
PAWP, pulmonary artery wedge pressure
PBMC, peripheral blood mononuclear cells
PCA, patient-controlled analgesia
PCI, percutaneous coronary intervention
PCP, phencyclidine

PCs-WB, platelet concentrates from whole blood
PCV, pressure-controlled ventilation
PCWP, pulmonary capillary wedge pressure
PD, physiologic derangement
PDE, phosphodiesterase
PDGF, platelet-derived growth factor
PDH, pyruvic dehygrogenesis
PDPH, post-dural puncture headache
PDR, plasma disappearance rate
PE, preeclampsia
PEA, pulseless electrical activity
PEEP, positive end-expiratory pressure
PEG, percutaneous endoscopic gastrostomy
PEP, pre-ejection period
PF, peak flow
PFI, peak flow index
PG, prosteoglycan
PGE2, prostaglandin E2
PGI_2, inactivate prostacyclin
PGNF, primary graft non function
PGs, proteoglycans
P_{ip}, Pulmonary interstitial pressure
PIRO, predisposing factors, infection, response, organ dysfunction
PKC, protein kinase C
PMN, polymorphonuclear leukocyte
PONV, postoperative nausea and vomiting
PPS, prognosis predicting score
PPV, pulse pressure variation
Pra, right atrial pressure
PROWESS, Protein C Worldwide Evaluation of Severe Sepsis
PSVT, paroxysmal supraventricular tachycardia
PT, prothrombin time
PTCA, percutaneous transluminal coronary angioplasty
PTT, partial thromboplastin time
PVB, premature ventricular beat
PVT, polymorphic ventricular tachycardia
P_{Vx}, partial pressure in mixed venous blood
PWI, perfusion-weighted imaging
R, resistance
RAAS, renin-angiotensin-aldosterone system
RANTES, regulated upon activation normal T cell expressed and secreted
RAP, right arterial pressure
RCA, right coronary artery
rCBF, regional blood flow
rCMRglc, regional cerebral metabolic rates for glucose
RCOG, Royal College of Obstetrics and Gynaecology
RCT, randomised clinical trial
REM, remifentanil
ROS, reactive oxygen species
ROSC, return of spontaneous circulation
rPAF-AH, recombinant platelet-activating factor acetylhydrolase
RPP, Reversed Pulsus Paradoxus
RR, recovery room
RSA, respiratory sinus arrhythmia
RSI, rapid sequence induction
RVEDP, right ventricular end diastolic pressure
RVEDVI, right ventricular end-diastolic volume index
RVSV, right-ventricular stroke volume
RVSWI, right ventricular stroke work index
SAA3, serum amyloid A3
SACs, stretch-activated channels
SAH, subarachnoid haemorrhage

SAN, sino-atrial node
SAP, systolic arterial pressure
SBP, systolic blood pressure
SCCM, Society of Critical Care Medicine
SCI, spinal cord injury
SERPIN, serine protease inhibitors
SIAARTI, Società Italiana di Anestesia, Analgesia, Rianimazione e Terapia Intensiva (Italian Society of Anaesthesia, Analgesia, Reanimation and Intensive Care)
SIRS, systemic inflammatory response syndrome
SIS, Surgical Infection Societies
SNP, sodium nitroprusside
SPECT, single-photon emission computed tomography
SPV, systolic pressure variation
SR, sarcoplasmic reticulum
STI, systolic time intervals
sTNFII, soluble TNF receptor type II
SUPPORT, Study to Understand Prognoses and Preferences for Outcomes and Risks of Treatment
SV, stroke volume
SvO_2, mixed venous oxygen saturation
SVT, supraventricular tachycardia
SVV, stroke volume variation
TBARS, thiobarbituric acid reactant substances
TBI, traumatic brain injuries
TBSA, total body surface area
TBW, total body water
TCDB, Traumatic Coma Data Bank
TD, thermodilution
TDP, Torsades de pointes
TEA, thromboendoartherectomy
TEB, thoracic electrical bioimpedance
TEE, transesophageal echocardiography
TETRO, technetium 99m tetrofosmin
TF, tissue factor
TFC, total fluid conductivity
TGF-ß, transforming growth factor-ß
TIBC, total iron binding capacity
TIMP, tissue inhibitors of metalloproteinases
TISS, trauma index severity score
TIVA, total intravenous anaesthesia
TNF, tumour necrosis factor
TNFR1, tumour necrosis factor receptor 1
TNF-α, tumour necrosis factor-α
TNM, tumour, node, metastases
TOF, train-of-four
TPA, tissue plasminogen activator
TPID, transpulmonary indicator dilution
TRALI, transfusion associated lung injury
TSVRi, indexed total systemic vascular resistances
TTP, thrombocytopoenic purpura
TXA_2, thromboxane A_2
UBS, unit of burned skin
UKPDS, UK Prospective Diabetes Study
UTI, urinary tract infection
V/Q, ventilation/perfusion ratio
VACs, volume-activated channels
VAP, ventilator associated pneumonia
V_{Dalv}, alveolar dead space
V_{Danat}, anatomical dead space
V_{Dphys}, physiological dead space
VET, ventricular ejection time
VF, ventricular fibrillation
VILI, ventilation-induced lung injury
VLC, videolaparoscopic cholecysthectomy

VLDL, very low-density lipoprotein
VLS, volume loading step
VR, vascular resistance
VS, vital support
VT, tidal volume
VT, ventricular tachycardia
WHO, World Health Organization
WP, wedge pressure
ΔZ, change in impedance
η, hysteresivity

PERIOPERATIVE MEDICINE

Preoperative assessment from a clinical point of view

M. Greher, H. Tschernich, M. Zimpfer

Perioperative management and care of a patient requiring surgery represents the single most complex and cooperative task in medicine. Considering the evolutionary concept of performing perioperative medicine instead of simply administering anaesthesia, every anaesthesiologist today is confronted with the unique challenge and chance of qualifying in this field. Optimal and efficient preoperative assessment of the patient is the crucial step at the beginning of this whole process, and is often decisive in determining what follows.

This paper focuses on the objective practice and impact of evidence-based preoperative assessment with a view to reducing perioperative morbidity and mortality on one side and to achieving cost containment on the other, reviews current guidelines and standards with the aim of providing an integrated approach and finally looks into the future of preoperative evaluation on the even more sophisticated level of functional genomics.

Perioperative risk

Recent decades have seen a lot of research focused on the assessment of perioperative risk: in 1954, a retrospective review [1] of approximately 600,000 anaesthetics identified the three major causes of perioperative mortality: anaesthesia, surgery and patient disease, with a respective primary contributory roles in mortality in 1 out of 2,680, 1 out of 420 and 1 out of 95 cases in this study. This three-component concept has been maintained in subsequent work [2], and multifactorial risk indices focusing on patient disease, the main contributor to poor outcome, have been developed [3-5]. Although discussed controversially [6], large studies [7] could underline the basic validity of these indices for predicting perioperative mortality when applied appropriately [8].

The high prevalence of cardiovascular diseases in western industrial countries and the increasing percentage of older patients presenting who are eligible for surgery imply an increasing challenge to anaesthesiology, since the major cause of morbidity and mortality after noncardiac surgery are cardiac complications. Coronary artery disease is the major risk factor for perioperative myocardial infarction [9] and is considered to be associated with preceding ischaemic episodes [10]. Patients undergoing major elective surgery, such as vascular surgery, experience perioperative cardiac death or nonfatal myocardial infarction in 1-6% of cases [11-13]. Risk rates in orthopaedic surgery are comparable [14]. Considering the large number of patients who are given anaesthesia each year (an estimated 27 million patients in the United States), the medical impact and the resulting cost are substantial (approx. $20 billion annually in the United States) [15].

Apparently there is no significant difference in the rate of perioperative myocardial infarction between patients with established prior myocardial infarction and patients only at risk of coronary artery disease (3.8% vs 1.5-5%). This underlines the importance of preoperative risk assessment.

Goals of effective preoperative assessment

To decrease perioperative morbidity and mortality and to increase the quality while reducing the cost of perioperative care is one of the two major goals of preoperative medical assessment of the patient. To educate the patient about anaesthesia [16], reduce anxiety and obtain informed consent is the second important goal, but this is not discussed here.

Reviewing pertinent medical records, performing a patient interview and a physical examination are the essential first steps in identifying anaesthesia-relevant specific preexisting conditions (e.g., age, smoking, previous myocardial infarction, difficult airway, pulmonary disease, functional capacity). Based on the results, further tests may be indicated, but automated screening should be discouraged because of cost considerations and the possibility of false-positive results. At the end of this complex process, which is summarized in Fig. 1 as a pyramid, the individual risk should be estimated, leading to one of the following strategies:

1. Perform surgery under specific anaesthetic considerations and intraoperative management (e.g., transoesophageal echocardiography)
2. Postpone surgery to optimise the patient's condition, or even cancel
3. Initiate a preoperative intervention procedure (e.g., coronary artery bypass graft, PTCA, stenting, insertion of a pacemaker)
4. Give perioperative medication as a possible method of reducing periope-

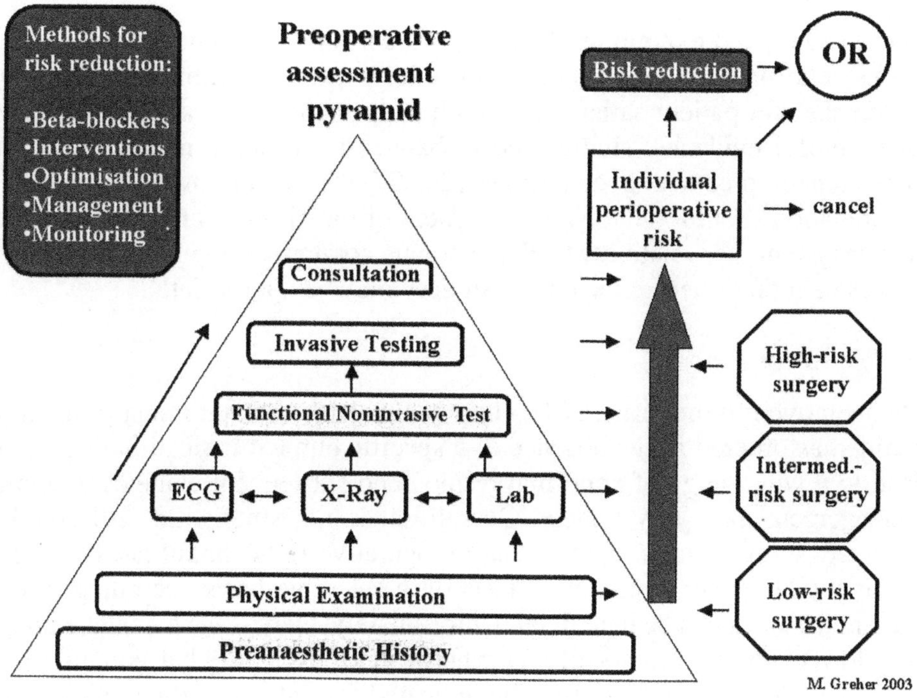

Fig.1 The "preoperative assessment pyramid", a functional flow chart visualizing the complex integrative process of preoperative decision making

rative risk (e.g., beta-blockers [17, 18], alpha-2 adrenergic agonists? [19], statins? [20])

Fortunately, recent years have seen an emphasis on strategies of reducing the risk [21, 22], rather than simply assessing it. However, the new knowledge is still surprisingly underutilised [23, 24], and its application should strongly be encouraged as a central objective of the preanaesthesia visit.

Guidelines and standards

Practice advisory for preanaesthesia evaluation

Last year, a 12 member task force appointed by the ASA published a useful practice advisory [25], issuing the following statements after a literature-based review of the current evidence.

Preanaesthetic history and physical examination

Interviewing and examining the patient is considered essential component of anaesthetic practice. Benefits may include, but are not limited to, improved outcomes and patient satisfaction. Although uncontrolled and not providing unequivocal evidence, studies show changes in resource management after detection of preexisting conditions [26, 27]. As a minimum, the physical examination should include an assessment of the airway, lungs and cardiovascular system. For relatively healthy patients not undergoing high-risk surgery, assessment on or before the day of surgery may be appropriate.

Preoperative tests

Preoperative routine tests (ECG, chest X-ray, labs tests, pulmonary function), defined as ordered in the absence of a specific clinical indication or purpose, lead to a wide range of abnormal results, and subsequent changes in clinical management may vary widely. Overall, since no benefit [28, 29] could be detected, the task force agrees, that preoperative tests should not be ordered routinely. However, performing tests on a selective basis according to each patient's history can be beneficial. Unfortunately, there is insufficient evidence to allow explicit rules specifying what test to order in what condition. For example, although an ECG may be indicated for patients with cardiovascular risk factors, age alone may not be an indication and no consensus was reached on a specific minimum age for performing an ECG. Interestingly, the only laboratory test considered indicated routinely is pregnancy testing for all female patients of childbearing age. Consensus was reached that test results obtained from the medical record within 6 months of surgery are acceptable if there is no significant change in a patient's history or symptoms or when the test plays a part in selection of specific techniques (e.g. regional anaesthesia in the setting of anticoagulation therapy).

At the University of Vienna, we advocate no preoperative tests for ASA 1 and 2 patients younger than 40 years except blood count and blood group if surgical blood loss is probable. For those over 40 an ECG is recommended, and in those over 75, chest X-ray and laboratory tests are performed in addition. In ASA 3 and higher, these tests are generally considered important regardless of age. With specific pathologies, individual decisions on tests have to be made according to the institution's standard procedures.

Cardiovascular assessment

The guidelines for perioperative cardiovascular evaluation in noncardiac surgery published by the American Heart Association in 1996 were updated last year under consideration of 400 new articles [30] and it is strongly recommended that these be read in detail. Figure 2 shows a comprehensive summary of the identified risk factors and provides an abbreviated clinically useful algorithm for risk stratification and decision making. It is important to note that clinical risk factors are classified as major (with immediate therapeutic consequences and postponement of elective noncardiac surgery), intermediate and minor (Fig.2). The traditional 3- and 6-month intervals after myocardial infarction were modified into a new concept of 7 days for acute and 30 days for recent infarction. Functional capacity is the second influential factor and is measured in METs (metabolic equivalents). The threshold seems to be a value of 4, corresponding to the ability to do light work in the house or to climb a flight of stairs. Finally, the third factor is surgery-specific risk, with a classification into high, intermediate and low (Fig.2).

Regarding supplemental preoperative evaluation, resting LV function was not found to be a consistent predictor of perioperative ischaemic events, while

Clinical predictors of increased perioperative cardiovascular risk (myocardial infarction, heart failure, death)

Major
Unstable coronary syndromes
• Acute (<7d) or recent (<31 d) myocardial infarction with evidence of important ischemic risk
•Unstable or severe angina (Canadian class III or IV)
Decompensated heart failure
Significant arrhythmias
• High-grade atrioventricular block
• Symptomatic ventricular arrhythmias (underlying heart disease)
• Supraventricular arrhythmias with uncontrolled ventricular rate
Severe valvular disease
Intermediate
Mild angina pectoris (Canadian class I or II)
Previous myocardial infarction by history or pathological Q waves
Compensated or prior heart failure
Diabetes mellitus (particularly insulin-dependent)
Renal insufficiency
Minor
Advanced age
Abnormal ECG (left ventricular hypertrophy, left bundle-branch block, ST-T abnormalities)
Rhythm other than sinus (e.g., atrial fibrillation)
Low functional capacity
History of stroke
Uncontrolled systemic hypertension

Adapted preoperative cardiac evaluation algorithm (ACC/AHA Guidelines 2002)

Questions:	If yes	If no
1. Urgent surgery ?	OR	Step 2
2. Coronary revasc.<5y?	OR if no symptoms or signs, else step 3	Step 3
3. Coronary evaluation <2y?	OR if favorable and no symptom change, else step 4	Step 4
4. Major clinical predictors ?	Cancel or delay, do angiography, evaluate	Step 5
5. Intermediate clinical predictors?	Step 6	Step 8
6. Functional capacity poor?	Noninvasive testing, if positive consider inv.test, if neg. OR	Step 7
7. High-risk surgery ?	Noninvasive testing, if positive consider inv.test, if neg. OR	OR
8. Functional capacity poor?	If high-risk-surgery, Step 9, else OR	OR
9. Noninvasive testing positive?	Consider invasive testing, if negative OR	OR

Cardiac risk stratification for noncardiac surgical procedures

High (Reported cardiac risk often greater than 5%)
• Emergent major operations, particularly in the elderly
• Aortic and other major vascular surgery
• Peripheral vascular surgery
• Anticipated prolonged surgical procedures associated with large fluid shifts and/or blood loss
Intermediate (Reported cardiac risk, generally less than 5%)
• Carotid endarterectomy
• Head and neck surgery
• Intraperitoneal and intrathoracic surgery
• Orthopedic surgery
• Prostate surgery
Low (Reported cardiac risk generally less than 1%)
• Endoscopic procedures
• Superficial procedure
• Cataract surgery
• Breast surgery
*Combined incidence of cardiac death and nonfatal myocardial infarction. Do not generally require further preoperative cardiac testing

M. Greher 2003

Fig. 2 An adapted preoperative cardiac evaluation algorithm, considering cardiovascular risk factors, functional capacity and type of surgery (following the ACC/AHA - Guidelines 2002)

stress testing is considered a class 1 indication for diagnosis of adult patients with intermediate pretest probability of coronary artery disease [31-37]. In another chapter, reviewing the impact of intraoperative management, the task force states that there appears to be no one best myocardium-protective anaesthetic technique, while effective postoperative pain management is emphasised.

The American College of Physicians has disseminated other guidelines [38], which are similar but show some differences in recommendations for preoperative tests [39].

Preoperative intervention procedures

Coronary artery bypass graft (CABG) surgery, percutaneous coronary intervention (PTCA), stenting or valve surgery may be indicated before noncardiac operations. However, the following statements can be made: clinically stable patients undergoing low- and intermediate-risk surgery will not benefit from extensive preoperative testing and revascularisation procedures [40]. A potential benefit exists for patients with prognostic high-risk coronary anatomy and noncardiac surgery. Timing of PTCA seems to be important, since a benefit could only be found with the intervention more than 90 days before noncardiac surgery [41]. Moreover, if urgent surgery is required, a patient with a recent stent implantation has to be considered at high risk [42]. In valvular heart disease, only patients with severe aortic stenosis (perioperative mortality of 10%) seem to benefit from replacement or valvuloplasty before noncardiac surgery [43].

Pulmonary assessment

Pulmonary complications such as pneumonia or respiratory insufficiency are common postoperative problems associated with substantial morbidity and mortality. After thoracotomies and laparotomies in general anaesthesia, vital and functional residual capacity are depressed to a large extent up to 2 weeks postoperatively. However, as with other preoperative examinations, routine lung function testing for all patients is not acceptable. Therefore, identification of the influential risk factors is crucial: patient anamnesis, auscultation, coughing, smoking history or dyspnoea may serve as indicators for additional tests, such as type of surgery does [44]. Arozullah et al. have developed a multifactorial risk index to predict postoperative pneumonia [45]. In another study, pulmonary complications after CABG were found to be associated with age over 70 years, productive cough, diabetes mellitus and positive cigarette smoking history in the last 8 weeks [46].

Additional areas of concern

Besides cardiovascular and pulmonary assessment, evaluation of hepatic, gastrointestinal, coagulatory, renal, metabolic, neurological and musculoskeletal diseases may have an influence on outcome.

Organisational considerations

Questionnaires [47] and computer-based evaluation systems [48] hold promise for simplification and standardised evaluation in a timely manner. An electronic record helps to ensure availability of the analysed information on the day of surgery, can offer immediate data dissemination through networking and is an important research tool. Moreover, algorithms can be implemented in the software and assist the anaesthesiologist in individual decision making.

In a cost-conscious medical system with cut-backs in reimbursement, same-day admissions are increasing, confronting the anaesthesiologist with a considerable organizational and medical challenge. Generally, centralised anaesthesia preoperative evaluation clinics represent an optimal solution with the ideal infrastructure for efficient preoperative assessment [49]. Cost reduction and a decrease in surgery cancellation are logical consequences of running such facilities, besides many other advantages [50-53]. Finally, anaesthesia preoperative evaluation clinics increase the awareness of the anaesthesiologists' clinical expertise and their central role in perioperative medicine.

Impact of guideline implementation

Guidelines for preoperative assessment are developed to improve outcome and to reduce the amount of unnecessary testing, as algorithms save money. Validation studies successfully confirm these intentions [54]. However, more effort has to be made to communicate these advantages and to train residents in preoperative evaluation [55].

Preoperative assessment in the future

With the introduction of functional genomics, a new age of perioperative risk factor identification has risen. Recently, Donahue et al. [56] have shown a linkage between the factor V Leiden polymorphism and a nearly 30% reduction in blood loss following cardiac surgery. An excellent review [57] of the influence of genotype on perioperative risk and outcome – including inflammation, infection, thrombosis or vascular reactivity – gives an insight into current knowledge and future implications for anaesthesiology. After further validation of these data in larger populations, recommendations for distinct preoperative routine genetic screening could result. With the increasing body of evidence in this field and an expanding number of variant alleles of predictive value for rational therapy, the development of evidence-based guidelines for genetic risk factor assessment will follow, by analogy with today's cardiovascular risk assessment guidelines [30]. These new tools have the potential to tremendously increase our understanding of individual untoward patient responses to surgery and could enable us to identify new patient groups at specific risk.

In summary, existing guidelines and practice advisories for preoperative assessment should be implemented increasingly in our clinical practice. Although they cannot guarantee any specific outcome or may be adapted according to clinical needs and constraints, they provide the best synthesis of expert opinion and evidence available today. Thus, we can enhance our perioperative performance, avoiding unnessessary and expensive tests while simultaneously increasing risk perception, leading to a decrease in perioperative morbidity and mortality. In this context we should, finally, always be aware of the additional obvious influence of anaesthesia provider characteristics on perioperative outcomes [58].

References

1. Beecher HK, Todd DP (1954) A study of death associated with anesthesia and surgery. Ann Surg 140:2-34
2. Lunn JN, Hunter AR, Scott DB (1983) Anaesthesia-related surgical mortality. Anaesthesia 38:1090-1096
3. Anesthesiologists ASA (1963) New classification of physical status. Anesthesiology 24:111.
4. Goldman L, Caldera DL, Nussbaum SR et al (1977) Multifactorial index of cardiac risk in noncardiac surgical procedures. N Engl J Med 297:845-850
5. Detsky AS, Abrams HB, Forbath N et al (1986) Cardiac assessment for patients undergoing noncardiac surgery. A multifactorial clinical risk index. Arch Intern Med 146:2131-2134
6. Heinisch RH, Barbieri CF, Nunes Filho JR et al (2002) Prospective assessment of different indices of cardiac risk for patients undergoing noncardiac surgeries. Arq Bras Cardiol 79:327--338
7. Prause G, Ratzenhofer-Comenda B, Pierer G et al (1997) Can ASA grade or Goldman's cardiac risk index predict peri-operative mortality? A study of 16,227 patients. Anaesthesia 52:203-206
8. Dupuis JY, Nathan HJ, Wynands JE (1991) Clinical application of cardiac risk indices: how to avoid misleading numbers. Can J Anaesth 38:1055-1064
9. Ashton CM, Petersen NJ, Wray NP et al (1993) The incidence of perioperative myocardial infarction in men undergoing noncardiac surgery. Ann Intern Med 118:504-510

10. Greher M, Wolrab C, Wildling E et al (1998) Perioperative myocardial ischemia and assessment of regional left ventricular function with transesophageal echocardiography (TEE). Acta Anaesthesiol Scand 42:181-184
11. Lee TH, Marcantonio ER, Mangione CM et al (1999) Derivation and prospective validation of a simple index for prediction of cardiac risk of major noncardiac surgery. Circulation 100:1043 -1049
12. Mangano DT (1990) Perioperative cardiac morbidity. Anesthesiology 72:153-184
13. Boersma E, Poldermans D, Bax JJ et al (2001) Predictors of cardiac events after major vascular surgery: role of clinical characteristics, dobutamine echocardiography, and beta-blocker therapy. JAMA 285:1865-1873
14. Mantilla CB, Horlocker TT, Schroeder DR et al (2002) Frequency of myocardial infarction, pulmonary embolism, deep venous thrombosis, and death following primary hip or knee arthroplasty. Anesthesiology 96:1140-1146
15. Fleisher LA, Eagle KA (2001) Clinical practice. Lowering cardiac risk in noncardiac surgery. N Engl J Med 345:1677-1682
16. Lee A, Chui PT, Gin T (2003) Educating patients about anesthesia: a systematic review of randomized controlled trials of media-based interventions. Anesth Analg 96:1424-1431, table of contents
17. Mangano DT, Layug EL, Wallace A et al (1996) Effect of atenolol on mortality and cardiovascular morbidity after noncardiac surgery. Multicenter Study of Perioperative Ischemia Research Group. N Engl J Med 335:1713-1720
18. Poldermans D, Boersma E, Bax JJ et al (2001) Bisoprolol reduces cardiac death and myocardial infarction in high-risk patients as long as 2 years after successful major vascular surgery. Eur Heart J 22:1353-1358
19. Wijeysundera DN, Naik JS, Beattie WS (2003) Alpha-2 adrenergic agonists to prevent perioperative cardiovascular complication: a meta-analysis. Am J Med 114:742-752
20. Poldermans D, Bax JJ, Kertai MD et al (2003) Statins are associated with a reduced incidence of perioperative mortality in patients undergoing major noncardiac vascular surgery. Circulation 107:1848-1851
21. Grayburn PA, Hillis LD (2003) Cardiac events in patients undergoing noncardiac surgery: shifting the paradigm from noninvasive risk stratification to therapy. Ann Intern Med 138:506--511
22. Goldman L (2003) Evidence-based perioperative risk reduction. Am J Med 114:763-764
23. VanDenKerkhof EG, Milne B, Parlow JL (2003) Knowledge and practice regarding prophylactic perioperative beta blockade in patients undergoing noncardiac surgery: a survey of Canadian anesthesiologists (table of contents). Anesth Analg 96:1558-1565
24. Warltier DC (1998) Beta-adrenergic-blocking drugs: incredibly useful, incredibly underutilized. Anesthesiology 88:2-5
25. ASA Task Force on Preanesthesia Evaluation (2002) Practice advisory for preanesthesia evaluation: a report by the American Society of Anesthesiologists Task Force on Preanesthesia Evaluation. Anesthesiology 96:485-496
26. Prause G, Ratzenhofer-Komenda B, Smolle-Juettner F et al (1998) Operations on patients deemed "unfit for operation and anaesthesia": what are the consequences? Acta Anaesthesiol Scand 42:316-322
27. McKee RF, Scott EM (1987) The value of routine preoperative investigations. Ann R Coll Surg Engl 69:160-162
28. Narr BJ, Warner ME, Schroeder DR et al (1997) Outcomes of patients with no laboratory assessment before anesthesia and a surgical procedure. Mayo Clin Proc 72:505-509
29. Schein OD, Katz J, Bass EB et al (2000) The value of routine preoperative medical testing before cataract surgery. Study of medical testing for cataract surgery. N Engl J Med 342:168-175
30. Eagle KA, Berger PB, Calkins H et al (2002) ACC/AHA guideline update for perioperative cardiovascular evaluation for noncardiac surgery – executive summary a report of the American College of Cardiology/American Heart Association Task Force on Practice Guidelines (Com-

mittee to Update the 1996 Guidelines on Perioperative Cardiovascular Evaluation for Noncardiac Surgery). Circulation 105:1257-1267
31. West JC, Napoliello DA, Costello JM et al (2000) Preoperative dobutamine stress echocardiography versus cardiac arteriography for risk assessment prior to renal transplantation. Transplant Int 13:S27-30
32. Takhtehchian DS, Novaro GM, Barnett G et al (2002) Safety of dobutamine stress echocardiography in patients with unruptured intracranial aneurysms. J Am Soc Echocardiogr 15:1401--1404
33. Sicari R, Ripoli A, Picano E et al (2002) Long-term prognostic value of dipyridamole echocardiography in vascular surgery: a large-scale multicenter study. Coron Artery Dis 13:49-55
34. Poldermans D, Bax JJ, Thomson IR et al (2000) Role of dobutamine stress echocardiography for preoperative cardiac risk assessment before major vascular surgery: a diagnostic tool comes of age. Echocardiography 17:79-91
35. Dhond MR, Nguyen TT, Sabapathy R et al (2003) Dobutamine stress echocardiography in preoperative and long-term postoperative risk assessment of elderly patients. Am J Geriatr Cardiol 12:107-109, 112
36. Das MK, Pellikka PA, Mahoney DW et al (2000) Assessment of cardiac risk before nonvascular surgery: dobutamine stress echocardiography in 530 patients. J Am Coll Cardiol 35:1647-1653
37. Bossone E, Martinez FJ, Whyte RI et al (1999) Dobutamine stress echocardiography for the preoperative evaluation of patients undergoing lung volume reduction surgery. J Thorac Cardiovasc Surg 118:542-546
38. (1997) Guidelines for assessing and managing the perioperative risk from coronary artery disease associated with major noncardiac surgery. American College of Physicians. Ann Intern Med 127:309-312
39. Gordon AJ, Macpherson DS (2003) Guideline chaos: conflicting recommendations for preoperative cardiac assessment. Am J Cardiol 91:1299-1303
40. Metzler H (2003) Lowering cardiac risk by preoperative interventions. Minerva Anestesiol 69:412-415
41. Posner KL, Van Norman GA, Chan V (1999) Adverse cardiac outcomes after noncardiac surgery in patients with prior percutaneous transluminal coronary angioplasty. Anesth Analg 89:553-560
42. Kaluza GL, Joseph J, Lee JR et al (2000) Catastrophic outcomes of noncardiac surgery soon after coronary stenting. J Am Coll Cardiol 35:1288-1294
43. Bonow RO, Carabello B, de Leon AC et al (1998) ACC/AHA Guidelines for the Management of Patients With Valvular Heart Disease. Executive Summary. A report of the American College of Cardiology/American Heart Association Task Force on Practice Guidelines (Committee on Management of Patients With Valvular Heart Disease). J Heart Valve Dis 7:672-707
44. Pate P, Tenholder MF, Griffin JP et al (1996) Preoperative assessment of the high-risk patient for lung resection. Ann Thorac Surg 61:1494-1500
45. Arozullah AM, Khuri SF, Henderson WG et al (2001) Development and validation of a multifactorial risk index for predicting postoperative pneumonia after major noncardiac surgery. Ann Intern Med 135:847-857
46. Hulzebos EH, Van Meeteren NL, De Bie RA et al (2003) Prediction of postoperative pulmonary complications on the basis of preoperative risk factors in patients who had undergone coronary artery bypass graft surgery. Phys Ther 83:8-16
47. Badner NH, Craen RA, Paul TL et al (1998) Anaesthesia preadmission assessment: a new approach through use of a screening questionnaire. Can J Anaesth 45:87-92
48. Essin DJ, Dishakjian R, deCiutiis VL et al (1998) Development and assessment of a computer-based preanesthetic patient evaluation system for obstetrical anesthesia. J Clin Monit Comput 14:95-100
49. van Klei WA, Moons KG, Rutten CL et al (2002) The effect of outpatient preoperative evaluation of hospital inpatients on cancellation of surgery and length of hospital stay (table of contents). Anesth Analg 94:644-649

50. Fischer SP (1996) Development and effectiveness of an anesthesia preoperative evaluation clinic in a teaching hospital. Anesthesiology 85:196-206
51. Pollard JB, Zboray AL, Mazze RI (1996) Economic benefits attributed to opening a preoperative evaluation clinic for outpatients. Anesth Analg 83:407-410
52. Pollard JB, Olson L (1999) Early outpatient preoperative anesthesia assessment: does it help to reduce operating room cancellations? Anesth Analg 89:502-505
53. Pollard JB, Garnerin P (1999) Outpatient preoperative evaluation clinic can lead to a rapid shift from inpatient to outpatient surgery: a retrospective review of perioperative setting and outcome. J Clin Anesth 11:39-45
54. Greer AE, Irwin MG (2002) Implementation and evaluation of guidelines for preoperative testing in a tertiary hospital. Anaesth Intensive Care 30:326-330
55. Tsen LC, Segal S, Pothier M et al (2000) Survey of residency training in preoperative evaluation. Anesthesiology 93:1134-1137
56. Donahue BS, Gailani D, Higgins MS et al (2003) Factor V Leiden protects against blood loss and transfusion after cardiac surgery. Circulation 107:1003-1008
57. Ziegeler S, Tsusaki BE, Collard CD (2003) Influence of genotype on perioperative influence and outcome. Anesthesiology 99:212-219
58. Silber JH, Kennedy SK, Even-Shoshan O et al (2002) Anesthesiologist board certification and patient outcomes. Anesthesiology 96:1044-1052

Intraoperative volume optimisation

M. Parrinello, L.M. Sá Malbouisson, J.O.C. Auler

Cardiovascular monitoring

The accurate estimation of effective intravascular volume is of great importance in patients after major vascular procedures. The main goal of achieving an adequate preload is to improve the ability of the left ventricle to cope with alterations in contractility or afterload and maintain cardiac output. Because major surgical procedures are associated with imperceptible fluid losses, blood loss, large amounts of intravenous fluids, and underlying cardiovascular pathology, patients may have either inadequate or excessive preload postoperatively. Volume status is particularly difficult to assess during the early recovery period during which mechanical ventilation is still necessary. There are several reasons why conventional haemodynamic monitoring may give a poor indication of changes in intravascular volume. During anaesthesia, hypovolaemia occurs frequently without being accompanied by tachycardia. This is because baroreflexes are depressed by anaesthetic agents and because the volume receptors in the right atrium are unloaded by the decreased venous return.

The kind of haemodynamic monitors used during a given surgical procedure must reflect a balance between invasiveness and the ability to obtain enough knowledge to manage haemodynamics, and the outcome of surgical patients can be improved following early recognition and treatment of haemodynamic problems. Haemodynamic monitoring should be able to provide direct measures or estimates of afterload, preload and contractility, which are components of Starling's law. According to this law, the relationship between preload and contractility is not linear but, rather, curvilinear. Thus, only if the ventricle works on the ascending portion of the relationship (preload-dependence) can an increase in preload increase the stroke volume. This mechanism provides a functional reserve (preload reserve) to the heart in situation of acute stress [1] and highlights the need to use haemodynamic monitors that can predict volume expansion efficacy in order to avoid fluid overload and differentiate between responder and nonresponder patients to fluid therapy. In this chapter, we will review some methods of assessing volume expansion efficacy and some aspects of the fluid solutions currently used to correct volaemia replacement during the intraoperative period.

Pulmonary artery catheter

The pulmonary artery catheter (PAC) was introduced into clinical practice three decades ago and its use has continued without definitive evidence of decreased morbidity or mortality [2]. In 1996, Connors et al. [3] examined the association between PAC use during the first 24 hours of intensive care and subsequent survival. In that study, PAC-monitored patients had increased mortality, longer hospital stay and higher costs. Recently, Sandham et al. [4] found no benefit in therapy directed by PAC over standard care in elderly, high-risk surgical patients requiring intensive care but there was a significant increase in the incidence of pulmonary embolism in the PAC group. However, the pulmonary artery catheter remains the most popular means of continuous monitoring of cardiac index, mixed venous oxygen saturation, pulmonary artery pressure and pulmonary capillary wedge pressure (PCWP).

The left and right cardiac filling pressures, central venous pressure (CVP) and PCWP are the parameters most frequently used to estimate ventricular preload and make decisions on volume expansion during the anaesthetic procedure. Central venous and pulmonary artery catheterisation are procedures that are easy to accomplish and are available in most surgical rooms. On the other hand, clinical studies have emphasised the low value of CVP and PCWP in predicting volume expansion efficacy [5]. Some conditions frequently present during an anaesthetic procedure, such as altered ventricular compliance, mechanical ventilation with PEEP, valvular regurgitation or stenosis, can induce bias in the interpretation of CVP and PCWP as well as its responses to fluid infusion.

An estimation of cardiac output (CO) is essential to quote cardiac function based on Frank-Starling diagrams. Nowadays, in the great majority of ICUs and operating rooms, CO is measured by injecting an exact amount of fluid (saline or dextrose) of known temperature into the right atrium and then using a thermistor in the pulmonary artery to detect the resultant change in blood temperature. CO is inversely proportional to the area under the temperature versus time curve.

Left ventricular end-diastolic volume (LVEDV) is not usually measured but estimated and is a major determining factor of CO. Thermodilution CO associated with radionuclide ejection fraction (and the calculation of LVEDV) is the most accurate method of determining cardiac performance in the ICU. However, this technique cannot be used as a bedside routine to assess LVEDV, owing to several limitations. New generation of PAC and volumetric assessment of end-diastolic volume (EDV) are designed to enable the monitoring of haemodynamic pressures and provide continuous cardiac output (CCO) and continuous right ventricular EDV, as well as mixed venous oxygen saturation (SvO_2). Continuous cardiac output measurements are made by periodically warming the blood in the right atrium or ventricle by 0.2 deg C each 30 seconds, the opposite procedure to that used during bolus thermodilution. Continuous volumetric data are calculated from CCO measurements and heart rate from a "salved" ECG signal. From the ejection fraction and CO measurements recorded by the volumetric PAC, stroke volume and systolic and diastolic volume of the right ventricle are estimated. Although in many clinical situations CCO catheter utilisation is growing, replacing traditional boluses for CO determination, some limitations should be considered. Poli de Figueiredo et cols. [6] found that CCO monitoring was not able to detect acute changes in cardiac output induced by haemorrhage and resuscitation in dogs when compared to cardiac output measured by an ultrasonic probe placed in the main pulmonary artery. The cardiac output presented a 3 to 5 minutes delay in response during acute haemodynamic changes.

Right ventricular end-diastolic volume (RVEDV) has also been proposed as an indicator of preload responsiveness in hypovolaemic patients. Data from clinical studies are conflicting as regards the usefulness of RVEDV versus PCWP as a parameter of fluid infusion responsiveness. Wagner and Leatherman [7] found that RVEDV was not a reliable predictor of the response to fluid in critically ill patients. As a predictor of fluid responsiveness PCWP was superior to RVEDV. On the other hand, Diebel and colleagues [8] also found in critically ill patients that RVEDV was a more accurate predictor of preload levels that would increase CO than was PCWP.

Continuous oesophageal Doppler

Recently, continuous oesophageal Doppler measurements of cardiac output have been proposed as a noninvasive alternative to PAC in critically ill patients [9]. Development of the transoesophageal ultrasound probe combining echographic flow meter (M-mode) and pulsed Doppler measurements has enabled a noninvasive approach to real-time and continuous monitoring of cardiac function. The primary value of measuring CO noninvasively and in real time with a transoesophageal ultrasound probe is the possibility of an immediate, complete, left-ventricular flow-based assessment of the net effects of changes in the haemodynamic components, i.e., stroke volume, heart rhythm, preload, contractility and afterload. The standard of operation is based on the simultaneous, independent, real-time ultrasound measurements of aortic cross section and blood velocity, to determine the instantaneous descending aortic blood flow, which is a measurement of CO. The oesophageal transducer is inserted into the patient's oesophagus, by either the oral or the nasal route, and its position is guided externally according to the aortic blood flow wave morphology. In the transoesophageal probe, one transducer is an M-mode echograph at 10 MHz, and the other is a pulsed Doppler transducer at 5 MHz, which measures blood velocity. The aortic blood flow is determined, in each cardiac cycle, by two simultaneous local measurements. Stroke volume can be calculated by multiplying this average blood velocity during a systolic cycle by the ejection time (stroke distance) and by the cross-sectional area through which the blood flows. Despite potential sources of error, a good correlation has been demonstrated between the CO measured by oesophageal Doppler and simultaneously by thermodilution and Fick methods [10, 11]. Aside from providing continuous real-time monitoring of CO, the characteristics of the Doppler flow-velocity waveform provide information on both cardiac preload and contractility. The peak-flow velocity that is readily identified as the apex of the waveform is a good indicator of myocardial contractility. Furthermore, the left ventricular ejection time (or flow-time) corrected for heart rate gives an index of preload. Based on these parameters, it is possible to construct preload versus cardiac output beat by beat. Singer et al. [12] demonstrated a good correlation between the corrected flow time (Ftc) and changes in preload when preload was increased from hypovolaemic states. On the other hand, factors such as aortic disease, probe displacement or even failure to reposition the probe prior to each measurement may lead to biased measurements of CO and poor conformity with other techniques [13].

Transoesophageal echocardiography

Transoesophageal echocardiography (TEE) is considered the principal tool for the assessment of left ventricular diastolic function during anaesthesia. Left ventricular filling and pulmonary venous Doppler flow parameters have been utilised to assess relaxation, stiffness and left ventricular filling pressure [14]. TEE is considered the "gold standard" instrument to evaluate the anatomic structure of the heart during cardiac surgery. Additionally, some authors suggest that the haemodynamic evaluation provided by TEE investigation bears more relation to the actual cardiovascular function than the data derived from haemodynamic measurements obtained using PAC [15]. In a recent cross-sectional survey among anaesthesiologists from USA and Canada, Jacka et al. [16] reported that the PAC is widely used during anaesthesia for cardiac and vascular surgery, while TEE is often employed in cardiac valve surgery. According to these authors, rather than simply replacing the PAC, TEE may currently be used to examine specific aspects of morphology and cardiovascular function and provide complementary information to the data obtained using the PAC. Aside from morphologic diagnosis of heart and great vessels, systolic function is quantitatively measured during the TEE evaluation, allowing computation of ejection fraction and myocardial fibre shortening fraction. Cardiac output can be obtained by the Doppler method, by multiplying the flow velocity time integral over mitral, aortic or pulmonary valve, valve area and heart rate. From evaluation of the transmitral and pulmonary venous flow pattern it is possible to estimate both diastolic compliance and filling pressures. Recently, it was shown that analysis of changes of the early filling wave velocity and its deceleration time during an acute change of cardiac load enabled the identification of patients with deficient length-dependent regulation of myocardial function [17]. In conjunction with a decreased dP/dtmax and an increase in end-diastolic pressure, these patients demonstrated a typically restrictive pattern (increased early to late filling wave velocity ratio in combination with a shortened deceleration time). Lattik et al. [18] demonstrated that the mitral flow Doppler measurement is superior to haemodynamic variables and two- dimensional echocardiography variables in prediction of the increase in CO after fluid challenge submitted to a cardiac surgery.

Preload can also be estimated using TEE through direct measurement from end-diastolic area or estimations of the LVEDV from cavity dimensions. It is also possible to estimate the PCWP from a color M-mode Doppler study of left ventricular filling and Doppler tissue imaging. However, there is no consensus on whether parameters derived from TEE can accurately estimate the correct preload necessary to improve CO. Tavernier et al. [19] have demonstrated that neither conventional PCWP nor end-diastolic area derived from TEE could guide fluid therapy in patients with sepsis-induced hypotension. A recent study [20] has shown that in patients with postoperative circulatory shock and acute lung injury, echocardiographic estimation of PCWP may not be accurate enough to be used for adjusting therapy.

Data obtained by echocardiography can have a significant impact on a patient's treatment, but this monitoring technique requires a high standard of training and experience, and the cost is very high in comparison to the other monitoring devices.

Systolic pressure variation

Systolic arterial pressure variations (SPV) through the respiratory cycle are assumed to be a dynamic indicator of the sensitivity of the heart to changes in preload conditions induced by pleural pressure changes. These respiration-induced changes in arterial pressure have also been proposed as good predictors of the response to volume loading. The magnitude of the respiratory changes in LV stroke volume could be a good indicator of biventricular preload dependence [21].

Left ventricular stroke volume is a major determinant of systolic arterial pressure. Analysis of respiratory changes in systolic pressure has been proposed to assess the respiratory change in LV stroke volume during mechanical ventilation. The movement of pressurised air inside the alveoli decreases preload and increases afterload of the right ventricle [22]. The inspiratory increase in pleural pressure decreases the venous return pressure gradient with a decrease in RV preload. Afterload increase is due to the elevation in transpulmonary pressure (alveolar minus pleural pressure). The inspiratory reduction in RV ejection leads to a decrease in LV filling, with a consequent decrease in LV stroke volume. Interestingly, a slight augmentation in LV stroke volume may be observed during the inspiratory phase. Two mechanisms may occur: firstly, blood squeezing out of alveolar vessels during mechanical lung inflation, which may lead to an increase in LV preload, and secondly, the inspiratory increase in pleural pressure, which may decrease LV afterload and thus facilitate LV ejection [23].

The systolic pressure variation (SPV) over a respiratory cycle presents two components: Δup and Δdown. Δup is the difference between the maximal value of systolic pressure over a single respiratory cycle and the reference systolic pressure obtained during a brief period of apnoea obtained by means of an end-expiratory pause. It reflects the inspiratory increase in systolic pressure and LV stroke volume, due to blood acceleration from alveolar vessels into LV. Δdown is the difference between the reference systolic pressure and the minimal value of systolic pressure over a single respiratory cycle. It reflects the transient decline of venous return and the expiratory decrease in LV preload and stroke volume related to the inspiratory decrease in RV stroke volume. Perel and colleagues [24] demonstrate that Δdown represents the main component of SPV. In hypovolaemia there is an increase in Δdown and, in contrast, volume expansion decreases. Recently, Δdown has been proposed as an indicator of fluid responsiveness. In patients with sepsis-induced hypotension, Tavenier et al. [19] found that the Δdown was significantly greater in volume infusion responders than in non-responders. These authors also reported that there was a positive and robust relationship between the baseline value of Δdown and the percentage of increase in stroke volume in response to volume expansion. They also suggest that Δdown is a more sensitive indicator of the response of CO to volume infusion than PCWP or end-diastolic area obtained by echocardiography. In contrast, Denault et al. [25] could not demonstrate, in anaesthetised cardiac surgery patients, any relationship between LV measured by transoesophageal echocardiography and SPV, proposing that changes in systolic pressure may reflect changes in airway pressure and pleural pressure rather than changes in LV haemodynamics.

Arterial pulse contour-PiCCO system

Wesseling et al. [26] describe continuous cardiac output measurement using the pulse contour cardiac output principle. This method measures the area under the systolic portion of the arterial wave tracing and is proportional to the stroke volume and inversely related to arterial compliance. Comparison of this technique with the conventional thermodilution technique was performed in cardiac surgery and intensive care unit patients [27]. Michard et al. [28] show that this technique can be used to predict adverse haemodynamic effects of PEEP. The pulse contour is not influenced by mechanical ventilation, because the change in pleural pressure affects both diastolic and systolic pressure. Recently Wiesenack et al. [29] have shown that SVV (stroke volume variation) derived from pulse contour analysis cannot serve as variable of fluid responsiveness in mechanically ventilated cardiac surgery patients. In contrast, Reuter et al. [30] have demonstrated the ability of this technique to predict myocardial responsiveness to volume administration, but they used a large tidal volume (15 ml/kg) which can possibly influence SVV assessment.

The continuous pulse contour analysis has also become available with the PiCCO system (Pulsion Medical System, Munich, Germany), which displays a SVV number that it evaluates from the variation in calculated LV stroke volume over a short time interval. The PiCCO system also calculates the arterial cardiac index, the global end-diastolic volume index, the intrathoracic blood volume index (ITBVI) and the extravascular lung water (EVLW) with the transpulmonary indicator dilution (TPID) using the single indicator dilution technique. Originally, ITBVI and EVLW measurements required the use of a double indicator technique that combined thermodilution and dye-dilution and required the simultaneous central venous injection of two indicators, one of which is distributed into the extravascular space while the other remains in the intravascular compartment. After bolus injection, the washout curves are detected in the femoral artery. With the PiCCO system these variables can now be obtained using thermodilution alone, needing only a central venous catheter for indicator injection and a thermistor-tipped femoral artery catheter for detection.

Perel et al. [31] have reported the successful use of an axillary artery catheter to make the thermodilution measurement. Some studies have demonstrated the ability of ITBVI and SVV to predict preload, particularly in cardiac surgery patients and in the critically ill setting [32, 33]. Della Rocca and colleagues evaluated the relationship between PCWP and the volume preload variable derived from the PiCCO system during lung transplantation. These authors conclude that the assessment of ITBVI by the TPID provides a valid index of cardiac preload that may be superior to PAWP [34].

Volume replacement

Adequate volume replacement is fundamental in the management of surgical patients. The main goal of achieving an adequate preload is to improve the ability of the left ventricle to cope with alterations in contractility or afterload and maintain cardiac output and oxygen transport. Absolute or relative blood volume deficit often occurs during surgery as result of bleeding and imperceptible fluid losses. Hypovolaemia with normal extracellular volume can also result from any disorder that alters the balance between the intravascular and extravascular fluid compartments by increasing vascular permeability. This condition is most frequently observed in patients with a systemic inflammatory response syndrome secondary to sepsis, trauma, shock or major surgical procedures such as cardiac surgery with cardiopulmonary bypass and major vascular surgery [35].

During hypovolaemic states, the organism attempts to compensate for the hypovolaemia-related perfusion deficits by redistribution of flow to vital organs (heart and brain), resulting in hypoperfusion of gut, kidneys, muscles and skin owing to activation of the sympathetic, renin-angiotensin-aldosterone and antidiuretic systems. These compensatory mechanisms cannot adequately compensate hypovolaemia. Systemic organ failure and death may occur as a consequence of sustained organic hypoperfusion.

Several kinds of fluid replacement solutions are available to treat intraoperative hypovolaemia. These solutions can be grouped into two broad categories: crystalloids and colloids. The choice between a colloid and a crystalloid solution is still controversial [36]. Arguments in favour of the use of crystalloids include the observation that postoperative organ function appears to be improved. Moreover, crystalloids can minimise the risk of anaphylactic reactions and they cost less than colloids, but crystalloids may predispose to pulmonary and peripheral oedema [37]. Colloid resuscitation requires less volume and time and has also been shown to improve oxygen transport, myocardial contractility and cardiac output [38]. Meta-analyses comparing colloids with crystalloids have reached divergent conclusions. Schierhout and Roberts [39] report that resuscitation with colloids is associated with an increased absolute risk of mortality of 4%. In a systematic review comparing crystalloids and colloids in fluid resuscitation, Choi et al. [40] did not demonstrate any differences in mortality, pulmonary oedema or length of stay between crystalloid- and colloid-treated patients. A trend suggesting lower mortality with crystalloids was not statistically significant. The controversy does not only concern the crystalloid vs colloid debate, but also what kind of crystalloid or colloid solution is best in the intraoperative period. Evaluating a postal survey questionnaire sent to 451 ICUs in Germany, Boldt and colleagues [41] show that there are no standards for volume therapy. Hydroxyethyl starch (HES) solution was the solution most often used for volume replacement (total: 193 ICUs, exclusively HES: 93 ICUs), crystalloids were next (crystalloids exclusively: 61 ICUs), and human albumin was rarely used as the first choice. Sepsis, coagulation disorders and renal and liver insufficiency were situations in which albumin solution was still used for volume replacement. Nonetheless, there is a large body of evidence in the literature suggesting that HES preparations have only a minor influence on coagulation [42].

Crystalloids

Crystalloids can be divided into hypotonic (dextrose in water), isotonic (lactate Ringer's solution) and hypertonic solutions (7.5% saline solution). Crystalloids can permeate freely across the vascular membrane and are therefore distributed in the plasma and interstitial or intercellular fluid compartments [43]. Taking into account the redistribution of fluid to extravascular spaces, a crystalloid volume approximately three to four times the intravascular volume deficit is required to correct hypovolaemia. This partitioning begins immediately after fluid infusion. Within 2 hours, less than 25% of the infused fluid remains within the intravascular space. Excessive administration of crystalloids is accompanied by a critical reduction in plasma colloid oncotic pressure with the risk of generalised oedema. Massive crystalloid resuscitation alone is less likely to achieve adequate restoration of blood flow and tissue oxygenation. Using an animal haemorrhagic shock model, Wang et al. [44] investigated the quality of fluid resuscitation by laser Doppler flowmetry. They conclude that lactated Ringer's solution is not able to restore microvascular perfusion correctly. These results are in accordance with those from Funk and Baldinger [45], who report that volume replacement with artificial colloids yields haemodynamic stability and adequate tissue oxygen supply, whereas administration of crystalloids alone jeopardises tissue perfusion and oxygenation. Although several authors argue that crystalloids alone appear to be less effective in restoring intravascular volume deficits in the hypovolaemic patient [42], controversy persists.

Hypertonic saline solutions

Hypertonic saline solutions are crystalloids that contain sodium in supraphysiological concentrations. They expand the extracellular space by exerting an osmotic effect that displaces water from the intracellular compartment to extracellular space. They mobilise endogenous fluid from endothelial cells, whereupon the plasma volume rapidly increases and so does microcirculatory blood flow. Human use of 7.5% NaCl solutions began with Felipe et al. [46], treating patients with refractory shock in a critical care unit and showing haemodynamic benefits. The cardiovascular improvement following hypertonic solution administration is observed immediately after infusion and has been attributed to plasma volume expansion, vasodilatation of vascular beds and a direct cardiac inotropic effect [47]. The addition of 6% dextrane-70 to the hypertonic solution (HSD) does not add to the initial plasma expansion; however, it does contribute to the maintenance of the fluid in the intravascular compartment for a longer period and exhibits an additive acute circulatory effect [48]. With the introduction of hypertonic saline solutions, the concept of small-volume resuscitation came into clinical practice. Defined as bolus infusion of 4 ml/kg of hypertonic solution within 2-5 minutes, a substantial clinical experience has been accumulated with small-volume resuscitation. In view of data from diverse controlled clinical trials, it has been demonstrated to be effective with respect to conventional fluid therapy for primary resuscitation of trauma patients [49]. Hypotensive patients after sustaining head injury who had Glasgow Coma Scale scores of 8 or less and who received hypertonic saline treatment presented higher survival to hospital discharge. This was demonstrated in a multicentre trial [50] as well as in a meta-analysis of individual patients from clinical trials [51]. This meta-analysis was conducted on the individual records of patients from controlled clinical studies on trauma and demonstrated a significant increase in survival favouring HSD over standard of care. Moreover, hypertonic saline resuscitation has been shown to reduce bacterial translocation, which has been attributed to prevention of gut hypoperfusion [52].

Some potential adverse effects of hypertonic saline solution use are acute hypernatraemia and its consequences and internal bleedings. The application of hypertonic saline/dextran solution has proved safe in patients, and in none of the controlled clinical trials have adverse effects been attributed to the colloid component; nor have anaphylactoid reactions been observed [53]. Clinical studies have not found severe side effects that could preclude the use of hypertonic solutions in clinical practice [48-51].

Colloids

Colloids can be divided into natural (albumin) or synthetic, artificial (polydispersed) colloids (dextran, gelatins, hydroxethyl starch solution). The ability of administered colloids to increase colloid osmotic pressure constitutes one mechanism by which colloids might reduce interstitial oedema. Because the barrier between the intra- and extravascular spaces is only partially permeable to the passage of these molecules, colloids tend to remain in the intravascular space for longer periods than do crystalloids.

Albumin

Albumin is the most commonly used colloid. It has a molecular weight of 66,000-69,000 and is available as a 5% or a 25% solution. The serum half-life of exogenous albumin is less than 8 hours, though less than 10% leaves the vascular space within 2 hours after administration. It increases intravascular volume to five times the administered quantity.

Although albumin is derived from pooled human plasma, there is almost no risk of disease transmission, as albumin is heated and sterilised by ultrafiltration. Moreover, albumin offers several advantages over artificial colloids, including less restrictive dose limitations, lower risk of coagulation impairment, absence of tissue deposition that could lead to prolonged pruritus and reduced incidence of anaphylactic reactions. The cost of albumin can limit its usage. Albumin also appears to be favoured in ICU patients with hypoalbuminaemia [41]. However, it has not been shown to have any beneficial effects on either morbidity or mortality [54]. A study by Sapijaszko et al. [55] has shown that serially measured low albumin concentration may be a predictor of complicated or prolonged weaning from mechanical ventilation. The Cochrane meta-analysis [56] has raised questions about the safety of albumin. It has found no evidence that albumin reduces mortality and a strong suggestion that it might increase the risk of death in patients with hypovolaemia, burns or hypoproteinaemia. However, the results of this review must be interpreted with caution, since the conclusions drawn were based on relatively small trials in which there were only a reduced number of deaths. Moreover, another well-conducted meta-analysis failed to find increased risk associated with albumin infusion.

Dextrans

Two forms of dextran are currently available: dextran 70 (90% of molecules have MW 25,000-125,000) and dextran 40 (90% have MW 10.000-80.000). The main difference concerns their influence on microcirculation. Dextran 40 has been reported to produce a greater increase in microcirculatory flow [57].

Anaphylactic reaction occurs in patients with high anti-dextran antibody titers. The incidence of reaction is between 0.03-5% [58]. Dextrans have well-documented negative effects on coagulation, resulting in an increased bleeding tendency [59]. The clinical effect is similar to the manifestations of von Willebrand's disease, the effects being greater with dextran 70 than with dextran 40. These colloids are not first choice fluids for volume replacement therapy because of their high incidence of side effects compared with the other colloid solutions.

Gelatins

Three types of modified gelatin are available: cross-linked (Gelofundiol), urea-linked (Haemaccel) and succinylated (Gelofusin). These preparations contain different concentrations of electrolytes. Because of the low average molecular weight (35 kDa), plasma half-life is short, so that repeated infusions are necessary to maintain adequate blood volume. Gelatins have also been considered to be free of any major negative influence on the coagulation process [60]. However, an in vitro study suggests that a significant inhibition of platelet aggregation may be induced by gelatin infusion [61]. Gelatins are associated with a relatively high incidence of anaphylactic reactions. These reactions appear to be more common with urea-linked gelatins than with other preparations [62]. Despite good availability, these synthetic colloids have been replaced by newer generation synthetic colloids, such as hydroxyethil starch, with lower side effect profiles.

Hydroxyethyl starch

Hydroxyethyl starch (HES) is a modified natural polymer of amylopectin with volume expansion proprieties. The degree of hydroxyethylation is the major determinant of circulating half-life, and its molecular weight (MW) determines colloidal activity. At equal plasma concentrations, the colloidal activity is inversely related to the MW. HES is classified according to its manufactured or in vitro MW into high MW (450-480 kDa), medium MW (200 kDa) and low MW (70 kDa) starch preparations. The rate of metabolisation depends mainly on the degree of hydroxyethyl substitution (ranging from 0.4 to 0.7) and the C2/C6 ratio of hydroxyethylation. A high degree of substitution and a high C2/C6 ratio lead to a slow metabolisation of HES, resulting in a large in vivo MW [63]. HES have been associated to coagulation disorders [64], although several studies have demonstrated that low-molecular-weight HES solution is associated with a limited risk of coagulation abnormalities [65]. The extravascular starch deposits frequently lead to severe protracted pruritus. Impairment of renal function has also been documented in association with HES usage [66]. Compared with albumin solutions, HES may have a higher incidence of side effects. On the other hand, Boldt et al. [67] do not show any superiority of albumin over HES: volume therapy with HES was shown to be superior to that with albumin in increasing cardiac index and oxygen delivery and consumption.

References

1. Braunwald E, Sonnenblinck EH, Ross J (1988) Mechanism of cardiac contraction and relaxation. In: Braunwald E (ed) Heart disease. WB Saunders, Philadelphia, pp 383-425
2. Cooper AB, Doig Gs, Sibbald WJ (1996) Pulmonary artery catheters in the critically ill: an overview using the methodology of evidence-based medicine. Crit Care Clin 12:777-794
3. Connors AF Jr, Speroff T, Dawson NV et al (1996) The effectiveness of right heart catheterization in the initial care of critically ill patients. JAMA 276:889-897
4. Sandham JD, Hull RD, Brant RF et al (2003) A randomized, controlled trial of the use of pulmonary-artery catheters in high risk surgical patients. N Engl J Med 348:5-14
5. Tousignant CP, Walsh F, Mazer CD (2000) The use of transesophageal echocardiography for preload assessment in critically ill patients. Anesth Analg 90:351-355
6. Poli de Figuerido LF, Malbouisson LM, Varicoda EY et al (1999) Thermal filament continuous thermodilution cardiac output delayed response limits its value during acute hemodynamic instability. J Trauma 47:288-293
7. Wagner GJ, Leatherman JW (1998) Right ventricular end-diastolic volume as a predictor of the hemodynamic response to a fluid challenge. Chest 113:1048-1054
8. Diebel NL, Wilson RF, Tagett MG et al (1992) End diastolic volume. A better indicator of preload in the critically ill. Arch Surg 127:817-822
9. Marik PE (1999) Pulmonary artery catheterization and esophageal Doppler monitoring in the ICU. Chest 116:1085-1091
10. Feinberg MS, Hopkins WE, Davila-Roman VG et al (1995) Multiplane transesophageal echocardiograhic Doppler imaging accurately determines cardiac output measurements in critically ill patients. Chest 107:769-773
11. Sinclair S, James S, Singer M (1997) Intraoperative intravascular volume optimization and length of hospital stay after repair of proximal femoral fracture: randomized controlled trial. BMJ 315:909-912
12. Singer M, Bennet ED (1991) Noninvasive optimization of the left ventricular filling by esophageal Doppler. Crit Care Med 19:1132-1137
13. Di Corte CJ, Latham P, Grellich PE et al (2000) Esophageal Doppler monitor determination of cardiac output and preload during cardiac operations. Ann Thorac Surg 69:1782-1786
14. Nishimura R, Abel M, Hatle L et al (1990) Relation of pulmonary vein to mitral flow velocities by transesophageal Doppler echocardiography. Circulation 81:1488-1497
15. Fontes ML, Bellows W, Ngo L et al (1999) Assessment of ventricular function in critically ill patients: limitation of pulmonary artery catheterization. J Cardiothorac Vasc Anesth 13:521-527
16. Jacka MJ, Cohen MM, To T et al (2002) The use of and preferences for the transesophageal echocardiogram and pulmonary artery catheterization. J Cardiothorac Vasc Anesth 94:1065-1071
17. De Hert S, Vander Linden P, Ten Broecke P et al (2000) Assessment of length-dependent regulation of myocardial function in coronary surgery patients using transmitral flow velocity patterns. Anesthesiology 93:374-381
18. Lattik R, Couture P, Denault A et al (2002) Mitral Doppler indices are superior to two dimensional

echocardiography and hemodynamic variables in predicting responsiveness of cardiac output to a rapid intravenous infusion of colloid. Anesth Analg 94:1092-1099
19. Tavernier B, Makhotine O, Lebuffe G et al (1998) Systolic pressure variation as a guide to fluid therapy in patients with sepsis induced hypotension. Anesthesiology 89:1313-1321
20. Bouhemad B, Nicolas-Robin A, Benois A et al (2003) Echocardiographic Doppler assessment of pulmonary capillary wedge pressure in surgical patients with postoperative circulatory shock and acute lung injury. Anesthesiology 98:1091-1100
21. Michard F, Teboul JL (2000) Using heart-lung interactions to assess fluid responsiveness during mechanical ventilation. Crit Care 4:282-289
22. Jardin F, Delorme G, Hardy A et al (1990) Revaluation of hemodynamic consequences of positive pressure ventilation. Anesthesiology 72:966-970
23. Pinsky MR, Matuschak GM, Klain M (1985) Determinants of cardiac augmentation by elevations in intrathoracic pressure. J Appl Physiol 58:1189-1198
24. Perel A, Pizov R, Colev S (1987) Systolic pressure variation is a sensitive indicator of hypovolemia in ventilated dogs subjected to graded hemorrhage. Anesthesiology 67:498-502
25. Denault AY, Gaisor TA, Gorcsan J et al (2000) Determinants of aortic pressure variations during positive-pressure ventilation in man. Chest 116:176-186
26. Wesseling KH, de Wit B, Weber JAP et al (1983) A simple device for the continuous measurement of cardiac output. Adv Cardiovasc Physiol 5:16-52
27. Godje O, Hoeke K, Lichtwarck-Aschoff M et al (1999) Continuous cardiac output by femoral arterial thermodilution calibrated pulse contour analysis: comparison with pulmonary arterial thermodilution. Crit Care Med 27:2407-2412
28. Michard F, Chemla D, Richard C et al (1999) Clinical use of respiratory changes in arterial pulse pressure to monitor the hemodynamic effects of PEEP. Am J Respir Crit Care Med 159:935-939
29. Wiesenack C, Prasser C, Rodig G et al (2003) Stroke volume variation as an indicator of fluid responsiveness using pulse contour analysis in mechanically ventilated patients. Anesth Analg 96:1254-1257
30. Reuter DA, Felbinger TW, Schmidt C et al (2002) Stroke volume variation for assessment of cardiac responsiveness to volume loading in mechanically ventilated patients after cardiac surgery. Intensive Care Med 28:392-398
31. Perel A, Berkenstadt H, Katzenelson R et al (1998) Cardiac output measurement using an axillary arterial thermodilution technique. Intensive Care Med 24:S50
32. Bindels AJ, van der Hoeven JG, Graafland AD et al (2000) Relationships between volume and pressure measurements and stroke volume in critically ill patients. Crit Care 4:193-199
33. Reuter DA, Felbinger TW, Kilger E et al (2002) Optimizing fluid therapy in mechanically ventilated patients after cardiac surgery by on-line monitoring of left ventricular stroke volume variations: comparison with aortic systolic pressure variations. Br J Anaesth 88:124-126
34. Della Rocca G, Costa MG, Coccia C et al (2002) Preload index: pulmonary artery occlusion pressure versus intrathoracic blood volume monitoring during lung transplantation. Anesth Analg 95:835-843
35. Thijs LG (1995) Fluid therapy in septic shock. In: Sibblad WJ, Vincent JL (eds) Clinical trials for the treatment of sepsis. (Update in intensive care and emergency medicine, vol 19) Springer, New York, pp 167-190
36. Vincent JL (1991) The colloid-crystalloid controversy. Klin Wochensch 69:S104-111
37. Rackow EC, Falk JL, Fein A et al (1983) Fluid resuscitation in circulatory shock: a comparison of the cardiorespiratory effects of albumin, hetastarch, and saline solution in patients with hypovolemic and septic shock. Crit Care Med 11:839-850
38. Hankein K, Radel C, Beez M et al (1989) Comparison of hydroxyethyl starch and lactated Ringer's solution on hemodynamics and oxygen transport of critically ill patients in prospective cross-over studies. Crit Care Med 17:133-135
39. Schierhout G, Roberts I (1998) Fluid resuscitation with colloids or crystalloids in critically ill patients: a systematic review of randomized trials. BMJ 316:961-964

40. Choi P, Yip G, Quinonez L et al (1992) Crystalloids versus colloids in fluid resuscitation: a systematic review. Crit Care Med 27:200-210
41. Boldt J, Lenz M, Kumle B et al (1998) Volume replacement strategies on intensive care units: results from a postal survey. Intensive Care Med 24:147-151
42. Strauss RG (1998) Volume replacement and coagulation: a comparative review. J Cardiothorac Anesth 2:24-32
43. Hillman K, Bishop G, Bristow P (1997) The crystalloid versus colloid controversy: present status. Baillieres Clin Anaesthesiol 11:1-13
44. Wang P, Hauptman JG, Chaudry IH (1990) Hemorrhage produces depression in microvascular blood flow which persists despite fluid resuscitation. Crit Shock 32:307-318
45. Funk W, Baldinger V (1995) Microcirculatory perfusion during volume therapy: a comparative study using crystalloid or colloid in awake animals. Anesthesiology 82:975-982
46. de Felippe J Jr, Timoner J, Velasco IT et al (1980) Treatment of refractory hypovolemic shock by 7.5% sodium chloride injections. Lancet II:1002-1004
47. Kreimeier U, Bruckner U, Niemczyk S et al (1990) Hyperosmotic saline dextran for resuscitation from traumatic-hemorrhagic hypotension: effect on regional blood flow. Circ Shock 32:83-99
48. Walsh JC, Kramer GC (1991) Resuscitation of hypovolemic sheep with hypertonic saline/dextran: the role of dextran. Circ Shock 34:336-343
49. Mols P, Robert P, Henry B et al (1999) Study on the feasibility and hemodynamic efficacy of intravenous administration of small 7.2% NaCl 6% hydroxyethyl starch 200/0.5 in trauma patients during the pre-hospital period: a pilot study. JEUR 3:99-104
50. Vassar MJ, Fisher RP, O'Brien PE et al (1993) A multicentre trial for resuscitation of injured patients with 7.5% sodium chloride. The multicenter group for the study of hypertonic saline in trauma patients. Arch Surg 128:1003-1111
51. Wade CE, Grady JJ, Kramer GC et al (1997) Individual patient cohort analysis of the efficacy of hypertonic saline/dextran in patients with traumatic brain injury and hypotension. J Trauma 42:S61-S65
52. Reed LL, Mangano R, Martin M et al (1991) The effect of hypertonic saline resuscitation on bacterial translocation after hemorrhagic shock in rats. Surgery 110:685-690
53. Kreimeier U, Frey L, Messmer K (1993) Small-volume resuscitation. Curr Opin Anaesth 6:400-408
54. Rubin H, Carlson S, de Meo M et al (1997) Randomized, double-blind study of intravenous human albumin in hypoalbuminemic patients receiving total parenteral nutrition. Crit Care Med 25:249-252
55. Sapijaszko MJA, Brant R, Sanham D et al (1996) Non–respiratory predictor of mechanical ventilation dependency in intensive care unit patients. Crit Care Med 24:601-607
56. Cochrane Injuries Group Albumin Reviewers (1998) Human albumin administration in critically ill patients: systematic review of randomized controlled trials. BMJ 317:235-240
57. Arfors KE, Buckley P (1997) Pharmacological characteristics of artificial colloids. Baillieres Clin Anaesth 11:15-47
58. Paull J (1987) A prospective study of dextran-induced anaphylactoid reactions in 5745 patients. Anaesth Intensive Care 15:165-167
59. Abramson N (1988) Plasma expanders and bleeding. Ann Intern Med 108:307-312
60. Karoutsos S, Nathan N, Lahrimi A et al (1999) Thromboelastogram reveals hypercoagulability after administration of gelatin solution. Br J Anaesth 82:175-177
61. Evans PA, Glenn JR, Heptinstall S et al (1998) Effects of gelatin-based resuscitation fluids on platelet aggregation. Br J Anaesth 81:198-192
62. Laxenaire M, Charpentier C, Feldman L (1994) Réaction anaphylactoides aux subsitutes colloidaux du plasma: incidence, facteurs de risque, mécanismes. Ann Fr Anesth Reanim 13:301-310
63. Treib J, Baron JF, Grauer MT et al (1999) An international view of hydroxyethyl starches. Intensive Care Med 25:258-268

64. Cope JT, Banks D, Mauney MC et al (1997) Intraoperative hetastarch infusion impairs hemostasis after cardiac operations. Ann Thorac Surg 63:78-82
65. Boldt J, Muller M, Heesen M et al (1996) Influence of different volume therapy on platelet function in the critically ill. Intensive Care Med 22:1075-1081
66. Citanova ML, Leblanc I, Legendre C et al (1996) Effect of hydroxyethyl-starch in brain-dead kidney donors on renal function in kidney-transplant recipients. Lancet 348:1620-1622
67. Boldt J, Muller M, Menteges D et al (1998) Volume therapy in the critically ill. Is there a difference? Intensive Care Med 24:28-36

News on muscle relaxants

C. MELLONI, F. ANTOLINI, F. SFOGLIAFERRI

The big news in the field of neuromuscular blocking agents is ... that there are no new drugs on the horizon. The shortage of money in the field of neuromuscular research derives from the simple fact that the pharmaceutical companies have no money to invest in market niches and perhaps from the perceived evidence that the drugs we have today are already highly sophisticated and there is no absolute need to improve them. Organon tried to launch a new fast-onset/fast-offset drug (rapacuronium), but it had dangerous side effects on the airways, especially a worrying incidence of bronchospasm and oxygen desaturations [1], and was therefore withdrawn from the formularies after a promising start. We are still short of a drug with clinical time actions similar to those of succinylcholine, and this is still a goal of pharmaceutical research in the field of the neuromuscular blocking agents, pushed by the continuous growth of day surgery/day anaesthesia.

Neuromuscular blocking agents are used as adjuvants in day-case anaesthesia to facilitate tracheal intubation and/or surgery; although the majority of day-case procedures are performed without the use of neuromuscular blocking agents, there are procedures, such as laparoscopic surgery, microsurgery, open-eye surgery, some ear, nose and throat procedures and some paediatric procedures, which may require neuromuscular blockade. Therefore, it is important that the drug possesses a short onset, a short clinical duration and a short recovery time, with or without reversal; ideally it should also lack histamine release, provide haemodynamic stability, and be competitively priced.

The alternatives have been:

1) To find a new drug (rapacuronium); attempts so far have been abortive.

2) Use currently available drugs, such as succinylcholine and mivacurium; as these are not ideal for many reasons this means studying strategies to reduce side effects.

3) Use low doses of an intermediate-acting neuromuscular block, such as rocuronium, atracurium or vecuronium.

Since succinylcholine and mivacurium have many drawbacks, many clinicians revert to point 3, where safety can be challenged on the basis of new findings following the studies by Baillard [2], who found an alarming high frequency (42%) of clinically significant residual block (TOF.7) in patients given vecuronium without the use of a nerve stimulator and without reversal, and Hayes [3], who confirmed that postoperative residual block is still a problem even after intermediate acting neuromuscular blocking drugs and notwithstanding the use of tactile and visual evaluation of the response to TOF nerve stimulation. Postoperative residual curarisation was investigated [4] after administration of either vecuronium or rocuronium with reversal by pyridostigmine in 602 consecutive patients without perioperative neuromuscular monitoring. On their arrival in the recovery room, neuromuscular function was assessed both by acceleromyography in a train-of-four (TOF) pattern and also clinically by the ability to sustain a head-lift for >5 s and the tongue-depressor test.

Postoperative residual curarisation was defined as a TOF ratio <0.7. Almost 20% of the 602 patients had a TOF <0.7 in the recovery room. There were no significant differences in the TOF ratios between 10 mg and 20 mg of pyridostigmine. The authors were able to recognise that patients with residual block several associated factors applied: the absence of perioperative neuromuscular monitoring, the use of pyridostigmine, which is less potent than neostigmine, a larger dose of vecuronium, shorter time from the last neuromuscular blocker to TOF monitoring, or peripheral cooling. Therefore it was concluded that significant residual neuromuscular block after vecuronium or rocuronium was not eliminated even with reversal by a large dose of pyridostigmine. This means that, without monitoring, the significant residual neuromuscular block after vecuronium or rocuronium is not eliminated even by reversal with a large dose of pyridostigmine and can still be a problem in the recovery room.

The problem is further compounded by the use of continuous infusions Camu et al. [5] found that after cisatracurium and rocuronium infusions for long-duration interventions without systematic antagonism residual block was a consistent finding in 30 patients undergoing major surgery who were paralysed with either rocuronium or cisatracurium during propofol anaesthesia. Infusions were discontinued at the beginning of surgical closure; spontaneous recovery of neuromuscular function was awaited in both groups. Neostigmine (50 microg/kg) was administered only when a patient started to wake without a TOF of 0.9. In the cisatracurium and rocuronium groups, 4 (27%) and 1 (7%) patients, respectively, had a TOF ratio ≥0.9 at the end of surgery. The TOF ratio in each group at that time was 51±32% for cisatracurium and 47±31% for rocuronium (P = 0.78). Six patients (40%) in the cisatracurium group and 7 (47%) in the rocuronium group required neostigmine. The TOF ratio at the time of reversal was 63±7% for cisatracurium and 40±19% for rocuronium (*P* =0.01). The time interval between the end of surgery and a TOF ratio of 0.9 was 10±9 min for cisatracurium and 18±13 min for rocuronium (n.s.). Patients receiving a cisatracurium or rocuronium infusion have a high incidence of postoperative residual curarisation when the block is not antagonised. When 'reversal' is not attempted, cisatracurium seems to be safer than rocuronium.

The other field that has received much attention in the last decade has been that of reversal agents; being unable to find a new nondepolarising drug having a fast onset/fast offset, it may well be that the research has focused on new fast-acting reversal agents, so that the need for a fast-onset/fast-offset drug could become less important if and when the antagonism was rapid and had no sequelae. If this is the case, new drugs have been synthesised either following the classic pharmacology, i.e. inhibition of the receptors of ACHE or according to a completely new concept: anionic cyclophanes and cyclodextrins.

In the first class, piperidinium and pyridinium agents as water-soluble acetylcholinesterase inhibitors were developed for the reversal of neuromuscular blockade [6]; these piperidinium and pyridinium agents contain a common structural fragment of 5,6-dimethoxybenzothiophene; they are a sort of water-soluble acetylcholinesterase inhibitors. Several compounds, for example 42 (AChE IC [50] 0.03 μM) have been found to reverse the neuromuscular blockade induced by vecuronium bromide in vitro and in vivo. Coupled with their high water solubility (up to 30-60 mg/mL), these compounds appeared potentially useful as intravenous reversal agents of neuromuscular blocking agents in surgical anaesthesia.

In another series of experiments [7], a series of carboxyl-containing cyclophanes were designed and synthesised as chemical chelators (or host molecules) of cationic muscle relaxant drugs (or guest molecules). Three of these cyclophane derivatives, 1-3, have been shown by NMR to form 1:1 complexes with the muscle relaxants pancuronium, and gallamine in D(2)O, with association constants up to 10(4) M(-1). When tested in an in vitro chick biventer muscle preparation, the cyclophanes reversed the neuromuscular block induced by pancuronium and gallamine, with the most effective reversal against pancuronium (EC(50) 40 μM.

According to these new routes of development, ciclodextrins appeared as reversal agents for NMB agents [8]; the authors developed a series of mono- and per-6-substituted cyclodextrin derivatives synthesised as synthetic receptors (or host molecules) of rocuronium bromide. By forming host-guest complexes with rocuronium, these cyclodextrin derivatives reverse the muscle relaxation induced by rocuronium in vitro and in vivo in 3 min. Because this supramolecular mechanism of action does not involve direct interaction with the cholinergic system, the reversal by these compounds, e.g. compound 14 (Org 25969), is not accompanied by cardiovascular side effects usually attendant on acetylcholinesterase inhibitors such as neostigmine. The structure-activity relationships are consistent with this supramolecular mechanism of action, and stereochemistry will be presented at the APICE meeting and include effects of binding cavity size and hydrophobic and electrostatic interaction with the reversal activities of these compounds.

The fact that cyclodextrins are devoid of any other pharmacological effects is particularly important, since classic anticholinesterases have been implicated in other adverse side effects, including nausea and vomiting, that are particularly troublesome in the practice of day-case anaesthesia, even though the meta-analysis of Fuchs-Buder [9] failed to link the administration of neostigmine conclusively with the PONV. At the same time, omitting reversal introduces a not inconsiderable risk of residual paralysis, an effect that is a particular cause for concern since the report by Berg et al. [10] on the relationship between residual paralysis and respiratory complications.

An improved understanding of the pathologic consequences of residual paralysis (i.e. impaired laryngeal and pharyngeal muscle function, alterations in hypoxic ventilatory control, reduced margin of safety) led to the establishment of more rigorous criteria for defining adequacy of neuromuscular recovery: a ratio of TOF ≥ 0.9 is now accepted as the index of adequate recovery of neuromuscular function. With this new definition, residual paralysis becomes a frequent adverse side effect. Neuromuscular recovery should therefore be routinely monitored in ambulatory patients and residual paralysis prevented by reversing neuromuscular block.

As a matter of fact, it should always be stressed that routine quantitative neuromuscular monitoring is in every way superior to the usual clinical practice of tactile or visual assessment. As shown by Kierkegard et al. [11], administration of neostigmine following cisatracurium at different levels of TOF tactile recovery never accomplished a complete reversal even after 30 min; therefore, in order to achieve rapid (within 10 min) reversal to a TOF ratio of 0.7 in more than 87% of patients, three or four tactile responses should be present at the time of neostigmine administration. However, we must stress that within 30 min it was impossible to achieve a TOF ratio of 0.9 in all patients, regardless of the number of tactile responses present at the time of neostigmine administration.

TOF < 0.95 correlates with clinical and objective measurements of impairment in the function of the respiratory muscles and of the muscles protecting the airways [12]: accelerometry of the adductor pollicis muscle (AP) predicts recovery of respiratory function from neuromuscular blockade; since accelerometric measurements predict the effects of residual paralysis on pulmonary and upper airway functions, accelerometry at the AP can be used instead of tests of pulmonary and pharyngeal function. However, the abover study was conducted on young healthy volunteers not subjected to any medication; the margin of safety of these measures can be much lower in anaesthetised patients, in whom there are at least two problems, residual paralysis and residual sedation. If only a 100% recovery of TOF ratio predicts an acceptable recovery of forced vital capacity, forced inspiratory volume in 1 s, and mean ratio of expiratory and inspiratory flow at 50% of vital capacity in 93%, 73%, and 88% of measurements (calculated negative predictive values), respectively in the abovementioned study, it seems highly probable that a TOFR of 100% at least should be present at the end of surgery or before discharge home for ambulatory patients! Here the correct choice of muscle relaxant could be of the utmost importance as far as complete recovery is concerned; for example, mivacurium has been accepted as superior to vecuronium in ENT paediatric practice since Lysakowski et al. [13] found that mivacurium-induced NMB is of very short duration in paediatric patients and residual paralysis is less frequent after mivacurium than after vecuronium; however, maintaining the neuromuscular block was more expensive after mivacurium than after vecuronium and required many additional boluses, so that the problem should be considered from many different points of view in addition to safety.

Another problem exposed by many authors concerns the sites suggested for the monitoring of neuromuscular function; the eye has been used frequently for accelerometry, but controversies arose concerning the exact site to be used for monitoring and result interpretation: Plaud [14] suggested that the medial site, i.e. corrugator supercilii, could be used as a surrogate measure of laryngeal adductor muscle blockade, but Henmmerling [15] showed that neuromuscular block at the diaphragm was much shorter than at the orbicularis oculi and corrugator supercilii. If I can draw some conclusion from these papers, the corrugator supercilii may be better suited for monitoring of onset of neuromuscular block at the larynx, while for recovery nothing is better than the adductor pollicis. Moreover, the relationship between orbicularis oculi and the adductor pollicis holds for normal patients and myasthenic patients presenting with the generalised type of the disease, i.e. neuromuscular block following vecuronium is less pronounced at the orbicularis oculi than at the AP, while at the time of extubation neuromuscular monitoring at the eye could be better since the orbicularis oculi is the most sensitive and recovers more slowly in the ophthalmic type of myasthenia [16]; by the same line of reasoning, the thumb can be the best muscle to monitor for adequate relaxation during abdominal surgery in myasthenic patients.

Two new sites were recently described for electromyographic monitoring; the larynx, where the recurrent laryngeal nerve was transcutaneously stimulated and the block of the laryngeal muscles measured through a disposable laryngeal electrode [17-19]; and the right sides of the T12/L1 or L1/l2 vertebrae [20, 21], where the lumbar diaphragm is inserted with its muscular crura, so that diaphragmatic electromyography can be performed with stimulation of the phrenic nerve in the neck. However, these new sites are used mainly for research purposes and do not seem amenable to everyday practice.

Last but not least, acoustic myography has been reported to correlate with the force responses of the small hand muscles, but Bellemare et al. [22] found that the time-course of relaxation using acoustic myography differed from the time-course of force relaxation, with the acoustic signal exhibiting a slower onset but a faster recovery than the force response.

References

1. White PF (2002) Rapacuronium: why did it fail as a replacement for succinylcholine? Br J Anaesth 88;163-65
2. Baillard C, Gehan G, Reboul-Marty J et al (2000) Residual curarization in the recovery room after vecuronium. Br J Anaesth 84:394-395
3. Hayes AH, Mirakhur RK, Breslin DS et al (2001) Postoperative residual block after intermediate-acting neuromuscular blocking drugs. Anaesthesia 56:312-318
4. Kim KS, Lew SH, Cho HY, Cheong MA (2002) Residual paralysis induced by either vecuronium or rocuronium after reversal with pyridostigmine. Anesth Analg 95:1656-1660
5. Camu G, de Baerdemaeker L, den Blauwen N et al (2002) Postoperative residual curarization with cisatracurium and rocuronium infusions. Eur J Anaesthesiol 19:129-134
6. Palin R, Clark JK, Cowley P et al (2002) Novel piperidinium and pyridinium agents as water-soluble acetylcholinesterase inhibitors for the reversal of neuromuscular blockade. Bioorg Med Chem Lett 12:2569-2572
7. Cameron KS, Fielding L, Mason R et al (2002) Anionic cyclophanes as potential reversal agents of muscle relaxants by chemical chelation. Bioorg Med Chem Lett 12:753-755
8. Adam JM, Bennett DJ, Bom A et al (2002) Cyclodextrin-derived host molecules as reversal agents for the neuromuscular blocker rocuronium bromide: synthesis and structure-activity relationships. J Med Chem 45:1806-1816
9. Fuchs-Buder T, Mencke T (2001) Use of reversal agents in day care procedures (with special reference to postoperative nausea and vomiting). Eur J Anaesthesiol Suppl 23:53-59
10. Berg H, Viby-Mogensen J, Roed J et al (1997) Residual neuromuscular block is a risk factor for postoperative pulmonary complications: a prospective, randomised and blinded study of postoperative pulmonary complications after atracurium, vecuronium and pancuronium. Acta Anaesthesiol Scand 41:1095-1103
11. Kirkegaard H, Heier T, Caldwell JE (2002) Efficacy of tactile-guided reversal from cisatracurium-induced neuromuscular block. Anesthesiology 96:45-50
12. Eikermann, M, Groeben H, Husing J, Peters J (2003) Accelerometry of adductor pollicis muscle predicts recovery of respiratory function from neuromuscular blockade. Anesthesiology 98:1333-1337

13. Lysakowski C, Fuchs-Buder T, Tassonyi E (2000) Mivacurium or vecuronium for paediatric ENT surgery. Clinical experience and cost analysis. Anaesthesist 49:387-391
14. Plaud B, Debaene B, Donati F (2001) The corrugator supercilii, not the orbicularis oculi, reflects rocuronium neuromuscular blockade at the laryngeal adductor muscles. Anesthesiology 95:96-101
15. Hemmerling TM, Schmidt J, Wolf T et al (2001) Intramuscular versus surface electromyography of the diaphragm for determining neuromuscular blockade. Anesth Analg 92:106-111
16. Itoh H, Shibata K, Yoshida M et al (2000) Neuromuscular monitoring at the orbicularis oculi may overestimate the blockade in myasthenic patients. Anesthesiology 93:1194-1197
17. Hemmerling TM, Schmidt J, Hanusa Q et al (2000) Simultaneous determination of neuromuscular block at the larynx, diaphragm, adductor pollicis, orbicularis oculi and corrugator supercilii muscles. Br J Anaesth 85: 856-860
18. Hemmerling TM, Schurr C, Walter S et al (2000) A new method of monitoring the effect of muscle relaxants on laryngeal muscle using surface laryngeal electromyography. Anesth Analg 90:494-497
19. Hemmerling TM, Schmidt J, Wolf T et al (2000) Comparison of succinylcholine with two doses of rocuronium using a new method of monitoring neuromuscular block at the laryngeal muscles by surface laryngeal electromyography. Br J Anaesth 85:251-255
20. Hemmerling TM, Schmidt J, Wolf T et al (2001) Intramuscular versus surface electromyography of the diaphragm for determining neuromuscular blockade. Anesth Analg 92:106-111
21. Hemmerling TM, Schmidt J, Hanusa C et al (2001) The lumbar paravertebral region provides a novel site to assess neuromuscular block at the diaphragm. Can J Anesth 48:356-360
22. Bellemare F, Couture J, Donati F (2000) Temporal relation between acoustic and force responses at the adductor pollicis during nondepolarizing neuromuscular block. Anesthesiology 93:646-652

Cerebral protection during anaesthesia

A.J. Sutcliffe

Primary brain injury is caused by disease, injury and infection. All too frequently, the damage is irreversible and leads to death or disability with significant consequences for the patient, the family and society. It is very important, therefore, to protect the brain from secondary damage. In clinical medicine, methods for providing cerebral protection are depressingly few in number and relatively crude. Animal experiments, however, offer the promise that in the future, targeted cerebral protection will be possible. This chapter describes the pathophysiological features of cerebral damage, defines the meaning of the term protection, reviews animal models of protection and discusses cerebral protection in clinical anaesthesia.

The pathophysiology of brain injury

Primary brain injury

Primary brain injury causes cellular disruption or death. Within the disrupted cell, metabolic processes cease to function normally and energy failure results. Both injury and energy failure cause terminal depolarisation of neurons and failure of ionic pumps. As a result, ionic homeostasis within neurons is lost. The neuron and its organelles swell, membranes are damaged and toxic molecules leak into the interstitium [1].

Secondary brain injury

Secondary damage is caused by excitotoxic neurotransmitters, calcium, expression of immediate early genes, nitric oxide, and oxygen free radicals. All brain pathologies are associated with reduced cerebral blood flow (CBF) and ischaemia. Consequently, in ischaemic areas, anaerobic metabolism produces increases in lactate and hydrogen ions.

Delayed brain injury

In common with other injuries, both primary and secondary brain injuries provoke an inflammatory response that, if uncontrolled, causes further damage. Also, immediate early genes stimulate processes that lead to programmed cell death, i.e. apoptosis. Finally, glial scarring occurs in areas of neuronal death. Although these processes do contribute to the eventual outcome, their effect is small compared with that caused by secondary brain damage [1].

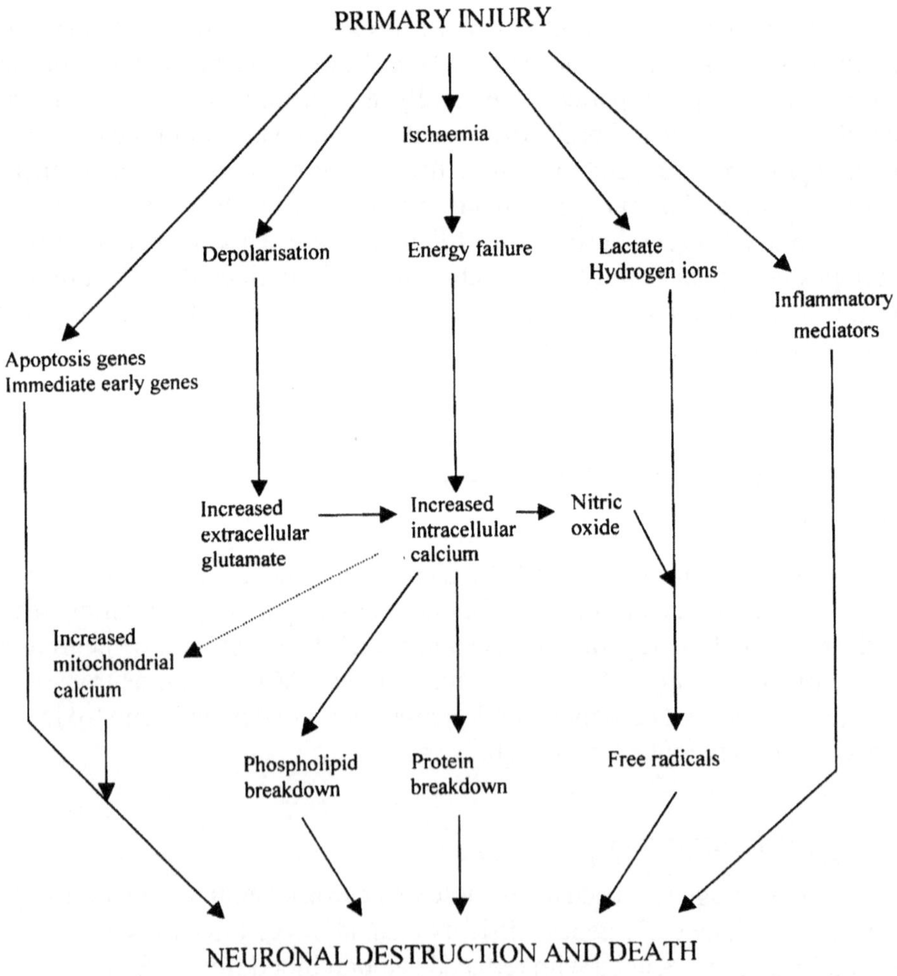

Fig. 1 Key events associated with brain damage

Key processes in brain damage

Figure 1 illustrates some of the biochemical mechanisms associated with brain damage. Multiple pathways are involved that might be amenable to treatment. Furthermore, certain chemical substances link the pathways and therefore represent key targets for investigation. For simplicity, these are described separately, but the fact that interaction exists may be one reason why successful animal studies cannot be translated into useful treatments for patients. Our understanding of the complex processes that result from primary brain damage is far from complete. It is possible, indeed probable, that targeting a single molecule or chemical cascade has unrecognised effects on related pathways that counteract the expected benefit.

Some key processes are summarised below. For more detailed explanations, readers are referred to an excellent review article by Wheeler and Menon [1].

Excitatory amino acids

Within the brain several amino acids function as neurotransmitters. Of these, the most important is glutamate. Normally, neuronal excitation causes glutamate release. Depolarisation following neuronal injury or energy depletion releases glutamate, and because reuptake mechanisms also fail, glutamate accumulates in the extracellular space. Extracellular glutamate stimulates surrounding cells, and they too depolarise and release more glutamate, setting up a vicious circle of escalating depolarisation around the area of damage. Depolarised cells suffer a huge influx of sodium and calcium which, if the ionic pumps fail, leads to cytotoxic oedema.

Ionic calcium

An increase of intracellular ionic calcium has multiple effects, which include the activation of protein kinase C, nitric oxide sythetase, phopholipases, endonucleases and proteases. All these enzymes catalyse reactions which destroy the cell and its membranes. In the mitochondria, calcium triggers the release of cytochrome C, which is one of the triggers for apoptosis.

Nitric oxide and free radicals

Nitric oxide causes vasodilatation, and thus its release, triggered by glutamate in the presence of calcium, should promote cerebral blood flow and tissue oxygenation. Unfortunately, nitric oxide combines with oxygen to form peryoxynitrile, which in turn breaks down into damaging free radicals. In excess, free radicals damage deoxyribonucleic acid by several mechanisms.

Immediate early genes

Activation of immediate early genes causes an alteration in the balance of secondary messenger enzymes that trigger yet more genes involved in cell survival, regeneration and apoptosis. The net effect in the injured brain is a trend towards apoptosis mediated by capsase and calpain proteases.

Cerebral protection, preservation and resuscitation

The verb "to protect" means to prevent harm. In theory, therefore, protection should be provided prior to an insult in order to prevent its harmful effects. In animal experiments, a large number of compounds, when given prior to brain injury, are protective. Of course, in the real world, disease and injury to the brain cannot be predicted. Thus, genuine protection is impossible. Sometimes, however, it is possible to intervene at the time of the insult, e.g. during surgery, or immediately afterwards, e.g. in the case of head injury. At this time, intervention is most correctly called cerebral preservation. Similarly, intervention some time after the insult is correctly called cerebral resuscitation. In clinical practice, cerebral preservation is the goal and cerebral resuscitation is sadly, the frequent reality. Nevertheless, researchers and clinicians continue to pursue the goal of cerebral protection, a term which is used loosely to describe all interventions which minimise the effects of primary brain damage.

It is also important to note that it is possible to protect against the effects of secondary insults that cause cerebral ischaemia, such as hypoxia, hypotension, raised intracranial pressure (ICP) and vasospasm. The first three should be preventable. Vasospasm is not always preventable but usually occurs some time after subarachnoid haemorrhage and is, therefore, predictable. Thus, genuine protection against the damaging effects of vasospasm is a clinical option.

Cerebral protection in animals

Experimentally, numerous compounds provide cerebral protection in animals. Examples include progesterone, which reduces oedema [2] and melatonin, which scavenges free radicals [3]. Cyclosporin A [4] improves function, and isoflurane appears to confer protection against ischaemic damage [5]. So far, none of these has an established clinical role in cerebral protection. However, progesterone, cyclosporin A and isoflurane must be candidates for further study because these agents are already used in clinical practice for other indications.

Why does successful cerebral protection in animals fail in humans?

One of the biggest disappointments of recent years has been the failure to translate successful animal techniques into clinical treatment. The reasons are complex. Perhaps the most important is incomplete knowledge of brain chemistry and normal neuronal function. Analysis of current knowledge, however, shows that most of the compounds that cause brain damage have a vital role in normal brain function if they are released in the right place, in the right concentration, at the right time. Given that brain damage is usually localised, it becomes clear that treatments which antagonise the effects of these compounds may be helpful in damaged brain but might cause significant, unwanted damaging effects in normal brain. Consequently, although protective of damaged brain, these drugs actually do more harm than good.

Many experimental studies are conducted in rodents. The rodent brain does not function in an identical manner to the human brain. The pharmacokinetics and pharmacodynamics of certain drugs may differ between rodents and humans. An interim step, which is being used increasingly more often, is the use of primates to test compounds that work in rodents prior to proceeding to human trials. The rationale is that the primate brain more closely resembles the human brain. Furthermore, extrapolating equivalent doses from rodents to humans is fraught with difficulty. Consequently, it is possible that in human trials, either suboptimal doses are being used or humans are being overdosed with a consequent increase in side-effects [6].

Finally, the management of brain-damaged patients is not the same as a controlled animal experiment. Humans receive drugs such as sedatives, analgesics and mannitol, which are known to affect cerebral metabolism and function. In animal experiments, only one drug is tested at a time and then under controlled conditions. This control means that secondary insults such as hypoxia and hypovolaemia do not occur and do not compromise results. It could be that the apparent failure of individual protective drugs in patients is due to interactions between the new drug and established treatments. It could also be that additional secondary insults occurring after completion of the protective treatment mask any prior benefit obtained from the trial drug. Furthermore, the need for informed consent prior to patient entry into a clinical trial leads to prolonged delays before treatment is started. Thus, during clinical trials of cerebral protection, the trial treatment is given during the resuscitation phase rather than the protection or prevention phases.

The following sections describe protective treatments that have been tested in humans. There seems to be a common pattern. First, small single-institution studies demonstrate a perceived improvement in outcome or a surrogate measure, such as ICP level. Then, large, multi-centre, randomised, controlled, double-blind studies fail to confirm initial results. In this age of evidence-based practice, failure of a large trial means that the treatment is abandoned. We should not forget, however, that sequential trials often demonstrate an improvement in outcome for both control and test groups when compared over a time span of many years. Improvements in survival following the adult respiratory distress syndrome are a classic example. The implication of this finding is that in institutions enthusiastic enough to undertake clinical trials there is a commitment to excellence that includes using existing treatments in an optimum way. Sadly, this trend is not apparent in trials relating to head injury management. Could this be because the initial brain injury has such an overwhelming effect on outcome?

Pharmacological approaches to cerebral protection in patients

Steroids

Steroids may inhibit lipid peroxidation and lipolysis, maintain normal CBF, maintain normal energy metabolism and reverse intracellular calcium accumulation. Dexamethasone reduces swelling around tumours. However, the evidence accumulated to date does not support the use of steroids for cerebral protection in head-injured patients [7]. There are still many neurosurgical centres where it is believed that high-dose methyl prednisolone could benefit head-injured patients, and a large trial is currently being performed in Europe [8]. The beneficial effect is thought to be independent of methylprednisone's glucocorticoid effect, but it is important to remember that methylprednisolone does increase blood glucose and that this may be undesirable in the presence of brain ischaemia (see below).

Super oxide dismutase to inhibit free radicals

Polyethylene-glycol-conjugated superoxide dismutase is a free radical scavenger. Unfortunately, in a large trial, benefit at 6 months following head injury was statistically insignificant [9].

Tirilazad mesylate to inhibit lipid peroxidation

Although successful in animal experiments, this compound has not been successful in clinical practice, probably because it does not cross the blood--brain barrier [10].

Modulators of arachidonic acid metabolism

Indomethacin and ibuprofen are cyclo-oxygenase inhibitors that improve CBF and cerebral metabolism in animals. These effects are also seen in patients, but without a beneficial effect on outcome [6].

Calcium channel blockers

Nimodipine improves outcome after subarachnoid haemorrhage [11]. This is probably because it genuinely protects the brain from vasospasm. Some benefit has also been demonstrated in patients with head injury complicated by subarachnoid haemorrhage [12]. Nimodipine can cause hypotension, particularly if given intravenously. Perhaps the reason for its success is that its side-effects are easily recognised and treated.

Neurotransmitter antagonists

Most research involves glutamate. Glutamate activity depends on at least four receptor sites, the most important of which is thought to be the *N*-methyl-D-aspartate (NMDA) receptor, which is coupled to a sodium-calcium channel. The effects of NMDA receptor antagonists are variable and in some cases are associated with hypotension and even cerebral toxicity [6]. Lesser, but still significant, side-effects are illustrated by the dissociative anaesthetic ketamine. Ketamine is a low-affinity NMDA antagonist.

Current cerebral protection in patients

The interventions described above are attractive because they target specific pathways that are associated with neuronal damage. Although current techniques of cerebral protection are crude and less specific, their benefits are clearer. Often, benefits have only been demonstrated in a particular diagnostic group of patients. However, given a lack of high-quality research for individual patient groups, it is probably acceptable to extrapolate between diagnostic groups if the pathologic processes are similar.

Common management goals for neurosurgical patients

Ultimately, all patients are managed in such a way that cerebral oxygenation is maintained. Multiple interventions include preventing hypoxia and hypovolaemia, controlling ICP, maintaining cerebral perfusion pressure (CPP) and hence CBF, and reducing cerebral metabolic demand for oxygen.

Hypotension and hypoxia

Hypotension and hypoxia significantly worsen outcome following head injury. Hypoxia alone has less impact than hypotension or combined hypoxia and hypotension [13]. This suggests that perfusion of brain tissues is crucial and that reduced perfusion pressure leads to reduced CBF and hence tissue ischaemia. Vasospasm after subarachnoid haemorrhage has the same effect and is also associated with poorer outcome.

Blood glucose

Hyperglycaemia is also associated with poor outcome after head injury. This association is stronger than the association of hypotension with poor outcome [14]. It is also clear that hyperglycaemia in the presence of hypotension has the worst prognosis. Some have argued that hyperglycaemia is merely part of the stress response to severe injury and that this alone explains the association. Others believe that hyperglycaemia is damaging. Soon after injury, adequate supplies of glucose to the brain may facilitate the maintenance of ionic gradients. However, as ischaemia develops, anaerobic metabolism produces increasing amounts of lactate and hydrogen ions. At this stage, increased supplies of glucose may augment anaerobic production of hydrogen ions and contribute to secondary brain damage. Microdialysis is a new technique that measures brain chemicals, particularly glucose, lactate and glycerol [15]. This technique will help to clarify the relationships between blood glucose and lactate in the ischaemic brain.

The Lund protocol

Established wisdom in most neurosurgical units is that ICP should be reduced by medical and surgical means and that CPP should be maintained at 70 mmHg [7]. Experience leads us to believe that even if ICP cannot be reduced below 20 mmHg, a good outcome is still possible if an adequate CPP is maintained. Thus, strenuous efforts are made to raise mean arterial pressure. In addition to restoration of circulating blood volume, this often requires large doses of inotropes.

In the Swedish centre of Lund, a radically different philosophy is practised. The Lund protocol is summarised in Table 1. Much greater efforts are made to reduce ICP and cerebral oxygen demand. Thiopentone is given routinely. Target CPP is still between 60 and 70 mmHg, but because ICP is much lower, this is easier to achieve. Furthermore, drugs are used to reduce capillary hydrostatic pressure and albumin is given to maintain colloid oncotic pressure. These interventions minimise the development of interstitial oedema and help to control raised ICP. Perusal of Table 1 will reveal an unexpected cocktail of vasoactive drugs. Some are vasodilators and tend to cause hypotension, while dihydroergotamine is a potent vasoconstrictor. At first glance, none of these drugs matches our expectations of drugs suitable for use in patients with raised ICP and reduced CBF. However, their combined effects achieve the stated goals and outcomes from Lund are impressive [16].

The Lund protocol has not been tested in a randomised, controlled trial. This may be the reason why it is not widely used. The important point illustrated by the Lund protocol is that it is vital to use a multi-faceted approach to control of ICP, CPP and cerebral oxygenation. As long as all interventions are balanced to achieve the desired goal, quibbles about their effect on a single parameter such as CBF become irrelevant.

Table 1 The Lund protocol

GOAL	TARGET	INTERVENTION
Decrease capillary hydrostatic pressure	CPP 60-70 mmHg	Metoprolol, clonidine, dihydroergotamine
Reduce cerebral blood volume	ICP < 25 mmHg	Thiopentone, dihydroergotamine
Reduce $CMRO_2$ and stress response	Sedation and analgesia	Benzodiazepines, fentanyl, thiopentone
Maintain blood volume and colloid osmotic pressure	Normal Hb and albumin, equal fluid balance	Albumin, furosemide, blood, nutrition
Intermittent CSF drainage	ICP < 25 mmHg	External ventricular drain

Hypothermia

Profound hypothermia has been used successfully for elective neurosurgery. Numerous animal experiments document its beneficial effects on ICP, CBF, glutamate levels and interleukin levels and, most importantly, its ability to depress cerebral metabolism and oxygen requirements. During elective neurosurgery, the role of hypothermia can be genuinely protective, although caution is necessary. A recent study showed that the link between cerebral metabolism and blood fow is uncoupled and that CBF falls to a greater extent than metabolism [17]. Following head injury, however, hypothermia has not improved outcome and this may be because it usually takes 8 to 10 hours before hypothermia is achieved. Thus, its role is limited to cerebral resuscitation.

An encouraging study from Pittsburgh demonstrated a beneficial effect of mild hypothermia (32°C) following head injury [18]. Unfortunately, a larger, multi-centre study failed to confirm the benefit [19]. These studies illustrate the problems of transferring animal work to humans. There is some evidence that the method of sedation used in animal experiments and failure to control for ambient temperature may have invalidated some animal work.

Although the incidence of major complications did not differ significantly between the groups in the largest clinical study [19], it is impossible to overlook the fact that unintended, mild postoperative hypothermia increases the incidence of cardiac complications following cardiac surgery, increases the volume of blood loss in orthopaedic procedures and prolongs time in hospital after colorectal procedures [20]. Thus, the perceived benefits of hypothermia to the brain may be outweighed by complications affecting other organ systems. Last but not least, the fact that a hoped-for benefit cannot be demonstrated should not detract from the need for detailed analysis of published results. Retrospective review of Marion's study [18] provoked by lack of concordance with Clifton's larger study [19] revealed that the hypothermic group had a mortality rate slightly better than that of the general severe head injury population. The difference in outcome was a result of a significantly higher mortality rate than would have been expected in the control group.

Titrated oxygen therapy

Most drugs are given in carefully controlled doses to achieve predetermined, delineated treatment goals. Oxygen is the exception to this rule. While hypoxia is feared and avoided, hyperoxia is accepted and even welcomed. Oxygen feeds the production of free radical species. Thus, in an environment where free radical damage is known to occur, perhaps more attention to oxygen therapy would be helpful. In relation to adult cerebral damage, oxygen therapy is not an area of active study. In many ways, spinal cord pathophysiology mimics cerebral pathophysiology. An interesting experiment has been performed in rabbits. Aortic clamping was used to cause ischaemic spinal cord damage. Following spinal cord injury, the animals were resuscitated (reperfused) in air or in a hypoxic environment. It is instructive to note that fewer animals in the hypoxic reperfusion group suffered permanent neurological damage than in the control, normoxic group [20]. This study shows that high concentrations of oxygen are not appropriate in all situations. In particular, where there has been a period of ischaemia, reperfusion with high concentrations of oxygen may be damaging. Perhaps the brain could be offered more protection if oxygen were used like all other drugs and the dose titrated to a specified arterial oxygen tension.

Cerebral protection during anaesthesia

Much of the discussion so far has been based on evidence obtained by studying patients in the critical care unit. These patients are frequently ventilated and often require complex cardiovascular support and numerous interventions to control ICP and maintain CPP, CBF and cerebral oxygenation. Furthermore, brain damage is usually already present and efforts to provide protection are limited in scope. In contrast, patients undergoing neuroanaesthesia are generally less ill and brain damage, if present at all, is localised. Some patients do so well that their postoperative course is entirely uneventful. Some people might argue, therefore, that neuroprotection during anaesthesia is either less necessary or less complex. Are these arguments valid?

The potential value of neuroprotection during neuroanaesthesia and surgery

Because many patients present for neurosurgery with minimal or absent neurological damage, any neuroprotection that can be provided has the potential to be of enormous value. Because anaesthesia is induced prior to surgery, protective strategies employed by anaesthetists are protective in the precise sense of the term. The use of profound hypothermia has already been mentioned. Although rarely used today, in the past it was used primarily for difficult operations when major haemorrhage with prolonged clamping of vessels was anticipated. Put simply, hypothermia was employed where CBF, CPP and cerebral oxygenation were expected to be impaired. Does this mean that with improved operative conditions provided by modern anaesthesia and advances in surgical technique, the need for routine cerebral protection is unnecessary? I believe that the answer to this question is no. Neuroanaesthesia and neuro-critical care are complementary, and management goals can and should be shared.

Specific pathophysiological effects associated with neurosurgery

In contrast to the pre- and postoperative periods, during surgery the skull is open and if full decompression occurs ICP is equivalent to atmospheric pressure. Furthermore, cerebrospinal fluid continuously leaks from the wound. Thus, because ICP is low, the MAP required to maintain CPP should also be lower. This may not be true. Many conditions requiring surgery are associated with reductions in CBF around the lesion [22]. Furthermore, surgical retractors cause demonstrable ischaemia [23]. Although total intravenous anaesthesia (TIVA) has potential benefits which include rapid recovery and reduced length of hospital stay [24], improved outcome has not been demonstrated. In everyday practice, TIVA can cause significant relative hypotension. This is also true of inhalational agents, such as isoflurane and sevoflurane. Advocates of inhalational agents for maintenance of anaesthesia point to animal experiments which suggest that vapours offer a protective effect against cerebral ischaemic insults [25]. There is no clear evidence that one technique is better than any other. At present, we should concentrate our efforts on reducing ICP to improve surgical access and increasing CPP to counteract the effects of reduced CBF around the lesion and surgical retraction.

Conclusions

Patients will be grateful for all medical interventions that prevent secondary cerebral injury and assist in achieving the best outcome that is compatible with the primary injury or disease. Although a "magic bullet" that blocks all damaging cascades is actively being sought, translating the results of animal experiments into useful, clinical protection is not straightforward. At present, better use of existing treatments guided by careful attention to the underlying pathophysiological processes may be a better approach.

References

1. Wheeler DW, Menon DK (2002) Secondary Neuronal injury mechanisms. Anaesth Intensive Care Med 3: 120-123
2. Wright DW, Bauer ME, Hoffman SW et al (2001) Serum progesterone levels correlate with decreased cerebral edema after traumatic brain injury in rats. J Neurotrauma 18: 901-909
3. Mesenge C, Margailli I, Verrecchia C et al (1998) Protective effect of melatonin in a model of traumatic brain injury in mice. J Pineal Res 25: 41-46
4. Sullivan PG, Thompson M, Scheff SW (2000) Continuous infusion of cyclosporin A postinjury significantly ameliorates cortical damage following traumatic brain injury. Exp Neurol 161: 631-637
5. Kapinya KJ, Lowl D, Futterer C et al (2002) Tolerance against ischemic neuronal injury can be induced by volatile anesthetics and is inducible NO synthase dependent. Stroke 33:1889-1898
6. Teasdale GM, Bannan PE (1997) Neuroprotection in head injury. In: Reilly P, Bullock R (eds) Head injury. Chapman and Hall, London, pp 423-438

7. Chesnut RM (1997) Guidelines for the management of severe head injury: what we know and what we think we know. J Trauma 42:S19-22
8. Gregson B, Todd NV, Crawford D et al (1999) CRASH trial is based on problematic meta-analysis. BMJ 319:578
9. Muizelaar JP, Marmarou A, Young HF et al (1993) Improving the outcome of severe head injury with the oxygen radical scavenger polyethylene glycol-conjugated superoxide dismutase: a phase 2 trial. J Neurosurg 78:375-82
10. Marshall LE, Marshall SB (1986) Pitfalls and advances from international tirilazad trial in moderate and severe head injury. J Neurotrauma 12:929-932.
11. Pickard JD, Murray GD, Illingworth R et al (1989) Effect of oral nimodipine on cerebral infarction and outcome after subarachnoid haemorrhage: British aneurysm nimodipine trial. BMJ 298:636-642
12. Harders A, Kakarieka A, Braakman R (1996) Traumatic subarachnoid haemorrhage and its treatment with nimodipine. German tSAH study group. J Neurosurg 85:82-89
13. Chesnut RM, Marshall SB, Piek J et al (1993) Early and late systemic hypotension as a frequent and fundamental source of cerebral ischemia following severe brain injury in the Traumatic Coma Data Bank. Acta Neurochir (Wien) 59:121-125
14. Walia S, Sutcliffe AJ (2002) The relationship between blood glucose, mean arterial pressure and outcome after severe head injury: an observational study. Injury 33:339-344
15. Reinstrup P, Stahl N, Mellergard P et al (2000) Intracerebral microdialysis in clinical practice: baseline values to chemical markers during wakefulness, anesthesia, and neurosurgery. Neurosurgery 47:701-709
16. Eker C, Asgeirsson B, Grande P-O et al (1998) Improved outcome after severe head injury with a new therapy based on principles for brain volume regulation and preserved microcirculation. Crit Care Med 26:1881-1886
17. Sato K, Sato K, Yashimoto T (2000) Systemic and cerebral haemodynamics during craniotomy under mild hypothermia in patients with acute subarachnoid haemorrhage. Acta Neurochir (Wien) 142:1013-1019
18. Marion DW, Penrod LE, Kelsey SF et al (1997) Treatment of traumatic brain injury with moderate hypothermia. N Engl J Med 336:540-546
19. Clifton GL, Miller ER, Choi SC et al (2001) Lack of effect of induction of hypothermia after acute brain injury. N Engl J Med 344:556-563
20. Harper CM, McNicholas T, Gowrie-Mohan S (2003) Maintaining perioperative normothermia. BMJ 326:271-272
21. Danielisova V, Marsala M, Chavko M et al (1990) Postischemic hypoxia improves metabolic and functional recovery of the spinal cord. Neurology 40:1125-1129
22. Sutcliffe AJ (2003) Neuroanaesthesia: key points during the perioperative period. Minerva Anestesiol (in press)
23. Yundt KD, Grubb RL, Diringer MN et al (1997) Cerebral hemodynamic and metabolic changes caused by brain retraction after aneurysmal subarachnoid hemorrhage. Neurosurgery 40:442--450
24. Sato K, Karibe H, Yoshimoto T (1999) Advantage of intravenous anaesthesia for acute stage surgery for aneurysmal subarachnoid haemorrhage. Acta Neurochir (Wien) 141:161-163
25. Engelhard K, Werner C, Reeker W et al (1999) Desflurane and isoflurane improve neurological outcome after incomplete cerebral ischaemia in rats. Br J Anaesth 83:415-421

Anaesthesia and splanchnic perfusion

N. Požar Lukanović

Despite advances in anaesthesia and intensive care, organ failure remains one of the common causes of postoperative morbidity and mortality [1].

Even after correctly performed surgery and uneventful anaesthesia, patient's condition may deteriorate considerably. Numerous studies have investigated the correlation between perioperative hypoxia of the gut mucosa and postoperative complications [2-7]. Anatomical and physiological characteristics of the gut mucosa render it sensitive to hypoxia that cannot be detected by routinely monitored haemodynamic parameters (blood pressure, heart frequency, hour diuresis) [8]. Any increase in oxygen demand or decrease of oxygen delivery can lead to gut mucosa hypoxia and acidosis, which may be present in 24–26% of patient during major surgery [9].

The gut mucosa is a barrier to the external milieu. Damaged gut mucosa permits bacterial and endotoxin translocation from the gut into the circulation. Smaller quantities of endotoxin and bacteria are regularly removed from the circulation by liver reticuloendothelial system-Kupffer cells. In hypoxic conditions translocation is abundant and Kupffer cells less efficient, which may lead to systemic bacteraemia and endotoxinaemia, postoperative infection and organ failure [10].

Anatomy and physiology of hepatosplanchnic circulation

Arterial blood reaches the abdominal organs through small splanchnic arteries, which, through capillary plexuses, provide blood for the gut, spleen, liver and pancreas. Venous blood from these plexuses is drained into the portal vein, which supplies the liver with most of its oxygen.

The liver receives its blood supply from two different systems, arterial and portal. Total liver blood flow is 1100–1800 ml/min, representing 25% of cardiac output at rest; 70% of the total liver flow is portal blood. Despite being partly deoxygenated (portal blood oxygen saturation is 65–75%), it provides the liver with more than 50% of oxygen in rest.

The liver's oxygen supply is uneven, because it is not dependent only on the oxygen in arterial blood; more than 50% of it is derived from the portal oxygen content. It is reduced if portal blood flow or oxygen content is decreased [10]. Decreased portal oxygen transport can be compensated by increased oxygen extraction and by increased arterial blood flow; this is known as reciprocal arterioportal blood flow and depends on local release of liver adenosine [11]. Portal blood flow can also adjust to arterial blood pressure in a reciprocal way. This phenomenon is known as the veno-arterial response and is dependent on intact sympathetic function.

Anatomy and physiology of gut wall

The gut wall consists of four concentric layers: the mucosa (lamina propria with numerous immune cells, muscular layer of mucosa), the submucosa, with nerves and vessels, the muscular layer and the adventitia. The gut receives 25% of the cardiac output, and 75% of that volume goes to the mucosa. Average flow in mucosa is four times that in the muscular layer, reflecting the fact that because of its absorptive and defensive function cell maturation and metabolism are greater than elsewhere in the body [10].

Countercurrent circulation in gut villi

In a gut villus, vein and lymph vessel are situated centrally, while one or two unbranched arteries lie submucosally and branch only near the tip of the villus to form a dense capillary network near the basal membrane. This arrangement improves absorption, but at the same time increases direct diffusion of oxygen from artery to vein, the distance between them at the basis of villus being only 20 μm.

The consequence of countercurrent circulation is lower tissue partial O_2 pressure at the tip of the villus [11].

Influence of sympathetic nervous system on gut circulation

Sympathetic stimulation increases vascular resistance in the mesenteric and liver arteries and the portal vein and reduces blood flow to the liver. The splanchnic region is abundantly supplied with vegetative nerves and responds intensely to stress. The α_1 adrenergic supply is dense, and splanchnic vasoconstriction is an early response to decrease of oxygen transport, resulting in redistribution of blood to the heart and brain. A decrease in blood volume in the splanchnic region is more intense than in other body regions in these circumstances. In an animal exsperiment it was proved that vascular resistance in the gut is four times the total vascular resistance in conditions of hypovolaemia [12].

In healthy volunteers in was found that a reduction in blood volume by 15% results in a 40% decrease in gut blood volume, while blood pressure and heart frequency remained unchanged [13].

Sympathetic activity regulates blood flow in the microcirculation. Capillary flow is regulated by vasomotor activity of muscles in metaarterioles and precapillary sphincters – the mechanism of selective opening and closing of precapillary sphincters.

During maximal contraction of precapillary sphincters, capillary flow is blocked completely. Sympathetic denervation impairs capillary sphincters' contractility leading to increased blood volume, blood flow velocity, and blood pressure in capillaries. These findings apply to the sympathetic block effect in skin and skeletal muscles. Its effect on gut capillary blood flow and countercurrent flow in gut villi is not known [14].

Influence of local factors on microcirculation

Vasodilatation of precapillary sphincters caused by sympathetic denervation is not complete. There is a residual arteriolar tone. The influence of cellular environment on vasomotor activity is well known. Endogenous vasoactive substances-NO, angiotensin II, and endothelin-1, are released in response to changes in regional blood flow [14].

Influence of hypoxic damage of gut mucosa on bacterial and endotoxin translocation

Gut wall permeability for bacteria and endotoxinis increases after ischaemia and mechanical and reperfusion damage. The most common causes of increased gut wall permeability resulting from insufficient blood flow are hypovolaemia and septic shock.

Hypoxia harms intracellular tight junctions, their permeability being energy dependent. Permeability for large molecules (endotoxin) is increased. In low-flow states the effect of countercurrent blood flow is amplified, damaging the tips of gut villi [16].

In recent years, numerous investigations have confirmed a correlation between increased gut mucosa permeability for endotoxin and the development of sepsis and multiorgan failure. It is crucially important to prevent states that may lead to hypoxic gut mucosa damage with consequent increased permeability [17-19].

Surgery and stress response

Surgery and trauma cause a complex inflammatory response. Numerous inflammation mediators are released from traumatised tissue: lysosome enzymes, histamin, kinin, serotonin, prostaglandins, leukotriens and others. These substances increase capillary permeability and activate complement and coagulation cascades. Activated immune cells secrete proinflammatory cytokines (Il-1, Il-6, TNF-α) that stimulate the thalamus to secrete corticotropin releasing factor (CRF) and activate the hypothalamo-hypophyse axis (HHA). At the same time, afferent vegetative and somatic nerve fibres transmit pain stimuli from the operative site and also stimulate hypothalamus. Emotions such as fear, dehydration, starvation, hypoxia, hypo- and hypercapnia and hyperthermia, also activate HHA. In the course of major surgery HHA stimulation is pulsatile and stress hormones are released in waves.

CRF stimulates hypophyse to release proopiomelanocortin (POMC), prolactin, vasopressin and growth hormone. CRF acts on brain stem nucleus-locus coeruleus, that in 50% of cases consists of noradrenaline releasing sympathetic neurons. ACTH stimulates the adrenal gland to release gluco- and mineralocorticoids and activates renin-angiotensin system.

The complex stress response is directed to mobilisation and transport of reconstructive substances to the site of injury. An exaggerated stress response after surgery leads to catabolism, degradation of body proteins, body weight loss and reduced ability to resist infections.

The majority of stress hormones (catecholamines, vasopressin, growth hormone, glucagon, angiotensin II) are vasoconstrictors that centralise blood flow and thus help the organism to survive the period immediately after trauma, but they reduce the blood flow to gut and kidneys, with consequent hypoxic damage and an increase in the incidence of complications after surgery [20].

The more extensive surgery is, the more abundant are the stress hormones released. In open heart surgery, a nine-fold increase in adrenaline is found relative to preoperative values [21]. Increased angiotensin II concentrations are found in a period of extracorporeal circulation [19]. In liver transplant patients, increased levels of β-endorfin are detected [22].

In aortic surgery, a positive correlation is found between intraoperative concentrations of catecholamines and postoperative renal and cardiac failure [23]. In liver surgery it is often necessary to block blood flow to the liver (Pringle manoeuvre) to prevent excessive bleeding from liver tissue. This manoeuvre causes stagnant hypoxia in the gut, with possible damage to the gut mucosa [24].

Influence of anaesthesia on stress response

The choice of anaesthetic technique influences the haemodynamics and modulates immune and metabolic perioperative changes.

Large doses of opioids efficiently reduce the release of stress hormones during surgery. Morphine in large doses reduces the initial endocrine and metabolic response in heart surgery [21], while fentanyl in large doses prevents the increase in stress hormone concentrations in patients during open heart surgery [22].

In major abdominal surgery postoperative catecholamine blood concentrations are similar to preoperative values in patients anaesthetised with a combination of general and thoracic epidural anaesthesia (TEA), while in patients anaesthetised with general anaesthesia only catecholamine concentration and oxygen consumption are significantly increased [25].

The last two investigations cited confirm that TEA with local anaesthetics reduces the metabolic response to surgery.

TEA to the level of T-3 prevents HHA stimulation through somatic and sympathetic nerve fibres. However, vagal fibres cannot be blocked, and nor can HHA stimulation, by inflammation mediators released from the site of surgery.

Complete stress response is not desirable, while the stress response is crucial to survival after damage. The goal of the correct choice of anaesthesia is to reduce an exaggerated response with its harmful effects in the postoperative period.

Several investigations show that the combination of TEA and general anaesthesia in major abdominal surgery reduces the need for transfusion, incidence of postoperative complications and the duration of ICU stay [29].

A large meta-analysis has demonstrated an overall reduction in mortality in patients with TEA [26]. There was a reduction in the incidence of myocardial infarction. In another recent meta-analysis, there was a reduction in myocardial infarction, and TEA was far superior to lumbar epidural anaesthesia in this respect [27].

Higher oxygen tension in the surgical wound is shown in patients treated with epidural anaesthesia and analgesia than in those who underwent major abdominal surgery under i.v. analgesia [28].

Effect of TEA on gut perfusion

Effect of TEA on gut blood flow is due to several interconnected mechanisms. Block of sympathetic nerve fibres produces vasodilatation and reduces arterial blood pressure and perfusion pressure in splanchnic region. Reduced HHA activation leads to lower levels of stress hormone concentrations. Decreased vascular resistance results in increased blood flow. Vasodilation increases the volume of blood per unit of tissue.

Sympathetic block prevents the rhythmic contractions of muscular components of precapillary sphincters, and residual tonus is dependent on local mediators (NO, endotelin, angiotensin convertase).

Vasodilation in the blocked area produces increased blood flow and oxygen transport. On the other hand, decreased arterial blood pressure and perfusion pressure also decrease oxygen transport. The end effect on oxygen delivery/consumption ratio is not clear.

The influence of TEA on splanchnic blood flow has mostly been investigated in animals. In rats TEA reduces blood flow measured with direct intravital microscopy in the tips of gut villi [29]. With the same technique it has been found that TEA attenuates haemorrhage-induced impairment of intestinal perfusion in rats [30]. In rabbits epidural anaesthesia retards intestinal acidosis and reduces the portal vein endotoxin concentration during progressive hypoxia [31].

TEA increases blood flow measured with laser Doppler spectrometry in the gut during gut resections in man [32]. In another study, a significantly lower proportion of patients with TEA developed low pH values of gastric mucosa [26].

Two clinical studies that measured gastric pH (pHi) came to opposite conclusions. In a study in which vascular filling was assessed only by arterial blood pressure, pHi values were higher in patients who received a combination of TEA and general anaesthesia than in patients who received general anaesthesia only [33]. In a second study, vascular filling was optimised by means of a pulmonary artery catheter, and no difference was found in pHi values between patients anaesthetised with TEA and general anaesthesia and with general anaesthesia only [34]. This could be because TEA could not improve gut perfusion which was already optimal, and in conditions of mild hypoperfusion TEA may protect the gut from hypoxic damage.

In a prospective, randomised investigation we studied the effect of TEA with a local anaesthetic, bupivacaine, on gut perfusion in liver resections. To prevent excessive blood loss, lower than optimal values of CVP (CVP=8–12 mmHg) were maintained (CVP=6±2 mmHg). Gut perfusion was assessed by partial pressure of oxygen (pO_2vp) and pH (pHvp) in the portal blood. In conditions of low CVP (6±2 mmHg), the correlation between pH and pO_2 in the portal

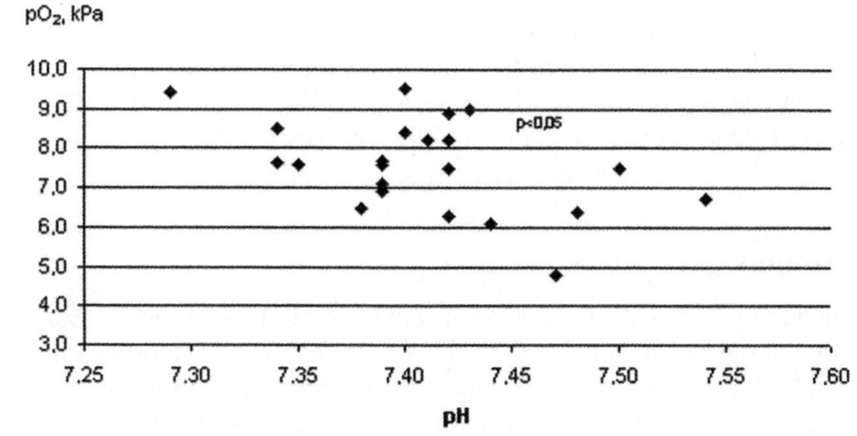

Fig. 1 Patients with combination of thoracic epidural anaesthesia (TEA) and general anaesthesia

blood in the TEA group was negative (r=–0.47) and statistically significant (P=0.027).

In the presence of low CVP (6±2 mmHg), the correlation between pH and pO_2 in the portal blood in the TEA group was negative (r=–0.47) and statistically significant (P=0.027).

In the group with general anaesthesia only, this correlation was lost (r=0.058).

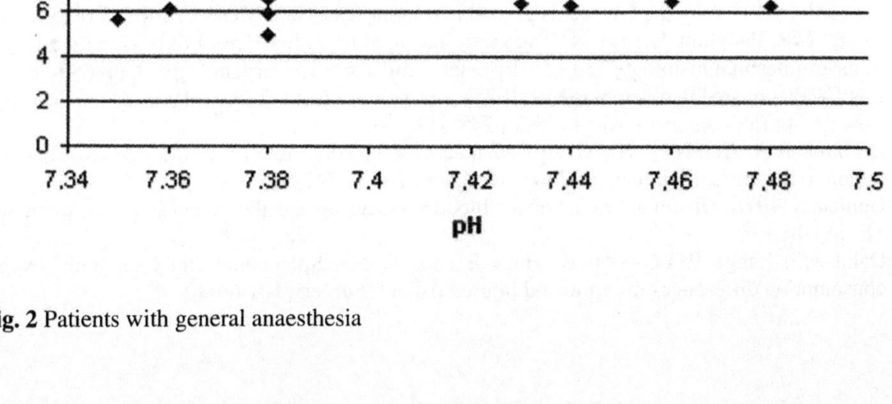

Fig. 2 Patients with general anaesthesia

The negative correlation between pHvp and pO_2vp confirmed the existence of oxygen shunt at the base of the gut villi in the TEA group of patients and also preserved the regularity of gut perfusion. We conclude that TEA has a protective role for gut mucosa in conditions of low CVP.

Conclusions

Knowledge of intestinal physiology has expanded in recent years. Besides its strong potential for preventing pain, TEA can also prevent hypoxic damage to vulnerable gut mucosa during major surgery. Early investigations found no influence of this type of anaesthesia on patient outcome. Only in recent years has this important evidence encouraged anaesthesiologists to use their skill to implement thoracic epidural blockade and in this way reduce the morbidity and mortality attached to complex surgical procedures.

References

1. Mythen MG, Webb AR (1994) The role of gut mucosal hypoperfusion in the pathogenesis of post-operative organ dysfunction. Intensive Care Med 20:203-209
2. Van Aken H, Rolf N (1999) Thoracic epidural anaesthesia. Baillieres Clin Anesthesiol 13:10-107
3. Peyton PJ, Myles PS, Silbert BS et al (2003) Perioperative epidural analgesia and outcome after major abdominal surgery in high-risk patients. Anest Analg Feb 96(2):548-554
4. Adeau A, Newell P, Dobbs BR et al (2002) Postoperative epidural analgesia following elective major abdominal surgery in high risk patients: a retrospective cohort study. N Z Med J 115:69-72
5. Rigg JR, Jamrozik K, Myles PS et al (2002) Epidural anaesthesia and analgesia and outcome of major surgery: a randomised trial. Lancet, Apr 13;359(9314):1276-1282
6. Holte K, Kehlet H (2002) Effect of postoperative epidural analgesia on surgical outcome. Minerva Anestesiol Apr;68(4):157-161
7. Rodgers A, Walker N, Schug S et al (2000) Reduction of postoperative morbidity and mortality with epidural or spinal anaesthesia: results from an overview of randomised trials. BJM 321:1493-1497
8. Lundgreen O (1989) Physiology of the intestinal circulation. In: Marston A, Bukley GB, Fiddian-Green RG, Haglund UH (eds) Splanchnic ischemia and multiple organ failure. Edvard Arnold, London, pp 29-40
9. Fink MP (1991) Why the GI tract is pivotal in trauma sepsis and MOF. Crit Ilness 6:253-276
10. Neutra MR, Padykula HA (1984) The gastrointestinal tract. In: Weiss I (ed) Modern concepts of gastrointestinal histology, 2nd edn. Elsevier, New York Amsterdam Oxford, pp 659-705
11. Lautt WW, Legare DJ, d'Almeida MS (1985) Adenosine as a putative regulator of hepatic arterial flow (the buffer response). Am J Phisiol 248: H331-338
12. Brinkmann A, Calzia E, Trager K, Rademacher P (1998) Monitoring the hepato-splanchnic region in the critically ill patient. Intensive Care Med 24:542-556
13. Gelman S (1976) Disturbances in hepatic blood flow during anesthesia and surgery. Arceh Surg 111:881-883
14. Dahn MS, Lange P, Lobodell K, Hans B et al (1987) Splanchnic and total body oxygen consumption differences in septic and injured patient. Surgery 101:69-80

15. Greene NM, Brull SJ (1993) Haemodynamic effects of spinal anaesthesia In: Physiology of spinal anaesthesia, 4th edn. Williams & Wilkins, Baltimore
16. Mythen MG, Barclay GR, Browne DA et al (1992) Endogenous anti-endotoxin-core antibodyes, gut mucosal perfusion and postoperative MODS. Int Care Med 18:S57
17. Kirton OC, Civetta JM (1997) Splanchnic flow and resuscitation. In: Civetta JM, Taylor RW, Kirby RR (eds) Critical care, 3rd edn. Philadelphia, Lippincot-Raven 443-455
18. Weismann C (1990) The metabolic response to stress: an overview and update. Anesthesiology 73:308-328
19. Roizen MF, Lampe GH, Benefiel DJ et al (1987) Is increased operative stress associated with worse outcome? Anesthesiology 67:A1
20. Kehlet H (1998) Modification of stress response to surgery by neural blockade: clinical implications. In: Cousins MJ, Bridenbough PQ (eds.) Neural blockade in clinical anesthesia and management of pain, Philadelphia, Lippincot-Raven, pp 129-175
21. Brandt MR, Korshin J, Prange-Hansen A et al (1978) Influence of morphine anaesthesia on the endocrine-metabolic response to open-heart surgery. Acta Anaesth Scand 31:243-247
22. Walsh ES, Paterson JL, O'Riordan JBA, Hall GM (1981) Effect of high-dose fentanyl anaesthesia on the metabolic and endocrine response to cardiac surgery. Br J Anaesth 53:1155-1165
23. Reves JG, Karp RB, Buttner et al (1982) Neuronal and adrenomedullary cathecholamine release in response to cardiopulmonary bypass in man. Circulation 66:49-55
24. Acosta F, Diaz J, Moreno J et al (1995) Relationship between β-endorphin release and surgical stress in orthotopic liver transplantation. Transplant Proc 27:2303
25. Hortgson PS (1999) Thoracic epidural anaesthesia and analgesia for abdominal surgery: effects on gastrointestinal function and perfusion. Baillieres Clin Anaesthesiol 13:9-22
26. Sutcliffe NP, Mostafa SM, Gannon J, Harper SJ (1996) The effect of epidural blockade on gastric intramucosal pH in the peri-operative period Anaesthesia. Jul;51(7):711
27. Beattie WS, Badner N, Choi P (2001) Epidural analgesia reduces postoperative myocardial infarction: a meta-analysis. Anesth Analg 93:853-858
28. Buggy DY, Doherty WL, Hart EM, Pallett EJ (2002) Postoperative wound oxygen tension with epidural or intravenous analgesia: a prospective, randomised, single –blinded clinical trial. Anesthesiology 98:952-958
29. Sielenkamper AW, Eicker K, Van Aken H (2000) Thoracic epidural anesthesia increases mucosal perfusion of rats. Anesthesiology 93:844-851
30. Adolphs J, Schmidt DK, Mousa SA et al (2003) Thoracic epidural anesthesia attenuates hemorrhage-induced impairment of intestinal perfusion in rats. Anesthesiology 99:685-692
31. Ai K, Kotake Y, Satoh T (2001) Epidural anesthesia retards intestinal acidosis and reduces portal vein endotoxin concentrations during progressive hypoxia in rabbits. Anesthesiology 94:263-269
32. Johansson K, Ahn H, Lindhagen J et al (1988) Effects of epidural anaesthesia on intestinal blood flow. Br J Anaesth 75:73-76
33. Vaisanen O, Parvianen I, Roukonen E et al (1998) Epidural analgesia with 5% bupivacaine does not improve splanchnic tissue perfusion after aortic reconstruction surgery. Br J Anaesth 81:893-898
34. Mallinder PA, Hall JE, Bergin FG et al (2000) A comparison of opiate- and epidural-induced alterations in splanchnic blood flow using intra-operative gastric tonometry. Anesthesia 55:659-665

Remifentanil+desflurane for inhalational induction without airway irritation and rapid post-anaesthetic recovery. Preliminary results in 100 patients

R. MUCHADA

Desflurane (DES)'s characteristics make this halogen an interesting product for the maintenance of general anaesthesia [1, 2], but it is an irritant for the upper airways during induction. To avoid this undesirable action a remifentanil (REM) infusion used in parallel with inhaled DES allows a smooth induction without airway irritation.

Anaesthetic protocol:

- Premedication: Hydroxyzine 50 mg-alprazolam 0.5 mg per os 1 h before the procedure.
- Induction: Pre-oxygenation, i.v. REM 1 μg kg^{-1} min-1 into a specific peripheral vein, until miosis, bradypnoea (5< RR <10) and the partial loss of palpebral reflex, in about 2 min. Then REM is reduced to 0.2 μg kg^{1} min^{-1} followed by metered DES at 6%, with a FiO_2=1, under initially spontaneous and then manual ventilation for 60 s. Curarisation with i.v. atracurium, 0.4 mg/kg. After 2 min of additional ventilation with DES at 6% tracheal intubation with xylocaine 5%, topical anaesthesia.
- Maintenance: Mechanical volumetric ventilation with 50% O_2/air. TV = 8 ml/kg, RR = 12 c/min. Flow for the re-breathing circuit 1.5 l/min of fresh gas. DES maintained at a Fe DES ~4%. REM perfusion at about 0.1 to 0.2 μg kg^{-1} min^{-1}.
- End of anaesthesia. Gas flow in the respirator is increased to 7-9 l/min. of 100%/O_2. DES closed and REM ended when Fe DES is near 1% and 2 min before awakening is expected.

Induction was always possible in our patients without respiratory tract irritation. Patients were under mechanical ventilation in 8±2 min after the beginning of induction. In most cases induction and early anaesthetic periods were characterised by bradycardia and hypovolaemic hypotension. No tachycardia over 90 b/min or hypertension was observed, even during intubation. Extubation was performed 240±45 s after the end of the REM infusion. The maximum Aldrete score was obtained in 10±2 min. This approach shows the possibility of using DES for inhalational induction of anaesthesia and maintenance as sole narcotic when it is associated with REM, without respiratory tract irritation and with correct haemodynamic stability and a rapid and pleasant recovery.

The characteristics of DES make it an inhalational agent that is interesting for maintenance of narcosis during general anaesthesia [1, 2]. Its low blood and tissue solubility and its low solubility coefficient [3] allow rapid modulation of the depth of anaesthesia [4].

The very low metabolic transformation [5] avoids the production of degradation product, which is potentially toxic for the patients.

From the cardiovascular point of view, DES differs from other halogens in having an intrinsic action that leads to an increase in the sensitivity of the cardiac beta receptors to the cathecholamine action [6, 7]. It also shares with other halogens some protective myocardial effects against hypoxy thanks to its preconditioning action [8, 9].

The rapid elimination of the agent when vaporisation is stopped and ventilation maintained allows recovery of the conscious state in a short period, generally with a calm and subjectively agreeable awakening [10-12]

Nevertheless, DES presents a major disadvantage in inhalational anaesthetic induction: it provokes an irritation of the airway and lung canalisation, where the manifestations are hypersecretion, cough, respiratory freezing or laryngeal spasm [13-15]. In these conditions, DES cannot be used for anaesthetic induction [16].

However, the irritant effects on respiratory airways seem to be partly decreased when morphine-like products are perfused by intravenous infusion preceding inhalational induction [17].

Based on this result, a protocol has been established for inhalational induction and maintenance of general anaesthesia with only one narcotic, whose current application would demonstrate the following elements:

- Feasibility of inducing inhalational anaesthesia under spontaneous ventilation, in combination with remifentanil (REM), an opiate with a short duration of action, without provoking irritant respiratory manifestations.
- Observation of the haemodynamic evolution during the maintenance of narcotic analgesia with these two products.

– Evaluation of the rapidity and quality of postanaesthesia recovery following the interruption of the two agents, characterised by their rapid elimination.

Patients and methods

The protocol has been applied in a collective of 100 patient classed as ASA 1 (67%) and ASA 2 (33%). The group was composed of 38 men and 62 women, whose average age was 62 ±18 years. The patients had undergone transabdominal gynaecological surgery in 41% of cases; laparotomic intraperitoneal surgery in 18%; orthopaedic surgery (in 12 for total hip replacement, 8 patients for total knee replacement) in 20%; and peripheral vascular surgery (arterial bypass in 10, varicose in 11 patients) in 21%.

The anaesthetic protocol used

Premedication

Hydroxizine 50 mg, alprazolam 0.5 mg by mouth administered 60 min before the beginning of anaesthesia.

Induction

Preoxygenation with $FiO_2 = 1$, under spontaneous ventilation; i.v. infusion of REM, 1 $\mu g\ kg^{-1}\ min^{-1}$ until the observation of miosis or bradypnoea (respiratory rate < 10 but > 5 c/min), and the diminution of palpebral reflex. These clinical signs appeared approximately 2 min after the beginning of REM perfusion. Thereafter, the dose of REM was reduced to 0.2 $\mu g\ kg^{-1}\ min^{-1}$.

Introduction of DES vaporised at 6%, always with $FiO_2 = 1$. Steady spontaneous ventilation followed by manual ventilation, without provoking any hyperpressure in the airways. After 1 min, curarisation with atracurium 0.4 mg/kg. following manual ventilation for 2 min with DES at 6%. At this point, oro-tracheal intubation was performed.

Maintenance

Controlled ventilation was then implemented (O_2 to 50% + AIR 50%, TV = 8 ml/kg, RR = 12 c/min). Concentration of DES on the vaporiser at 6%. When Fe DES arrived to 4%, the circuit was semiclosed with a fresh gas flow at 1.5 l/min. The DES vaporiser was set at 5% to maintain a Fe DES between 4% and 4.5%.

A continuous perfusion of REM was given, with a dose between 0.1 and 0.30 μg kg^{-1} min^{-1}. The amount of REM was regulated according to the variation in heart rate (HR). If HR was < 60 b/min, reduction by steps of 0.05 μg/kg every 3 min. If FC was > 80 b/min increase by steps of 0.05 μg/kg every 3 min.

Curarisation was never routinely used.

End of anaesthesia

At the beginning of the cutaneous surgical incision closing and about 5 min before the expected end of the operation the respiratory circuit was opened. Controlled mechanical ventilation was maintained with a $FIO_2 = 1$. The DES vaporiser was closed. The REM perfusion was stopped. Stop of the DES was < 1%.

Postoperative analgesia was insured with morphine 5 to 10 mg. by sub cutaneous way (s.c.) and Proparacetamol 1 g i.v. injected 30 min before the end of anaesthesia.

Monitoring

Haemodynamic monitoring comprises a transoesophageal Doppler echo (HemoSonic 100, Arrow – USA), a three-derivation electrocardiogram and a non-invasive oscillometric method to measure arterial pressure.

Respiratory monitoring on a Julian (Draeger, Germany) comprised, in addition to conventional ventilation parameter control (TV, RR, airway pressure), capnometry, pulse oximetry, FiO_2 and FeO_2, the analysis of halogen inspiratory and expiratory concentration.

Correction of haemodynamic modifications

An injection of atropine i.v. 0.2 to 0.5 mg was used when HR was lowered to under 55 b/min.

On the other hand, when volaemia-dependent arterial hypotension was diagnosed by means of haemodynamic criteria, a filling test with 500 ml of hydroxy methyl starch was done.

In the case of hypotension, depending on the vascular situation 10 to 15 mg of ephedrine by i.v. injection was used.

If haemodynamic monitoring allowed suspecting a systolic decrease of left ventricle performance Dobutamine, 3 to 5 mg/Kg/min was infused.

Results

Induction was possible in 100% of patients without respiratory irritation or discomfort.

The time between the beginning of REM infusion and the start of controlled ventilation was 8±2 min. The average operating time was 72±27 min (minimum = 28 min – maximum = 158 min).

In15% of patients, moderate muscular rigidity was observed before curare action. Even so, ventilation using a facial mask was always possible. In 2 patients, a decrease in haemoglobin saturation (HbO_2 sat) at 90% was observed but very rapidly corrected with manual ventilation. The average dose of REM needed to maintain analgesia was 0.15±0.07 μg kg^{-1} min^{-1}. Fe DES was maintained at a minimum of 3.8% and a maximum of 4.5%

From the haemodynamic point of view, the modifications most frequently observed during anaesthetic induction or immediately after the end of mechanical ventilation were:

- Bradycardia in 39% of patients. Twenty-three of these received atropine 0.25 mg i.v. and 0.5 mg was used for the other 16, when HR fell to under 55 B/min.
- Mean arterial pressure (MAP) was lower than 70 mmHg in 35 patients. In 29 patients, hypotension was accompanied by an indexed aortic blood flow (ABFi) of 2.2 l/m^2 (normal 2.5 to 4 l/m^2), a maximal blood speed (Vmax) lower than 50 m/s (normal 55 to 75 m/s), indexed total systemic vascular resistances (TSVRi) between 1850 and 2800 dyn.s.cm^{-5}/m^2 (normal value 1600 to 2600 dyn.s.cm^{-5}/m^2), an indexed stroke volume (SVi) of under 35 ml/m^2 (normal value 40-60 ml/m^2), an intra-aortic blood acceleration (Acc) superior to 18 m.s.s. (normal value 9-15 m.s.s.).

In these conditions, a filling test with 500 ml of hydroxymethyl starch allowed recovery of an average arterial pressure over 70 mmHg and balance of the other haemodynamic parameters in 27 patients.

In 2 patients, the persistence of hypotension after the filling test necessitated the injection of ephedrine, 10 mg i.v.

Six other patients had MAP lower than 70 mmHg, but with TSVRi lower than1500 dyn.s.cm^{-5}/m^2. In these patients, a dose of 10 to 15 mg of ephedrine repeated once per 5-min interval in 3 of them allowed us to balance MAP and TSVRi.

Twelve patients had episodes of MAP over 125 mmHg. These episodes were corrected by adjustment of the REM dose. No patients received hypotensive drugs. Diastolic arterial pressure (DAP) was always kept over 40 mmHg.

A drop in systolic left ventricle performance was observed in only 3 ASA

2 patients. A fall in ABFi to under 2 l min^{-1} m^{-2} was observed, a fall in SVi to under 25 ml, and a value of Acc lower than 8 mss. These 3 patients received a dobutamine perfusion at 3.5±0.5 μg kg^{-1} min^{-1} for 20±7 min.

No episodes of tachycardia with over 90 b/min were observed, even during tracheal intubation manoeuvres.

HR, after correction of the initial bradycardia, was maintained between 60 and 80 b/min throughout the period of general anaesthesia.

Maximum inspiratory pressure was 22±4 mmHg, and mean inspiratory pressure in the respiratory airway was 9±3 mmHg.

After discontinuous REM, spontaneous ventilation was restored in 120±15 s in 93% of patients. Extubation was possible in 93 patients in 240±45 s. In 4 other patients, extubation was possible after neutralisation of the residual curare action. Finally, in 3 other patients, extubation was possible in 420±125 s.

Most (95%) of the patients reached their highest awakening Aldrete score in 10±2 min; 5 patients took over 10 min to reach this maximum, but always less than 15 min.

The time needed for recovery was not influenced by the duration of anaesthesia.

Awakening was calm and subjectively agreeable.

A supplementary dose of 3 to 5 mg morphine i.v. was necessary in the first 15 min of the postoperative period in 5 patients to complete a comfortable analgesia.

Conclusions

These results allow us to say that strict adherence to the proposed protocol makes it possible to use DES as an inhalational narcotic induction agent under spontaneous ventilation and without any manifestations of respiratory irritation. DES was used as the only narcotic agent throughout general anaesthesia.

From a haemodynamic point of view, bradycardia, already described under REM, was the effect most frequently observed [18-20]. The utilisation of atropine in 39% of case raises the question of preventive atropinisation, but in all cases, bradycardia introduced a limitation to this technique, in any case of contraindication to the use of atropine.

No episodes of tachycardia over 90 b/min and/or hypertension were observed during induction or during tracheal intubation, even though the latter was sometimes laborious. The absence of tachycardia and arterial hypertension during mechanical stimulation of the pharyngo-laryngeal region could be a beneficial protection, especially for patients in whom the effect of an adrenergic reaction needs to be avoided [21-23].

Only 3% of patients, all ASA 2, presented a haemodynamic profile evoking a reduction of the systolic performance of the left ventricle compatible with an anaesthetic-induced myocardial depression. Correction was rapidly obtained with a low perfused dose of β1 stimulation over a limited time. The weak impact of the myocardial alteration and its rapid recovery could have been linked to β1 receptors sensitised to the intrinsic action of DES. On the other hand, it has been shown that direct myocardial depression determined by DES was concentration dependent [24]. Using DES associated with REM a synergic increased action of the first is obtained [26], allowing inhalation of a low concentration of DES under a MAC. With a Fe DES around 4% in an air- O_2 fresh gas flow, DES concentration was always under 1 MAC (approximately 0.7) [25] during the general anaesthesia maintenance period. This low concentration of DES could be considered as a collateral factor preserving the inotropic function of the heart during general anaesthesia.

All haemodynamic modifications were observed during the induction or immediately after the beginning of mechanical ventilation. They were rapidly corrected with an adapted therapy. They had not apparently had any important consequences for the good progress of the intervention or for rapid post-anaesthetic recovery. Variations linked to surgical events were observed secondarily. In this case supplementary adapted therapy was necessary.

Alveolar perioperative ventilation was done with a mixed air-O_2 flow. N_2O was not used. Despite this, approximately 4% Fe DES was enough to obtain adequate narcosis, without any other narcotic associated. N_2O elimination of the anaesthetic circuit could not only have an economic impact but also be important for environmental preservation and to avoid pollution of operating theatres [27, 28]

The use of curare was conditional, in all patients, on the kind of surgical intervention applied or used to facilitate oro-tracheal intubation. If, for surgical reasons, recurarisation was necessary within the 20 min before the end of intervention, the action was reversed to allow a rapid recovery of spontaneous ventilation.

The short half-life of REM means that correct analgesia is not ensured after the interruption of product infusion. The use of paracetamol i.v. and s.c. morphine 30 min before the end of the intervention [29] seems a good compromise, allowing correct postoperative analgesia in 95% of patients, monitored with the visual evaluation pain scale showing a mean value of <4.

To avoid postoperative discomfort particular attention must be paid to the relationship between postoperative residual curarisation and postoperative pain. Reversal of curarisation and improvement of the degree of analgesia need to be used if necessary, because rapid recovery allows patients to repress any recollection of a disagreeable experience.

The very rapid recovery after general anaesthesia and the few haemodynamic modifications observed in the postoperative period are elements to point out. These could allow shortening of the patient's postoperative stay in the recovery room and reduce the time in day hospital.

In conclusion, and with reference to the three initially proposed objectives it seems that:

1. Rigorous application of this protocol allows use of DES as the only inhalational narcotic for the induction and maintenance of general anaesthesia.
2. The main haemodynamic modifications observed at the beginning of anaesthesia were bradycardia and hypovolaemic hypotension. During maintenance only modest cardiovascular variations depending on anaesthetic effect were observed. Left ventricular function was very rarely impaired.
3. The postanaesthetic recovery was very rapid, and in all patients subjectively agreeable.

This approach to the induction and maintenance of anaesthesia with the combination of DES and REM should be used in a larger collective of patients to verify the apparently interesting anaesthetic results observed in this series, as well as to allow a more rigorous evaluation of secondary phenomena that could be dependent on this technique.

References

1. Yasuda N, Lockhart SH, Eger EL II et al (1991) Kinetics of desflurane, isoflurane and halothane in humans. Anesthesiology 74:489-498
2. Lochead KM, Karash ED, Zager RA (1991) New advances in anesthesia. Nurs Clin North Am 6:451-461
3. Grundmann U, Risch A, Kleinschmidt S et al (1990) Desflurane animal and human pharmacology: aspect of kinetics, safety, and MAC. Anesth Analg 71:340-348
4. Yasuda N, Targ AG, Eger EL II (1989) Solubility of I-653, sevoflurane, isoflurane and halothane in human tissues. Anesth Analg 69:370-373
5. Joones RM, Koblin DD, Gruenke LD et al (1991) Fluoride metabolites after prolonged exposure to volunteers and patients to desflurane. Anesth Analg 73:180-185
6. Gueugniaud PY, Hanouz JL, Vivien R et al (1997) Effects of desflurane in myocardium: comparison with isoflurane and halothane. Anesthesiology 87:599-609
7. Hanouz JL, Massetti M, Guesne G et al (2000) In vitro effects of desflurane, sevoflurane, isoflurane and halothane in isolated human right atria. Anesthesiology 92:116-124
8. Hanouz JL, Yvon A, Massetti M et al (2002) Mechanism of desflurane-induced preconditioning in isolated human right atria in vitro. Anesthesiology 97:33-41
9. Pirriou V, Chiari P, Lhuiller F et al (2002) Pharmacological preconditioning: comparison of desflurane sevoflurane isoflurane and halothane in rabbit myocardium. Br J Anaesth 89:486-491
10. Behene M, Wilke HJ, Lishcke V (1999) Recovery and pharmokinetic parameters of desflurane, sevoflurane and isoflurane in patients undergoing urologic procedures. J Clin Anesth 6:460-465
11. Nathalson MH, Fedman B, Smith I, White PF (1995) Sevoflurane versus desflurane for

outpatient anesthesia: A comparison of maintenance and recovery profiles. Anesth Analg 81:1186-1190
12. Beaussier M, Deriaz H, Abdelhim Z et al (1998) Comparative effects of desflurane and isoflurane on recovery after long lasting anesthesia. Can J Anaesth 45:429-434
13. Klock PA, Czeslic EG, Klafta JM et al (2001) The effect of sevoflurane and desflurane on upper airway reactivity. Anesthesiology 94:963-967
14. Wrigley SR, Faifield JE, Jones RM, Black AE (1991) Induction and recovery characteristic of desflurane in day cases patients: a comparison with propofol. Anaesthesia 46:615-622
15. Taylor RHI, Lerman J (1992) Induction maintenance and recovery characteristics of desflurane in infants and children. Can J Anaesth 39:6-13
16. Lebenbom-Mansour MH, Pandit SK, Kothary SP et al (1993) Desflurane versus propofol anesthesia: a comparative analysis in outpatients. Anesth Analg 76:936-941
17. Kong CF, Chew STH, Ip-Yam PC (2000) Intravenous opioids reduce airway irritation during induction of anaesthesia with desflurane in adults. Br J Anaesth 84:364-367
18. Egan TD, Lemmens JM, Fiset P et al (1993) The pharmacokinetics of the new short acting opioid remifentanil (G187084B) in healthy adult male volunteers. Anesthesiology 79:881-892
19. Alexander R, Olufolabi AJ, Booyh J et al (1999) Dosing study of remifentanil and propofol for tracheal intubation without use of muscle relaxant. Anaesthesia 54:1037-1040
20. Feiss P (1997) Rémifentanil; avantages cliniques en per opératoire. Cah Anesthesiol 3:223-227
21. Krumholz HM, Radford MJ, Wang Y et al (1999) Early beta-blocker therapy for acute myocardial infarction in elderly patients. Ann Intern Med 131:648-654
22. Schmidt M, Lindenauer PK, Fitzgerald JL, Benjamin EM (2002) Forecasting the impact of clinical practice guideline to perioperative β-blockers to reduce cardiovascular morbidity and mortality. Arch Intern Med 162:63-69
23. Zaugg M, Tagilente T, Lucchinetti E et al (1999) Beneficial effects from β-adrenergic blockage in elderly patients undergoing non-cardiac surgery. Anesthesiology 91:1674-1686
24. Weiskopf RB, Cahalan MK, Ionescu P et al (1991) Cardiovascular actions of desflurane with and without N_2O during spontaneous ventilation in humans. Anesth Analg 75:1103-1114
25. Rampil IJ, Lokhart SH, Zwass MS et al (1991) Clinical characteristic of desflurane in surgical patients: minimum alveolar concentration. Anesthesiology 74:429-433
26. Ghouri AF, White PF (1991) Effects of fentanyl and nitrous oxide on the desflurane anesthetic requirement. Anesth Analg 72:377-381
27. Henderson KA, Raj N, Hall JE (2002) The use of nitrous oxide in anaesthesia practice; a questionnaire survey. Anaesthesia 57:1155-1158
28. Byhahn C, Wilk H-J, Strouhal U et al (2000) Occupational exposure to nitrous oxide and desflurane during ear-nose-throat surgery. Can J Anaesth 47:984-988
29. Muñoz HR, Guerrero ME, Brandes V, Cortínez LI (2002) Effect of timing of morphine administration during remifentanil based anaesthesia on early recovery from anaesthesia and post operative pain. Br J Anaesth 88:814-818

Perioperative b-adrenergic blocking drugs: from concept to applications

R. MUCHADA

Beta blockers (BB) are selective and competitive antagonists of beta adrenergic receptors. They oppose with their action, to the stimulant effect of the sympatho-adrenergic system. Since the differentiation of alpha and beta adrenergic receptors by Alhquist [1], pharmacologists have not ceased to create agonist molecules or increasingly selective antagonists. These molecules are designed to produce the desired action with the least possible secondary effect.

The discovery of propanolol by Sir James Black in 1964 opened the way to the utilisation of BB. The list of products has not ceased to increase. They have been progressively introduced into current therapeutic peri-anaesthetic use [2-5].

Their short half-life and their rapid action aimed at the induction of a pharmacological coma, which is quickly reversible, characterise these anaesthetic drugs. The integration into the therapeutic arsenal of some cardio-vasoactive products to be used during the entire anaesthetic period needs to respect the two preceding conditions: rapid, short and quickly reversible actions.

It is for this reason that the interest for BB use in per anaesthetic period acquired some more interest with the therapeutic introduction of molecule (Esmolol) [6, 7], able to be injected by i.v. way, having a very short duration of action and without marked collateral effect.

Sites of action

The beta visceral receptors are classically divided into two groups: β1 receptors that have cardiac predominance and the β2 receptors that are essentially extracardiac, being localized at the levels of bronchi, vessels, the digestive tract and the uterus.

The actions of a newly described β3 [8] receptor now seem to be arousing some interest in the cardiac action that its stimulation and blockage can determine.

During the peri-anaesthetic period the principal advantage of using BB is concentrated around the ß1 cardiac receptor block.

Effects of the stimulation and the blockage of β1 receptors

The beta myocardial membrane receptors are stimulated by the catecholamines liberated for the postganglion sympathetic neurons and for the suprarenal glands. This results in a trans-membrane action with endocellular activation of the adenylcyclase. This last transforms the ATP to cyclic AMP. The cyclic AMP phosphorilyses, the protein component of the potential-dependent calcium channels. An increase in the number of potential-dependent calcium channels opened during the depolarisation follows where the calcium penetration is more important. This fact is responsible of the cardio-stimulant effects released by the activation of the beta receptors.

With the same level of stimulation, the end-result depends on the number, the sensitivity and the capacity for response of the beta receptors, the last partly influenced by the up- and down-regulation phenomena.

If the number can remain constant, the sensitivity and the reply are largely influenced by the action of BB. The blocking action is achieved by way of a competitive action over the site of action. The presence of beta blocking on the site renders stimulation impossible [9].

What are the aims of BB use in the peri-anaesthetic period?

At present, the researched effects of BB are fundamentally those that concern cardiac activity. For this reason the preference of the choice has to be focused on products having β1 cardioselectivity (β1-receptor block) preponderant [10, 11].

In the peri-anaesthetic period an increase in cathecolamine secretion is frequently observed conditional on a β1 stimulation whose effects increase the inotropism, the chronotropism, the dromotropism and the bathmotropism.

In some conditions, this β1-stimulation can be a risk factor for the patient, when this stimulation is too extreme to allow a response from a heart that is in failure or has a nonadapted coronary perfusion [12, 13].

The entire advantage of utilising BB lies in the possibility of modulating the endogenous β1-stimulation and the excessive response to it, thanks to their fundamentally negative chronotropic, inotropic and bathmotropic actions [9].

On the other hand, excessive β1-cardiostimulation can compromise the myocardial diastolic relaxation by way of a lusiotropic negative effect [14, 15].

Cardioblocking could be opposed to this action, and not only to preserve but also to improve the altered diastolic function [16].

Indications for BBs in the peri-anaesthetic period

From the notion that the cardiac effects of the cathecholamine actions can be modulated with the β1-blockers during the peri-anaesthetics, their use and the indications for them derive from this fact.

Protection against myocardial ischaemia and cardiac failure can be analysed from several points of view:

Negative chronotropic effect

Thanks to this action, the reduction of the heart rate (HR) implies a reduction of the MVO_2 and of the cardiac work and a lengthening of the diastolic time, favouring the duration of the coronary filling time [17-19].

The reduction of the HR can be obtained when a peri-anaesthetic sino-atrial tachycardia or a supraventricular arrhythmia (auricular fibrillation or flutter) are diagnosed

Of course, before proceeding to introduction of a BB to treat a peri-anaesthetic tachycardia, its origin must be identified. It is necessary to diagnose and control the tachycardia dependent on an acute cardiac failure, a respiratory or ventilatory trouble, a hypovolaemia, or an insufficient narcosis or analgesia level.

Antihypertensive action

The treatment of an episode of hypertension during the peri-anaesthetic time with BB [20] merits a certain reflection.

The measured value of arterial pressure (AP), is directly dependent on the temporal variation of two parameters: vascular resistance (VR) and cardiac output (cO).

Starting from this mathematical relationship, the interpretation of the AP modifications remains subjective and user dependent.

The therapeutic goal of antihypertensive drugs is to treat the cause of the pressure modification. The cardioselective BBs, when used for acute therapy, have no action on peripheral vascular resistances or on adrenergic secretion reduction. The only possible way of reducing the AP will be by way of a cO decrease.

In this case, the real physiopathological therapeutic indication of a BB during an acute peri-anaesthetic hypertension syndrome is to reduce the cO, depending on an adrenergic hyperkinetic syndrome.

The beta blockade will be able to reduce the β1-cardiac adrenergic stimulation but in any case will determine a vasodilation with diminution of the afterload.

The desired myocardial protection will be obtained only by means of a myocardial energy consumption reduction secondary to the break imposed to the catecholamine action.

An interesting fact in relation to AP modification with BB is that the Delta systolic AP decrease is 4 to 5 times that in the diastolic AP [21]. The preservation of the Diastolic AP could be another myocardial protection mechanism, because during the diastolic period the coronary filling is diastolic AP dependent.

Positive lusiotropic action

Diastolic ventricular dysfunction, especially in the left ventricle, is a frequently identified alteration [22-25]. It is observed in cardiac patients subjected to continuous and prolonged endogenous adrenergic stimulation and in cases where an acute stimulation (exogenous or endogenous) appears.

This dysfunction could have three important consequences :

1. Reduction of the diastolic ventricular capacity.
2. Reduction of the systolic shortening of myocardial fibres.
   These two determine a decrease in the stroke volume (SV) and compromise the maintenance of an adequate cO, whose compensation is generally achieved by an increase of the HR.
3. Persistence of the ventricular wall tension with reduction of the best coronary filling conditions.

In contrast to the adrenergic stimulation, BB have the capacity to change this situation and to improve a myocardical failure thanks to reactivation of the lusiotropic conditions [26, 27].

This improvement of the ventricle diastolic function could explain and justify the utilisation, frequently recommended, of BB in the case of a diastolic-dependent cardiac failure syndrome.

Whilst BB are generally used in monotherapy, in the peri-anaesthetic period they could be combined with some other cardioactive drugs to modulate the contractility even when a complex acute peri-anaesthetic haemodynamic syndrome is observed [28-32].

Preventive or curative BB utilisation during the peri-anaesthetic period?

Preventive use of BB has been widely recommended by several authors [33-35] in patients with cardiac or coronary risks.

The antecedents of the patients, the pre-anaesthetic treatment with BB and the possibility of increasing the risk with a peri-anaesthetic adrenergic discharge could lead to protection.

This is the case in patients under BB therapy arriving in the operation theatre with a tachycardia of 90 b/min. Reducing the HR to about 60 and 80 b/min could be attempted [36] before induction of the anaesthesia.

Nowadays such a preventive action is easier done because it is possible to proceed in the immediate pre-anaesthetic period to a careful infusion of a preferably short-action BB [37].

But despite the generally positive arguments advanced, the widespread systematic use of BB for prophylaxis, using the argument of a myocardio-protective action in patients over particular age, has received some consistent criticisms that are leading to a review of this kind of indication [38-40].

Three other indications have been recommended for BB peri-anaesthetic utilization:

1. The prevention of the access of tachycardia and hypertension frequently observed during the airway intubation [41, 42]. Actually it is very difficult to adhere to this proposition, because the incidents described are sufficiently worrying to be taken into account. On the other hand, some current anaesthetic techniques allow the adrenergic airway problems to be overcome without using collateral products
2. Hyperthroidism
3. Phaeochromocytoma

These two last specific indications are not dealt with in this text.

A curative therapeutic action of BB has been recommended for treatment of the hypertensive crisis, but for the reasons explained above this indication could have a beneficial result especially in the situation of a hypertension that is cO dependent. Even so, the combination of BB with vasodilators could be interesting because BB action could prevent the baroreflex reaction, avoiding the tachycardia after AP decrease or in controlled hypotension [43, 44].

On the other hand, all the potential benefit of BB has to be exploited in patients exposed to a real risk during their episodes of tachycardia, atrial fibrillation [45] or hyperkinetic cardiac syndrome [46].

Monitoring of BB actions

How is it possible to monitor BB action in the peri-anaesthetic period with a simple technique?

According to what has been said previously, the principal actions of β1-blockers are focused on the negative chronotropic and inotropic effects.

A simple surveillance of the efficiency of BB can be made by:

- Observing the HR variation and adapting the perfused dose to obtain a value between 60 and 80 b/min.
- Deducing the appreciation of the negative inotrope action by following the modification of the systolic AP.

The arterial pressure depends on the cO and VR. Taking into account that the β1-blockers have no action on VR, the reduction in AP is necessarily linked to a decrease in the cO. With a stabilized HR, a non-modified afterload and stable preload, the cO is directly dependent on the inotropic status.

The decrease in AP can be an indirect way of giving information on the negative inotropic action. The excessive negative inotropic action could lead to an extreme reduction of the cO that can compromise the vital organ perfusion in certain patients at risk.

Of course the utilisation of some other haemodynamic monitoring systems is, obviously, recommended because more information can be obtained [47, 48]. These systems allow, for example, continuous cO or the aortic blood flow measurement and appreciation of the systolic left ventricle function, following up the variations of a haemodynamic profile. Information about the pre-ejection period, the systolic blood acceleration, ejection fraction, wall moving, etc. are clearly useful to the user. A real appreciation of the balance between moderation of the chronotropism and quality of the inotropism can then be obtained.

Is it possible to evaluate the necessity for BB therapy in the peri-anaesthetic period by a simple method?

The fundamental objective of the action BB is to preserve cardiac function thanks to the protection against any excessive increase of the MVO_2 and to preserve an adequate condition of the coronary perfusion. The tachycardia, the shortening of the diastolic period and the poor myocardial diastolic relaxation are the three factors favouring heart muscle dysfunction. These three factors could be modified by a correct therapeutic with BB.

From a physiological point of view, the coronary flow depends, partly, on the time of coronary filling, meaning the duration of the diastolic period and the level of the diastolic AP value.

To detect the risk of myocardial suffering following an imbalance between DMO_2/VMO_2, calculation of the "double product" has been proposed [49], which means, the relationship between the HR multiplicator for the systolic AP.

The product of these two parameters allows the introduction of a scale for a evaluation risk.

Once again it is necessary to insist on the fact that the Δ pressure depends on ΔCO × Δ resistance. The interpretation of the "double product" result obtained when the AP modification are predominant can be radically different if the changes of the AP are determined for either cO or for VR modifications.

Instead of using the double product variations it would be more interesting to observe modification of the quotient diastolic AP/HR [50], because it takes into account the factor diastolic pressure, the frequency, and indirectly the duration of the diastolic time.

A quotient diastolic AP/HR of between 0.7 and 1 or >1 makes the possibility of a peri-anaesthetic coronary event unlikely.

A quotient between 0.5 and 7 alerts the practitioner.

Under 0.5 would lead to consideration of a corrective BB therapy to avoid an imbalance between the MDO_2 and the MVO_2.

Of course, this quotient has some limits that need to be respected:

- The quotient can be established for a diastolic AP varying between 40 and 90 mmHg.
- The HR has to be over 80 b/min.

In any case, the decision on the better solution for acting on diastolic AP or HR sequences is left to the practitioner.

It is important to signal that a low HR <60 b/min could be badly supported for some patients having a ventricular capacity limited to compensate the cO frequency dependent on an increase in the SV.

Evaluation of this phenomenon necessitates methods allowing monitoring or calculation of the value of the SV beat for beat.

This monitoring could also allow appreciation of the beneficial effect of a BB on the lusiotropic function. When there is a decrease in the HR and the diastolic period is longer, the ventricular filling is facilitated. If the mechanism of Starling is not exceeded, the ventricular contraction can be improved. This does not mean increasing the ejection fraction, but SV is increased thanks to a greater telediastolic volume.

Choice of BB for the peri-anaesthetic period

The necessary characteristics of a BB to be used during the peri-anaesthetic period are:

a) Suitability for administration by intravenous route.
b) Administration in a bolus or in a continuous infusion.
c) Specificity of β1-action.
d) Rapid regulation of the dose looking for the desired effect by way of the monitored parameters.
e) Short duration of action.
f) Rapid metabolism.
g) Absence of secondary effects of the metabolised product.

Several BB are currently administered intravenously.

Propanolol and sotalol can be administered in a bolus, but they do not have a β1-cardiospecificity; the hepatic metabolism for the first and the renal elimination for the second determine a long half-life (>4 h and to 10 h respectively) do not make them products of choice for the peri-anaesthetic period.

The i.v. route can be used for acebutalol and for metropolol, as a bolus for both or in a continuous infusion for the first. They have β1-cardio specificity, but their half-life is long (>3 h) determined by renal elimination for acebutalol and by hepatic metabolism for the metropolol.

Esmolol (Brevibloc) presents some interesting characteristics that can make of it a product of choice for a preventive action or curative peri-anaesthetic therapy [51, 52].

Administration i.v. as a bolus or continuous infusion is possible. It has cardio β1-selectivity. The product has a very short half-life (9 min) because it is metabolised for the esterases (probably arilsterase) contained on the e-rythrocytes. The degradation products are an acid metabolite (ASL-8123) and methanol. The first has a BB power 1/1,500 that of esmolol. It is eliminated via the kidney. The metanol, does not have a BB action and follows the hepatic degradation way. Only a fraction (>2%) of esmolol is eliminated unchanged in the urine.

Another product presenting similar characteristics to esmolol, landiolol [50], seems to have a more powerful action on chronotropism but a less significant action on inotropism.

Doses recommended

A vigilant attitude has to be maintained when making a decision to use and administer a BB.

In the first place, the indication has to be precise, based on the physiopathologic analysis and on the cardiovascular alterations interpreted in the light of the parameter variations shown for the haemodynamic monitoring.

Secondly, any other peri-anaesthetic alterations, directed at explaining a cardiovascular modification for anaesthetic or surgical facts, needs to be corrected with the adapted action before initiation of the BB therapy.

Thirdly, the therapeutic objective has to be clearly specified (reduction of the tachycardia, treatment of a hyperkinetic syndrome, cardio-ß-modulation, preventive action, etc.).

Fourthly, the individual reaction to the action of BB has to be calibrated, with low doses at the beginning, increased gradually under cardiovascular monitoring until the research goal is reached.

If esmolol is retained as the product of choice the treatment must begin with a dose of 0.25 mg/kg, which could be doubled every 5 min according to the patient reaction, without exceeding 1 mg/kg per dose.

Thereafter, if a continuous perfusion is decided upon it can begin with 20 $\mu g\ kg^{-1}\ min^{-1}$ with a progressive 10- to 20-$\mu g\ kg^{-1}\ min^{-1}$ increase, every 3 min, without exceeding 150 $\mu g\ kg^{-1}\ min^{-1}$.

Contraindications for esmolol

Relative

Systolic arterial hypotension, latent cardiac failure, severe renal insufficiency, state of hypoglycaemia, especially in diabetic patients, venous fragility (risk of endothelial aggression), age less than 12 years.

Absolute

Bradycardia <50 2 b/min, cardiogenic shock, cardiac failure not controlled with treatment, auriculo-ventricular blocks of 2nd and 3rd degrees without pacemaker, atrial or atrioventricular sinuous sicknesses, asthma, bronchospasm and chronic obstructive pulmonary disease, medication with sultopride, hypersensitivity to esmolol are absolute contraindications.

Particular attention is necessary in the case of combination of esmolol with calcium inhibitors, amiodarone and anti-arrhymics, such as propafenone, because some electrophysiological intracardiac conduction and inotropic negative additive effects can be observed.

References

1. Ahlquist RP (1948) A study of adrenotropic receptors. Am J Physiol 153:586-600
2. Piriou V, Aouifi A, Lehot JJ (2000) Intérêt des bêta-bloquants en médecine périopératoire. Can J Anaesth 7:653-663
3. Jones KG, Powell JT (2000) Slowing the heart saves lives: advantages of perioperative ß blockade. Br J Surg 84:689-690
4. Roysler RL (2002) Perioperative beta-blockade can reduce morbidity and mortality. APSF Newslett 17:21-23
5. Raby KE, Brull SJ, Timimi F et al (1999) The effect of heart rate control on myocardial ischemia among high-risk patients after vascular surgery. Anesth Analg 88:477-482
6. Coloma M, Chiu JW, White PF, Armbruster SC (2001) The use of esmolol as an alternative to remifentanil during desflurane anesthesia for fast-track outpatient gynecologic laparoscopic surgery. Anesth Analg 92:352-357
7. Johansen JW, Schneider G, Windsor AM, Sebel PS (1998) Esmolol potentiates reduction of minimum alveolar isoflurane concentration by alfentanil. Anesth Analg 87:671-676
8. Moniotte S, Kobazik L, Feron O et al (2001) Up regulation of b3 adrenoceptors and altered contractility response to inotropic amines in human failing myocardium. Circulation 103:1649-1655
9. Zaugg M, Schaub MC, Pasch T, Sphan DR (2002) Modulation of ß adrenergic receptors subtype activities in perioperative medicine: mechanisms and sites of actions. Br J Anaesth 88:101-123
10. Gheorghiade M, Colucci S, Swedelberg K (2003) ß Blockers in chronic heart failure. Circulation 107:1570-1575
11. Peterzen B, Lonn U, Babi'c A et al (1999) Anesthetic management of patients undergoing coronary artery bypass grafting with the use of an axial flow pump and a short-acting beta-blocker. J Cardiothorac Vasc Anesth 13:431-436
12. Poldermans D, Boeresma E, Bax JJ et al (1999) The effect of bispropolol on perioperative mortality and myocardial infarction in high-risk patients undergoing vascular surgery. Dutch Echocardiographic Cardiac Risk Evaluation Applying Stress Echocardiography Study Group. N Engl J Med 341:1789-1794
13. Auerbach AD, Goldamn L (2002) Beta blockers and reduction of cardiac events in non cardiac surgery. JAMA 287:1435-1444
14. Angeja BG, Grossman W (2003) Evaluation and management of diastolic heart failure. Circulation 107:659-663
15. Vasan RS, Benjamin EJ (2001) Diastolic heart failure – no time to relax. N Engl J Med 1:56-58
16. Kim MH, Devlin H, Das SK et al (1999) Effect of β adrenergic blocking therapy on left ventricular diastolic relaxation proprieties in patients with dilated cardiomiopathy. Circulation 100:729-735
17. Nagatsu M, Spinale FG, Koide M et al (2000) Bradycardia and the role of β blockade in the amelioration of left ventricle dysfunction. Circulation 101:653-659
18. Lechat P, Hulot JS, Escolamo S et al (2001) Heart rate and cardiac rhythm relationships with bispropolol benefit in chronic heart failure in CIBIS II trial. Circulation 103:1428-1433
19. Landesburg G, Zhou W, Aversano T (1999) Tachycardia–induced subendocardial necrosis in acutely instrumented dogs with fixed coronary stenosis. Anesth Analg 88:973-979
20. Pasternack PF, Imparato AM, Bauman FG et al (1987) The hemodynamics of beta blockade in patient undergoing abdominal aortic aneurysm repair. Circulation 76 (Suppl III):1-7
21. Fita G, Gomar C, Rovira I (1999) Esmolol en anestesiología: farmacología e indicaciones. Rev Esp Anestesiol Reanim 46:404-414
22. Grossman W (2000) Defining diastolic dysfunction. Circulation 101:2020-2021
23. Banerjee P, Banerjee T, Khand A et al (2002) Diastolic heart failure: neglected or misdiagnosed? J Am Coll Cardiol 39:138-141
24. Zile MR, Brutsaert DL (2002) New concepts in diastolic dysfunction and diastolic heart failure: part I. Circulation 105:1387-1393

25. Zile MR, Brutsaert DL (2002) New concepts in diastolic dysfunction and diastolic heart failure: part II. Circulation 105:1503-1508
26. Bristow MR (1997) Mechanism of action of beta-blocking agents in heart failure. Am J Cardiol 80:26L-40L
27. Krum H (1999) ß blockers in heart failure. The "new wave" of clinical trials. Drugs 58:203-210
28. Muchada R (2002) Cardio beta modulation with dobutamine – esmolol simultaneous perfusion. Anesthesiology 96:A635
29. Muchada R (1999) Non invasive hemodynamic diagnostic of hyperkinetic septic shock treated with β blocker. Intensive Care Med 25 Suppl 1:142
30. Shakar SF, Abrham WT, Gilbert EM et al (1998) Combined oral positive inotropic and β blockers therapy for treatment of refractory class VI heart failure. J Am Coll Cardiol 31:1336-1340
31. Bristow MR, Shakar SF, Linseman JV et al (2001) Inotropes and β–blockers: is there a need for new guidelines? J Cardiac Failure 72 (Suppl 1):8-12
32. Bristow M (2003) Antiadrenergic therapy of chronic heart failure. Surprises and new opportunities. Circulation 107:1100-1102
33. Magnano DT, Layug EL, Wallace A et al (1996) Effect of atenolol on mortality and morbidity after non cardiac surgery. Multicenter study of perioperative research group. N Engl J Med 335:1713-1720
34. Harwood TN, Butterworth J, Prielipp RC et al (1999) The safety and the effectiveness of esmolol in the perioperative period in patients undergoing abdominal aortic surgery. J Cardiothorac Vasc Anesth 13:555-561
35. Frishman WH, Cheng A (1999) Secondary prevention of myocardial infarction: role of beta adrenergic blockers and angiotensin converting enzyme inhibitors. Am Heart J 137:S25-S34
36. Palatini P, Casaglia E, Julius S, Pessina AC (1999) High heart rate: a risk factor for cardiovascular death in elderly men. Arch Intern Med 159:585-592
37. Barbier GH, Shettigar UR, Appunn DO (1995) Clinical rationale for the use of an ultra short acting beta-blocker; esmolol. Int J Clin Pharmacol Ther 33:212-218
38. Leug JM, Manku K (2000) Prophylactic therapy of preoperative myocardial ischemia. Curr Anesthesiol Rep 2:77-85
39. Howell SJ, Sear JW, Foex P (2001) Peri-operative β-blockade a useful treatment that should be greeted with cautious enthusiasm. Br J Anaesth 2:161-164
40. Kleiman B (2002) Perioperative beta-blockade requires further study – not standard of care. APSF Newslett 17:55
41. Manigaux C, Guignard B, Adam F et al (2002) Esmolol prevent movement and attenuates BIS response to orotracheal intubation. Br J Anaesth 89:857-862
42. Than PH, Yang LC, Shih HC et al (2002) Combined use of esmolol and nicardipine to blunt the haemodynamic changes following laryngoscopy and tracheal intubation. Anaesthesia 57:1195-1212
43. Scott DB, Buckley FP, Drumond GB et al (1978) Cardiovascular effect of labetalol during halothane anaesthesia. Br J Anaesth 3 (Suppl):817-821
44. Edmonson R, Del Valle O, Sha N et al (1989) Esmolol for potation of nitroprusside-induced hypotension: impact on the cardiovascular adrenergic and rening angiotensin systems in men. Anesth Analg 69:202-206
45. Gold MI, Sacks DJ, Grosnoff DB et al (1989) Use of esmolol during anesthesia to treat tachycardia and hypertension. Anesth Analg 68:104-104
46. Seltzer JL, Ritter DE, Starsnic MA, Marr AT (1985) The hemodynamic response to traction on the abdominal mesentery. Anesthesiology 63:96-99
47. Muchada R (2001) Mesure du débit aortique par méthode non invasive. In: Dalens B (ed) Traité d'anesthésie générale, vol 4. Arnette, Rueil-Malmaison, pp 2-18
48. Peterson GE, Brickner E, Reimold SC (2003) Transesophageal echocardiography. Clinical indications and applications. Circulation 107:2398-2402
49. Askenazi J, MacCosbe PE, Hoff J et al (1987) Hemodynamic effects of esmolol, an ultrashort-acting beta blocker. J Clin Pharmacol 27:567-573

50. Buffington CW (1985) Hemodynamic determinants of ischemia myocardial disfunction. Anesthesiology 63:655-662
51. Menkaus PG, Reves JG, Kissing Y et al (1985) Cardiovascular effects of esmolol in anesthetized humans. Anesth Analg 64:327-334
52. Reilly CS, Wood M, Kosakii RP, Wood AJ (1985) Ultra-short-acting-blockade: a comparison with conventional beta-blockade. Clin Pharmacol Ther 38:579-585
53. Sasao J, Tarver SD, Kindscher JM et al (2001) In rabbits, landiolol, a new ultra-short-acting β-blocker exert more potent negative chronotropic effect and less effect on blood pressure than esmolol. Can J Anaesth 48:985-989

Beta blockers in premedication of the cardiac patient – a must in 2003?!

M. Klimek

Myocardial cardiac events are the most common medical complication of surgery, occurring in 2-5% of patients undergoing noncardiac surgery and as many as 30% of patients undergoing vascular surgery. Perioperative cardiac events are associated with a mortality rate of nearly 60% per event, prolonged hospitalisation, and high costs [1, 2]. One study found that postoperative ischaemia increased the odds of postoperative myocardial events 21-fold [3].

The perioperative use of beta-blocking agents has been discussed among anaesthesiologists, cardiologists and surgeons for more than 30 years. Neither several early reports showing the danger of cessation of beta-blocker treatment but a benefit of adding beta blockers to the premedication in at-risk patients nor the extended randomised controlled trials of the late 1990s could change the fact that even today beta blockers are "incredibly underutilised" [4]. Hence you find the "!" after the "?" in the title. This essay aims to promote the use of beta blockers in the premedication of cardiac patients undergoing all kinds of surgery. The author will guide the reader on a path from the historical background via the present state of knowledge to the future perspectives and will also give some advice on implementation of a perioperative beta-blocker protocol in the hospital setting.

The observational years: 1973-1995

In 1973 a reduction of the incidence of perioperative myocardial ischaemia by beta blockers given preoperatively was reported [5]. During the 1980s too, there were several reports showing beta blockers to be effective in reducing perioperative cardiac morbidity and mortality [6-8]. However, at that time antihypertensive treatment with beta blockers was considered to threaten circulatory homeostasis during the procedure. Therefore beta-blocking agents were often stopped before surgery, but there were also some warning comments about propranolol-withdrawal syndromes with episodes of severe hypertension [4, 9, 10].

In the studies of Slogoff and Keats [7, 8] continuation of a chronic treatment with beta blockers in patients undergoing cardiac surgery was associated with less preoperative myocardial ischaemia. In 1987 Pasternack et al. presented a nonrandomised trial on the prophylactic use of metoprolol in abdominal aortic aneurysm repair with a reduction of postoperative myocardial infarction in the treatment group [11]. In the same year Cruickshank et al. published a randomised double blind study in brain trauma patients, showing less myocardial infarction and arrhythmias in patients receiving prophylactic atenolol [12].

Stone demonstrated, in a prospective randomised trial in patients with mild hypertension undergoing noncardiac surgery, that a small amount of beta blocker given with premedication decreased the incidence of perioperative myocardial ischaemia significantly. He failed, however, to show an effect on the cardiac outcome of these patients [13].

Yeager et al. performed a retrospective study in patients undergoing vascular surgery to evaluate possible risk factors of perioperative myocardial infarction and found a risk reduction of 50% in patients taking preoperative beta blockers [14]. However, even in the group of patients receiving beta-blocking agents a 30% incidence of perioperative myocardial infarction was reported, which seems quite high.

The breakthrough

After these more or less observational studies, the breakthrough for the perioperative use of beta blockers in cardiac patients came in the second half of the 1990s.

In 1996 Mangano et al. published the first extended randomised controlled trial [15, 16]. Two hundred patients with or at risk of coronary artery disease who underwent noncardiac surgery showed significantly lower overall mortality among the group receiving atenolol than in the placebo group. This effect was not seen at discharge from the hospital, but built up during the 2 years after hospital discharge. Mangano et al. treated their patients from 2 days before until the 7th day after the procedure and tried to keep the heart rate at about 55-65 bpm and the systolic blood pressure at about 100-110 mmHg.

This study was the subject of some controversy, but a second multivariate analysis of the data confirmed the finding that perioperative atenolol increases survival among patients suffering from diabetes mellitus by 75% [17].

Based on the findings of Mangano, in 1997 the American College of

Physicians presented a guideline on perioperative risk management, recommending atenolol in patients with or at risk of coronary artery disease [18].

Poldermans et al. showed that in high-risk patients undergoing vascular surgery, perioperative bisoprolol reduced postoperative cardiac mortality by 80% and cardiac morbidity by 90% [19].

Their patients had one or more risk factors of coronary artery disease (age >70 years, old myocardial infarction, angina pectoris, history of myocardial decompensation, treated ventricular arrhythmia, hypertension or diabetes mellitus) and a positive dobutamine stress echocardiography. Of 846 patients enrolled based on their risk profile, 173 had positive results on dobutamine echocardiography: 59 of these patients were treated 7 days preoperatively with 5 or 10 mg bisoprolol p.o., aiming for a heart rate of 60 bpm. Intraoperatively metoprolol was given when the heart rate exceeded 80 bpm, whilst 53 patients received standard care without beta blockade. Patients excluded from the study were 53 chronically treated with beta blockers and 8 with extensive wall motion abnormalities.

The same group recently presented another impressive study assessing the effects of perioperative beta blockers in more than 1,300 patients at different risk levels undergoing major vascular surgery. They demonstrated the beneficial effect of perioperative beta blockade in all patients irrespective of risk category: in low-risk patients the rate of cardiac complications was 0.8% with beta blockers vs 2.0% in the control group; in intermediate- and high-risk patients 2.0% of the patients with beta blockers and 10.6% of the placebo group had cardiac complications [20].

In recent years new studies from different groups using different beta blockers in different groups of patients have supported the findings of Mangano and Poldermans.

Raby et al. showed beneficial effects of esmolol on the frequency of perioperative myocardial ischaemia in patients undergoing vascular surgery, but provided no data on the long-term outcome of these patients [21].

Urban et al. also used prophylactic esmolol, but only postoperatively, in patients after total knee arthroplasty. They also found a reduction of perioperative ischaemic events but no improvement of the cardiac outcome [22].

For geriatric patients additional advantages associated with the use of beta blockers were found: patients receiving beta blockers could be detubated earlier, consumed smaller amounts of analgesic drugs and were postoperatively more alert [23].

There is a tendency towards "cautious enthusiasm" in the recent literature about perioperative beta blockers [24]. However, there are still some studies showing little or no effect of perioperative beta-blocker treatment [25-29]. In none of these papers are any data provided to show how effective the beta blockade was accomplished. Giving beta blockers without reducing heart rate seems not to be effective in preventing cardiac morbidity.

In 1999 Sutton and Rock postulated [30]: "Beta blockers should be used in all patients undergoing vascular surgery!" Not only from this author's point of view, in 2003 there is enough evidence available to go even further: *Beta blockers should be used in all patients who are at risk of perioperative myocardial ischaemia and in whom there are no contraindications to the use of beta blockers!* [31-36]

How do beta blockers reduce cardiac risk?

It is frequently postulated that beta blockers suppress the stress response. However, there is no real evidence on this point, since the study of Zaugg et al. showed no alteration of the endocrine response to perioperative stress when beta blockers were given [23]. However, even when the amount of circulating catecholamines is the same, their actions on beta-adrenergic receptors are suppressed.

In a recent study on patients undergoing coronary surgery, the authors thought the protective effect might be based on the better cardiac function or fewer concomitant diseases of patients taking beta blockers. However, in their group of patients these factors were not found [37].

Another theory states that beta blockers reduce the shearing forces on the atherosclerotic plaques in the coronary vessels of the patient, making plaque ruptures and consequent coronary thrombosis with ischaemia less probable [38].

There is also some scientific support for the theory that beta blockers take effect by improving the oxygen supply-demand balance in the myocardium by different mechanisms [4, 39].

The reduced heart rate prolongs diastolic filling of the ventricle, increases the time of coronary perfusion and so increases the time for oxygen delivery. The reduced heart rate and inotropic state are associated with decreased oxygen consumption, but the myocardial metabolism might be improved by other mechanisms, too [14, 40]. Also there are some beta blockers that are known to shift the oxygen dissociation curve to the right, which additionally improves tissue oxygenation.

Another important effect of the beta blockers is their suppression of dysrhythmias, which also has an impact on long-term mortality [41, 42].

Finally, the concept of remodelling of the left ventricle, which is known from patients with chronic heart failure, must also be considered as one possible mechanism improving outcome of perioperative patients [43].

It is necessary to differentiate between patients having acute and chronic treatment with beta blockers, because in the second group an up-regulation of the beta-1 receptors takes place, causing a reduced drug effect. Additionally, the expression of beta-2 receptors might be increased, also causing a reduced effect of the beta blockers [44]. Animal experiments have demonstrated that chronic beta blockade induces a special kind of "inverse agonism", which can also explain the lack of efficiency in chronically treated patients [45].

There is a genetic predisposition determining the efficiency of beta-blocker treatment. This must be given due consideration in comparisons of different populations of patients [46].

Perioperative beta blockers in daily practice

We recommend the use of selective beta-1-receptor blocking agents as these have a lower incidence of side effects than nonselective beta blockers. Peripheral vascular disease is not worsened by using beta blockers [19, 47]. Allergic airway disease is not a contraindication to the use of beta blockers, and especially patients with chronic heart failure (NYHA class II and III) should be treated with beta blockers if necessary [48, 49]. In this second group beta blockers have been shown to improve quality of life and to reduce the frequency of admissions to hospital [50-52].

The known side effects, such as feeling tired or impotence, should be accepted by the patient [35]. However, severe bradycardia and hypotension might lead to a dose reduction or to antagonism with atropine or catecholamines. This happens in about 10-15% of patients [13, 15, 16].

Last but not least, an important reminder: in daily practice in the operating room (OR) one must be aware that a patient under the influence of beta blockers will not react with tachycardia in moments of pain or hypovolaemia. On the other hand, one should not start treating tachycardia by injecting beta blockers in a given patient without having excluded hypovolaemia, hypoxia and hypercapnia [53]. Therefore, especially in patients using beta blockers close monitoring by an alert and skilled anaesthesiologist must be guaranteed.

How to implement a protocol of perioperative beta blockade?

Various regimens of perioperative beta blockade have become established and published. All have grown out of the local situation in the hospital they come from. Therefore, no simple, universal solution can be provided.

1. When is the patient seen by the anaesthesiologist for the first time? Is the anaesthesiologist the right one to start the beta blocker treatment in a certain patient?
2. Who decides whether a patient is at risk of coronary artery disease and has no contraindications? When is this decision taken?
3. Is there close cooperation with the family practitioner? Can the patient start treatment long before elective procedures and continue the treatment afterwards at home?
4. Who is responsible for prescribing the drugs? The surgeon or the anaesthesiologist? Who is responsible for dosing faults and complications?
5. Is there a medical/cardiology department in house caring for these risk patients on the wards? Can additional examinations (e.g. dobutamine echocardiography) be done at short notice?
6. Which i.v. and/or p.o. beta blockers are available in this hospital? Do we prefer a simple, universal or an elaborated, individual approach? Do we prefer an oral or an i.v. regimen? Are the nurses trained and allowed to give beta blockers i.v.? At the moment efficiency is proven for bisoprolol, atenolol, esmolo, labetalol, oxprenolol and metoprolol [54].
7. When should the beta blockers be started and how long should they be continued? Should they be started at home weeks before the procedure p.o. or i.v. with the induction of anaesthesia? Is 2 days after the procedure, the day of discharge from hospital or after 1 year the time to stop, or should they be continued for the rest of the patient's life?
8. Do we use a standard dosage or do we try to keep the patient below a certain heart rate by titrating the drugs? Do we have enough trained manpower to adopt an individual approach, aiming to keep each patient's heart rate at <60 bpm, or do we rely on the efficiency of 5 mg bisoprolol p.o. to reach this aim in the majority of patients?

These are only a few examples of legal and logistical questions that must be considered when such a protocol is introduced.

Auerbach and Goldman recently published a paper summing up the results of their literature review in a clinical algorithm, a set of patient selection criteria and a list of selected medications, routes, and dosages [55]. A large selection of guidelines from different departments is also available on the internet, e.g. http://libraryinfo.bhs.org/secure/bblock.pdf.

How long is it necesary to continue beta blockers?

One of the crucial topics in establishing a beta-blocker protocol is the question of whether, and if so when, a successful beta blocker treatment must be stopped? It may be postulated that withdrawal symptoms and rebound hypertension will not occur if a patient is treated for only a few days [13, 16, 19].

However, there are some data showing increased mortality in patients in whom a long-term beta-blocker treatment has been stopped perioperatively [56]. On the other side, mortality can be reduced by 86% if beta-blocker treatment is continued postoperatively for a year [57].

Close cooperation with the department of internal medicine / cardiology and with the patient's family practitioner is mandatory for a successful implementation of regimen [58, 59].

Open questions

Certainly there is enough evidence to treat patients at risk with beta blockers perioperatively. However, there is also a lack of evidence on some practical aspects of further optimising this treatment [36]:

1. Which group of patients has the greatest advantages from beta blockade?
2. What is the most effective level of beta blockade?
3. Must the heart rate be kept below 70 or 60 or 55 bpm?
4. What are the most effective times for starting and stopping treatment?
5. How many patients develop symptoms of beta-blocker withdrawal even after short-term treatment?
6. Can/may/should beta-blockers be combined with other sympatholytic drugs (e.g. clonidine)?
7. What about beta blockers in patients receiving thoracic epidural anaesthesia?
8. If beta blockers are so effective in reducing risk, do we still need a risk stratification protocol with extensive preoperative testing?

Even when these questions are answered another challenging question will remain:

It is known that surgical high-risk patients have an improved outcome after preoperative optimisation using beta-stimulating agents. How can it be possible that beta-blocking agents also improve the outcome of these patients?

From the author's point of view, preoperative optimisation is all about optimising oxygen transport, creating haemodynamic stability and, last but not least, keeping the patient adequately filled. If these requirements are met, beta blockers will help to balance the oxygen demand-supply ratio and can exert their beneficial effects in preventing plaque rupture at the coronary endothelium.

References

1. Mangano DT, Wong MG, London MJ et al (1991) Perioperative myocardial ischemia in patients undergoing noncardiac surgery. I. Incidence and severity during the 1st week after surgery. The Study of Perioperative Ischemia (SPI) Research Group. J Am Coll Cardiol 17:851-857
2. Mangano DT, Browner WS, Hollenberg M et al (1990) Association of perioperative myocardial ischemia with cardiac morbidity and mortality in men undergoing noncardiac surgery. The Study of Perioperative Ischemia Research Group. N Engl J Med 323:1781-1788
3. Landesberg G, Luria MH, Cotev S et al (1993) Importance of long-duration postoperative ST segment depression in cardiac morbidity after vascular surgery. Lancet 341:715-719
4. Warltier DC (1998) Beta-adrenergic-blocking drugs: incredibly useful, incredibly underutilized. Anesthesiology 88:2-5
5. Prys-Roberts C, Foex P, Biro GP et al (1973) Studies of anaesthesia in relation to hypertension. V. Adrenergic beta- receptor blockade. Br J Anaesth 45:671-681
6. Smulyan H, Weinberg SE, Howanitz PJ (1982) Continuous propranolol infusion following abdominal surgery. JAMA 247:2539-2542
7. Slogoff S, Keats AS (1986) Further observations on perioperative myocardial ischemia. Anesthesiology 65:539-542
8. Slogoff S, Keats AS (1985) Does perioperative myocardial ischemia lead to postoperative myocardial infarction? Anesthesiology 62:107-114
9. Atkinson RS, Rushman GB, Lee JA (1987) A synopsis of anaesthesia, 10th edn. Wright, Bristol
10. Zaugg M, Jamali NZ, Lucchinetti E et al (2000) Norepinephrine-induced apoptosis is inhibited in adult rat ventricular myocytes exposed to volatile anesthetics. Anesthesiology 93:209-218
11. Pasternack PF, Imparato AM, Baumann FG et al (1987) The hemodynamics of beta-blockade in patients undergoing abdominal aortic aneurysm repair. Circulation 76:III1-III7
12. Cruickshank JM, Neil-Dwyer G, Degaute JP et al (1987) Reduction of stress/catecholamine-induced cardiac necrosis by beta 1- selective blockade. Lancet II:585-589
13. Stone JG, Foex P, Sear JW et al (1988) Myocardial ischemia in untreated hypertensive patients: effect of a single small oral dose of a beta-adrenergic blocking agent. Anesthesiology 68:495-500
14. Yeager RA, Moneta GL, Edwards JM et al (1995) Reducing perioperative myocardial infarction following vascular surgery. The potential role of beta-blockade. Arch Surg 130:869-872
15. Mangano DT, Layug EL, Wallace A et al (1996) Effect of atenolol on mortality and cardiovascular morbidity after noncardiac surgery. Multicenter Study of Perioperative Ischemia Research Group. N Engl J Med 335:1713-1720
16. Wallace A, Layug B, Tateo I et al (1998) Prophylactic atenolol reduces postoperative myocardial ischemia. McSPI Research Group. Anesthesiology 88:7-17
17. Mangano DT (1997) Effect of atenolol on mortality and cardiovascular morbidity after noncardiac surgery. N Engl J Med 1997;336:1453-1454
18. American College of Physicians (1997) Clinical guideline I. Guidelines for assessing and managing the perioperative risk from coronary artery disease associated with major noncardiac surgery. Ann Intern Med 127:309-312
19. Poldermans D, Boersma E, Bax JJ et al (1999) The effect of bisoprolol on perioperative mortality and myocardial infarction in high-risk patients undergoing vascular surgery. Dutch Echocardiographic Cardiac Risk Evaluation Applying Stress Echocardiography Study Group. N Engl J Med 341:1789-1794
20. Boersma E, Poldermans D, Bax JJ et al (2001) Predictors of cardiac events after major vascular surgery: role of clinical characteristics, dobutamine echocardiography, and beta-blocker therapy. JAMA 285:1865-1873
21. Raby KE, Brull SJ, Timimi F et al (1999) The effect of heart rate control on myocardial ischemia among high-risk patients after vascular surgery. Anesth Analg 88:477-482
22. Urban MK, Markowitz SM, Gordon MA et al (2000) Postoperative prophylactic administration of beta-adrenergic blockers in patients at risk for myocardial ischemia. Anesth Analg 90:1257-1261

23. Zaugg M, Tagliente T, Lucchinetti E et al (1999) Beneficial effects from beta-adrenergic blockade in elderly patients undergoing noncardiac surgery. Anesthesiology 91:1674-1686
24. Howell SJ, Sear JW, Foëx P (2001) Perioperative β-blockade: a useful treatment that should be greeted with cautious enthousiasm. Br J Anaesth 86:161-164
25. Sear JW, Howell SJ, Sear YM et al (2001) Intercurrent drug therapy and perioperative cardiovascular mortality in elective and urgent/emergency surgical patients. Br J Anaesth 86:506-512
26. Sear JW, Foex P, Howell SJ (2000) Effect of chronic intercurrent medication with beta-adrenoceptor blockade or calcium channel entry blockade on postoperative silent myocardial ischaemia. Br J Anaesth 84:311-315
27. Higham HE, Sear JW, Sear YM et al (2000) Does perioperative silent myocardial ischaemia predict long-term adverse outcome in surgical patients. Br J Anaesth 85:651P-652P
28. Howell SJ, Sear YM, Yeates D et al (1999) β-Blockers and perioperative cardiovascular risk. Br J Anaesth 82:458P
29. Sear JW, George S, Sear YM et al (1999) Can we predict the development of postoperative cardiovascular complications in non-cardiac surgical patients? Br J Anaesth 82 Suppl I:4
30. Sutton T, Rock P (1999) Pro: beta-blockers should be used in all patients undergoing vascular surgery. J Cardiothorac Vasc Anesth 13:490-495
31. Böttiger BW, Martin E (2000) Prevention of perioperative myocardial ischemia - an update. Anaesthesist 49:174-186
32. Piriou V, Aouifi A, Lehot JJ (2000) Perioperative beta-blockers. 2. Therapeutic indications. Can J Anaesth 47:664-672
33. Jones KG, Powell JT (2000) Slowing the heart saves lives: advantages of perioperative beta-blockade. Br J Surg 87:689-690
34. Selzman CH, Miller SA, Zimmerman MA et al (2001) The case for beta-adrenergic blockade as prophylaxis against perioperative cardiovascular morbidity and mortality. Arch Surg 136:286-290
35. Lee TH (1999) Reducing cardiac risk in noncardiac surgery. N Engl J Med 341:1838-1840
36. Damen J (2001) Perioperatieve myocardischemie en niet-cardiale chirurgie. III. Preventie van myocardischemie en cardiale complicaties: een conceptrichtlijn. NVIC Monitor, 2001:4-18
37. Ten Broecke PWC, de Hert SG, Mertens E et al (2003) Effect of preoperative beta-blockade on perioperative mortality in coronary surgery. Br J Anesth 90:27-31
38. Rabbani R, Topol EJ (1999) Strategies to achieve coronary arterial plaque stabilization. Cardiovasc Res 41:402-417
39. Piriou V, Aouifi A, Lehot JJ (2000) Perioperative beta-blockers. 1. Fundamentals. Can J Anaesth 47:653-663
40. Guvendik L, Davies M, Parker DJ (1986) Oral beta-blockade with hypothermic potassium cardioplegia in cardiac surgery. Is there an additive protective effect? Thorac Cardiovasc Surg 34:25-29
41. CIBIS II Investigators and Committees (1999) The cardiac insufficiency bisoprolol study. II. (CIBIS-II): a randomised trial. Lancet 353:9-13
42. Bühler, FR, Bolli P (1980) The concept of beta-adrenoreceptor blockade in the primary and secondary prevention of cardiac mortality and morbidity. Triangle 19:35-45
43. Szabo BM, De Graeff PA (2000) Beta-blockers bij hartfalen. Geneesmiddelbulletin 34:65-70
44. Yndgaard S, Lippert FK, Berthelsen PG (1997) Are patients chronically treated with beta 1-adrenoceptor antagonists in fact beta-blocked? J Cardiothorac Vasc Anesth 11:32-36
45. Milligan G, MacEwan DJ, Mercouris M et al (1997) Inverse agonism at adrenergic and opioid receptors: studies with wild type and constitutively active mutant receptors. Receptors Channels 5:209-213
46. Gottlieb S (2001) β-Blocker response may have gene link. BMJ 322:814
47. Hansson L, Zanchetti A, Carruthers SG et al (1998) Effects of intensive blood-pressure lowering and low-dose aspirin in patients with hypertension: principal results of the Hypertension Optimal Treatment (HOT) randomised trial. HOT Study Group. Lancet 351:1755-1762

48. Tafreshi MJ, Weinacker AB (1999) Beta-adrenergic-blocking agents in bronchospastic diseases: a therapeutic dilemma. Pharmacotherapy 19:974-978
49. Bristow MR (2000) Beta-adrenergic receptor blockade in chronic heart failure. Circulation 101:558-569
50. Abraham WT (2000) Beta-blockers: the new standard of therapy for mild heart failure. Arch Intern Med 160:1237-1247
51. Hjalmarson A, Goldstein S, Fagerberg B et al (2000) Effects of controlled-release metoprolol on total mortality, hospitalizations, and well-being in patients with heart failure: the Metoprolol CR/XL Randomized Intervention Trial in congestive heart failure (MERIT-HF). MERIT-HF Study Group. JAMA 283:1295-1302
52. Bonet S, Agusti A, Arnau JM et al (2000) Beta-adrenergic blocking agents in heart failure: benefits of vasodilating and non-vasodilating agents according to patients' characteristics: meta-analysis of clinical trials. Arch Intern Med 160:621-627
53. Böttiger BW, Martin E (2001) Beta-Rezeptorenblocker verbessern postoperatives Überleben koronarer Risikopatienten. Dtsch Arzteblatt 198:A 1896-1898
54. Park KW (2003) Preoperative cardiology consultation. Anesthesiology 98:754-762
55. Auerbach AD, Goldman L (2002) Beta-Blockers and reduction of cardiac events in noncardiac surgery (scientific review). JAMA 287:1435-1444
56. Shammash JB, Trost JC, Gold JM et al (2001) Perioperative beta-blocker withdrawal and mortality in vascular surgical patients. Am Heart J 141:148-153
57. Martinez EA, Kim LJ, Faraday N et al (2000) Postoperative use of beta-blockers reduces mortality at one year in high risk surgical patients. ASA Abs: A-238
58. Fonarow GC, Gawlinski A, Moughrabi S et al (2001) Improved treatment of coronary heart disease by implementation of a Cardiac Hospitalization Atherosclerosis Management Program (CHAMP). Am J Cardiol 87:819-822
59. Armanious S, Wong DT, Etchells E et al (2003) Successful implementation of perioperative beta-blockade utilizing a multidisciplinary approach. Can J Anaesth 50:131-136

Interactions of anaesthetic drugs with herbal medicines

J. RUPREHT, K. LEENDERTSE-VERLOOP, R. RUPREHT

Interactions and incompatibilities of anaesthetic drugs account for a considerable part of an anaesthetist's training, the aim being safer and predictable course of anaesthesia also in patients with unusual medical background. Smooth, safe and generally trouble-free anaesthesia depends heavily on the choice of anaesthetic drugs and methods of using them in the majority of appropriately prepared patients, as well as on anaesthetists' experience. No one single anaesthetic approach has been successful for all patients, because of medical, pharmacological or organisational interactions and incompatibilities. Some examples follow to illustrate the tricky field of anaesthetic drug interactions with the specific circumstances of an individual patient.

Anaesthetists are well aware of the unsuitability of barbiturates for patients suffering from porphyria. Suxamethonium or halothane must not be used in malignant hyperpyrexia patients, and pethidine interacts badly with some antidepressants. In some patients, opiates cause severe and protracted nausea and vomiting, an interaction with the patient's opiate-receptor system that is better prevented or avoided. Prolonged exposure to nitrous oxide of patients who are treated with cytostatic drugs should be avoided because the cytostatic effect may be dangerously enhanced. Organisational interactions and incompatibilities are just as important as the better acknowledged pharmacological ones. It is unwise to administer long-acting agents in the fast-track anaesthesia approach of day-case surgeries. Conversely, it may be unwise to schedule a severely hypothyroid patient for fast-track day-case anaesthesia. Similarly, a degree of anticoagulation may preclude local or regional anaesthetic blocks. Organisationally, day-case anaesthesia is permissible and compatible only when reliable home after-care has been arranged for the first postoperative night. Contemporary anaesthesiologists are trained to deal with a plethora of anaesthetic drug interactions and with all sorts of medical organisational interference, some of which are declining in importance while others are here to stay.

Not surprisingly, another new field of anaesthetic drug interactions has now been established in patients using herbal medicines [1-4]. Anaesthesiologists and patients should be alerted to the need to communicate about the use of herbal medicines, to be aware of potential interactions in the perioperative period and of the possible need to stop the use of herbs long enough before anaesthesia [5, 6] and surgery.

Prevalence of preoperative use of herbal medicines

Herbal medicines have been ubiquitously used since prehistoric times and have successfully survived the introduction of the scientifically developed drugs of modern medicine. Moreover, recent upheaval about the supposed goodness of all that is called natural has led to indiscriminate acceptance of herbal medicines, often without the slightest critical assessment. In China, traditional medicine continues to thrive splendidly along with the western medicine. The main reasons for use of herbal medicines are the same the world over: management and prevention of chronic disorders, enhancement of general wellbeing and cognitive function and hopes of longevity [7]. In some circumstances, lack of access to formal medicines plays a part. When faced with the surgeon or the anaesthesiologist, many patients fail to consider any herbal treatment as medication and do not report it. The prevalence of herbal use is thought to be high, but seems to be under-reported even in cases where the patients are specifically asked about the intake. It is generally thought that Chinese and U.S. citizens are great consumers of alternative medical treatments, including herbs [2, 8]. Californian investigators estimated that about 40% of surgical patients use alternative medicines and that of these items 67% are herbs. The doctor was not consulted in 44% of cases, and in 56% the use of herbs was not reported to the anaesthetist. Half of the users discontinued their intake of herbs before surgery [8].

A British survey disclosed that only 4.8% of presurgical patients self-administered herbal medicines, and the conclusion was drawn that health care providers must know of this because of potential for side effects and anaesthetic drug interactions [4]. The use of herbal medicines has traditionally been high in Germany. Herb-drug interactions have been recognised in several branches of medicine and counselling of patients about the consequences of concomitant intake demands a tactful and non-judgemental approach [9]. Physicians need to know the basics of the pharmacological actions of herbal medicines in order to warn patients at risk against the concurrent use of incompatible prescription medicines with certain herbal products. For example, patients taking anticoagulation therapy should not touch preparations based on ginkgo, papaya, garlic or ginger. Patients taking several chronic medications should avoid using St. John's wort (*Hypericum perforatum*) as this drug may prime the patient's enzymes for trouble in regard to established chronic medication.

Mechanisms of anaesthetic and herb-drug interactions

Herb-drug intake paves the way to difficulties in the perioperative period in several distinct ways, but the underlying mechanism for the trouble has been elucidated for only a few compounds [1, 10]. Three major mechanisms of interference can cause a disturbance of blood coagulation, diminish the effect of anaesthetic drugs or enhance and prolong anaesthesia. Most reports on anaesthetic drugs interaction with herbal compounds deal with eight commonly used herbal medicines. Limitation of discussion to these eight is misleading because a large number of herbal compounds may be potentially hazardous in the perioperative setting and in emergencies.

Echinacea

Used for generally improving health and for its immunostimulatory effects, echinacea may counteract immunosuppressive medication when taken for shorter periods. Patients awaiting organ transplantation should be advised to avoid taking echinacea. When taken for prolonged periods, e.g. several months or more, echinacea may in fact cause more postsurgical infectious complications. It has been suggested that echinacea may increase the risk of allergic reactions in patients with an allergic constitution [11].

Ephedra

This Eurasian plant species producing the ephedrine alkaloids has been used as a general tonic, as a slimming agent and against respiratory tract dysfunction. Ephedrine alkaloids easily cause a sympathetic overactivity leading to many reported cardiac and cerebral fatalities [12] based on hypertension and vasoconstriction. There is an increased risk of cardiac arrhythmias when ephedrine and volatile anaesthetics act simultaneously, especially in the presence of catecholamine infiltration during surgery. In patients using monoaminooxidase inhibitors it is hazardous to administer ephedrine, as this may result in life-threatening hyperpyrexia, hypertension and coma. Long-term use of ephedra-based-medicines results in perioperative cardiovascular instability due to depletion of endogenous cathecholamines.

Garlic (Allium sativum)

Garlic is one of the 4G herbs causing disturbance of blood coagulation. The other three are ginkgo, ginger and ginseng. Garlic is an essential element in good cooking and in folk medicine. Its historical antihelmintic use has somehow been forgotten, and at present the malodorous herb is promoted for its antiatherosclerotic effects. Unfortunately, dose-dependent inhibition of platelet aggregation accompanies the excessive use of garlic, and this may potentiate the inhibitory effect of prostacyclin or indomethacin on platelet aggregation.

Ginkgo (Ginkgo biloba)

Gingko preparations have been used against senility and age-related afflictions, the beneficial effects supposedly being based on improved blood circulation and an antioxidant effect of ginkgo flavonoids and terpenoids. The anti-platelet-activation effect is worrying in the perioperative period, because many reports of spontaneous bleeding have been attributed to ginkgo [1].

Ginseng

From the famed Asian herb (*Panax ginseng*), but also produced from the Canadian ginseng herb, ginseng has been widely used as a wonder tonic drug to improve adaptation and reduce stress responses [13]. Several decades of research have failed to completely elucidate many of the actions of the ginseng herb. Of importance is a postprandial fall in blood sugar level, an effect which may cause unintended hypoglycaemia in fasting patients. Furthermore, platelet-aggregation inhibition after ginseng use may be irreversible and may cause unpredictable disturbance of perioperative coagulation [14].

Kava

Medicine derived from the dried root of *Piper methysticum*, kava has recently become popular as an anxiolytic and sedative. The kava lactones may act as an antiepileptic and sedative through the GABA-neuroinhibitory effect and prolong barbiturate-induced sleep. A case of coma has been attributed to alprazolam-kava interaction [15]. It is not clear how profoundly a recent intake of kava could potentiate anaesthetic drugs and whether tolerance to kava could result in withdrawal symptoms or a diminished effect of anaesthetics.

Valerian

From *Valeriana officinalis*, valerian has been universally used as a sedative and hypnotic. It apparently acts through GABAneurotransmission [16] and can be expected to potentiate the sedative effects of anaesthetics. Also of importance in the perioperative period is the risk of benzodiazepine-like withdrawal after abrupt discontinuation of valerian. This can easily occur when the use of the drug has not been mentioned and recorded. Benzodiazepines can be used to treat acute valerian withdrawal [17].

Hypericum primes patients for trouble

Hypericum perforatum produces hypericin and hyperforin, the compounds responsible for the antidepressant effect [18], the mechanism being inhibition of serotonin, dopamine and noradrenaline re-uptake. The drug has not been found to improve major depressive states [19]. The drug is nowadays famous for its capacity to induce or trigger the body's defence against chemical toxins, rendering many other drugs less potent [10]. St John's wort induces hepatic metabolism of drugs through activation of the pregnane X receptor (PXR), which serves as a key regulator of cytochrome P 450 (CYP)3A4 [20]. This latter CYP3A4 is a mono-oxygenase involved in the metabolism of many alien compounds which reach the liver. The list of medical drugs that are broken down extra quickly in users of hypercine is very long and contains an impressive number of compounds that are relevant in the perioperative period. Cyclosporine levels decrease in organ recipients and several organ transplant rejections have been ascribed to the hyperactive liver previously primed for trouble by the hypericum drug [1, 10, 21]. The activated CYP3A system also seriously disturbs the therapeutic levels of theophylline, alfentanil, midazolam, lidocaine, calcium--channel blockers and warfarin. Many other drugs may be affected by the concomitant use of hypericum. It has been suggested that several unwanted pregnancies have resulted from inadequate action of the pill during use of hypericum [10].

Perioperative counselling concerning herbal medicine and drug use

During the preoperative assessment and planning for surgery the use of herbal medicines must be checked and, sometimes, stopped. Based on the duration of activity of substances in various herbs it has been advised that use of ephedra and kava be stopped 24 h before surgery. Garlic, ginseng and hypericum should be stopped 7 days preoperatively, and ginkgo 2 days before an operation. No advice has been given for valerian and echinacea [1], but the Hong Kong anaesthesiologists recommend that, in case of doubt, herbal medicines should be stopped 2 weeks prior to anaesthesia and surgery [2]. The accumulated knowledge of the potentially worrying and serious consequences of herbal drug use in the perioperative course has stimulated the American Society of Anaesthesiologists to issue guidelines in a newsletter [22]. The potential risk of herbal medicines has also been the force behind the Swedish and UK efforts to provide information to health professionals and patients [23].

Grey zone of herb use and anaesthetic interaction

Most authors limit their analysis of herbal medicines and anaesthetic drug interactions to 8 or at most to 12 herbal drugs, also including *Glycyrrhiza glabra* (liquorice root) and ginger root [2]. There is still a huge area of illicit drug use, which does not differ at all from the permissive intake of herbal medicines in causing trouble. Anaesthetists should be aware of the possible use of anticholinergic compounds in asthma cigarettes, the use of psilocybe mushrooms, and the widespread use of cannabis or cocaine. All of these and many other nonprescription substances may interact with anaesthetics, a possibility that the anaesthetist should consider.

Furthermore, we hope that special chapters will be included in standard textbooks of anaesthesia, surgery, emergency medicine and intensive care, describing the aspects of interference and trouble caused by the use of biologically active herbal compounds.

References

1. Ang-Lee MK, Moss J, Yuan CS (2001) Herbal medicines and perioperative care. JAMA 286:208-216
2. Cheng B, Hung CT, Chiu W (2002) Herbal medicine and anaesthesia. Hongkong Med J 8:123-130
3. Tsen LC, Segal S, Pothier M et al (2000) Alternative medicine use in presurgical patients. Anesthesiology 93:148-151
4. Skinner CM, Rangasami J (2002) Preoperative use of herbal medicines: a patient survey. Br J Anaesth 89:792-795
5. Dorman T (2001) Herbal medicine and anaesthesia (editorial) Curr Opin Anesth 14:667-669
6. Hodges PJ, Kam PCA (2002) The peri-operative implications of herbal medicines. Anaesthesia 57:889-899
7. Ness J, Sherman F, Pan C (1999) What the data say about common herbal therapies. Geriatrics 54:33-38

8. Leung JM, Dzankic S, Manku K, Yuan S (2001) The prevalence and predictors of the use of alternative medicine in presurgical patients in five California hospitals. Anesth Analg 93:1062--1068
9. Fugh-Berman A (2000) Herb-drug interactions. Lancet 355:134-138
10. Vogel G (2001) How the body's "garbage-disposal" may inactivate drugs. Science 291:35-37
11. Mullins RJ (1998) Echinacea-associated anaphylaxis. Med J Aust 168:170-171
12. Nightingale SL (1997) From the Food and Drug Administration. JAMA 278:15
13. Brekham II, Dardimor IV (1969) New substances of plant origin which increase nonspecific resistance. Annu Rev Pharmacol 9:419-430
14. Janetzky K, Morreale AP (1997) Probable interaction between warfarin and ginseng. Am J Health Syst Pharm 54:692-693
15. Almeida JC, Grimsley EW (1996) Coma from the health food store: interaction between kava and alprazolam. Ann Intern Med 125:940-941
16. Houghton PJ (1999) The scientific basis for the reputed activity of valerian. J Pharm Pharmacol 51:505-512
17. Garges HP, Varia J, Doraiswamy PM (1998) Cardiac complications and delirium associated with valerian root withdrawal. JAMA 280:1566-1567
18. Gaster B, Holroyd J (2000) St John's wort for depression: a systematic review. Arch Intern Med 160:152-156
19. Shelton RC, Keller MB, Gellenberg A et al (2001) Effectiveness of St. John's wort in major depression. JAMA 285:1978-1986
20. Moore LB, Goodwin B, Jones SA et al (2000) St. John's wort induces hepatic drug metabolism through activation of the pregnane X receptor. PNAS 97:7500-7502
21. Ernst E (2002) St. John's wort supplements endanger the success of organ transplantation. Arch Surg 137:316-319
22. Leak JA (2000) Herbal medicines: what do we need to know? ASA Newslett 64
23. Henderson L, Yue QY, Bergquist C et al (2002) St. John's wort *(Hypericum perforatum)*: drug interactions and outcomes. Br J Clin Pharmacol 54:349-356

Awareness during anaesthesia: incidence and clinical and legal aspects

C. Ori, A. Roncarati, S. Rizzi

Until the early 1940s, before the introduction into clinical practice of neuromuscular blocking drugs, the adequacy of the depth of anaesthesia could be assessed by observing patients' reactions to surgical stimuli in terms of gross movements, breathing activity, reflexes, and muscular tone. Furthermore, the use of highly soluble volatile agents made it possible to distinguish clearly between different levels of anaesthesia, which were accomplished quite slowly. In those circumstances, an excessive depth of anaesthesia was the main danger.

With the use of neuromuscular blocking drugs, gross movements in response to surgical stimuli can be blunted in spite of a light level of anaesthesia. Therefore, the major risk is now centred on shallow anaesthesia, that is incomplete unconsciousness in a paralysed patient. Consequently, the monitoring of anaesthesia depth is very important to avoid undesired lightening of anaesthesia and intraoperative awareness.

Monitoring depth of anaesthesia

Several techniques and instruments have been proposed to evaluate depth of anaesthesia. Simply watching patients' movements is obviously an inadequate means of monitoring anaesthesia level, this being only an approximate decurarisation index and not necessarily related to inadequate anaesthesia, but rather representing a spinal reflex. A method developed from this elementary evaluation is the isolated arm technique [1-3]: the forearm is excluded from blood circulation with a tourniquet before muscle relaxants are administered and the anaesthesiologist instructs the patient to move this forearm to order. There is weak relation between movements, narcosis and postoperative recollection of intraoperative events. Neurovegetative disorders (hypertension, tachycardia, mydriasis, perspiration, lacrimation and salivation) are not very reliable indices of anaesthesia depth because they are masked by anaesthetics and, possibly, other drugs administered intraoperatively [4].

The lower oesophageal contractility test [5] is based on the assumption that neuromuscular blocking drugs do not influence smooth muscle and on the observation of a close relation between frequency and amplitude of muscle contraction and anaesthetic concentration. Unfortunately, however, there is wide individual variability in anaesthetic agents, other drugs administered during anaesthesia, and type of surgery, so that the method has low value.

In the same way, wide individual variability precludes basing the evaluation of anaesthesia depth on electromyographical activity of frontal muscle [6], which is innervated by visceral fibres of the VIIth cranial nerve and shows low sensitivity to neuromuscular blocking drugs.

Cortical electric activity is unanimously considered the most reliable index of anaesthesia depth [7]. However, intraoperative recording of an EEG requires cumbersome apparatus and specialised knowledge, so that its routine use seems unreasonable; on the other side, the introduction of microchip technology has allowed elaboration of the EEG signal and its transformation into simple numerical parameters currently used as anaesthesia depth indices: "spectral edge frequency", "median frequency", "zero-crossing frequency", and "bispectral index (BIS)" [2, 8].

Of those techniques, BIS has received most attention and is the only one currently approved by the FDA [9-10]. BIS is based on bispectral analysis, a statistical method used to investigate nonlinear phenomena such as metereological events, oceanic waves and seismic activity.

BIS is the result of the elaboration of data on power, frequency and signal phase plus the analysis of EEG sinusoidal basic elements. The data obtained are subsequently compared with a database collected from healthy anaesthetised volunteers and turned into in a dimensional number ranging from 100 (awake patient) to 0 (no EEG activity) [11-15].

An alternative to EEG-based indices is the use of medium-latency auditory evoked potentials (MLAER) and their related index (AAI) [16-25]. The latter index is obtained by analysing medium-latency evoked responses (presumably located between the medial geniculate body and primary auditory cortex) to acoustic stimulation of the VIIIth cranial nerve. Various reports suggest that MLAER can effectively discriminate between anaesthesia state and consciousness; nevertheless, they are not, or only poorly, affected by some drugs, e.g. opioids, midazolam and ketamine [8]. Regional cerebral metabolism studies emphasise that anaesthesia is related to global cortical and variable subcortical depression, with volatile agents and endovenous drugs having different behaviours [26, 27]. Human studies used positron emission tomography [28, 29], which involves an expensive and bulky device that cannot be used for intraoperative vigilance; however, it could be used in validating BIS and MLAER software.

Conscious awareness and narcosis

Monitoring narcosis depth is not an easy task. In fact, finding a suitable monitoring system able to take into consideration all the variables relating to consciousness and cognition is extremely difficult. Some authors ascribe conscious awareness to particular neural populations, while others believe in the fundamental importance of particular organisations of neural activity consisting in regenerative and self-sustaining processes. These theories are not necessarily mutually exclusive, and most modern research techniques are not able to answer the question [30, 31].

At present, narcosis is explained by hypotheses invoking suppression of neural signal production, blockade of neural signal transmission or disruption of the coherence of neural signs. The paradoxical condition of cortical elevated discharge rates and loss of conscious awareness in propofol or chloralose anaesthesia is compared with the unconscious state resulting from excessive epileptic bombardment producing a blockade of integrative function of the systems that are critical to conscious awareness. Because of our incomplete knowledge of the mechanisms of consciousness and anaesthesia, it is difficult to evaluate and define how cognitive function change with anaesthesia depth; we certainly know that memory function, that is the ability of recall past events, is strictly related to awareness [31].

Many authors distinguish explicit memory, which allows the recall of acquired information and concerns awareness (wakefulness), from implicit memory, which does not allow conscious recollection, belongs to the unconscious sphere and reveals itself in dreams or nightmares related to intraoperative events. During anaesthesia, explicit memory fails first, while implicit memory is deleted slowly. Presumably, there is a transition time in which, without wakefulness, conscious recollection persists [13, 32-34]. The speed of explicit memory loss appears to be related to cognitive ability (speed of memorisation and mental processes) [4].

Incidence and clinical remarks

The issue of awareness during anaesthesia has been reviewed in recent years, and many authors have underlined its relatively high incidence, i.e. about 0.2-0.7% [2, 35-38]. The incidence is considerably higher if we take account of the types of surgery, such as cardiac (1.5%) [39], emergency and trauma (11-43%) [39], or obstetric (0.4%), in which light anaesthesia is required [39]. Moreover, the growth of day surgery has disclosed a large new group of patients exposed to intraoperative awareness, even though different opinions have been formulated [37, 40, 41].

Inadequate dosage of anaesthetic agents, equipment failure, administration of muscle relaxant prior to induction agents and prolonged intubation attempts are frequent causes of awareness during anaesthesia. The main problem with awareness is the morbidity linked to episodes of explicit or implicit memory [3, 10, 39], which becomes manifest in serious emotional injury and post-traumatic stress disorder.

Patients might remember intraoperative events immediately after the recovery from anaesthesia or after 2 days or more. Experiences reported by patients involve sensations of fear and helplessness, sometimes recalled as dreams or nightmares and only rarely associated with acute pain sensations. Other patients describe auditory perceptions (sounds and conversations in the operating room, comments about their body habit, etc.) [39, 42]. Symptoms such as sleep disturbances, dreams, nightmares, anxiety, depression, difficulty in concentrating, irritation, attacks of panic, flashbacks, feelings of fear and anxiety about death are frequent complaints. They are worse in paralysed than in nonparalysed patients and if intraoperative pain is recalled there are more neurotic symptoms [35-37, 39, 43-53].

Legal aspects

At present, few patients file a medical malpractice claim as a result of injuries related to awareness during anaesthesia. This attitude is caused by fear of being considered insane and by the difficulty of demonstrating emotional injury and quantifying its severity, since there is no physical injury. Moreover, low payment for emotional injury may deter plaintiff attorneys from pursuing claims for intraoperative awareness. The recent trend to higher claims for recall during general anaesthesia in the 1990s, compared with the 1970s, may represent an increase in public knowledge about intraoperative recall rather than an increase in incidence [53].

At the moment there is no medicolegal regulation or generally accepted legal opinion. The USA and UK experiences stand out in the world.

In USA, the **ASA Closed Claims Project** counted awareness claims: their incidence was 1.8% of total claims, similar to that for burns, aspiration pneumonitis, myocardial infarction, hepatic dysfunction and renal failure [39, 53]. Compared with all other claims, awareness claims more frequently involved women, patients under 60, and patients undergoing elective surgery.

Claims for awareness in the Closed Claims Database fall into two categories: *awake paralysis* and *recall under anaesthesia* [39, 53].

The first (*awake paralysis*) occurs in the pre-induction or induction period for accidental administration of the muscle relaxant instead of the hypnotic agent. This accident is usually promptly recognised and appropriately managed. Its incidence has remained relatively constant for years. Injury is acknowledged in 96% of events, but is considered slight and compensated with relatively low payments, although anaesthesiologist malpractice and substandard anaesthesia care are always admitted [39].

The second situation (*recall under anaesthesia*) appears during the maintenance phase of anaesthesia and is not always attributed to substandard anaesthesia care. In the research examined, anaesthesia was judged appropriate in 33%, inadequate in 44% and impossible to judge in the remainder of claims. Claims for recall under anaesthesia have increased in frequency in recent years, but the restoration injuries rate is about 56% because it cannot always be related to malpractice or substandard anaesthesia care [39].

The amounts paid are similar in both cases, with average sums of around $20,000 as against average payments of $105,000 for all other claims. Higher payments are related to the presence of additional injuries (aspiration pneumonia with substandard care) [39, 53].

In the USA, legal evaluation of standard anaesthesia care gives importance to halogenated administration, because a volatile anaesthetic level higher than 0.8 MAC certainly reduces recall during anaesthesia [54]. Benzodiazepine premedication has low legal importance [28].

In the United Kingdom, claims of awareness are much more frequent (12.5% of all claims) [55]. This may be a result of differences in anaesthetic technique, but it may alternatively relate to the fact that low-value claims are more likely to be pursued if the patient is able to obtain all legal costs from the state than if the risk of litigation is assumed by plaintiff's lawyer, whose reimbursement is restricted if the outcome is a low settlement (as in the United States).

In the rest of Europe claims for awareness during anaesthesia have remained rare and account of a similar proportion to that in USA, although this issue has not been extensively investigated.

References

1. Tunstall ME (1997) Detecting wakefulness during general anaesthesia for caesarean section BMJ 21:1321
2. Coupland TG (2003) Awareness under anaesthesia is a synonym for inadequate anaesthesia. Anaesth Intensive Care 31:235-236
3. St Pierre M, Landsleitner B, Schwilden H et al (2000) Awareness during laryngoscopy and intubation: quantitating incidence following induction of balanced anesthesia with etomidate and cisatracurium as detected with the isolated forearm technique. J Clin Anesth 12:104-108
4. Munte S, Munte TF, Mitzlaff B et al (2001) Postoperative reading speed does not indicate implicit memory in elderly cardiac patients after propofol and remifentanil anaesthesia. Acta Anaesthesiol Scand 45:750-755
5. Evans JM, Davies WL, Wise CC (1984) Lower oesophageal contractility: a new monitor of anaesthesia. Lancet I:1151-1154
6. Chang T, Dworsky WA, White PF (1988) Continuous electromyography for monitoring depth of anaesthesia. Anesth Analg 67:521-525
7. Schultz B, Schultz A (2002) EEG monitoring improves quality and safety of TIVA. Anaesth Intensive Care 30:817-818
8. Muncaster AR, Sleigh JW, Williams M (2003) Changes in consciousness, conceptual memory, and quantitative electroencephalographical measures during recovery from sevoflurane- and remifentanil-based anesthesia. Anesth Analg 96:720-725
9. Lehmann A, Karzau J, Boldt J et al (2003) Bispectral index-guided anesthesia in patients undergoing aortocoronary bypass grafting. Anesth Analg 96:336-343
10. Bergman IJ, Kluger MT, Short TG (2002) Awareness during general anaesthesia: a review of 81 cases from the Anaesthetic Incident Monitoring Study. Anaesthesia 57:549-556
11. Rosenblatt M, Van Ness Jw (1972) Estimation of the bispectrum. Ann Math Stat 36:1120-1136
12. Rampil IJ (1998) A primer for EEG signal processing in anaesthesia. Anesthesiology 89:980-1002
13. Kerssens C, Lubke GH, Klein J et al (2002) Memory function during propofol and alfentanil anesthesia: predictive value of individual differences. Anesthesiology 97:382-389
14. Drover DR, Lemmens HJ, Pierce ET et al (2002) Patient State Index: titration of delivery and recovery from propofol, alfentanil, and nitrous oxide anesthesia. Anesthesiology 97:82-89
15. Luginbuhl M, Schnider TW (2002) Detection of awareness with the bispectral index: two case reports. Anesthesiology 96:241-243
16. Thornton C, Sharpe RM (1998) Evoked responses in anaesthesia. Br J Anaesth 81:771-781
17. Bailey AR, Jones JG (1997) Patients' memories of events during general anaesthesia. Anaesthesia 52:460-476
18. Schwender D, Klasing S, Madler C et al (1993) Effects of benzodiazepines on mid-latency auditory evoked potentials. Br J Anaesth 71:622-628
19. Schwender D, Klasing S, Madler C et al (1993) Effects of increasing doses of alfentanil, fentanyl and morphine on mid-latency auditory evoked potentials. Can J Anaesth 40:1148-1154
20. Schwender D, Klasing S, Madler C et al (1993) Mid-latency auditory evoked potentials during ketamine anaesthesia in humans. Br J Anaesth 71:629-632
21. Aceto P, Valente A, Gorgoglione M et al (2003) Relationship between awareness and middle latency auditory evoked responses during surgical anaesthesia. Br J Anaesth 90:630-635
22. Absalom AR, Sutcliffe N, Kenny GN (2001) Effects of the auditory stimuli of an auditory evoked potential system on levels of consciousness and on the bispectral index. Br J Anaesth 87:778-780
23. Loveman E, Van Hooff JC, Smith DC (2001) The auditory evoked response as an awareness monitor during anaesthesia. Br J Anaesth 86:513-518
24. Maattanen H, Anderson R, Uusijarvi J et al (2002) Auditory evoked potential monitoring with the AAITM-index during spinal surgery: decreased desflurane consumption. Acta Anaesthesiol Scand 46:882-886
25. Ghoneim MM, Block RI, Dhanaraj VJ et al (2000) Auditory evoked responses and learning and

awareness during general anesthesia. Acta Anaesthesiol Scand 44:133-143
26. Ori C, Dam M, Pizzolato G et al (1986) Effects of isoflurane anaesthesia on local cerebral glucose utilization in the rat. Anesthesiology 65:152-156
27. Dam M, Ori C, Pizzolato G et al (1990) The effects of propofol on local glucose utilization in the rat. Anaesthesiology 73:499-505
28. Alkire MT, Haier RJ, Barker SJ et al (1995) Cerebral metabolism during propofol anaesthesia in humans studied with positron emission tomography. Anaesthesiology 82:393-403
29. Alkire MT, Haier RJ, Shah NK, Anderson CT (1997) Positron emission tomography study of regional cerebral metabolism in humans during isoflurane anaesthesia. Anesthesiology 86:549-557
30. John ER (2002) The neurophysics of consciousness. Brain Res Brain Res Rev 39:1-28
31. Cariani P (2000) Anesthesia, neural information processing, and conscious awareness. Conscious Cogn 9:387-395
32. Barr G, Anderson RE, Owall A, Jakobsson JG (2001) Being awake intermittently during propofol-induced hypnosis: a study of BIS, explicit and implicit memory. Acta Anaesthesiol Scand 45:834-838
33. Ori C, Meroni M, Innocente F (2002) Valutazione della profondità dell'anestesia. In: Gullo A (ed) Medicina perioperatoria, terapia intensiva, emergenze. Springer Italia, Milan, pp 189-198
34. Ghoneim MM (2000) Awareness during anesthesia. Anesthesiology 92:597-602
35. MacClaurin SC (2002) Awareness under TIVA. Anaesth Intensive Care 30:816
36. Ranta SO, Hynynen M, Rasanen J (2002) Application of artificial neural networks as an indicator of awareness with recall during general anaesthesia. J Clin Monit Comput 17:53-60
37. Wennervirta J, Ranta SO, Hynynen M (2002) Awareness and recall in outpatient anesthesia. Anesth Analg 95:72-77
38. Palm S, Linstedt U, Petry A et al (2001) Dose-response relationship of propofol on mid-latency auditory evoked potentials (MLAEP) in cardiac surgery. Acta Anaesthesiol Scand 45:1006-1010
39. Spitellie PH, Holmes MA, Domino KB (2002) Awareness during anaesthesia. Anesthesiol Clin North Am 20:555-570
40. Leslie K, Lee L, Myles PS, Lerch N et al (2003) Patients' knowledge of and attitudes towards awareness and depth of anaesthesia monitoring. Anaesth Intensive Care 3163-3168
41. Spitellie PH, Holmes MA, Domino KB (2002) Awareness during anesthesia. Anesthesiol Clin North Am 20:317-332
42. Yli-Hankala A (2000) Operating theatre – the patient is listening. Acta Anaesthesiol Scand 44:131-132
43. Enlund M, Hassan HG (2002) Intraoperative awareness: detected by the structured Brice interview? Acta Anaesthesiol Scand 46:345-349
44. Lennmarken C, Bildfors K, Enlund G et al (2002) Victims of awareness. Acta Anaesthesiol Scand 46:229-231
45. Ho AM (2001) 'Awareness' and 'recall' during emergence from general anaesthesia. Eur J Anaesthesiol 18:623-625
46. Schou J (2000) Awareness during anaesthesia. Lancet 13:1723
47. Gilston A (2000) Awareness during anaesthesia. Lancet 13:1722
48. Buerkle H, Wuesten R (2000) Awareness during anaesthesia. Lancet 13: 1721-1722
49. Downie P, Avidan M (2000) Awareness during anaesthesia. Lancet 13:1721
50. Sandin RH, Enlund G, Samuelsson P et al (2000) Awareness during anaesthesia: a prospective case study. Lancet 26:707-711
51. Simini B (2000) Awareness of awareness during general anaesthesia. Lancet 26:672-674
52. Metz S (2000) Awareness during cardiac surgery. J Cardiothorac Vasc Anesth 14:107-108
53. Domino KB, Posner KL, Caplan RA et al (1999) Awereness during anaesthesia: a closed claims analysis. Anesthesiology 90:1053-1061
54. Ghoneim MM (2000) Awareness during anaesthesia. Anesthesiology 92:597-602
55. Domino KB, Aitkenhead AR (2001) Medicolegal consequences of awareness during anesthesia. In: Goneim MM (ed) Awareness during anaesthesia. Butterworths, London, pp 155-172

Infection control in operating theatres

K.M. Woodhead

Operating theatre infection control practice in UK has remained largely unaffected by evidence and is to a great extent based on behaviours and rituals which have been practised for many years.

In order to provide clear guidance for the multidisciplinary teams involved, an extensive review of the available English language literature was undertaken over a 2-year period by an expert working party of the Hospital Infection Society and was published at www.his.org.uk in July 2002. My role was to lead the subgroup, specifically looking at behaviours and rituals in operating room practice. This paper will highlight some of the findings and describe recommendations made to influence practice using epic categories to emphasise the strength of the evidence.

Of all patients admitted to hospital, 48% undergo a surgical intervention, and although it is very difficult to identify the specific role that each part of the surgical continuum plays in the acquisition of hospital-acquired infection, it is clear that a high proportion may in some way be attributable to operating theatre practice. Some of that practice will directly relate to the nature of the surgery, to the individual patient, to surgical technique and to other factors, but equally some will be directly related to infection control practice in the operating department. There are no statistics which enable us to define more closely what that direct relationship is, and indeed many patients return so quickly to their homes that follow-through of the exact numbers of post-operative infections for day surgery patients are currently unavailable. Hospital infection surveillance has not been undertaken consistently or comprehensively until the last 2 years, and data has yet to be published. The last available data came from a survey by Public Health Laboratory Service of surgical site infections in 70 acute hospitals undertaken in England, in 1997-1998, which indicated that 4% of patients suffered some kind of wound infection [1].

A National Audit Office report in 2000 stated that it is possible that currently 30% of hospital-acquired infection could be prevented by better application of existing knowledge and implementation of realistic infection control policies [2].

It was within this political and strategic focus on hospital-acquired infection that the group of microbiologists, theatre and infection control nurses, engineers and surgeons met to review practice in perioperative environments.

Practice is heavily influenced by "the way it has always been done", which may be due to the layout of the department and the profile of infection control practice in the hospital. It is not uncommon for orthopaedic theatres to have completely different practices from the general surgical theatre next door. This is usually done on the basis of history rather than evidence or rationale, and may be very confusing for staff, often anaesthetists and nurses, working in different theatres on different days of the week. Rituals develop and get embedded into "the way things are done".

In England and Wales, there has never been clinical policy on infection control determined by central recommendations, which means that each hospital had freedom to devise its own policies and until HIV/Aids became a reality there was very little agreement about core practice. Professional organisations, such as those for theatre nurses and infection control nurses and the Hospital Infection Society have produced guidance, which influences practice but does not determine it locally.

When bloodborne diseases came to the fore and started to influence practice recommendations, the concept of universal precautions was introduced and is widely practised in operating theatres in the United Kingdom. With the advent of variant von Creutzfeldt Jacob disease, practitioners were encouraged to practise standard precautions, where in addition to assuming that all patients had an underlying reason for caution all patients should be assessed individually for potential risks.

Sadly, this is not the situation generally, and the message to move from universal precautions to the specifics of standard precautions has fallen largely on stony ground. It seems that the prevailing hospital culture and awareness of financial imperatives has stopped staff from thinking rationally about their own safety. There are many theatres where personal protective equipment is available, such as eye protection, and is just not used. It is reported that many "old school" staff say that if they have done themselves harm over the last 25 years then wearing goggles now will make no difference. Some of this is due to laziness and some just foolhardiness, but as role models these people do not encourage staff at the beginning of their careers to make their own safety part of everyday practice.

The first recommendation in the behaviours and rituals document is related to universal precautions and is a category 3 recommendation, indicating that there is limited scientific evidence, but uses expert sound infection control and common sense derived from national and international publications. The recommendation states that a standard set of precautions be established for every invasive procedure, with additional risk assessment of every patient to determine extra and specific precautions that may be appropriate.

Other practice is dictated by surgeons who have beliefs about practice, which are rarely challenged, and if they are, there are as many scientific papers to support their practice as to challenge it. Rarely is reference made to the hospital microbiologist to guide or update knowledge. Much depends to the individual department culture as to whether staff are able, or willing to challenge practice. The working party recognised that team members influence much of operating theatre practice, but they rely on all members of the team having similar standards of understanding and knowledge.

Rituals in practice are based on many imponderables. Ford and Walsh wrote extensively of rituals in practice, likening the myths that evolve as becoming parts of the identified tradition [3]. Wicker describes situations which may be more efficiently handled, particularly if they are unpleasant, by standardised behaviour [4]. Others write of the comfort and familiarity of ritualistic behaviour, enabling staff to standardise processes and systems of care. Redfern in 1998 reported from a study she undertook in Australia that only 12% of practitioners based their infection control practice in operating theatres on evidence [5].

The current practice of divesting patients of all their clothing prior to their operation was the next issue identified. A small study in Canada reported no raised infection rates in patients undergoing day case cataract surgery [6] when they were admitted to the operating theatre fully clothed, even with their ordinary outdoor shoes. This reflects much everyday practice in UK ophthalmic units, but written evidence substantiating the Canadian study appears sparse.

Patients in many hospitals in UK are asked to wear a paper hat as part of their theatre "dress" – no evidence could be found for patients' hair as the cause of an increase in infection risk, and so the document suggests that this practice, which is humiliating to patients, be stopped. Patients are often asked to remove their underwear when they come to the operating theatre. Brown [7] described this as the "most illogical of rituals" and suggests that it be stopped, as it causes embarrassment to the patient and serves no useful purpose.

The document therefore recommends that more work is required to confirm these practices, but that the current practice of divesting patients of all their clothes may be unnecessary as a category 3 recommendation.

Pre-operative shaving is the next topic, and unlike the previous two recommendations is assigned a category 1 recommendation, which signifies generally consistent findings from a range of evidence derived from a majority of acceptable studies.

It has long been practice that the patient should be shaved pre-operatively, in the belief that removal of the hair reduces the incidence of wound infection. Shaving was traditionally done on the night prior to operation. This method of hair removal can injure the skin, however, and such injury may cause an increased risk of infection by producing microscopic infected lacerations by the time of operation. The benefit of the use of depilatory creams was demonstrated in 1973 by Cruise and Foord [8]. They found an infection rate of 2.3% in patients who were shaved but of only 1.7% in patients who were not shaved but had their hair clipped, whilst in those patients who were neither shaved nor clipped the infection rate was 0.9%. Seropian and Reynolds [9], in a study of 406 clean wound operations, reported patients shaved had a 5.6% incidence of infection whereas in those who underwent no depilation or in whom a depilatory cream was used the incidence of infection was 0.6%. The hard, chitinous surface of a hair is easier to clean with the skin preparation solution than the skin on which it grows.

A study by Alexander et al. [10] examined infection rates in over 1,000 patients undergoing elective surgery who had their hair removed by either clipping or shaving the night before or on the morning of operation. Fewer infections were found both at discharge and 30 days after surgery in the group that had undergone hair removal by clipping on the morning of surgery.

The recommendation of the document reads "Only the area to be incised needs to be shaved and, if this cannot be done by depilatory cream the day before operation, it should be done in the anaesthetic room immediately pre-operatively using clippers rather than a razor. Shaving brushes should not be used."

1. Avoid shaving if at all possible
2. Use depilatory cream; if this is not possible, use clippers
3. Only shave if other options are not open

Studies relating to the efficacy of pre-operative showering to reduce postoperative wound infections were also examined. Repeated chlorhexidine showers appear to reduce the bacterial count from the skin, and particularly that of staphylococci, but there is little evidence that this makes a significant reduction to the incidence of postoperative infection and it has not been found to be cost effective in the UK. In one study of vascular surgery patients [11] there was a higher incidence of postoperative wound infection in the group that used chlorhexidine than in those who used soap, but this may be related to the distal infection in the leg and contamination of the wound via lymphatics. The statement in category 1 is that there is no evidence that chlorhexidine showers reduce the incidence of postoperative infection.

There is no universal agreement on how long a surgical scrub should be or what type of antiseptic should be used, although it is recognised that it is important for the scrub team to wash their hands before operating.

No agent or method of skin decontamination which causes skin abrasions should be used, and using a scrubbing brush on the skin is not recommended. Dineen [12] found no significant difference between a 5- and a 10-minute handwash. Rehork and Ruden [13], using a 5-minute initial wash, found that if the operation was of less than 1 hour's duration the wash prior to the next operation need only be for 1 minute, but for operations of more than 1 hour the results were inconclusive and a longer wash may be required. Perira, Lee and Wade [14] compared a 3-minute wash and a 30-second subsequent wash with a 5-minute initial and a 3-minute subsequent wash. They also compared 4% chlorhexidine gluconate with 7.5% povidine-iodine. Their optimal regimen was 5 minutes initially followed by the 3-minute wash using chlorhexidine gluconate. Washing for 2 minutes is at least as effective as the 10-minute wash in reducing hand bacterial colony counts, but the optimal duration of washing is not known [15]. The first wash of the day should include a thorough clean under the fingernails. A brush or orange stick can be used.

Alcoholic hand rubs are increasingly available as alternative products for hand hygiene for ward use [16]. The application of alcohol as a gel, foam, or liquid to clean hands is highly effective at destroying micro-organisms on skin surfaces. Ethanol or isopropanol, 60-80%, are even more effective than detergents or antiseptic soaps, if applied to clean hands. These products may be considered by infection control teams for specific situations within operating theatre practice [17]. A British Medical Journal editorial recommended that alcohol hand rubs should replace washing as the recommended method of hand hygiene on the wards [18], and their use is considered adequate in the operating theatre between cases where the surgeons hands are clean and have already been decontaminated by conventional methods.

Hand decontamination is an important contributor to reducing infections. There is no evidence that more than a 2-minute wash using aqueous disinfectants is required, before any procedure regarded as 'sterile'. Alcoholic hand rubs are an acceptable alternative to repeated washing. The recommendation by the HIS document is a category 3 recommendation.

Skin preparation of the operation site was the next topic on which the evidence was surveyed, and the ideal antiseptic described as follows:

- The spectrum of activity should be broad, with rapid and persistent effects against Gram-negative and Gram-positive bacteria and against fungi and viruses which are resistant to some antiseptics.
- It should be resistant to inactivation by organic materials, such as blood and faeces.

- There should be no toxicity or allergic reaction.
- It should be cosmetically acceptable.

Ideally, antiseptics should be supplied at ready-for-use dilution in small, single-use containers with dispensers attached where necessary. Multiple-use containers are liable to contamination each time they are opened, and the re-use of hand pumps and topping up of half-used containers has been implicated in outbreaks of infection by resistant organisms that can multiply in antiseptic solutions [19]. Antiseptic 'cocktails' should not be used because many antiseptics are mutually inactivating. For this reason, if several consecutive applications are made to the same body site, the same agent should be used.

Gross contamination at the site of incision should be removed before the antiseptic skin preparation [20]. The antiseptic skin preparation should be performed in concentric circles moving away from the proposed incision site to the periphery allowing sufficient prepared area to accommodate an extension to the incision or new incisions or drain sites to be made [21]. Sufficient time must be allowed for alcohol-based skin preparation to dry thoroughly before commencing the procedure to ensure that all combustible ingredients have evaporated.

A category 2 was given to this recommendation.

Gloves play a dual role: to give a barrier for personal protection from patients' blood and exudates and to prevent bacteria from the surgeon's hands from entering the surgical site.

Randomised studies within various surgical specialities have shown that wearing two pairs of gloves decreases leaks by 3- to 9-fold in water permeability tests, compared with wearing one pair of gloves [22]. Double gloving may be uncomfortable, reducing manual dexterity and tactile sensitivity, but it provides increased protection from penetration of needlestick injuries [23]. The use of double gloves also reduced the percentage of hand contamination [24]. "Scrub" team members should wear sterile gloves donned after the sterile gown. A fresh pair of sterile gloves should be worn for each procedure. It has been traditional teaching that gloves should be changed promptly if punctured [25]. However, Dodds et al. demonstrated no increase in bacterial contamination of the surgeons' hands or the outside of the surgical gloves in operations where gloves were shown to be punctured and could find no association between glove perforation and postoperative wound infection [26].

The recommendation made within the document is in category 1.

"Wearing double gloves at surgical procedures helps to protect the wearer from viral transmission. There is no evidence that perforated gloves increase the incidence of infection and needle puncture of a glove is not an indication to change gloves. If any action is taken it is preferable to don a second pair of gloves to protect the operating surgeon or individual undertaking the procedure."

Recent UK practice has changed significantly, so that in many specialities masks are no longer worn by all team members, those not in the immediate scrub team being excused. Orthopaedic and neurosurgery are the two main specialities unaffected by this change to everyday practice. Observation in operating theatres in many other parts of the world shows that this practice has not been adopted elsewhere – so what is the evidence? It is possible that UK operating theatres have changed practice too quickly without due respect for the evidence?

The use of masks to reduce post-operative wound infections is questionable. Orr [27] reported that there was no increase in infection rate when masks were not worn for general surgery. Bacterial shedding onto the operative field was found by Berger et al. [28] to be significantly higher when no masks, as compared to full masks, were worn. However, a relationship between contaminant density and wound infection rate was not established. Oral microbial flora dispersal by unmasked male and female volunteers standing 1 metre from the table failed to contaminate exposed settle plates placed on the operating table. Mitchell and Hunt [29] suggested, therefore, that the wearing of face masks by nonscrubbed staff working in an operating room with plenum ventilation appears to be unnecessary.

A controlled, prospective study by Tunevall [30] recorded incidence of wound infection in 3,088 patients over a 2-year period in acute and general surgery. The study design randomised patients into weeks during which staff were "masked" and "unmasked". Results were statistically insignificant, the 1,537 "masked" operations having an infection rate of 4.7% compared with 1,551 "unmasked" operations with an infection rate of 3.5%. However, McLure et al. [31] demonstrated that facemasks significantly reduced the number of bacterial colonies on the operating field.

Masks provide not only a barrier for airborne organisms but also protection for the wearer against blood and body fluid splashes. Risk assessment of such invasive procedures indicates the need for personal protective equipment to be worn by any member of the team undertaking a sterile procedure [32]. There is also a need for staff to be protected from inhalation of surgical smoke and laser plumes [33].

A mask (with a filter size 0.1 μm) may be worn over the mouth and nose by all members of the scrub team, with a visor or goggles as desired, for protection. A fresh mask should be worn for each operation, and masks that become damp should be replaced. Whilst there is no evidence to prove the point either way, it seems reasonable for the scrub team to continue to wear masks when performing prosthetic implant operations. In vertical laminar flow theatres a mask should be worn during prosthetic implant surgery. Although there is no evidence on which to base the recommendation, it seems reasonable that surgeons with beards should wear a facemask.

To summarise the evidence, the document suggests that category 2 should apply to the following recommendation.

"Risk assessment should be undertaken and if necessary masks should be worn for the protection of the wearer; however there is insignificant evidence to support the continued wearing of masks to prevent wound infection. The HIS group accepts that it would be prudent for the 'scrub' team to wear a facemask for prosthetic implant operations. If worn, the mask should be changed after each operation or if deemed to have become contaminated or saturated."

A number of other ritualistic practices were identified as commonly practised in UK operating theatres, which are generally perpetuated by staff, and were examined in order to offer the catalyst for changes in practice. The first of these is jewellery worn by staff. Recommendations by the UK and US professional associations for perioperative nurses are quoted as recommendations as there is little scientific evidence related to the wearing of jewellery in theatres.

A small study by Nicolai et al. [34] found multiple perforations at the base of the gloved ring finger in surgeons who wore a wedding ring during major joint replacement operations and recommended that these be removed.

In the absence of evidence, therefore, a category 3 recommendation was made stating that "necklaces, ear-rings and rings with stones be removed but wedding rings may continue to be worn by 'scrub' and 'nonscrub' staff although surgeons may be advised to remove these, particularly if working with metal prostheses."

Among modern cosmetic practices of staff, that of wearing false nails was identified as needing guidance related to infection control. Hedderwick et al. [35] have shown that false finger nails harbour pathogens, and the longer they are worn the more likely it is that a pathogen will be isolated. They confirm the recommendation that false nails should not be worn in the operating theatre.

Insufficient evidence was found to support the continued wearing of cover gowns, or a covering often untied and barely covering the scrub suit underneath. There is little or no research-based evidence to show that wearing surgical attire outside the theatre and returning to the theatre without changing into clean theatre suits increases surgical wound infection rates. However, in a small study Copp et al. [36] reported that reduced levels of contamination were found on theatre suits when cover gowns were worn outside the operating room. Practice varies in the USA: there is no recommendation restricting the use of scrub suits to the operating suite or for covering the suit when its wearer is outside of the operating suite, whilst in the UK, the National Association of Theatre Nurses recommend that "all personnel should change into outer clothes when leaving the perioperative environment and don a new set of theatre attire upon their return." It was agreed therefore that the recommendation should be based locally on hospital requirements to meet aesthetic and disciplinary requirements.

Footwear in the operating theatre environment was examined next, and two relevant studies were found although the recommendation was set at category 3. Humphreys et al. [37] illustrated that the use of plastic overshoes led to a significant increase in floor colony counts rather than a decrease. Carter [38] also showed that hands became contaminated when overshoes were put on or removed.

The floor surface of the operating theatre should be kept clean, but the effect this has on infection rates remains uncertain. Studies of bacterial contamination of operating theatre corridor floors indicate that any change of footwear should occur as far from the operating theatre as possible [39]. Well-fitting footwear with impervious soles should be worn and regularly cleaned to remove splashes of blood and body fluid. All footwear should be cleaned after every use, and procedures should be in place to ensure that this is undertaken at the end of every session.

A number of environmental issues were identified and sources of evidence for their current practice examined.

Visitors to the operating department are subject to much discussion when perioperative nurses get together; however one aspect of practice is rarely discussed: the ritual of dressing parents and carers in gowns, hats and overshoes before they accompany a child into the anaesthetic room. There is no evidence to support this practice, and overshoes have been shown to positively increase contamination risks to the wearer, as previously stated. If the visitor is to enter the operating theatre itself then they should change into theatre suits.

The influence that this piece of work has had on the workplace and on practice has yet to be determined; however it has been widely published and discussed at international and national meetings. It has certainly raised some interesting further questions and, as ever, has identified the need for further studies. It was also discovered at the discussion following presentation to the 5th International Conference of the Hospital Infection Society in Edinburgh last year that had the group been able to read Swedish additional evidence would have been available!

There has been gathering momentum to provide evidence-based infection control policies for operating departments, and this document has been significantly referenced and used.

Acknowledgements

I gratefully acknowledge the other members of the subgroup, their expertise and their significant contributions to the work.

References

1. Public Health Laboratory Service (1999) Analysis of a year's surveillance in English hospitals 1997-1998. PHLS Colindale, London
2. National Audit Office (2000) Acute infection control in acute hospitals in England. Audit Commission, London
3. Ford P, Walsh M (1994) New rituals for old. Butterworth Heinemann, Oxford
4. Wicker P (1997) Sacred cows and sound practice. Br J Theatre Nurs 7: 31-34
5. Redfern S (1998) Myths and rituals in the operating suite. MSc Dissertation, Monash University, Australia
6. Editorial (1997) OR Manager 13:8
7. Brown GH (1993) The sacred cow contest. Can Nurse 89:31-33
8. Cruise PJ, Foord R (1973) A five-year prospective study of 23,649 surgical wounds. Arch Surg 107:206-210
9. Seropian R, Reynolds BM (1971) Wound infections after preoperative depilatory versus razor preparation. Am J Surg 1971 121:251-254
10. Alexander JW, Fischer JE, Boyajian M et al (1983) The influence of hair removal methods on wound infections. Arch Surg 118:347-352
11. Earnshaw JJ, Berridge DC, Slack RC et al (1989) Do preoperative chlorhexidine baths reduce the risk of infection after vascular reconstruction. Eur J Vasc Surg 3:323-326
12. Dineen P (1969) An evaluation of the duration of the surgical scrub. Surg Obstet 129:1181--1184
13. Rehork B, Ruden H (1991) Investigations into the efficacy of different procedures for surgical hand disinfection between consecutive operations. J Hosp Infect 19:115-127
14. Pereira LJ, Lee GM, Wade KJ (1990) The effect of surgical handwashing routines on the microbial counts of operating room nurses. Am J Infect Control 18:354-364
15. O'Shaughnessy M, O'Malley VP, Corbett G et al (1991) Optimum duration of surgical scrub time. Br J Surg 78:685-686
16. Larson EL (1995) APIC guideline for handwashing and hand antisepsis in healthcare settings. Am J Infect Control 23:251-269
17. Babb RJ (1992) The action of disinfectants and antiseptics and their role in surgical practice. In: Infection in surgical practice. Taylor EW (ed) Oxford Medical Publications, Oxford, pp 56-67
18. L Teare, Cookson B, Stone S (2001) Hand hygiene. BMJ 323: 411-412
19. Ayliffe GAJ, Fraise AP, Geddes AM et al (2000) Control of hospital infection, 4th edn. London, Arnold
20. Recommended practices subcommittee AORN (1982) Proposed recommended practices for preoperative skin preparation of patients. AORN J 35: 918-923
21. Hardin WD, Nichols RL (1997) Handwashing and patient preoperative skin preparation. In: Malangoni MA (ed) Critical issues in operating room management. Lippincott-Raven, Philadelphia, pp 133-149
22. Doyle PM, Alvi S, Johanson R (1992) The effectiveness of double gloving in obstetrics and gynaecology. Br J Obstet Gynaecol 99:83-84
23. Patterson JM, Novak CB, Mackinnon SE et al (1998) Surgeons concern and practices of protection against blood-borne pathogens. Am Surg 228:266-272

24. Fisher MD, Reddy VR, Williams FM et al (1999) Biochemical performance of latex and non-latex double glove systems. J Biomed Mater Research 48:797-806
25. Eckesley JRT, Williamson DM (1990) Glove punctures in an orthopaedic trauma unit. Br J Accident Surg 21: 177-178
26. Dodds RD, Guy PJ, Peacock AM et al (1988) Surgical glove perforation. Br J Surg 75:966-968
27. Orr NW (1981) Is a mask necessary in the operating theatre? Ann R Coll Surg Engl 63: 390-392
28. Berger SA, Kramer M, Nagar H et al (1993) Effect of surgical mask position on bacterial contamination of the operative field. J Hosp Infect 23:51-54
29. Mitchell NJ, Hunt S (1991) Surgical face masks in modern operating rooms – a costly and unnecessary ritual? J Hosp Infect 18:239-242
30. Tunevall TG (1991) Postoperative wound infections and surgical face masks in a controlled study. World J Surg 15:383-388
31. McLure HA, Tallboys CA, Yentis SM et al (1998) Surgical face masks and downward disposal of bacteria, Anaesthesia 53:624-626
32. Hedderwick SA, McNeill SA, Lyons MJ et al (2000) Pathogenic organisms associated with artificial fingernails worn by healthcare workers. Infect Control Hosp Epidemiol 21:505-509
33. Copp G, Mailho CB, Zaler M et al (1986) Cover gowns and the control of operating room contamination. Nurs Res 35:263-268
34. Humphreys H, Marshall RJ, Ricketts UE et al (1991) Theatre overshoes do not reduce operating theatre floor bacterial counts. J Hosp Infect 17:117-123
35. Carter R (1990) Ritual and risk. Nurs Times 86:63-64
36. Nagai I, Kadata M, Takechi M et al (1984) Studies on the mode of bacterial contamination of the operating theatre corridor floor. J Hosp Infect 15:50-55

Perioperative medicine: organisation of operating theatres and recovery room

Y. LEYKIN, S. MILESI

The emergence from the drug-induced coma necessary during surgery is the most critical phase in the post-operative period. At present, 50% of deaths correlated with surgery occur in the first hours of recovery [1]. Patients need observation after any anaesthetic procedure. The level of monitoring may differ according to type of surgery, anaesthetic, patient's conditions and possible complications. Careful and intensive monitoring cannot be achieved in a busy surgical ward, but on the other hand not all patients need to be transferred to the intensive care unit (ICU). The recovery room (RR) can be a satisfactory answer to the needs of post-operative patients.

The RR is defined by the Society of Anaesthesiology of Great Britain and Ireland as "the place where the patient coming from the operating theatre stays till recovery of consciousness and haemodynamic and respiratory steady-state" [2].

The first RR was described in the UK in 1801, while in the USA first RR was opened in 1873 at the Massachusetts General Hospital in Boston [3]. During World War II the RR gained more importance, and specifically trained staff were allocated to this special ward. In the late 1980s, the need for RR increased as "day hospital" procedures became more popular.

At the beginning of the 1990s most anaesthesiological societies elaborated guidelines on the postoperative management of the patient.

Guidelines

The anaesthesiological societies of most countries regulate post-operative surveillance. In France, the "Société Francaise d'Anestésie et de Réanimation" published guidelines to surveillance and post anaesthetic care of the patient in 1990 and 1994. These guidelines served as the basis of a law approved by the Government in 1994 [4]. In 1990, the American Society of Anesthesiology indicated the "standards" for post-operative monitoring, which are the following [5]:

1. All patients undergoing anaesthesia of any kind need adequate post-operative monitoring.
2. The anaesthesiology department bears the medical responsibility for the RR.
3. Clinical conditions of the patients should be recorded on their admission to the RR and monitored periodically.
4. The patients should be accompanied to the RR by the anaesthesiologist with adequate clinical and instrumental monitoring.
5. The RR staff should receive adequate information on the patient.
6. The anaesthesiologist is responsible for discharging or transferring the patient from the RR.

Other countries, such as Australia, Canada, Germany, have also published guidelines on this topic.

The Italian guidelines were written by the Commission on Safety in Anaesthesiology and Intensive Care of the "Società Italiana di Anestesia, Analgesia, Rianimazione e Terapia Intensiva (SIAARTI)" [6, 7]. These are recommendations on optimisation of post-operative care in an equipped area. This document takes into account the inhomogeneous Italian situation, in terms of medical and nursing staff, location and equipment. The recommendations should therefore be seen as a goal, and any department can choose its own way to achieve it, depending on its local situation.

SIAARTI guidelines differ from those of the other countries in the following points:

- Post-operative surveillance may take place in the operating room area or in a dedicated room.
- It is not specified whether the anaesthesiologist accompanies the patient to the RR.
- No specific RR record is foreseen.
- Instrumental monitoring is divided into suggested and optional equipment.
- There is no specific indication on ambulatory anaesthesia.

Organisation (location, equipment, staff)

The RR should be close to the operating theatre, and access to the laboratory and radiology should be rapid and easy. The number of bays in the RR should be 1.5 per theatre, but if the throughput is rapid, as in a day-surgery unit, more will be needed. The temperature should be 21-22°C and relative humidity 38-45% [8].

The bays should be surrounded by a large area (standard floor area is about 9 m^2, but a larger area, e.g. 18 m^2, may be useful for patients needing a higher level of monitoring or mechanical support) to guarantee easy access to the head of the patient and the positioning of emergency carts, ECGraphs, echographs, medication carts etc.

An efficient RR should be equipped with patient **trolleys** or beds which should each have the following characteristics [2]:

- Oxygen cylinder with key, gauge, flowmeter, tubing, suitable oxygen masks.
- Rapid availability of head-down tilt operated from the head end.
- Mounting sites for infusion poles.

Every recovery bay should be equipped with:

- Oxygen supply with a set of facial masks and ventilation bags.
- Suction device.
- ECG, pulse oximeter, invasive and non-invasive blood pressure monitor.

Respiratory equipment

- Respiratory device with adequate monitoring (capnography).

The personnel working in the RR should be highly **professionally trained**. The nurses should be able to promptly recognise any sign of impairment of the vital signs and provide adequate support to the patients until the anaesthesiologist arrives. There should be one nurse to every two patients, unless the clinical conditions require a higher or a lower nurse-to-patient ratio. An anaesthesiologist should be always at reach [7].

Objectives

The stay in the RR has the following goals:

1. Recovery from effects of anaesthetic drugs
2. Stabilisation of cardio-pulmonary system and body temperature
3. Control of hydro-electrolyte balance
4. Intensive care support in case of acute complications
5. Definition of adequate post-operative analgesia
6. Recovery of motor activity after regional anaesthesia

Admission criteria

In the literature, little is mentioned about the admission criteria to the RR, because in most hospitals all surgical patients are observed there. In those cases where there is a patient selection, the admission criteria take into consideration the following:

1. Type and duration of surgery
2. Intraoperative course
3. Condition of the patient
4. Type of anaesthesia

Reception of the patient

When the patient arrives, both the anaesthesiologist and the nurse accompanying him or her give a full report to the colleagues in charge in the RR. It should include:

1. The patient's name and age
2. The clinical conditions and drugs administration before surgery
3. The surgical procedure performed
4. The anaesthetic technique used and its duration
5. The blood loss and fluid balance
6. The final monitoring record
7. Any complication encountered during anaesthesia
8. The number and type of drains and catheters
9. Post-anaesthetic requirements for positioning, oxygen therapy, intravenous fluid, drug therapy and analgesia

The patient should be immediately monitored and routinely observed, at least every 15 min, with records kept of

- Consciousness
- Respiratory function
- Cardiovascular function
- Body temperature, if below 36°C at admission
- Bleeding
- Pain
- Motor block, if regional anaesthesia

Normal recovery from general anaesthesia

The physiological recovery from general anaesthesia is not completed either in the operating or in the recovery room. It can be subdivided into three steps:

- Phase 1, **early recovery**: from the end of administration of anaesthetic drugs until the recovery of reflexes and conscience. This takes minutes.
- Phase 2, **intermediate recovery**: recovery of movement and thinking ability. This takes hours.
- Phase 3, **late recovery**: complete recovery of psychomotor ability. This takes days or weeks [2].

The duration of these three phases actually depends on the elimination time of all given medications and the condition of the patient.

The volatile agents are excreted unmodified by the lungs. Their elimination half-life is proportional to their solubility. Sevoflurane and desflurane have a faster elimination than isoflurane. The rate of metabolism of the gases used at present is very low.

The intravenous hypnotic drugs more used are propofol, thiopentone and ketamine. The rate of elimination of these drugs is faster for propofol and longer for thiopentone and ketamine.

Muscle relaxants have very different times of action, but all non-depolarising muscle relaxant agents are reversed by anticholinesterase (neostigmine). Their duration can be prolonged by low body temperature. Succinilcholine and mivacurium are metabolised by pseudocholinesterase, a lack of which results in a slower metabolism in the liver. This may last for several hours.

At the end of the anaesthesia a good analgesic level should be present, to allow a faster recovery of the patient. This is important especially when rapidly metabolised opioids are used.

Normal recovery from regional anaesthesia

When the patients are selected, they are generally admitted to the RR after combined epidural and general anaesthesia or after complications encountered during regional procedures. They all recover from motor block and start post-operative analgesia.

The recovery from regional anaesthesia is completed by the following steps:

- Cardiovascular stabilisation
- Sensitivity recovery
- Motor block disappearance (Table 1) [9]

Table 1 Bromage scoring system

Score	Block	Residual movement
iv	None	Complete knee and foot flexion
iii	Partial	Knee flexion still possible
ii	Almost complete	Foot flexion still possible
i	Complete	Knee and foot immobile

Discharge criteria

In the RR there is no minimum recovery time requirement, but discharge is possible when the criteria are met. The patient can be discharged to a ward or to the intensive care unit, or in the case of day surgery he/she can return home.

Before the patient is discharged, the RR staff must be sure that:

- The patient is fully conscious and reflexes have returned so s/he can protect his/her airway;
- Breathing is adequate and blood saturation is satisfactory;
- Cardiovascular system is stable;
- Pain is well controlled;
- No blood loss is ongoing.

Patients who are inappropriately prematurely discharged are more likely to have post-operative complications or to suffer injuries due to psychomotor impairment, while an inappropriate delayed discharge may occupy beds that could be used for other patients.

To help timely discharge many scoring systems have been adopted. One of the earliest was Aldrete's [10]. It mimics the Apgar scoring system and is useful for evaluating recovery of patients transferred to a ward (see Table 2). It is not appropriate for ambulatory patients.

To specifically address the intermediate recovery phase of the ambulatory patient, the Postanaesthesia Discharge Scoring System (PADSS) was developed. It assesses vital signs, activity and mental status, pain, nausea, vomiting, surgical bleeding, intake and output (see Table 3) [11].

PADS allows patients to be discharged significantly earlier than those assessed by clinical criteria alone and also gives a medicolegal documentation.

Since intake and voiding were not accepted as universal criteria, PADS was modified (Chung 1995) and these two requirements deleted. (See Table 4 [12]).

Patients whose recovery from anaesthesia is prolonged or complicated should be transferred to the ICU directly from the operating theatre or after admission to the RR.

Table 2 Aldrete scoring system

Parameter	Score
Motility (voluntary or on command)	
Four limbs	2
Two limbs	1
No	0
Respiration	
Deep breathing and active cough	2
Dyspnoea, superficial breathing	1
Apnoea	0
Circulation (systolic blood pressure)	
± 20% of preanaesthetic value	2
± 20-50% of preanaesthetic value	1
± 50% of preanaesthetic value	0
Conscience	
Awake	2
Awakable on calling	1
Not awakable	0
Colour	
Normal	2
Pale	1
Cyanotic	0

Table 3 Postanaesthesia Discharge Scoring System[a]

Vital signs	
Within 20% of preoperative value	2
20% to 40% of preoperative value	1
40% of preoperative value	0
Ambulation and mental status	
Oriented ×3 and has a steady gait[b]	2
Oriented ×3 or has a steady gait	1
Neither	0
Pain or nausea and vomiting	
Minimal	2
Moderate	1
Severe	0
Surgical bleeding	
Minimal	2
Moderate	1
Severe	0
Intake and output	
Has had oral fluid and has voided	2
Has had oral fluid or has voided	1
Neither	0

[a] Maximum score is 10; patients scoring 9 or 10 are considered fit for discharge home.
[b]×3 means that the patient is oriented sufficiently to know his name, his location and the time

Table 4 Modified Postanaesthesia Discharge Scoring System[a]

Vital signs	
Within 20% of preoperative value	2
20% to 40% of preoperative value	1
40% of preoperative value	0
Ambulation and mental status	
Steady gait/no dizziness	2
With assistance	1
No ambulatory or dizziness	0
Nausea and vomiting	
Minimal	2
Moderate	1
Severe	0
Pain	
Minimal	2
Moderate	1
Severe	0
Surgical bleeding	
Minimal	2
Moderate	1
Severe	0

[a] Maximum score is 10; patients scoring 9 or 10 are considered fit for discharge home

RR management and day surgery

Ambulatory anaesthesia care is constantly gaining in popularity because it may allow high volume, fast turnover and overall cost savings, compared with in-patient care. The choice of anaesthetic agents and techniques can improve OR efficiency and utilisation and reduce the amount of RR staff and amount of supplies needed to treat patients recovering from anaesthesia [13].

Home discharge criteria include:

1. Patient awake and alert
2. Stable vital signs
3. Able to ambulate (consistently with preoperative conditions and surgical effects)
4. No active bleeding
5. Adequate control of pain and nausea
6. Oral intake optional
7. Requirement to void pre-discharge only if indicated by surgery or anaesthetic technique (spinal/epidural anaesthesia, pelvic gynaecological/urological or hernia surgery)
8. Availability of a responsible adult

RR costs

The RR expenses are 3.2% of the cost of a patient's hospitalisation and treatment. Two thirds of the entire costs are independent of the actual presence of the patient, because they are due to the furniture, monitoring, staff, etc. More than 90% is accounted for by staff costs. Only 2% is due to the costs of the drugs [14].

The RR in Pordenone

Organisation

The organisation of the RR in Pordenone Hospital is based on the suggestions in the published guidelines, other RRs visited and an analysis of the actual local conditions. The RR is located in the middle of the area of the 10 operating theatres. It has 6 beds, 3 of which are equipped with mechanical ventilators. It is open from 8:00 a.m. to 8:00 p.m. from Monday to Friday.

Clinical model

Patients requiring clinical postoperative monitoring for less than 1 h are observed in the reception ward by the anaesthesiologist and the anaesthetics dedicated nurse working in the operating theatre, while patients needing a longer period of monitoring and care are transferred to the RR. The patients are transferred on a mobiliser; they are accompanied by the anaesthesiologist and by the nurse, vital signs are monitored (ECG and SpO_2), oxygen therapy is administered, and body temperature is maintained. Emergency drugs that may be used during transfer should be ready.

Records are taken from the operating theatre to the RR.

From opening (8:00 a.m.) until the arrival of the first patient, the RR staff prepares the patients (positioning of epidural and central venous catheters) who are to undergo major surgery on the following day. The staff is composed of an anaesthesiologist and two nurses whenever the RR is open.

The main duties of the anaesthesiologist are to:

- Receive the full report on the patient from the colleague in the operating theatre.
- Decide on post-anaesthetic requirements (oxygen, fluid, blood, analgesia), as suggested by the colleague and according to clinical examinations, laboratory tests and instrumental examination.
- Decide on discharge or transfer to the ICU.

- Manage any complication.

The main duties of the nurses are to:

- Receive the full report.
- Position the patient.
- Monitor and record vital signs at least every 30 min.
- Assist mechanical ventilated patients.
- Administer prescribed therapies.
- Psychologically support the patients.
- Prepare the patient for discharge.

The patient can be discharged to the ward by the anaesthesiologist when the following conditions are satisfied:

- The patient is awake.
- Vital parameters are stable.
- No respiratory depression.
- No bleeding.
- No nausea and vomiting.
- Good analgesia.
- Recovery from regional block.

Should any problem arise or the clinical condition be unstable, the patient is transferred to the ICU.

All clinical and instrumental information and the therapy administered to the patient in the RR are recorded.

Special attention is given to post-operative pain control. Different protocols are applied for at least 48-72 h after surgery. The goal is to maintain a score of 3-4 on the Visual Analogue Scale. The patients are monitored from admission to the RR until the end of the analgesic treatment by the nurses on duty in the RR, supervised by the Anaesthesiologist [15].

The mean cost of the RR in Pordenone hospital is about Euro 185,000.00 (without personnel costs).

Results

The first 2 years of activity

In the first 2 years of activity of the RR of S. M. degli Angeli Hospital, Pordenone, from July 1999, 22,363 operations were performed, 11,626 during the first year and 5.3% less in the second. Most (90.2%) of the patients were monitored in the reception ward. During the first year 9.04% were admitted to the RR and 0.95% (111 patients) to the ICU. During the second year 8.94% of patients were sent to the RR and 0.49% (55 patients) to the ICU.

The characteristics of the patients admitted to the RR differed from the first to the second year. Patients aged 61-80 accounted for 50% in the first and 53% in the second year. In the first and second year, respectively, ASA 2 patients accounted for 53.6% and 46.7%, ASA 3 for 28.4% and 41.8%, and finally ASA 4 for 0.48% and 2.34% (see Fig. 1).

As far as the characteristics of the surgical procedures are concerned, major surgery increased from 52.6% in the first to 61.8% in the second year (see Fig. 2).

The patients submitted to general versus combined (epidural and general) anaesthesia were 56.8% and 30.6% in the first and 51.8% versus 38.4% in the second year.

The numbers of patients arriving in the RR mechanically ventilated were 213 (20.3%) in the first and 49 (5%) in the second year.

The numbers of patients transferred to the RR were 111 (0.95%) and 55 (0.49%) in the first and second years, respectively.

The average stay in the RR was 3 h 49 min in the first and 5 h 30 min in the second year.

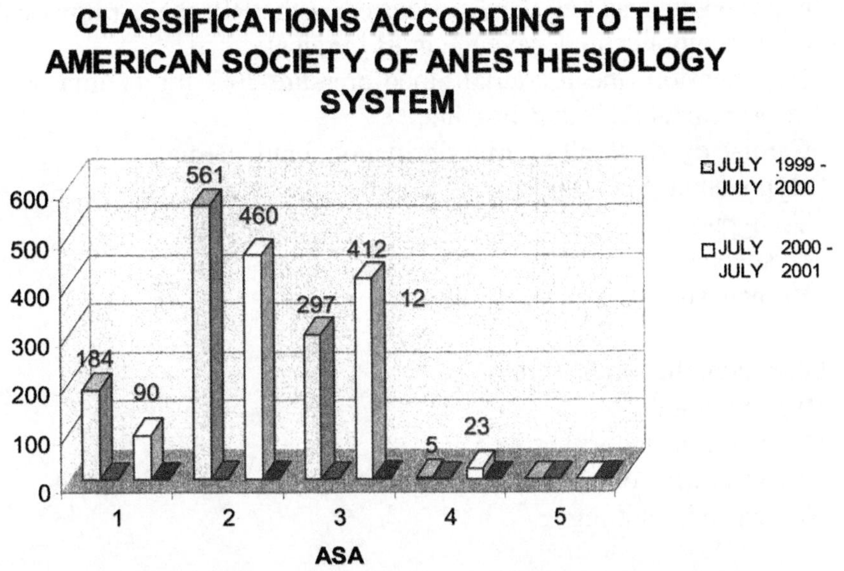

Fig. 1 ASA classification of the patients admitted to the recovery room (RR) in the first 2 years

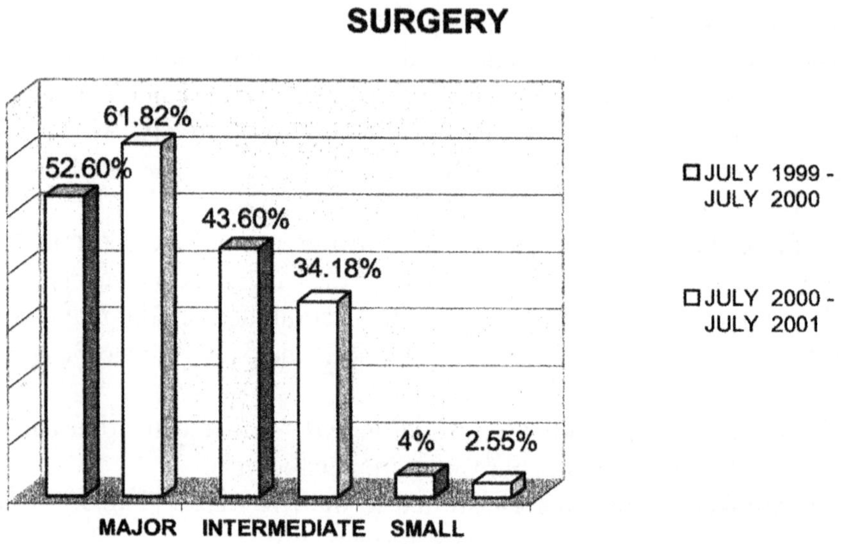

Fig. 2 Level of surgery performed at Pordenone Hospital in the first 2 years of activity of the RR

Complications

In the period analysed no deaths occurred in the RR, the cardiovascular and respiratory complications were the most frequent:

- Hypertension (mean arterial blood pressure 20% for 15 min or a single measurement 50% than baseline);
- Cardiac dysrhythmias (atrial fibrillation, bradycardia)
- Hypoxemia (SpO_2 90%)
- Tachypnoea
- Dyspnoea
- Bronchospasm

Other complications were:
Hyperthermia
Hypothermia and shivering
Oliguria (urine output < 0.5 ml kg^{-1} h^{-1})
Nausea and vomiting

All data are reported in Figs. 3 and 4.

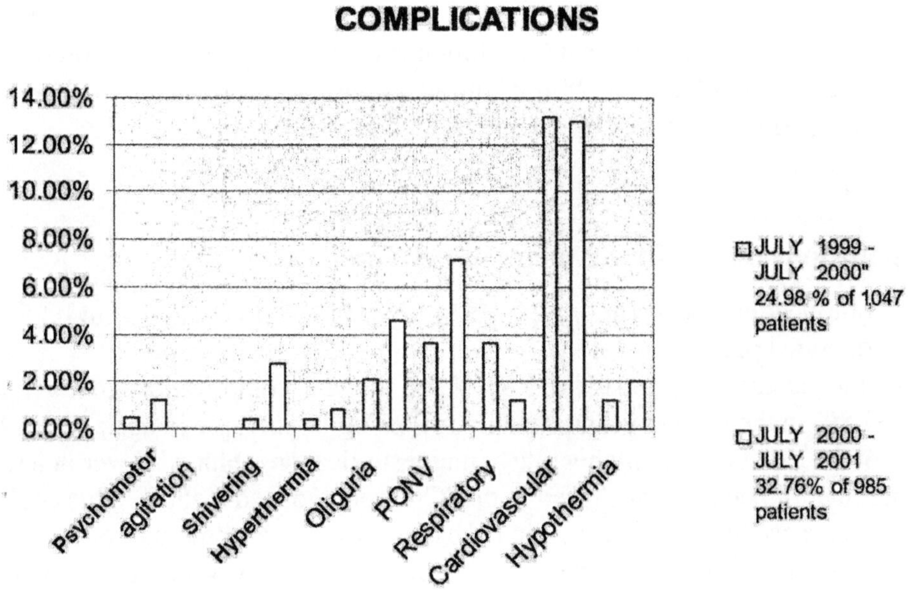

Fig. 3 Overall complications occurring in the RR in the first 2 years of activity

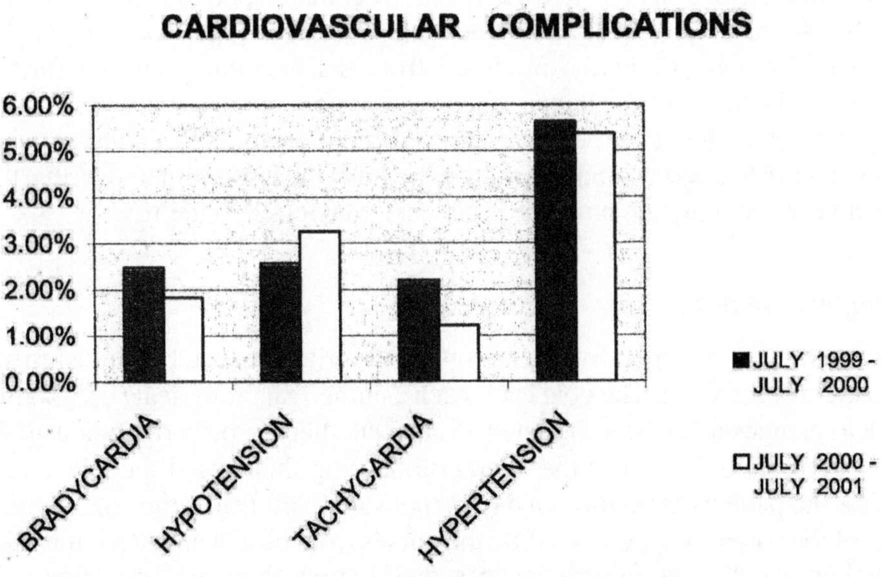

Fig. 4 Cardiovascular complications in the first 2 years of activity of the RR

During the second year, 32 patients underwent operation of major surgery longer than 7 h. They were monitored in the RR for less than 2 h, and then transferred to the ward. In the 48 h following surgery they were monitored for postoperative complications. Minor complications only were recorded: 4 became hyperthermic and 4 lost blood and needed blood transfusion.

Conclusions on the first 2 years of activity

The complications occurring in the RR of Pordenone Hospital affected 2.5% of all operated patients.

Of the patients admitted to the RR, 24.9% showed complications in the first and 32.8% in the second year, probably following an increase in age and ASA class of the patients and a higher rate of major surgical procedures. Nevertheless, the number of patients transferred to the ICU were reduced by 50%. This could happen because of the improved clinical experience of the whole staff of the RR.

The drastic reduction in the number of mechanically ventilated patients arriving in the RR followed the evidence that extubating the patient in the RR did not shorten the interval between operations. Therefore, only patients clinically requiring a longer recovery time from anaesthesia were extubated in the RR during the second year.

The presence of PONV in RR was much lower than reported in the literature, probably due to a high level of attention to the treatment of post-operative pain.

i) The RR was efficiently organised from the beginning, and no further increase in the turn-over of the patients was possible in the second year.

ii) Increased clinical experience allowed monitoring and treating patients with higher ASA scores and submitted to more invasive surgery during the second year, reducing the number of patients transferred to the ICU.

Post-operative pain

Good control of post-operative pain is one of the criteria needed for transferring any patient to the ward. The goal is to reach a numerical rating scale of 3-4 after efficient analgesia has been initiated. Analgesia therapy prescriptions usually cover the first 48-72 h after the operation. During this period the RR nurses monitor the patients three times a day in the wards, informing the anaesthesiologist of the patient's progress, while the nurses from each ward check the VAS throughout the day and inform the anaesthesia nurse about any problems.

During the night the anaesthesiologist and the anaesthesia nurse have the responsibility for postoperative analgesia problems.

Continuous analgesia, beginning in the operating theatre and continuing in the RR and in the designated ward, assures better control over the post-operative pain.

The structure of the RR allows us to apply more invasive analgesia methods (continuous epidural infusions, PCA, use of major opioids, peripheral nerve blocks), to supervise the patient until stabilised by therapy and to treat any side-effect in a better way.

The third year of activity

During the third year of the RR activity the total number of the operations performed was 10,941, 1,093 (9.9%) of which were on patients who were followed in the RR. Fifty-nine patients (0.5% of the total, 5.9% of the RR population) developed complications in the immediate post-operative period. The total number of complications was 163 (1.48% of the total and 14.9% of the RR population). The distribution of the complications is illustrated in Table 5.

Table 5 Type and frequency of the complications occurring in the RR (third year of activity)

Cardiovascular	20.22
PONV	6.40
Oliguria	5.95
Respiratory	5.67
Psychomotor agitation	2.65
Shivering	1.28
Hyperthermia	0.37
Hypothermia	0.00
Other	11.34
Total	100.00

The clinical course of these 59 patients was investigated from the pre-operative period until their discharge from the hospital. Twenty-four patients (41%) were visited by the anaesthesiologist 10-14 days before surgery. Of these, 19 (79% of 24 patients) received further cardiological staff visits. It is important to note that only 1.5% of the over 4,000 patients visited in the pre-anaesthetic clinic are scheduled for a further cardiological visit. Thirteen patients (54% of 24 patients) developed cardiological complications in the post-operative period.

Table 6 illustrates the characteristics of the patients who developed post-operative complications compared to the total population of the RR.

The operations which had a higher rate of complications were: videolaparoscopical cholecystectomy (VLC) (12%, while 7.1 % of the patients in the RR underwent this operation), carotid thromboendoarterectomy (TEA) (12%, 5.9% in RR) and femoral endoprosthesis (8%, 6.6% in RR).

Table 6 Characteristics of the patients with complicated surgery compared with those of the entire population of the RR

	Percentage of patients with complications (n=59)	**Percentage of patients** in RR (n=1,093)
Age 61-80	55.9	54.7
ASA 3-4	63.0	41.0
Emergency	29.0	6.8
Election	71.0	93.2
Major surgery	55.9	57.9
Mean surgery	38.9	39.4
Minor surgery	6.7	3.5
General surgery	47.4	50.4
Orthopaedic surgery	16.9	13.6
ENT surgery	18.1	2.5
Urological surgery	7.0	17.0
Obst-gynaecological surgery	5.0	7.8
Maxillary surgery	0.8	1.1
General anaesthesia	78.0	60.0
Combined anaesthesia	15.2	29.0
Regional anaesthesia	6.7	21.0

The mean length of stay of patients in RR was 3 h 25 min. 74.6% of the 59 patients were transferred to the surgical ward, while 25.4% to the ICU; of these 1 patient died after 6 days in the ICU from multi-organ failure syndrome. The mean stay of patients in the ICU was 3 days 9 h.

The mean hospitalisation time for complicated VLC was 9.6 days, while that for noncomplicated VLC was 2.5 days. Complicated TEA required hospitalisation for 5.8 days, versus 3 days for the noncomplicated variant. Finally, for a femoral endoprosthesis hospitalisation was 11.6 days versus 7-10 days.

One quarter of the patients with complications were discharged with a drug therapy tailored to the postoperative complication.

Conclusions on the third year

The data need further analysis, but some conclusions are possible.

1. The importance of perioperative medicine in the identification of the patient at risk and the reduction of the final postoperative risk for this patient.
2. The ASA class seems to be predictive for the risk of the postoperative complication.
3. Emergency surgery presents higher postoperative risks.
4. General anaesthesia technique presents higher postoperative risks.
5. Postoperative complications, even if not severe, prolong the total hospitalisation period.
6. Major surgery does not increase the postoperative risk.

References

1. Hatfield A, Tronson M (2001) The complete recovery room book. Oxford University Press, Oxford
2. Eltringham R, Casey W, Durkin M (1998) Post-operative recovery and pain relief. Springer, London
3. Zuck D (1995) Anaesthetic and postoperative recovery rooms. Anaesthesia 50:435-438
4. Decree no. 94-1050 du Décembre
5. A.S.A. Standards for Postanesthesia Care (approved by House of Delegates on October 12, 1988 and last amended on October 23, 1990)
6. Torri G (2000) Ruolo della PACU nel postoperatorio. Atti del congresso S.I.A.A.R.T.I, Naples, 25-28 October 2000
7. S.I.A.A.R.T.I. Raccomandazioni per la sorveglianza post-anestesiologica, 8/1994
8. www.virtualcongress.racs.edu.au/open/index.htm 'Virtual Congress of the Royal Australians College of Surgeons', 1999 .
9. Gauthier-Lafaye P, Muller A (1998) Anestesia locoregionale e trattamento del dolore. Masson, Milan p 246
10. Aldrete JA, Droulik D (1970) A postoperative recovery score. Anesth Analg 49:924
11. Chung F (1995) Discharge criteria a new trend. Can J Anaesth 42:1056-1058
12. Chung F (1995) Are discharge criteria changing. J Clin Anesth (Suppl 1):645-685
13. Kapur PA (2002) Challenges in the PACU Annual refresher course of the American Society of Anesthesiology, vol. 265. ASA Orlando Fla, pp 1-7
14. Dexter F, Tinker JH (1995) Analysis of strategies to decrease postanaesthesia unit costs. Anesthesiology 82:94-101
15. Leykin Y, Costa N, Gullo A (2001) Recovery room. Aspetti clinici ed organizzativi. Minerva Anestesiol 67:539-544

Perioperative cardiac anaesthesia: anaesthesia for off-pump coronary artery bypass graft

J.O.C. Auler, S. Almeida de Oliveira

During the last four decades coronary artery bypass grafting (CABG) has been an important weapon in the treatment of patients with coronary artery disease (CAD).

Cardiopulmonary bypass (CPB) was formerly used in the vast majority of patients operated on. This circulatory support created conditions making coronary artery revascularisation possible even in patients with severe and complex lesions and significant left ventricular impairment. Using CPB with correct myocardial protection by cardioplegia, it was possible to induce cardiac arrest in order to obtain a motionless operative field, free of blood, allowing the construction of a high-quality anastomosis.

More recently, with best medical control of CAD and with the progress in percutaneous coronary intervention (PCI), coronary artery revascularisation remains the best option of treatment for patients with more severe disease.

On the other hand, CPB is one of the most important determinants of perioperative morbidity, mainly as a consequence of the blood circulation through a nonendothelial surface.

CABG preformed in a beating heart without the use heart and lung machine (off-pump CAB) was used sporadically since the 1960s [1, 2] new interest in this technique was observed in the 1980s, especially in Brazil [3] and Argentina [4].

In 1995 Benetti et al. [5] reported a successful anastomosis of the left internal mammary artery to the left anterior descending coronary artery through a small left thoracotomy.

This new operation met with great enthusiasm among both surgeons and patients. After this, a large number of manoeuvres and devices were developed to allow better performance of a reliable and secure off-pump CAB through a mini-access. Meanwhile, these facilities have been extended to off-pump coronary artery revascularisation through a median sternotomy.

Spurred on by the awareness of the morbidity related to CPB, and by the possibility of complete revascularisation in off-pump procedures, the application of this technique has increased dramatically [6]. The necessity for reducing the cost of surgical treatment and for shorter stay in hospital were other factors that stimulated the application of this technique.

The evolution of off-pump CAB was then resumed in two phases. In the first phase the revascularisation was limited, being restricted to a few coronary arteries, and in most cases only vein grafts were used. In the second, after the development of technical details and devices for heart exposure, regional coronary artery stabilisation and intracoronary artery shunts, complete revascularisation, even using arterial grafts, was possible in a growing number of cases.

Many observational studies and prospective and randomised trials have been done recently in order to establish the real benefit of off-pump CAB over conventional on-pump CABG [7, 8].

There is considerable evidence showing that judicious application of correctly performed off-pump CABG does reduce cost and length of hospital stay, minimising the morbidity resulting from CPB use and permitting complete revascularisation with a comparable patency rate to bypasses [9, 10].

Graft patency results for off-pump CABG surgery

Complete revascularisation is considered the gold standard for CAGB, in spite of the surgical access and the use or not of CPB. A point of paramount importance for the success of myocardial revascularisation is the number of grafts that remain patent. Early graft patency depends directly on the technical quality of the anastomosis, a point that has been raised in attempts to compare surgery in beating versus arrested heart. The new advances in technology have made multivessel myocardial revascularisation possible without CPB, with good conditions. However, to construct a coronary anastomosis adequately, the surgeon also needs a bloodless field, which requires that the flow of the recipient coronary artery be temporarily interrupted. Vessel snares or vascular clips are used proximally and often also distally during coronary arteriotomy. Since this procedure promotes a bloodless field it provokes myocardial ischaemia and may sporadically cause arrhythmia and haemodynamic instability, sometimes requiring immediate CPB as a support. Before the use of coronary shunts, the regional ischaemia can be minimised by means of ischaemic preconditioning. This concept was obtained in experimental data, indicating that 5-min periods of coronary artery occlusion followed by reperfusion preceding a long period of occlusion markedly diminished the area of myocardial infarction [11]. This problem can be partially solved by placing an intracoronary shunt or seal during the anastomosis. The clinical values of this shunt need to be confirmed, since the flow through the device is only 30-50% and may be a factor in endothelial damage and can be associated with the development of late luminal narrowing [12]. Some data from graft patency investigations are presented in Table 1.

Table 1 Graft patency rates in various series

Author	Number of patients studied	Time after surgery	Percent of grafts that were patent
Oliveira [9]	102	0-7 days	98.1% of all grafts
Calafiore [10]	67	33 days	98.9% of all grafts 100% of left anterior descending artery grafts 98.2% of circumflex artery grafts
Puskas [13]	167	Before discharge	98.8% of all grafts 100% of left internal mammary artery grafts
Bhan [14]	96	Before discharge	95% of all grafts 97.9% of left internal mammary artery grafts
Wiklund [15]	84	0-5 days	96% of all grafts
Jansen [16]	86	6 months	95% of all grafts

In view of the high rates of anastomosis patency and the fact that such an anastomosis can be constructed with enough surgical comfort, it is not surprising that the technique has augmented the number of off-pump bypass operations from a negligible number in 1995 to 10% in 1999, which is expected to rise to 50% compared with traditional CAGB by 2005 [17].

Anaesthesia management of beating heart coronary artery surgery

Anaesthesia management for OPCGB includes the standards of conventional CAGB with CPB: hypothermia during the procedure should be a problem. The literature has shown that an increased rate in postoperative infection [18] in hypothermic patients as well as hypothermia itself causes some delay in extubation. To minimise body temperature losses during the procedure, the patient should be positioned on a water-heated mattress, and an additional heating system is also recommended. Warm fluids administered by the venous route and into the pleural space by the surgeon may also be used during the surgery to minimise the fall of body temperature. A twelve- or five-channel ECG should be continuously displayed, associated with ST segment trend analysis. The ECG waveform may be distorted during displacement of the heart by reduction of the amplitude and a tendency for false minimisation of ST segment changes. Peripheral and pulmonary artery cannulation (PAC) are also recommended, though routine use of PAC remains controversial. Standard gas exchange and respiratory mechanics monitoring are also indicated. Some groups also utilise transoesophageal echocardiography to detect wall motion abnormalities and optimise preload during the procedure. Although transoesophageal echocardiography rapidly demonstrates regional wall motion irregularity, which may indicate regional ischaemia, the displacement of the heart may make its interpretation very difficult [19]. Aspects of fast track anaesthesia, such as use of short-acting agents, aggressive pain control to permit rapid extubation, short stay in the ICU and early hospital discharge should also be considered. In our practice, an association of short-duration muscle relaxant, isoflurane, propofol as a hypnotic for induction and small boluses of sufentanil have been found to confer adequate haemodynamic stability. Slowing the reduction in heart rate is useful during the procedure and can be obtained by using a small bolus of sufentanil.

Depending on the surgical access, for instance a minithoracotomy incision, a single lung ventilation to facilitate heart exposure, caused by inflation and deflation of the left lung, may be considered. Heart access by conventional sternotomy requires single tracheal intubation. The consensus from the Oxford conference about minimally invasive CAGB surgery was also that a median sternotomy incision, besides permitting excellent access for LAD (left anterior descending), for RCA (right coronary artery) and marginal branches of the circumflex artery, was also associated with low morbidity [20]. To facilitate surgical anastomosis, exposure, stabilisation and immobilisation techniques have been introduced to permit access to the lateral, posterior and inferior walls of the heart. Exposure involves the use of retraction sutures in the inferior part of the pericardium to rotate and vertically displace the apex of the heart. Trendelenburg position and rotation of the operating table may also allow better exposure of the heart [21]. Stabilisation of the heart is necessary to facilitate the anastomosis. The immobilisation of the area for anastomosis may be possible utilising pharmacological agents to induce bradycardia by means of calcium or α-blockers, or even high thoracic epidural anaesthesia associated with mechanical devices [22]. In our hospital most of the patients referred for OPCAGB are treated preoperatively with calcium or β-blockers, and during the procedure for the heart immobilisation the surgeon's only option is to use mechanical devices. The stabilisation techniques involve the use of either suction or a compression device. Suction stabilisers utilize a vacuum system to lift the epicardium and pull the tissue to immobilise the local of anastomosis. Compression devices push downward at the selected site to compress the myocardium and restrict its motion, facilitating the surgical procedure.

Heparin 1 to 2 mg /kg is used during anastomotic phase to prevent clotting in the occluded native coronary arteries and arterial conduits. It is important to consider that coagulation is not compromised as it is during CPB, and thrombogenicity may be enhanced owing to the inflammatory response caused by the surgery itself. It must be considered that we antagonise heparin partially with protamine, and some centres recommend postoperative antithrombotic medications [23].

It is important for vasoactive drugs to be prepared and ready for administration, since the occurrence of cardiovascular deterioration is rapid and needs prompt interventions. In general small boluses of epinephrine (10 to 20 μg) are enough to restore cardiac contractility. The challenge in OPCAGB is the duality between circulation and myocardial oxygen consumption. Except in patients with compromised cardiac function or evidence of low cardiac output, β-mimetic agents such as dopamine, norepinephrine, dobutamine and epinephrine should not be regularly infused. On the other hand, the systemic circulation must be preserved within a certain limit in order to avoid hypoperfusion. Systolic arterial pressure is a good index to follow and should be maintained above 100 mmHg or not lower than 20% of baseline. In patients who have a PAC, an early signal of cardiac deterioration is a rapid and progressive elevation of the values. Continuous cardiac output (CCO) is provided by some monitors and may be useful as an indicator of the impact of the heart displacement on cardiac function, though the CCO value displayed in the monitor is few seconds behind the real value. Anaesthesiologists should be aware of this fact to avoid delay in any necessary intervention. Singh et al. compared intermittent cardiac output (ICO) with CCO and static cardiac output (SCO) in 20 patients undergoing off-pump minimally invasive direct coronary artery surgery [24]. They observed 400 pairs of CO during anastomosis of the left internal mammary artery to the left anterior descending artery. They observed a statistically significant decrease in mean arterial pressure and cardiac output; these parameters returned to baseline 1 min after completion of the anastomosis. They also reported excellent correlation among the three methods of the measuring CO at the time of anastomosis [24]. The response time for CCO monitoring is too slow for use as a monitor during manipulation and tilting of the heart, but is useful as a trend monitor during surgery. On-line continuous mixed venous saturation (SVO_2) monitoring reflects changes earlier than CCO variation and is excellent for detecting abrupt changes in CO caused by surgical manipulation of the heart [19].

The mechanisms of haemodynamic changes during off-pump CABG have been a matter of great interest. Haemodynamic changes can be explained as due to manipulation and stabilisation of the heart, or to myocardial ischaemia occurring during coronary occlusion. Anterior heart displacement (90° anterior) and compression of the right ventricle to a greater degree than the left ventricle are responsible for hypotension when suction type stabilisers are used [25]. Compression of the left ventricular outflow tract and difficult diastolic expansion secondary to direct anatomical deformation of the left ventricular geometry are potential mechanisms for haemodynamic alterations. The diminution of CO during OPCAB surgery is due to both left *and right* ventricular dysfunction and may be greater when the heart is positioned for the anastomosis of the circumflex artery. The torsion of the heart initially promotes outflow obstruction of the right ventricle, causing elevation of central venous pressure and decreasing CO. If left ventricular function is not affected by ischaemia, pulmonary arterial pressures remain unchanged or are decreased, as occurs with pulmonary wedge pressure. Progressive elevation of pulmonary artery pressure may reflect severe left ventricular deterioration resulting from ischaemia. Hypotension caused by outflow obstruction of the right ventricle may be reversed by placing the patient in a 30° head-down tilt and implementing an aggressive preload increased by previous volaemic expansion. When the situation persists, additional fluids may be infused and or a vasoconstrictor agent administered to increase preload and preserve cardiac output. Severe pulmonary hypertension requires anti-ischaemic therapy or immediate reversion of the heart position, or even conversion from an off-pump technique to bypass support [19, 26].

Communication between the anaesthesiologist and the surgeon is decisive to the success of OPCAB surgery. The anaesthesiologist must keep the surgeon informed about the use of or necessity for inotropes or vasopressors, ST segment or rhythm alterations, and the patient's general condition. Parameters, such as systolic arterial pressure and data from PAC, pressure levels, CO and SVO_2 if available, are also very important. Information from the surgeon should be transmitted too, such as the moment of heart displacement, when a coronary artery is occluded, and whether a shunt is necessary.

In summary, the principal aspects of anaesthesia management during off-pump CAGB are:

- Wall myocardial motion must be restrained enough to permit meticulous anastomosis, with minimal interference in the mechanical contraction.
- Deterioration of cardiac output during heart displacement needs to be diminished, identified and adequately treated.
- Possible regional ischaemia during recipient artery clamping should be minimised and promptly recognised.
- The extension of monitoring should be individualised according to the number of grafts and anatomic site, as well as previous cardiac function.

– Principles of fast track anaesthesia should be considered to promote shorter hospital stay.

In conclusion, OPCAGB has been demonstrated to be safe and effective, and early outcomes and graft patency rates appear to be of at least as good as those seen with traditional CAGB utilising CPB. Certain high-risk groups may be better referred for OPCAGB, but its advantages and disadvantages need to be evaluated in large randomised studies in order to verify the safety and efficacy of these new techniques in terms of long-term graft patency and reduced morbidity. Studies suggest that PTCA and OPCAGB offer exciting new research horizons and this new surgical technique promises to mature rapidly in the near future.

References

1. Goetz RH, Robman M, Haller JD et al (1961) Internal mammary-coronary artery anastomosis. A nonsuture method employing tantalum rings. J Thorac Cardiovasc Surg 41:378-386
2. Kolessov VI (1967) Mammary artery-coronary artery anastomosis as method of treatment for angina pectoris. J Thorac Cardiovasc Surg 54:535-544
3. Buffolo E, Andrade JC, Succi J et al (1985) Direct myocardial revascularization without cardiopulmonary bypass. Thorac Cardiovasc Surg 33:26-29
4. Benetti FJ (1985) Direct coronary surgery with saphenous vein bypass without either cardiopulmonary bypass or cardiac arrest. J Cardiovasc Surg 26:217-222
5. Benetti FJ, Ballester C (1995) Use of thoracoscopy and a minimal thoracotomy, in mammary-coronary bypass to left anterior descending artery, without extracorporeal circulation. Experience in 2 cases. J Cardiovasc Surg 36:159-161
6. Mack MJ (2003) Introduction. Semin Thorac Cardiovasc Surg 15:44
7. Nathoe HM, van Dijk D, Jansen EW et al (2003) A comparison of on-pump and off-pump coronary bypass surgery in low-risk patients. N Engl J Med 348:394-402
8. Puskas JD, Williams WH, Duke PG et al (2003) Off-pump coronary artery bypass grafting provides complete revascularization with reduced myocardial injury, transfusion requirements, and length of stay: a prospective randomized comparison of two hundred unselected patientes undergoing off-pump versus conventional coronary artery bypass grafting. J Thorac Cardiovasc Surg 125:797-808
9. Oliveira SA, Lisboa LA, Dallan LA et al (2002) Minimally invasive single-vessel coronary artery bypass with the internal thoracic artery and early postoperative angiography: midterm results of a prospective study in 120 consecutive patients. Ann Thorac Surg 73:505-510
10. Calafiore AM, Teodori G, Di Giammarco G et al (1999) Multiple arterial conduits without cardiopulmonary bypass: early angiographic results. Ann Thorac Surg 67:450-456
11. Murry CE, Jennings RB, Reimer KA (1986) Reconditioning with ischaemia: a delay of lethal cell injury in ischaemic myocardial. Circulation 7:1124-1136
12. Grundy S, Romano M, Shattuck O et al (1998) Seven-year follow-up of coronary artery bypasses performed with and without cardiopulmonary bypass. J Thorac Cardiovasc Surg 115:1273-1278
13. Puskas JD, Thourani VH, Marshall J et al (2001) Clinical outcomes, angiographic patency, and resource utilization in 200 consecutive off-pump coronary bypass patients. Ann Thorac Surg 71:1477-1484
14. Bhan A, Choudhary SSK, Mathur A et al (2000) Surgical myocardial revascularization without cardiopulmonary bypass. Ann Thorac Surg 69:1216-1221

15. Wiklund L, Johansson M, Grandup-Wongnsen G et al (2000) Difficulties in the interpretation of coronary angiogram early after coronary artery bypass surgery on the beating heart. Eur J Cardiothorac Surg 17:46-51
16. Jansen EWL, Borst C, Lahpor JR et al (1998) Coronary artery bypass grafting without cardio-pulmonary bypass using the Octopus method: results in the first one hundred patients. Ann Thorac Cardiovasc Surg 116:60-67
17. de Jaegere P, Suyker WJL (2002) Off-pump coronary artery bypass surgery. Heart 88:313-318
18. Sessler DI, Akca O (2002) Nonpharmacological prevention of surgical wound infections. Clin Infect Dis 11:1397-1404
19. Heames RM, Gill RS, Ohri S et al (2002) Off pump coronary artery surgery. Anaesthesia 57:676-685
20. Westaby S, Benetti FJ (1996) Less invasive coronary surgery: consensus from the Oxford meeting. Ann Thorac Surg 62:924-931
21. Subramanian V, McCabe JC, Geller CM (1997) Minimally invasive direct coronary artery bypass: two year clinical experience. Ann Thorac Surg 64:1648-1655
22. Nierich PA, Diephuis J, Jansen WLE et al (1999) Embracing the heart: perioperative management of patients undergoing off-pump coronary artery bypass grafting using the octopus tissue stabilizer. J Cardiothorac Vasc Anesth 13:123-129
23. Mariani MA, Gu YJ, Boonstra PW et al (1999) Procoagulant activity after off-pump coronary operation: is the current anticoagulation adequate? Ann Thorac Surg 67:1370-1375
24. Singh A, Junja R, Mehta Y et al (2002) Comparison of continuous, stat, and intermittent cardiac output measurements in patients undergoing minimally invasive direct coronary artery bypass surgery. J Cardiothorac Vasc Anesth 16:186-190
25. Couture P, Denault A, Limoges P et al (2002) Mechanisms of hemodynamic changes during off-pump coronary artery bypass surgery. Can J Anaesth 49:835-849
26. Vassiliades TA, Nielsen JL, Lonquist JL (2002) Hemodynamic collapse during off-pump coronary artery bypass grafting. Ann Thorac Surg 73:1874-1879

Perioperative paediatric anaesthesia

P. Busoni

The term perioperative is defined as the period of time and those areas of a patient care facility in which the patient preparation for, performance of, and recovery from surgical procedures occur [1]. It is evident that an efficient perioperative clinical information system becomes mandatory. An efficient perioperative clinical information system is now recognised as an indispensable clinical, financial and administrative management tool for the surgical services department. Surgical processes should be analysed beyond the narrow focus of the intraoperative anaesthesia. It is therefore necessary to address the information collection, documentation and management requirements of the entire perioperative period. Important modules of the perioperative process are the following:

- Surgery scheduling and support
- Tracking support
- Preoperative support
- Intraoperative support
- Postoperative support
- Pain management support
- Clinical support
- Administrative support
- Financial support

It is evident that anaesthesia occupies a crucial central position throughout the entire process. Anaesthesiology is changing and the economic marketplace is changing as well. There is an evident shift away from anaesthesia administered in the operating room to pain management and perioperative medicine practice in outpatients. No one has a better understanding of the perioperative process than anaesthesiologists, who will therefore be prepared to lead or assist in process management and redesign so that efficiency, cost savings, and enhanced quality, safety and customer satisfaction can be realised. Consideration of factors such as patient safety and outcomes and costs is essential for any clinical decision to be made. The optimal choice of anaesthesia management depends on maximising the positive aspects of health, function and satisfaction while minimising the negative aspects of mortality, morbidity and expense.

Perioperative medicine is a multidisciplinary environment, and anaesthesiologists can acquire advantages by taking perioperative leadership roles and designing the changes needed to promote safe, personalised and reasonably priced anaesthesia care. The focus of value-based anaesthesia on safety and outcomes ensures public confidence in anaesthesiology. The inclusion of costs in value-based anaesthesia care ensures its worth. The promotion of value-based anaesthesia care creates many opportunities for anaesthesiologists, who are the logical managers of expensive operating room resources and coordinators of perioperative services.

Patient care facility and medical staff policies

There should be a written policy designating and categorising the types of paediatric operative, diagnostic, and therapeutic procedures requiring anaesthesia on an elective and emergency basis, and indicating the minimum number of cases required in each category for the facility to maintain its clinical competence in their performance [1].

The categories should identify patients at increased anaesthetic risk and should include patient age procedures for which postoperative intensive care is anticipated and patients with special anaesthetic risks based on coexisting medical conditions [1]. Neonates are at higher risk than are older infants, and in turn older infants are at greater risk than paediatric patients older than 2 years of age [2]. Annual minimum case volume for anaesthesiologists to maintain clinical competence is an important issue [3]. Surgeons and anaesthetists should not undertake occasional paediatric practice. It is felt that at least one or two lists per month are indispensable for appropriate skills to be maintained [4].

Pain management

There should be a patient care facility for effective paediatric pain treatment in the perioperative anaesthesia environment. Pain management strategies need to be tailored to the types of surgical procedures, the individual variation of pain perception, and the options available for analgesic intervention. Parents of infants and children undergoing operative procedures on outpatient basis should receive instruction on pain management at home [5].

Patient Care Units

A separate preoperative unit or an area within a general preoperative unit should be available and dedicated to the accommodation of paediatric patients and their families.

Operating Room

An anaesthetist with paediatric anaesthesia experience should be responsible for the organisation of the paediatric anaesthesia services. Specialists who take responsibility for the care of children (particularly in district general hospitals and single specialty hospitals) must keep up to date with the management of children. Acquisition of the necessary experience could be a problem with local hospital practitioners. The necessary skills may be lost as a result of the centralisation of paediatric services. However, basic resuscitation skills are always required. Continuing experience can be augmented, if necessary, by visits to the local specialist centre to gain further "hands on" experience, particularly in the intensive care environment.

Nurse and technical personnel involved in the care of infants and children should be trained and experienced in routine and emergency paediatric perioperative care. Important considerations in the training of such personnel include: (1) the ability to formulate drugs and infusions in appropriate doses, concentrations, and volumes for paediatric patients; and (2) expertise in the methods of respiratory therapy administration appropriate for infants and children. Clinical laboratory and radiological services should be available at all times when patients are being cared for in the facility. The clinical laboratory must have the capability to provide haematological and chemical analyses on small samples.

Paediatric anaesthesia equipment and drugs

There should be a full selection of equipment available for use in paediatric patients. This equipment should be easily accessible and well maintained. A resuscitation cart with equipment appropriate for paediatric patients of all ages, including paediatric defibrillator paddles, is required. The anaesthesiologist should be trained in the recognition of cardiac dysrhythmias, have equipment for accurate recording of abnormal cardiac rhythms, and know how to use defibrillators that can deliver paediatric doses of energy accurately [6]. Resuscitation cardiac drugs should be available in appropriate paediatric concentrations. A written paediatric dose schedule for these drugs should be immediately available [1].

Other necessary items include:

1. Airway equipment for all ages of paediatric patients, including bronchoscopes
2. A separate, fully stocked "difficult airway cart" containing specialised equipment for management of the difficult paediatric airway, including emergency cricothyrotomy
3. Positive-pressure ventilation system appropriate for infants and children
4. Devices for the maintenance of normothermia
5. Intravascular fluid administration equipment and devices for intraosseous administration
6. Noninvasive monitoring equipment for the measurement of electrocardiography, blood pressure, pulse oximetry, capnography including anaesthetic gas concentrations, temperature, and inhaled oxygen concentration
7. Equipment for the measurement of arterial and central venous pressure in infants and small children

Postanaesthesia care unit

Postanaesthesia recovery nurses with paediatric training and experience who have special knowledge of intraoperative paediatric anaesthesia management are required. Paediatric Advanced Life Support course certification is recommended. An anaesthesiologist should be immediately available to evaluate and treat any child in distress. The paediatric anaesthesia equipment specified above must be available in this area as well. Every child admitted to the postanaesthesia care unit should have her/his vital signs monitored. A respiratory oxygen delivery system and an oxygen monitoring system should be available for use in transporting infants and children from the operating room to the postanaesthesia care room and/or postoperative intensive care unit when medically indicated.

Procedures performed outside the operating room

Increasing numbers of paediatric patients have anaesthesia or heavy sedation induced outside the operating room. Experienced anaesthetists and nursing staff are required, and in these locations there should be a reliable source of oxygen adequate for the length of the procedure. Suction apparatus that meets operating room standards is strongly encouraged. Other facilities (i.e. self-inflating hand resuscitator bag, adequate anaesthetic drugs, adequate monitoring equipment) are obviously recommended. An emergency cart with a defibrillator, emergency drugs and other equipment adequate to provide cardiopulmonary resuscitation should be immediately available in areas outside the operating room when anaesthesia or sedation are performed there.

Achieving optimal value

Value, in mathematical terms, is simply quality divided by cost. Thus, as costs rise, as they have in medicine, quality must improve by an equal amount if the value of a service is to stay the same. Quality in anaesthesia practice has two essential elements: quality of medical care and quality of services. Quality of services relates not only to patient-specific concerns, such as decreasing operating room turnover times and improved overall outcomes, but also to organisational concerns such as cooperation with one's group or hospital to reduce intensive care unit time or pharmacy cost. Optimal values are achieved by simultaneously maximising quality (the positive aspects of health, function and satisfaction) and minimising cost (the negative aspects of mortality, morbidity and expense).

When considering value-based anaesthesia with reference to the perioperative period and using information management techniques, anaesthesiologists need to look at many areas, including [7]:

- Preoperative laboratory testing – How much is needed?
- Outpatient versus inpatient surgery – Outpatient surgery is often cheaper and faster.
- Local regional versus general anaesthesia – Recovery and outcomes may be better with a combination of these two techniques.
- Selection of anaesthetic agents – Is there really a difference in outcome?
- Choice of muscle relaxants – Many, with marked cost differences, are available; is there a difference in outcome?
- Choice of narcotics – Marked differences in cost appear not be reflected in differences in outcome.
- Antiemetic therapy – Many studies show little difference in outcome with different antiemetics.
- Recovery requirements – These can greatly affect costs and satisfaction.

Perioperative anaesthesia involves much more than just the selection and interpretation of laboratory tests. Another area of opportunity for achieving good value is pain management. Anaesthesiologists, with their technical expertise and knowledge of clinical pharmacology and physiology, should be actively engaged in this area.

Paediatric anaesthesia is now considered a subspecialty. If we are proactive, if we strive to achieve better value for all, if we continue to expand our horizons outside the operating room, and if we develop our information system and management skills, we will have the opportunity to enhance the importance of our specialty and ensure our own survival and worth.

References

1. American Academy of Pediatrics (1999) Guidelines for the pediatric perioperative anesthesia environment (RE9820). Pediatrics 103:512-515
2. Cohen MM, Cameron CB, Duncan PG (1990) Pediatric anesthesia morbidity and mortality in the perioperative period. Anesth Analg 70:160-167
3. Yaster M, Krane RF, Cotè CJ et al (eds) (1997) Pediatric pain management and sedation handbook. Mosby, St Louis
4. Lunn JN (1992) Implications of the National Confidential Inquiry into Perioperative Deaths for paediatric anaesthesia. Paediatr Anaesthesiol 2:69-72
5. Tomlison A (2002) Anaesthesia and care of the critically ill child (editorial). Anaesthesia 58:309-311
6. American Hearth Association/American Academy of Pediatrics (1997) Cardiac rhythm disturbances. In: Chameides L, Hazinski MF (eds) Pediatric advanced life support. AHA/AAP, Elk Grove Village
7. Silber JH, Williams SV, Keakauer H, et al (1992) Hospital and patient characteristics associated with death after surgery. A study of adverse outcomes and failure to rescue. Med Care 30:615-627

Continuous peripheral nerve blocks in paediatrics

G. IVANI, A. SARTI, V. MOSSETTI

The control of long-term pain in children is a real problem for the paediatric anaesthesiologist. The ideal pain treatment would provide complete pain relief without interference with the daily life of the child, and the techniques and drugs would cause as few side effects as possible. For this reason, in recent years, there has been a renaissance in regional anaesthesia in children, in part because of a greater concern about postoperative pain management in young patients, and in part because of technical advances in equipment needed to perform the blocks. In fact, several techniques and routes can be used for pain treatment, but all have side effects. The intramuscular approach should be avoided in children not only from a psychological point of view (fear of needles, pain) but also because drug absorption is unpredictable. Intravenous opioid infusions are widely used, but their use for long-term pain control can lead to important side effects, such as nausea and vomiting, pruritus, urinary retention, gastrointestinal impairment and respiratory depression, so that doses must be titrated and managed; they must be limited to selected cases when no other options are available. An epidural infusion may be an alternative but can have such side effects as motor block, urinary retention and anaesthesia/analgesia also in the contralateral leg.

Central blocks, such as caudal blocks, and a very few peripheral blocks, such as penile blocks or ilioinguinal / iliohypogastric blocks, already have an established place in paediatric anaesthesia, mainly as techniques of postoperative analgesia, but generally speaking peripheral nerve blocks are not yet so popular; recently interest has been growing due to their safety, efficacy and well limited localisation of analgesia [1]. In 1996 Giaufré et al. reported the results of a prospective study on the practice of paediatric regional anaesthesia by the Association des Anésthesistes Réanimateurs Pédiatriques d'Expression Française. Data from 24,409 regional blocks were collected. With 15,013 central blocks only 23 complications were reported, and certainly none with sequelae, whereas out of 4,090 peripheral blocks none had complications. This survey report shows that regional anaesthesia in children is safe, and the zero incidence of complication after peripheral nerve blocks should encourage paediatric anaesthesiologists to use them, when appropriate, instead of a central block, as they have very few disadvantages, such as major technical demand, larger volume of anaesthetic solution required and longer onset time; moreover the use of a nerve stimulator, when appropriate, greatly increases the success rate of some of these blocks.

Central or peripheral approaches, if performed as single-shot analgesia, even with the addition of adjuvants, are not enough for long-term surgery and long-term pain; the continuous infusion, in fact, still remains the technique of choice for a prolonged operation or intense postoperative pain.

Performing regional anaesthesia in children requires expertise and knowledge of particular characteristics (anatomy and physiology) and problems only existing in children.

Combined regional and general anaesthesia

Children have a great fear of needles, so that performing a block in an awake child who can move and cry is not only not ethical but also dangerous, because we cannot control the correct position of our needle and it can damage the delicate nervous structures. Before executing a block it is good practice to anaesthetise or sedate the child [2, 3].

Obviously both anaesthesia and deep sedation have their own implications, whether during induction or maintenance of or recovery from anaesthesia, and these are due to circulatory or respiratory failure. Even sedation is not free from risks. Adverse events can occur even though drugs are administered within acceptable dosing limits [4].

Moreover, performing a block on an anaesthetized or deeply sedated child could be dangerous: any warning signals of something going wrong could easily be missed. Therefore, deep anaesthesia or heavy sedation should be avoided. A light general anaesthesia, without muscle relaxation or injection of narcotics, guarantees immobility and ensures that dangerous side effects related to respiratory and circulatory failures and the adverse events that can result from a faulty technique, such as excruciating pain or convulsions or tachycardia, are not hidden.

Differences between adults and children

Before continuous peripheral blocks are performed in children some differences from the practice in adults have to be considered.

Anatomy

The first obvious anatomical difference between adults and children is the size of the patients, which means the practitioner must locate peripheral nerves with slow movements and use microadjustments for precision. Then the anatomical landmarks are slightly different because the anatomical relationships vary depending on age; the bony growth is not the same for long, short, or flat bones, and the variations of body fluids influence skin thickness; therefore, the length of the needle should be the shortest that can easily reach the nerve to be blocked. Despite the potential difficulties that may arise from the anatomical differences in children, there are also anatomical advantages in the developing child. One is the ease with which nerves are blocked by local anaesthetics owing to their thin myelin sheaths, small fibre diameter, and short internodal distances. This allows lower concentrations of local anaesthetic agents to produce an adequate surgical block in infants and younger children. Another anatomical benefit in the paediatric patient is the presence of loose connective tissue around neuroaxial structures centrally and of nerve sheaths that are only loosely attached to the nerve trunks peripherally. These factors should lead to an improved spread of local anaesthetic without the dense anatomical barriers that may be present in adults .

Pharmacokinetics of local anaesthetics

We must consider that in small children there is a lower level of alpha-1-glycoprotein, which means a higher fraction of free local anaesthetic; then there are considerable individual variations and little information available on diffusion, protein binding and local metabolism; moreover, local spread is easier in children and fat is less dense. As in adults, the absorption depends on the site of injection and increases in the following order: proximal nerve blocks of lower extremity; brachial plexus blocks; caudal blocks; epidural blocks; intercostal blocks; topical laryngeal applications.

Monitoring

Safe continuous peripheral nerve block requires continuous monitoring, dedicated paediatric tools and strict observation of drugs guidelines. It must be executed by an expert anaesthesiologist, in an operating room and with the same monitoring as a general anaesthesia. As with any regional anaesthetic technique, an IV line must be in place. Monitoring includes electrocardiogram (ECG), noninvasive blood pressure and pulse oximetry and capnography if the child is sedated or anaesthetised. All resuscitation drugs and all the equipment required for immediate handling of possible complications should be on hand.

Indications

The full range of peripheral nerve blocks used in adults can also be used in paediatric patients. The indications for placement of a catheter for a continuous peripheral nerve block are: major orthopaedic procedures; procedures scheduled to last more than 2 hours; congenital malformation of foot or hand; fracture reduction; traction of femur fracture; need for postoperative pain therapy lasting for several days; painful physical therapy.

The commonly performed continuous peripheral blocks in children are the brachial plexus block (parascalene or axillary) for shoulder, forearm and hand surgery and for revascularisation. The femoral nerve block for femoral fractures, femoral osteotomies, femoral elongation, exostosis, quadriceps muscle biopsy; the *fascia iliaca* block with the same indications for the femoral nerve block plus the knee surgery. The technique could also be used after large soft tissues of the thigh surgery, thigh skin graft, and, as in adults, knee trauma or surgery (ligamentoplasty). The sciatic nerve block with the lateral approach for fibular osteotomy, club foot repair, the remove of plantar foreign bodies; the sciatic nerve block with the popliteal approach for Achilles tendon elongation, toe amputation, tibial osteotomy, ankle fractures or ankle osteosyntesis and exostosis.

Contraindications

There are no particular contraindications to peripheral nerve block in children except the "usual" lesions of the skin at the site of injection, severe generalised infection, allergy to the local anaesthetics (very rare), psychological disorders and refusal of the parents. The presence of a plaster is not a proper contraindication, but needs specific postoperative monitoring to identify any sign of compression. The management of patients with peripheral neuropathy is controversial: there are no scientific data that suggest that a peripheral nerve block can worsen the illness, but there could be legal problems.

Complications

Actually the disadvantages of this technique are very few if these blocks are implemented by expert hands. The complications are: inadequate block, usually because of incorrect placement of the catheter or because the catheter is introduced too deeply; nerve damage, which depends on the size and type of the needle (only use the paediatric set); infection, depending on the duration of placement (but we have implemented a continuous peripheral block of the sciatic nerve and left the catheter in place for 21 days with no sign of infection) [5]; haematoma, especially of the external jugular vein or subclavian artery; complications attributable to the catheter, such as a cut sustained on insertion or breakage on removal.

Data from the literature

Although continuous infusion can provide effective analgesia, optimising drug administration and pain management, and the technical difficulties have been overcome and paediatric tools for peripheral continuous infusions are now available, data on continuous peripheral nerve blocks in children show only a limited number of approaches [6].

In 1979 Rosenblatt et al. described the use of an axillary approach in a young boy 15 years old following a finger amputation and multiple lacerations of tendons. In this case the authors used an 18-G Teflon cannula 5 cm long with a 22-G spinal needle 8.75 cm long connected with an electrical stimulator inside [7]. The operation took place after positioning of the catheter and injecting of a mixture of 20 ml of bupivacaine 0.75% and chlorprocaine 3%. Subsequently the anaesthetics team started a continuous infusion of bupivacaine 0.25%, which ran at a speed of 10 ml/h for 48 hours. This report seems to be the first to describe the use of continuous infusion of a local anaesthetic with a volumetric pump. The plasma levels were checked in that case and showed that this infusion speed produces plasma levels of bupivacaine lower than the toxic levels. In 1994 Fewtrell et al. described the use of an axillary catheter for continuous blockade of the brachial plexus in a child of 11 months [8]. They used an insulated 18-G needle connected to a neurostimulator to detect the plexus, injected 3 ml of bupivacaine 0.25% diluted with 10 ml of saline solution, and then introduced the catheter for 4 cm. In 1994 Johnson published data on 23 children from 15 months to 14 years old with traumatic femur fracture who were treated with a continuous infusion of bupivacaine 0.25% at a speed of 0.3 ml kg^{-1} h^{-1} through a femoral catheter [9]. From 1994 to 1998 Matuszczak's group performed 162 axillary blocks in children aged between 6 and 16 years for postoperative pain relief following hand surgery for trauma or congenital hand anomalies [10]. Paut et al. described the use of a continuous block of the iliac fascia for postoperative pain relief after femur fracture in 23 children, while Sciard et al. described the use of a continuous block of lumbar plexus in 2 children of 2 and 4 years [11, 12].

In the last 2 years our group has also performed several continuous peripheral nerve blocks, particularly axillary, femoral and sciatic, for major orthopaedic surgery and trauma.

We had two particularly interesting cases with continuous sciatic blocks performed in two 3-year-old boys, each of whom underwent semiamputation of a foot. In these two cases we left in place the catheter for 15 and 21 days without any complications and with no need for rescue [5].

Drugs

Local anaesthetics are tertiary amines and are divided into esters, which are metabolised by plasma cholinesterases (neonates and infants up to 6 months have half the adult levels of this enzyme), and amides, which are metabolised by the liver and bound by the plasma proteins; neonates and infants up to 3 months have a reduced hepatic blood flow and immature degradation pathways. This means that much larger amounts of anaesthetic agents remain unmetabolised and active than in adults; moreover, neonates and infants are at greater risk of toxic effects due to lower levels of albumin and alpha glycoprotein. As the fibres are small and myelination is not complete, the minimum concentration necessary to obtain nerve block can be reduced and we can recognise the importance of using lower concentration of local anaesthetic. The toxic effects of local anaesthetics are dependent on the total dose of drug administered and on the rapidity of absorption into the bloodstream. Few local anaesthetics have been systematically studied and/or approved for use in the paediatric age group. Local anaesthetics such as mepivacaine, lidocaine and bupivacaine are still widely used, but even though adequate dose guidelines are available, case reports describing toxic plasma concentration (mainly about bupivacaine) have appeared [13, 14]. Recently two new aminoamide local anaesthetics, ropivacaine and levobupivacaine, have been introduced, which have interesting properties in children, owing to their lower affinity and toxicity to heart and nerves and a differential sensory/motor block duration [15-19].

The starting bolus dose administered before the continuous infusion depends on the target: 0.4-0.6 ml/kg of a low concentration (i.e. 0.2% ropivacaine) is used if only postoperative analgesia is needed, while a higher concentration (i.e. 0.5% ropivacaine) is used when intraoperative pain control is required [6]. Also, an association of 1.5% lidocaine and 0.2% ropivacaine can be used for the bolus [10]. The continuous infusion is administered with 0.125-0.25% bupivacaine or 0.2% ropivacaine, the usual dosage ranging from 0.1-0.3 to 0.2-0.4 mg kg^{-1} h^{-1}. A 25-30% reduction of dose of local anaesthetics is recommended in infants <6 months of age to avoid the risk of local anaesthetic plasma accumulation.

In our institution, we use a bolus dose of 0.5-1 ml/kg (depending on the nerve to be blocked) of ropivacaine 0.2% or levobupivacaine 0.25% with clonidine 2 μg/kg, and then in infants older than 6 months and children we use a continuous infusion of 0.1-0.3 ml kg^{-1} h^{-1} of 0.2% ropivacaine or 0.25% levobupivacaine with clonidine 3 μg kg^{-1} day^{-1} for 48-72 hours. For older children doses and concentrations are usually the same as are used in adults.

Materials

Earlier there was a lack of specific equipment for the performance of such techniques in infants and children. Radial artery catheterisation sets, epidural kits and central venous catheter sets were used [9, 20, 21].

Recently, a specially designed set for paediatric continuous peripheral nerve blockade (Contiplex D set, B Braun, Melsungen, Germany) has been developed. It is composed of a 20-G needle, 33 or 55 mm long, with a short bevel (15°) and conducting ensheathed in a plastic cannula and a 22- to 24-G catheter 400 mm long. It can be used for different approaches in infants and children younger than 10-12 years old. In older children it is possible to use adult sets.

General technique

In the operating room, first monitor and sedate the patient with an inhalational or intravenous technique. Arrange the patient in the correct position and detect the landmarks. Since the plexuses in children are quite superficial, especially the brachial one at the axilla, before introducing the needle try to detect the position of the plexus with the transcutaneous technique, i.e. to obtain the twitches with the tip of the neurostimulator only without the needle [22]. Sterilise the area thoroughly and introduce the insulated needle surrounded by the cannula; the length of the needle depends on the depth of the plexus to be blocked. The needle must not be introduced exactly over the landmark, as for a single-shot block, but some centimetres from the landmark and at an angle of

15°, so as to obtain minimum tunnelisation of the catheter. After introducing the tip of the needle connect it to the neurostimulator and set it to stimulate at a frequency of 2 Hz with a current of 1.5 mA; the needle is then advanced until distinct contractions of the region to be blocked are noted. The optimum nerve location is achieved by adjusting the cannula so that these contractions are still visible with currents of 0.6 mA. It is now possible to withdraw the needle from the cannula and to insert the catheter through the cannula and leave it in place. The catheter tip has to be advanced 2 cm beyond the tip of the cannula, which is removed at this point. The catheter is fixed to the skin with transparent tape. Make a negative aspiration of blood before injecting the local anaesthetic of choice. During the injection of the bolus dose, control the ECG continuously to detect any accidental intravascular injection; this could cause elevation of the ST tract, modifications of the T wave and later increase of the blood pressure and tachycardia (often preceded by bradycardia). The injection of the bolus dose has to be slow (no more than 10 ml/min) since the toxicity depends on the peak plasma concentration more than on the quantity of local anaesthetic injected.

In order to check the catheter position it is possible to perform an X-ray with 2 ml of radiopaque dye.

Specific techniques

Continuous sciatic nerve block

Since children are sedated during performance of the block, the approach to the sciatic nerve is different from that in adults because placing the patient in the prone position makes monitoring ventilation very difficult and it is impossible to maintain spontaneous ventilation. For this reason it is better to use the lateral approach both at the trochanter level and at the popliteal level, since in this way the child is in the supine position and can breathe properly.

Lateral trochanter approach: The landmark is the great trochanter and the site of puncture is immediately below it in the lateral face of the thigh. The block needle is inserted horizontally, perpendicular to the skin. The needle is advanced until twitches in the entire foot are obtained. The conducting needle is then removed and the catheter is introduced through the plastic cannula and advanced 2 cm into the sciatic nerve sheath.

Lateral popliteal approach: The lower leg is elevated on a pillow. The landmark is the biceps femoris tendon, which can be easily palpated; the tendon is then traced upward for about 3 to 5 cm. The insulated needle is inserted immediately below the tendon in a horizontal plane with a cephalad angulation and advanced until it is possible to observe a plantar or dorsiflexion of the foot. This confirms correct placement of the needle. Dorsiflexion or eversion of the foot identifies the common peroneal nerve, and plantar flexion of the foot is required to identify the tibial nerve. An elicited inversion of the foot, as recently demonstrated by Benzon et al., is the best predictor of a complete sensory blockade of the foot after a sciatic nerve block at the popliteal level [23]. The conducting needle is then removed and the catheter is introduced through the plastic cannula and advanced 2 cm into the sciatic nerve sheath.

There are specific contraindications, such as popliteal tumour, local infection and progressive demyelinating nerve disease. Except for postoperative technical problems (kinked or prematurely dislodged catheter), no complications have been described.

Continuous brachial plexus block

In children, since the structures surrounding the brachial plexus are very close together, it is not recommended that this block is performed with the same approaches as are used for adults, especially the supraclavicular, the infraclavicular and the interscalene approaches. The approaches most commonly used for a continuous block in infants and children are the parascalene and the axillary.

Parascalene approach: This is the safest approach to the supraclavicular part of the brachial plexus. The patient is placed in the supine position with the arm to be blocked lying along the body and the head turned to the side opposite to the block. A sheet is placed under the shoulders and the nape of the neck in order to expose the brachial plexus components. The landmarks are the middle part of the clavicle and the cutaneous projection of the Chassaignac tubercle sited at the insertion of the posterior edge of the sternocleidomastoideum muscle with the plane crossing the cricoid cartilage. The needle is inserted vertically, in the anteroposterior direction until the appearance of twitches of the forearm or of the hand.

Axillary approach: The patient is placed in the supine position with the arm to be blocked supinated and abducted at a 90° angle to the chest. The landmarks are the pectoralis major muscle, the coraco-brachialis muscle, and the axillarybrachial artery. The site of puncture is just above the arterial pulsation. The needle is then inserted at 15° to the skin and advanced until it elicits twitches in muscles supplied by one of the three terminal nerves of the brachial plexus (median, ulnar, or radial). The conducting needle is then removed and the catheter is introduced through the plastic cannula and advanced 2 cm into the plexus sheath.

The main indication for continuous brachial plexus block in infants and children is major painful or long-lasting procedures on the shoulder, hand, forearm or elbow, such as correction of congenital hand malformation, major trauma, or reimplantation of fingers. It can also be used to treat acute vascular insufficiency [24].

Specific contraindications are the presence of axillary large lymph nodes or tumour, local infection, and progressive demyelinating nerve disease. In infants and children, axillary and parascalene brachial plexus blocks are virtually free of complications. Accidental arterial puncture is the worst hazard and may result in transient vascular insufficiency or compressive haematoma.

Continuous femoral nerve block and fascia iliaca block

It is possible to perform two kind of continuous blocks in this area, the femoral nerve block, which is done in adults, and the fascia iliaca block. The latter is an interesting alternative technique, especially when a neurostimulator is not available, which makes it possible to block all the anterior part of the thigh and also the knee.

Femoral nerve block: The patient is placed in the supine position, preferably with the thigh slightly abducted and externally rotated. The landmarks are the inguinal ligament and the femoral artery, which are easily identified by palpation. The block needle is inserted at 30° to the skin in a cephalad direction, 1-2 cm distal to the inguinal ligament and lateral to the femoral artery. The needle is advanced until twiches of the quadriceps muscle are obtained. Then the catheter is introduced through the plastic cannula and advanced 3 to 7 cm into the femoral nerve sheath.

Fascia iliaca block: The patient lies supine. The site of puncture is located 1 cm below the junction of the lateral one fourth of a line drawn from the pubic tubercle to the anterior superior iliac spine. The needle is inserted at 40° to the skin in a perpendicular direction. It is advanced until two pops (passage through the fascia lata and iliaca) are felt. The catheter is then inserted 3 to 7 cm into the fascial sheath.

Specific contraindications are the presence of inguinal large lymph nodes or tumour, local infection or peritoneal infection. Complications are very rare. The only real risk is puncture of the femoral artery resulting in intravascular injection or local haematoma.

Conclusions

The use of continuous peripheral nerve catheters in children still requires research and validation, and their use should be restricted to anaesthetists who have a special understanding of the anatomy of infants and small children and who are comfortable with basic paediatric nerve blocks.

This technique should be widely used for the treatment of paediatric postoperative limb pain, since it is safe and easy to perform and as efficient as parenteral opioids and epidural analgesia, and it has fewer side effects than other techniques.

References

1. Giaufrè E, Dalens B, Gombert A (1996) Epidemiology and morbidity of regional anaesthesia in children: a one-year prospective survey of the French-language society of pediatric anaesthesiologists. Anesth Analg 83:904-912
2. Bosenberg A, Ivani G (1998) Regional anaesthesia: children are different (editorial). Paediatr Anaesth 8:447-450
3. Krane JE (2002) The ethics of regional anesthesia in anesthetized children. TRAPM 6:90-94
4. Coté CJ, Karl HW, Notterman DA et al (2000) Adverse sedation events in pediatrics: analysis of medications used for sedation. Pediatrics 4:633-644
5. Ivani G, Codipietro L, Gagliardi F et al (2003) A long term infusion via a sciatic catheter in a 3-years-old-boy. Paediatr Anaesth (in press)
6. Singelyn FJE (2002) Continuous peripheral nerve blocks in infants and children. TRAPM 6: 108-114
7. Rosenblatt R (1980) Continuous femoral anesthesia for lower extremity surgery. Anesth Analg 59:631-632
8. Fewtrell MS, Sapsford DJ, Herrick MJ et al (1994) Continuous axillary nerve block for chronic pain. Arch Dis Child 70:54-55
9. Johnson CM (1994) Continuous femoral nerve blockade for analgesia in children with femoral fractures. Anaesth Intensive Care 22:281-283
10. Matuszczak M,Sciard D, Gebhard R et al (2001) Upper extremity continuous perineural block in children. Anesthesiology 95:A1236
11. Paut O, Sallabery M, Schreiber-Deturmeny E et al (2001) Continuous fascia iliaca compartment block in children: a prospective evaluation of plasma bupivacaine concentrations, pain scores, and side effects. Anesth Analg 92:1159-1163
12. Sciard D, Matuszczak M, Gebhard R et al (2001) Continuous posterior lumbar plexus block for acute postoperative pain control in infants. Anesthesiology 95:1521-3
13. Berde CB (1993) Toxicity of local anesthetics in infants and children. J Pediatr 122:14-20

14. Wood CE, Goresky GV, Klassen KA et al (1994) Complications of continuous epidural infusions for postoperative analgesia in children. Can J Anaesth 41:613-20
15. Ivani G (2002) Ropivacaine: is it time for children? Paediatr Anaesth 12:383-387
16. Ivani G, DeNegri P, Conio A (2002) Comparison of racemic bupivacaine, ropivacaine, and levo-bupivacaine for pediatric caudal anesthesia: effects on postoperative analgesia and motor block. Reg Anesth Pain Med 27:157-161
17. Ivani G, De Negri P, Lonnqvist PA et al (2003) Comparison of three different concentrations of levobupivacaine for caudal block in children. Anesth Analg 97:368-371
18. Morton NS (2000). Ropivacaine in children. Br J Anaesth 85:344-346
19. Gunter J B (2002) Benefit and risks of local anesthetics in infants and children. Pediatr Drugs 4:649-672
20. Tan T, Watcha M, Safavi F et al (1995) Cannulation of the axillary brachial plexus sheath in children. Anesth Analg 80:640-641
21. Tobias J (1994) Continuous femoral nerve block to provide analgesia following femur fracture in a pediatric ICU population. Anaesth Intensive Care 22:616-618
22. Bosenberg A, Raw R, Boezaart (2002) AP Surface mapping of peripheral nerves in children with a nerve stimulator. Paediatr Anaesth 12:398-403
23. Benzon HT, Kim C, Benzon HP et al (1997) Correlation between evoked motor response of the sciatic nerve and sensory blockade. Anesthesiology 87:547-552
24. Audenaert S, Vickers H, Burgess S (1991) Axillary block for vascular insufficiency after repair of radial club hands in an infant. Anesthesiology 74:368-370

Suggested further reading

Dalens B (1995) Regional anesthesia in infants, children and adolescents. William & Wilkins, Baltimore

Regional analgesia in children: which drug? which block?

C. Dell'Oste, G. Ivani, A. Sarti

In recent years there has been a trend towards increasing use of regional anaesthetic techniques in infants and children. This increasing use of any regional technique has modified both the standards of practice in paediatric anaesthesia and the management of postoperative pain. New long-acting local anaesthetics, such as ropivacaine and levobupivacaine, have become available. Catheter techniques have become routine practice for peripheral nerve blocks, improving the quality of postoperative analgesia.

The advantages of lightening the level of general anaesthesia are now well established. They include early extubation and effective pain relief [1]. This is especially important for day-stay (ambulatory and outpatient) surgery, because analgesic requirements are reduced and early discharge is allowed [2]. Neonates are not excluded from regional techniques, and even some cardiac surgery procedures are performed under combined general and regional techniques. [3, 4].

Small, peripheral blocks have been "rediscovered". Most regional anaesthetic procedures are reliable and safe. However, no method is free of adverse effects, and the potential for complications must be carefully considered preoperatively [5]. To prevent any major undesirable side effects and complications many aspects should be considered, such as patient selection, accurate selection of the most appropriate regional technique and of local anaesthetic solutions, careful attention to pain control, insertion routes, and block procedures, in association with adequate monitoring of vital parameters.

The aim of this paper is to review the literature on the role of ropivacaine and levobupivacaine in paediatric practice and the choice of the more appropriate technique between a central and a peripheral block for a wide range of common surgical procedures.

Which drug for which block?

The selection of a local anaesthetic drug depends on the surgery planned, the expected duration of postoperative pain, and the pharmacological characteristics of the drug itself [6]. Two new long-acting local anaesthetics, ropivacaine and levobupivacaine, are reported both to have a better safety profile than bupivacaine and to pose less risk of central nervous system and cardiac toxicity [7, 8]. Ropivacaine is an aminoamide local anaesthetic, the first one to be formulated as a pure *S*-enantiomer. In many aspects, ropivacaine appears to represent an improvement for paediatric patients, especially in adolescents and older children. However, there are some concerns about its use in neonates and infants, although local anaesthetic toxicity is extremely rare in paediatric patients [9]. Several publications have reported a slower systemic absorption of ropivacaine than of bupivacaine from the epidural space in infants [10]. T_{max} of ropivacaine is significantly higher in infants less than 2 years of age; it decreases with age but adult values are not achieved before 8 years of age [11]. C_{max} too is concomitantly increased in infants [11]. Additionally, both drugs have a larger distribution volume and a greater clearance in children than in adults. After a single injection, the distribution volume of bupivacaine decreases considerably whilst that of ropivacaine remains unaffected or even tends to increase [12]. At the same time, the clearance of bupivacaine, which is not affected by the patient's age after single injection procedures, decreases considerably in the case of continuous infusion [13]. On the other hand, the clearance of ropivacaine increases slightly with patient's age after a single injection but remains unchanged in case of continuous infusion.

Levobupivacaine is the most recent long-acting local anaesthetic introduced in the clinical practice. This drug, the *S*(-)-enantiomer of racemic bupivacaine, is safe and effective for epidural and spinal anaesthesia in adults, but few studies are available to date in children [14, 15]. In patients undergoing major lower abdominal surgery, epidural levobupivacaine 0.75% resulted in a similar mean onset time of sensory and motor block to bupivacaine, but a significantly longer duration of action was shown (onset of action: 13.6 [5.6] min vs 14.0 [9.9] min; P=0.78; duration of action: 9.1 [1.4] h vs 8.4 [1.2] h; P=0.02) [14]. A comparison between bupivacaine 0.25%, ropivacaine 0.2% and levobupivacaine 0.25%, each administered as a single caudal injection in children showed that each provided apparently similar postoperative analgesia [16]. In this report, both ropivacaine and levobupivacaine were said to be associated with less motor blockade in the early postoperative phase than racemic bupivacaine. In a two-centre open-label study of 49 children under 2 years undergoing circumcision, herniorrhaphy or orchidopexy repair, levobupivacaine 0.25% (2 mg kg^{-1}) was shown to provide satisfactory postoperative analgesia in almost 90% of children (mean time to request for analgesia 7.6 h) [17].

In conclusion, for single-shot injections in infants and young children, there is no strong evidence to support a switch from bupivacaine to ropivacaine. Use of ropivacaine requires that infants be monitored for a longer period than following use of bupivacaine. Conversely, for continuous techniques, ropivacaine represents a significant improvement over bupivacaine and consistently enhances the overall safety of the procedures. On the basis of current evidence, levobupivacaine seems to be effective and safe, but additional studies with a much larger sample size are required to confirm the preliminary findings.

Combined anaesthesia: inhalation or intravenous?

Since the introduction of local anaesthetic skin preparations, painless venipuncture has become a reality and has increased the use of i.v. induction for paediatric anaesthesia. The eutectic mixture of lidocaine and prilocaine cream EMLA must be applied for at least 60 min to achieve painless venous cannulation.

Both the i.v. and the inhalation routes of induction are suitable in paediatric surgery. The choice depends on the needs of the individual child and now a smooth and nontraumatic induction can best be achieved. Whichever technique is used, a parental presence at induction can be very helpful for the child and also for the anaesthetist [18].

Inhalational induction is particularly suitable for infants and young children, needle-phobic patients and children with difficult venous access. Sevoflurane is now the first-choice volatile agent for this purpose in the USA and Europe. It is used either alone in oxygen-air or with nitrous oxide. There is a tendency toward less use of nitrous oxide, for both maintenance and induction. Sevoflurane has a pleasant smell, nonirritating airway properties and a rapid onset of action [19].

Inhalational induction is routinely used in many paediatric hospitals, but there is some evidence that i.v. induction may be less psychologically disturbing to children than inhalation methods [20]. The choice of the intravenous induction agent is generally between thiopental and propofol, singly or in association with ketamine. To limit haemodynamic alterations, a benzodiazepine, such as midazolam, often associated with ketamine, may be considered for unstable patients.

A maintenance technique using sevoflurane results in a greater incidence of emergence agitation than propofol-based maintenance. Total i.v. anaesthesia (TIVA) using propofol has definite advantages for some paediatric procedures. For patients at high risk of vomiting, propofol maintenance has been shown to have very significant antiemetic effects [21, 22]. Rapid and smooth awakening is particularly beneficial after day-case procedures [23].

In clinical practice, all paediatric blocks are performed in lightly anaesthetised children: perfect immobility of the child, as permitted by general anaesthesia, is mandatory [5, 24] for good results and the safety of the procedure.

Regional anaesthesia techniques for inguinal surgery

Caudal epidural anaesthesia

Caudal anaesthesia is the most popular and commonly used regional block in children, small infants and neonates. It is a safe and reliable technique, easy to perform, which provides effective intra- and postoperative analgesia [25]. However, as with any other central technique, caudal blocks are not without risks.

Advantages

Careful attention to pain control is actually required for successful surgery. Although the mean duration of analgesia provided by a single-shot technique is limited, the addition of other drugs, such as clonidine, ketamine or opioids, to local anaesthetic solutions enhances the duration and improves the quality of postoperative analgesia [2, 26, 27]. A caudal block is performed in high-risk children and ex-prematures in order to reduce the risk of postoperative apnoea, which seems to increase after general anaesthesia [28]. In neonates and young babies, a caudal catheter can be easily inserted and moved upward into the epidural space to the desired lumbar or thoracic level [29]. Cardiocirculatory stability, at least in children under 8 years of age, is well documented in regional anaesthesia [30].

Disadvantages

Major complications of central blocks have been described. These include systemic toxicity stemming from overdosing or intravascular injection, respiratory complications, usually following opioid use, undesired spread of the block causing a total spinal or a high level of motor blockade, CNS toxicity and bacterial complications. Some of these complications can be dramatic and, very rarely, may lead to major morbidity and death [5, 31, 32].

Spinal anaesthesia

Spinal anaesthesia is less widely used than caudal block in children.

Advantages

The spinal block is a rapid and easy technique, though more difficult to perform in small children, which provides surgical anaesthesia and muscle relaxation with a very small dosage of local anaesthetic. It is primarily indicated for short procedures of the lower abdomen in premature and ex-premature infants [33, 34]. Cardiovascular stability, with minimal changes in heart rate and arterial blood pressure even with high thoracic spinal blockade, has been demonstrated in children under 5 years of age [30].

Disadvantages

The complications of central blocks also apply for spinal anaesthesia, although smaller, 25-G needles are generally used. In spinal anaesthesia, the sensory block is unfortunately of short duration, lasting between 60 and 110 min, with no prolonged pain relief. Effective postoperative analgesia requires a balanced approach using wound infiltration with local anaesthetic and NSAID, often combined with an opioid such as codeine. Postdural puncture headache (PDPH) has not been considered a significant problem in paediatric patients. In a randomised study on 57 children ranging in age from 8 months to 15 years who underwent 98 spinal taps using different type of needles, the incidence of PDPH was 15% in the Quincke group and 9% in the Whitacre group (difference not statistically significant), irrespective of age: 8 out of 11 PDPH occurred in children less than 10 years of age [35]. While the needle bevel design influences the incidence of PDPH in adults, this seems not to be so in children; therefore, this rare complication cannot be prevented or anticipated, as no clinical symptom allowing identification of children prone to development PDPH has so far been identified [36].

Peripheral nerve blocks

Inguinal block

Ilioinguinal-iliohypogastric block provides effective analgesia of the ipsilateral inguinal area. Owing to its excellent risk/benefit ratio, this block is tending to progressively replace caudal anaesthesia for surgery in the inguinal area in some centres.

Penile block

This block is becoming the favoured local analgesic technique for circumcision, minor distal hypospadias surgery and other penile procedures. Various techniques for blocking the dorsal penile nerves have been described, including midline and paramedian approaches [37]. Both methods involve depositing 0.5% bupivacaine without epinephrine deep to Buck's fascia at the base of the penis.

The subcutaneous ring block (Broadman's technique) is suitable and very safe for circumcision, whereas block of the penis via the subpubic space (Dalen's technique) may be considered for other surface operation on the penis, such as hypospadias repair. This block can be repeated at the end of surgery to provide long-lasting pain relief. Excellent results have been shown with these techniques, with no reports of significant complications [38, 39].

Regional anaesthesia for lower limb surgery

Peripheral blocks or alternatively central blocks can be used for lower limb surgery. The study carried out by ADARPEF has established the overall safety of regional anaesthesia in paediatrics (24 accidents, all during central block procedures, with no sequelae or deaths and no legal proceedings among 24,409 procedures), and particularly the safety of peripheral nerve blocks (no significant problems following 9,396 procedures) [5]. Recently, the introduction into clinical practice of new devices allowing both easy and safe location of mixed nerve and fascial planes has prompted a revival of peripheral block techniques in children. These techniques are considered for intra- and postoperative pain control in localised areas, as either single-shot procedure or continuous procedures with placement of re-injection catheters [40, 41]. Selection of the devices is of the greatest importance. Conduction blocks of plexus nerves or mixed nerve trunks should be performed by nerve stimulation, with an adequate nerve stimulator delivering adequate current intensities. For most peripheral block procedures, a 35-mm-long needle is appropriate; other blocks, such as sciatic nerve or direct lumbar plexus blocks, require longer needles (up to 150 mm long) in large patients.

A nerve stimulator can also be used for mapping the path of peripheral nerves to avoid any puncture in children. This method has proved particularly useful for brachial plexus, axillary, ulnar and median nerve blocks in the upper limb and femoral and popliteal nerve blocks in the lower limb [42].

The fascia iliaca compartment block aims at blocking the lumbar plexus supplying the thigh. The main indication for the technique is pain in children with a fractured femoral shaft [43]. The block should be performed as early as possible to improve patient comfort during transport, radiological examinations and orthopaedic procedures. The placement of a catheter below the fascia iliaca allows repeated and continuous infusion of local anaesthetic, thus providing for long-lasting pain relief. The technique is also recommended for elective surgery of the soft tissues of the thigh [44, 45].

The lumbar plexus nerve blocks can be approached percutaneously within the psoas compartment: it represents a valid and safer alternative to epidural anaesthesia for the proximal part of the lower limb surgery if the placement of a catheter allows long-lasting pain relief [46, 47].

Specific femoral nerve blocks and sciatic nerve blocks are also considered for use in children.

Regional anaesthesia for upper limb surgery

The brachial plexus nerve block is a popular technique. The local anaesthetic solution is injected into the fascial envelope surrounding the plexus, either above the clavicle (interscalene) or in the axillary sheath. Axillary blocks should be preferred for elective and emergency surgery on the forearm and the hand. Supraclavicular approaches are considered when the operative field involves the upper arm or the shoulder or when the limb cannot be positioned for performance of an axillary blockade, whether because of the pain or of the lesion [48]. A continuous technique with a catheter allows safe and long-lasting pain management [49].

Metacarpal blocks and digital nerve blocks are indicated for any surgery on the relevant digit (traumatic or elective).

All these blocks require sound knowledge of anatomy, especially anatomical relationships.

Conclusions

It is our opinion that the choice of block depends on accurate patient selection, the type of surgery and an analysis of risk/benefit ratio for any particular procedure. Safety and effectiveness are major concerns, but costs should be also considered.

For instance, an ilioinguinal block is effective and safe for a unilateral hernia repair but if the repair is bilateral a caudal block will provide analgesia for both sides without a great difference in the total volume of local anaesthetic needed. On the other hand, the risk of complications is higher with a caudal than with a peripheral block, and this should be borne in mind particularly in tha case of an inexperienced operator.

In general, a light inhalation or intravenous general anaesthesia combined with a peripheral block is preferable for routine surgery in many cases, whereas central continuous blockades are indicated for large abdominal operations and prolonged pain relief.

We believe the anaesthetist should always plan to apply the safest effective technique for each particular procedure, keeping in mind the specific characteristics of every single patient.

References

1. Vas L, Naregal P, Sanzgiri S et al (1999) Some vagaries of neonatal lumbar epidural anaesthesia. Paediatr Anaesth 9:217-223
2. Klimscha W, Chiari A, Michalek-Sauberer A et al (1998) The efficacy and safety of a clonidine/bupivacaine combination in caudal blockade for pediatric hernia repair. Anesth Analg 86:54-61
3. Hammer GB (1999) Regional anesthesia for pediatric cardiac surgery. J Cardiothorac Vasc Anesth 13:210-213
4. Peterson KL, DeCampli WM, Pike NA et al (2000) A report of two hundred twenty cases of regional anesthesia in pediatric cardiac surgery. Anesth Analg 90:1014-1019
5. Giaufrè E, Dalens B, Gombert A (1996) Epidemiology and morbidity of regional anesthesia in children – a one-year prospective survey of the French-Language Society of Pediatric Anesthesiologists (ADARPEF). Anesth Analg 83:904-912
6. Eyres RL (1995) Local anesthetic agents in infancy. Paediatr Anaesth 5:213-218
7. Knudsen K, Beckman SM, Blomberg S et al (1997) Central nervous and cardiovascular effects of i.v. infusions of ropivacaine, bupivacaine and placebo in volunteers. Br J Anaesth 78:507-514
8. Mazoit JX, Boico O, Samii K (1993) Myocardial uptake of bupivacaine. II. Pharmacokinetics and pharmacodynamics of bupivacaine enantiomers in the isolated perfused rabbit heart. Anesth Analg 77:477-482
9. Gunter JB (2002) Benefit and risks of local anesthetics in infants and children. Paediatr Drugs 4:649-672
10. Karmakar MK, Aun CS, Wong EL et al (2002) Ropivacaine undergoes slower systemic absorption from the caudal epidural space in children than bupivacaine. Anesth Analg 94:259-265
11. Lonnqvist PA, Westrn P, Larsson BA et al (2000) Ropivacaine pharmacokinetics after caudal block in 1-8 year old children. Br J Anaesth 85:506-511
12. Luz G, Innerhofer P, Haussler B et al (2000) Comparison of ropivacaine 0.1% and 0.2% with bupivacaine 0.2% for single-shot caudal anaesthesia in children. Paediatr Anaesth 10:499-504
13. Meunier JF, Goujard E, Dubousset AM et al (2001) Pharmacokinetics of bupivacaine after continuous epidural infusion in infants with and without biliary atresia. Anesthesiology 95:87-95
14. Kopacz DJ, Allen HW, Thompson GE (2000) A comparison of epidural levobupivacaine 0.75% with racemic bupivacaine for lower abdominal surgery. Anesth Analg 90:642-648
15. Burke D, Kennedy S, Bannister J (1999) Spinal anesthesia with 0.5% S(-)-bupivacaine for elective lower limb surgery. Reg Anesth Pain Med 24:519-523
16. Ivani G, De Negri P, Conio P et al (2002) Comparison of racemic bupivacaine, ropivacaine, and levo-bupivacaine for pediatric caudal anesthesia: effects on postoperative analgesia and motor block. Reg Anesth Pain Med 27:157-161

17. Eyres RL, Chalkiadis G, Taylor R (1999) Efficacy and safety of levobupivacaine as caudal anaesthesia in paediatric surgery. Inter Monitor Reg Anaesth 11:31A
18. Hannallah RS (1994) Who benefits when parents are present during anaesthetic induction in their children? Can J Anaesth 41:271-275
19. Conran AM, Hannallah RS (1997) Pediatric outpatient anesthesia and perioperative care. Curr Opin Anesthesiol 10:205-208
20. Kotiniemi LH, Ryhanen PT (1996) Behavioural changes and children memories after intravenous inhalation and rectal induction of anaesthesia. Paediatr Anaesth 6:201-207
21. Watcha MF, Simeon RM, White PF (1991) Effect of propofol on the incidence of postoperative vomiting after strabismus surgery in pediatric outpatients. Anesthesiology 75:204-209
22. Sarti A, Busoni P, Dell'Oste C, Bussolin L (2003) Incidence of vomiting in susceptible children under regional analgesia with two different anaesthetic techniques. Paediatr Anaesth (in press)
23. Morton NS (1998) TIVA in paediatrics: advantages and disadvantages. Paediatr Anaesth 8:189-194
24. Dalens B, Mansoor O (1994) Safe selection and performance of regional anesthetic techniques in children. Curr Opin Anesthesiol 7:257-261
25. Berde C (1994) Epidural analgesia in children. Can J Anaesth 41:555-560
26. Krane EJ, Jacobsen LE, Lynn AM (1987) Caudal morphine for postoperative analgesia in children: a comparison with caudal bupivacaine and intravenous morphine. Anesth Analg 66:647-653
27. Lee HM, Sanders GM (2000) Caudal ropivacaine and ketamine for postoperative analgesia in children. Anaesthesia 55:798-810
28. Spear RM, Desphande JK, Maxwell LG (1988) Caudal anaesthesia in the high-risk infant. Anesthesiology 69:407-409
29. Bosemberg AT, Bland BAR, Schulte-Steinberg O et al (1989) Thoracic epidural anesthesia via caudal route in infants. Anesthesiology 69:265-269
30. Dohi S, Naito H, Takahashi T (1979) Age related changes in blood pressure and duration of motor block in spinal anesthesia. Anesthesiology 50:319-323
31. Flantin-Blét y C, Barrier G (1995) Accidents following extradural analgesia in children. The results of a retrospective study. Paediatr Anaesth 5:41-46
32. Berde C (1992) Convulsions associated with pediatric regional anesthesia. Anesth Analg 75:164 166
33. Mahe V, Ecoffey C (1988) Spinal anesthesia with isobaric bupivacaine in infants. Anesthesiology 68:601-603
34. Krane EJ, Haberkern CM, Jacobson LE (1995) Postoperative apnoea, bradycardia, and oxygen desaturation in formerly premature infants: prospective comparison of spinal and general anesthesia. Anesth Analg 80:7-13
35. Kokki H, Salonvaara M, Herrgard E et al (1999) Postdural puncture headache is not an age-related symptom in children: a prospective, open-randomized, parallel group study comparing a 22-gauge Quincke with a 22-gauge Whitacre needle. Paediatr Anaesth 9:429-434
36. Kokki H, Heikkinen M, Turunen M (2000) Needle design does not affect the success rate of spinal anaesthesia or the incidence of post-puncture complications in children. Acta Anaesthesiol Scand 44:210-213
37. McNicol LR (1994) Peripheral nerve blocks. In: Morton NS, Raine PA (eds) Paediatric day case surgery. University Press Oxford, Oxford, pp 38-53
38. Broadman LM, Hannallah RS, Belman B et al (1987) Post circumcision analgesia – a prospective evaluation of subcutaneous ring block of the penis. Anesthesiology 67:399-402
39. Dalens B, Vanneuville G, Dechelotte P (1989) Penile block via the subpubic space in 100 children. Anesth Analg 69:41-45
40. Taras JS, Behrman MJ (1998) Continuous peripheral nerve block in replantation and revascularization. J Reconstr Microsurg 14:17-21
41. Sutherland ID (1998) Continuous sciatic nerve infusion: expanded case report describing a new approach. Reg Anesth Pain Med 23:496-501

42. Bosenberg AT, Raw R, Boezzart AP (2002) Surface mapping of peripheral nerves in children with a nerve stimulator. Paediatr Anaesth 12:398-403
43. Dalens B, Vanneuville G, Tanguy A (1989) Comparison of the fascia iliaca compartment block with the 3-in-1 block in children. Anesth Analg 69:705-713
44. Longo SR, Williams DP (1997) Bilateral fascia iliaca catheters for postoperative pain control after bilateral total knee arthoplasty: a case report and description of a catheter technique. Reg Anesth 22:372-377
45. Paut O, Sallabery M, Schreiber-Deturmeny E (2001) Continuous fascia iliaca compartment block in children: a prospective evaluation of plasma bupivacaine concentrations, pain scores, and side effects. Anesth Analg 92:1159-1163
46. Johnson CM (1994) Continuous femoral nerve blockade for analgesia in children with femoral fractures. Anesth Intensive Care 22:281-283
47. Tobias JD (1994) Continuous femoral nerve block to provide analgesia following femur fracture in a paediatric ICU population. Anesth Intensive Care 22:616-618
48. Dalens B, Vanneuville G, Tanguy A (1987) A new parascalene approach to the brachial plexus in children: comparison with the supraclavicular approach. Anesth Analg 66:1264-1271
49. Scott DA, Schweitzer SA, Selander DE (1997) Continuous axillary brachial plexus block for postoperative pain relief. Intermittent bolus versus continuous infusion. Reg Anesth 22:357-362

Ketamine, a general anaesthetic agent and more. A review on its use in and out the clinical setting

C. Ori, M. Dalsasso, U. Freo

Ketamine is a non-competitive NMDA receptors antagonist with potent general anaesthetic and analgesic effects. NMDA receptors are involved in nociceptive modulation, in the wind-up phenomenon, in peripheral receptive fields expansion, in primary and secondary hyperalgesia, and in neuronal plasticity, a process implicated in central sensitisation of pain [1]. Ketamine also acts on nicotinic and muscarinic receptors, blocks sodium channels and interacts with μ, δ and κ opioid receptors.

The anaesthetic state produced by ketamine has been termed "dissociative anaesthesia" in that it appears to selectively interrupt association pathways of the brain before producing somaesthetic sensory blockade [2]. In particular, ketamine produces a cataleptic state with nystagmus and intact corneal and light reflexes with, eventually, hypertonus or vocalisation. Ketamine deeply affects the EEG pattern, causing a reduction of alpha wave activity, while theta, delta and beta wave activity increases. Ketamine causes cerebral vasodilation with increases of CBF (up to 60%), ICP and $CMRO_2$.

The analgesic and anaesthetic effects, as well as the "dissociative" phenomena observed during the recovery, are the result of the interaction to PCP site mediating inhibition of excitatory aminoacid transmission at NMDA receptors. The excitatory effect observed at higher doses, however, may be mediated by the haloperidol sensitive sigma receptor [3].

Ketamine effects are well known: it produces a state of "dissociative anaesthesia" and amnesia still maintaining the respiratory drive effective and supporting the systemic arterial blood pressure by increasing heart rate, systemic arterial pressure, systemic vascular resistance, pulmonary arterial pressure, and pulmonary vascular resistance [4]. The extensive review of White et al. [5] and the cardiovascular review of Reves et al. [6] are broad in their scope and have advanced the understanding of dissociative anaesthesia.

Since the first published report of its clinical use nearly forty years ago [7], advantages and disadvantages of dissociative anaesthesia have been reported in many studies [8]. When administered to adult patients as a sole anaesthetic agent, ketamine frequently causes emergence reactions characterized by anxiety, nightmares, and hallucination. Moreover, ketamine shows cardiovascular stimulant properties, increases salivary and bronchial secretions, and may increase intracranial and pulmonary pressures. All of those features have been advocated as limitations for its usefulness. Moreover, based on these considerations, ketamine is usually not administered as sole anaesthetic agent. In fact, in order to reduce or prevent emergence reactions and simpaticomimetic responses to intravenous ketamine, a wide number of drugs, including benzodiazepines and clonidine, have been proposed.

On the other hand, some characteristics might be desirable in particular circumstances, like during induction of burned or shocked patients, when stabilisation of blood pressure can be guaranteed by ketamine, or in asthmatic patients, because of its capability to alleviate bronchospasm.

Despite being suitable for inducing anaesthesia, sedation, analgesia, and amnesia, racemic ketamine and S(+)-ketamine have only been used in certain surgical subspecialties, like paediatrics and plastic, or in limited fields like war surgery, calamities and burns [9]. There are, however, sparse mentions of its use in general surgery for adults [10].

General surgery

Ketamine was introduced as a general anaesthetic for humans nearly forty years ago. Ketamine is now considered obsolete and, indeed, it has never been widely employed. Its use has been limited to paediatric patients and short surgical or diagnostic procedures, always in association with drugs able to contain its collateral effects. However, the knowledge of the complex and peculiar properties of ketamine and the modulation of its effect, obtained by the combination with other drugs, could permit an effective use in many other clinical situations.

The association with other drugs, like benzodiazepines, while minimising collateral effects, allows carrying out of deep or general anaesthesia in the absence of respiratory depression, provides high cardiovascular stability and adequate analgesia during surgery time and for a long period after the end of operation, with low incidence of nausea and vomiting.

There are sparse mentions of its use as a general anaesthetic for laparotomy and laparoscopy [10], reportedly with good results. Few other studies demonstrate that ketamine-based general anaesthesia is suitable for a wide range of different surgical intervention, like orthopaedic [13], and cardiothoracic [14].

During the last ten years, the interest for analgesic properties of ketamine at subanaesthetic doses [14] and the increasing importance recognized to pre-emptive analgesia have produced a large number of publications [15-19]. Pre-emptive analgesia is based on the concept that analgesia started before surgical stimulation achieves better results than analgesia initiated afterwards. Experimental studies show that afferent nociceptive impulses produce alterations of central nervous system function, particularly at the spinal dorsal horn level, defined central sensitisation and resulting in allodynia, hyperalgesia, wind-up, and eventually secondary hyperalgesia. The biochemical basis of central sensitisation has not been completely elucidated but it is known that excitatory amino acid (e.g. NMDA) and neuropeptide (e.g. substance P) neurotransmitters play a fundamental role and, actually, central sensitisation associated with nociception is limited by blockade of the related receptors. Ketamine, which is an NMDA receptor blocker, can therefore modulate central sensitisation [20] and this capability, associated with careful postoperative administration, allows providing effective analgesia for a long period after major surgery without psychotomimetic side effects and neurological disorders [21].

Paediatric anaesthesia

Ketamine is a water-soluble agent and is therefore especially useful for intramuscular, oral, nasal and rectal inductions in patients like children, in whom intravenous access is unavailable.

Ketamine, given orally with midazolam, improves anxiolysis and sedation and achieves better premedication, acceptance of parental separation and acceptance of face mask for induction of anaesthesia [24, 25]. Mild sedation with quiet spontaneous ventilation becomes possible in children with difficult venous access, in very anxious children and in those who are not aware of the necessity of treatment.

Ketamine produces a unique anaesthetic state, dissociative anaesthesia, which safely and effectively enables treatment of the uncooperative paediatric patients undergoing minor surgery, even short-lasting ophtalmic procedures, intraocular or extraocular [26, 27]. Furthermore, ketamine seems the ideal anaesthetic for most diagnostic procedures [28], permitting the immobility for long periods in the absence of respiratory problems. For the same reasons, ketamine is indicated in paediatric radiation therapy and in any procedure requiring short- or long-term immobilisation.

Caudal anaesthesia, usually associated to general anaesthesia, is one of the most frequently used regional techniques in paediatric anaesthesia, and is performed in healthy children to provide post-operative pain control. Drugs administered for caudal blocks should be free of severe side effects, and in this respect only clonidine and S(+)-ketamine are considered useful additives to local anaesthetics in paediatric caudal anaesthesia [29]. In fact, caudal administration of ketamine 0.5 mg.kg-1, with or without alfentanil, produces satisfactory postoperative analgesia without respiratory depression or other side effects [30].

Ketamine is the ideal agent for inducing anaesthesia in children with unstable haemodynamic conditions, burns and with cardiac defects connected with reduced lung perfusion.

Finally, when administered in low doses and combined to midazolam, ketamine may be used for sedation in intensive care patients not suffering from inflammatory and septic diseases [31].

Obstetrics

The most frequent indication for caesarean section is failure to progress, foetal distress, cephalopelvic disproportion, and prior uterine surgery or caesarean section. General anaesthesia is the method of choice for emergency caesarean section when regional anaesthesia is refused or contraindicated, in case of actual risk of profuse haemorrhage, or when uterine relaxation is required.

Ketamine is almost certainly the anaesthetic of choice for obstetric patients with hyperreactive airways or in case of hypovolaemia/haemorrhage, during caesarean section performed on a critically ill patient or under critical conditions. Moreover, some reports point out that ketamine can be safely utilised for rapid-sequence intubation in parturients undergoing caesarean section [32], when the difficulty or failure to intubate the trachea remains a major cause of maternal morbidity and mortality.

Although well known for its haemodynamic and respiratory favourable properties, ketamine is not only suitable for emergency caesarean section. Many papers report that, compared to other general anaesthetics and continuous epidural block for elective caesarean section [33], ketamine mediates specific antinociception without negative maternal or foetal effects, causing minimal cardiovascular disturbances, absence of intraoperative arrhythmia, low blood loss and better quality of anaesthesia and recovery scores. The psychotomimetic effects associated with ketamine administration are quite infrequent and usually prevented by the administration of benzodiazepines. Stress protection and haemodynamic responses are well balanced and usually there are no intraoperative recalls or negative dream reactions. In comparison with spinal anaesthesia, nausea and vomiting are less frequent [34]. Ketamine analgesic properties permit to extend into the postoperative period a reduced sensitisation to pain even if used for anaesthesia induction [35]. Ketamine can be administered intramuscularly to induce anaesthesia in parturients when pre-operative intravenous access proves impossible [36].

Ketamine has also been used as a sedative at subanaesthetic dosage in case of retained placenta if a regional anaesthetic is not in place, or as a sole agent in association with benzodiazepine for caesarean section performed in tropical surgery where the lack of instrumentations and trained personnel do not allow performing intubation, general or regional anaesthesia [37]. The same good results have been obtained in peripartum general anaesthesia without tracheal intubation [38].

The lack of toxicity, favourable labour response, and minimal effects on the foetus and mother make ketamine a suitable anaesthetic agent for obstetric and gynaecologic analgesia and anaesthesia [39], whose main indications are intravenous and intramuscular induction of anaesthesia for caesarean section, shock, asthma patients, short elective operations, and painful diagnostic procedures [40].

Office-based and one-day surgery

Office-based and one-day surgery are made possible by the introduction of new powerful and short-acting general anaesthetics.

In low-medium algic component interventions, performed in ambulatorial or one-day surgery, the ideal anaesthetic agent should provide adequate sedation, hypnosis, analgesia, amnesia, and muscle relaxation during surgery followed by quick recovery from anaesthesia. However, the ideal anaesthetic technique should also provide good intraoperative stability and recovery free from collateral effects, in particular pain, nausea and vomiting, and guarantee quick return to preoperative psychophysical conditions, rapid dismissal, and patient's personal satisfaction with anaesthesia.

Ketamine administration combined with propofol, benzodiazepines, or clonidine allows taking advantage of the analgesic action of subanaesthetic doses of ketamine while avoiding the side effects typical of opioids, i.e. high incidence of post-operative nausea and vomiting and respiratory depression.

Furthermore, the advantages of the ketamine-benzodiazepines association include high cardiovascular stability and adequate analgesia during surgery, absence of respiratory depression, rapid awakening and return of cardiovascular parameters to basic values, low incidence of nausea and vomiting and good persistence of analgesic effects in the immediate postoperative period.

Many studies testify the satisfactory use of ketamine anaesthesia in office-based surgery [41-44]. The results of these studies are of particular interest for outpatient surgery requiring appropriate surgical technique, careful anaesthesia, good postoperative pain control without opioids, and absence of postoperative nausea and vomiting.

During the last ten years, the interest for ketamine analgesia at subanaesthetic dosage [46] and the increasing importance attributed to pre-emptive analgesia produced a large number of publications [15-19], whose results were often dissimilar [47, 48]; remarkably, opioids were the main analgesic drugs employed in all studies.

In other studies, clonidine administered before or during anaesthesia contributed to ensure good intraoperative analgesia and limit cardiovascular and phsycotomimetic effects of ketamine [49-52]. The literature widely reports the effectiveness of benzodiazepines in preventing ketamine phsycotomimetic effects, probably through their effect on GABA receptors. In particular midazolam may be preferable to diazepam, because of similar pharmacokinetic properties to ketamine and a shorter recovery time [53]. Moreover, the use of continuous infusion of ketamine during outpatient procedures seems to achieve a smoother anaesthesia [54].

These experiences point out that ketamine, if accurately employed (i.e. adequate dosage and association with other drugs), might represent a suitable alternative to the use of opioid or volatile agents in day surgery regimen.

Regional anaesthesia

The epidural and intrathecal administration of opioids became popular among anaesthesiologists during recent years. The interaction of ketamine at opioid receptors level generated some investigations on its epidural and spinal administration. The first publication on the epidural administration of ketamine in humans appeared in 1982 [55] and, since then, several studies on clinical use, pharmacology, and toxicology of ketamine by epidural and intrathecal routes have been published.

Data on the neurotoxicity of ketamine after intrathecal administration are confusing. Spinal ketamine might be neurotoxic, and "balanced spinal analgesia", using a combination of low doses of drugs with separate but synergistic mechanisms of analgesic action, might produce the best results [56].

While neurotoxic effects have not been observed in baboons, primates and rabbits [57], they were in rats and monkeys. Those conclusions were based on uncontrolled data and could rather be the result of other factors such as faulty puncture technique or neurotoxicity of co-administered drugs.

It clearly appears that systemically administered ketamine interacts with different neurotransmitter systems and may even act as a local anaesthetic when used for intravenous regional anaesthesia [58]. The results of several studies in animals suggest that ketamine can cause complete sensory and motor blockade after intrathecal administration, due to a high concentration in the cerebrospinal fluid. The binding to local opiate receptors seems to play only a partial role, whereas any significant analgesia after even low doses of ketamine is the result of its action on NMDA receptors. In vitro and in vivo studies also suggest an involvement of the descending inhibitory pathways, mainly through inhibition of the reuptake of neurotransmitters. One study, investigating the effects of ketamine after epidural administration in humans, showed motor and sensory blockade of limited duration only after high doses, i.e. 50 mg [59].

After epidural administration, doses up to 30 mg did not give adequate pain relief after surgery in controlled studies, but had some analgesic effect in patients with chronic pain syndromes. When doses of 30 mg and more were used, postoperative analgesia was generally well achieved [55, 58].

Actual knowledge on epidural and intrathecal neurotoxicity of ketamine suggests that further studies are mandatory to evaluate its usefulness and side effects.

Chronic pain management

Interest in the utilisation of low doses ketamine for cancer and non-cancer chronic pain has grown recently. Control of malignant pain and related symptoms is fundamental in the care of patients with cancer. Till now, several classes of drugs have been used to treat cancer pain: nonsteroidal anti-inflammatory drugs (in particular COX-2 inhibitors), opioid analgesics, ketamine, and bisphosphonates, the latter prescribed for pain from bone metastases [60].

Current evidence is inadequate to definitely establish the benefits and harms of ketamine as an adjuvant to opioids for cancer pain relief, and more randomised controlled trials are mandatory. However, some recent trials concluded that ketamine improves the effectiveness of morphine in the treatment of cancer pain. During the treatment, based on the association ketamine-morphine or morphine alone, some patients experienced hallucinations successfully treated with diazepam, but no other serious adverse effect has been reported [61]. Ketamine is an adjuvant analgesic for the treatment of cancer-related pain when other agents either fail or reveal intolerable. Accordingly, there are several factors that may prevent adequate pain control by opioids and, therefore, alternative analgesics should be considered. Potential exists for ketamine as an adjuvant analgesic in appropriate and collaborative patients [62].

It has been reported that a low dose of ketamine per os (0.5 mg/kg body weight three times daily, added to the existing drug regimen) are effective in the management of intractable neuropathic pain of patients with advanced cancer. The oral route of administration seemed to be preferable on the bases of the poor relevance of adverse effects (i.e. nausea and vomiting or loss of appetite, drowsiness, sedation and "feeling of unreality"), associated with intravenous or intramuscular administration. None of the patients included in this study reported visual or auditory hallucinations [63].

Low or subanaesthetic doses of ketamine may be effectively used as either a primary analgesic or adjuvant analgesic in a variety of chronic or acute pain syndromes, including central post-stroke pain with allodynia and hyperalgesia, generally refractory to conventional pain treatments. The route of administration may be both intravenous and oral.

Chronic pain syndromes have been successfully managed by using low dose parenteral ketamine as an adjuvant to the principal analgesic, but were also treated using low doses of ketamine alone. Known side effects, including dysphoria, hallucinations, and paranoid feelings are commonly attenuated by benzodiazepines. Noteworthy, anedoctical reports state that equianalgesic doses of oral ketamine could be lower than the parenteral doses [64, 65].

Although not yet recommended for consistent clinical use, some experiences suggest that epidural infusion of ketamine at doses from 5 mg to 20 mg with lidocaine or bupivacaine could alleviate postherpetic neuralgia, representing an effective and useful alternative treatment in a patient with refractory postherpetic neuralgia [66].

Critically ill patients

The use of ketamine in general anaesthesia and sedation is quite limited, but its role becomes pivotal for the induction and maintenance of anaesthesia, even as a sole agent, in critically ill patients.

Ketamine is often employed in haemodynamically compromised patients because it increases heart rate and blood pressure through the release of endogenous catecholamines. These properties play an important role in patients with hypovolaemia, constrictive pericarditis, pericardial tamponade, and cardiogenic shock. Ketamine may therefore be advantageous in patients with unknown volaemic status, especially in war surgery and in catastrophic setting, when wounded and burns patients are the large majority. Ketamine by intravenous infusion has been recommended for military emergency surgery [67, 68].

Ketamine only mildly depresses respiratory rate and tidal volume, has minimal effect on responsiveness to hypercarbia, and minimally depresses laryngeal protective reflexes, unlike other intravenous anaesthetics. The combined effects on respiratory and cardiovascular systems permit to perform high stability anaesthesia in extreme circumstances, such as high altitude and third world surgery [37], where poor conditions, inadequate instrumentations and equipments, and the scarcity of trained personnel put the patient in a *per se* critical situation. There is real need for effective anaesthetic technique in high altitude and remote third-world areas, and ketamine represents a safe and effective anaesthetic agent for all these high-risk conditions [69]. Experience in war/tropical settings suggests that this technique could be useful in civilian contexts such as outdoor life-saving emergency surgery or in mass casualties where amputation and rapid extrication might be required [37].

White [70] considers unsafe the use of ketamine in shock status; in such a circumstance, ketamine might increase hypotension acting as a myocardial depressant if administered in the presence of autonomic nervous system blockade.

In burned patients, both adult and paediatric [71], ketamine permits surgical cleaning and repeated painful medication. Although its repeated use may lead to tolerance, increasing doses allow a safe and standard use [72].

Since its introduction into clinical practice, ketamine proved to be able to reduce airway resistance and increase lung compliance in the asthmatic patient. COPD and asthmatic patients, paediatrics included, take advantage from ketamine anaesthesia induction or maintenance due to its capacity to alleviate bronchospasm by a sympaticomimetic effect [73, 74].

Several studies have investigated bronchodilator properties of ketamine, producing discordant results. It has been stated that limited evidence is available in the literature to support administration of ketamine in severe exacerbation of asthma [75]. These studies report that intravenous bolus and infusion of ketamine did not produce greater bronchodilatory effect compared with standard therapy during exacerbations of asthma in adults [76]. On the other hand, in many reports the use of ketamine turned out to be successful as adjuvant or sole bronchodilator agent if administered in subanaesthetic doses in status asthmaticus, whereas conventional bronchodilator therapy failed to relieve acute refractory bronchospasm [77].

In order to avoid artificial ventilation, a continuous intravenous infusion of low dose ketamine, to avoid dysphoric reactions, has been used successfully.

The low incidence of side effects made acceptable its use when all other treatment failed. Different mechanisms of action have been hypothesised for the bronchodilator effect of ketamine: sympathomimetic effect, direct relaxant effect, antagonism to histamine and acetylcholine, and membrane stabilising effect [78]. In conclusion, ketamine is considered a useful drug in the intensive treatment of status asthmaticus in adult patients and should be tried before a decision is taken to start mechanical ventilation [79]. Ketamine-treated patients showed an improvement in physiological parameters like pO_2 and pCO_2, suggesting that ketamine might be useful in the treatment of bronchospasm during mechanical ventilation [80].

Ketamine may be useful as bronchodilator in paediatric patients too. Several studies report that addition of continuous infusion of ketamine to standard therapy is associated with improved indices of acute asthma severity, improving airway obstruction even in mechanically ventilated infant patients [81, 82]. Side effects, such as increased secretions, were transitory and comparable to those reported in other studies [83]. Hence, it can be stated that continuous infusion of ketamine in mechanically ventilated paediatric patients with refractory bronchospasm significantly improves gas exchange and dynamic compliance of the chest [84].

Analgesia and sedation are essential in the care of head injured patients to avoid secondary brain damage. Although the vascular and respiratory characteristics of ketamine may be desirable for an anaesthetic drug, its effects on cerebral metabolism cause an increase of $CMRO_2$ and consequently CBF and ICP grow. For those reasons ketamine is infrequently used in neuroanaesthesia. However, other studies did not confirm an increase in ICP when controlled ventilation and additional sedation were applied to obtain normocapnia and a stable blood pressure.

Other recent studies in animals have demonstrated the role and protective effect of neuroexcitatory NMDA-receptors in ischaemic and traumatic brain damage [85]. Also, the drug has proved to have an anticonvulsant effect in clinically applied doses. These recent acknowledgments have introduced new perspectives for the use of ketamine as a neuroprotective drug. Moreover, the potential neurotoxicity attributed to extremely high ketamine doses is scarcely understood. Hence, the role of ketamine and its more potent enantiomer S(+)-ketamine in combination with other neuroprotective measures deserve further investigations [86].

Treatment of alcoholism and heroin addiction

Ketamine, in subanaesthetic doses, produces profound psychedelic experiences and hallucinations. This effect of ketamine might represent the mechanism of ketamine-assisted psychotherapy for alcoholism. The observation that the frightening experience of delirium tremens induces alcoholics to moderate their alcohol intake suggested that the "psychotomimetic" experience produced by ketamine could be used to treat alcoholism [87].

Controlled clinical trials demonstrated a considerable increase in the efficacy of standard alcoholism treatment when supplemented by psychedelic therapy based on ketamine [88]. A narcopsychotherapeutic technique called "affective counterattribution" improves the effectiveness of alcoholism treatment through the association of strong pharmacogenic negative emotional experience with bright hallucinatory images to notions of alcohol and alcohol-related stimuli. Supposingly, this psychotherapeutic approach makes patients emotionally concerned about their disease and tends to make them more suggestible of alcohol intolerance. In many patients, alcoholic dependence was reduced and the pathological traits of personality were corrected [89, 90]. A number of well-controlled trials have indicated that hallucinogen-assisted psychotherapy is safe and effective.

The same approach has been used in adjunct to psychotherapy for heroin addiction, producing a significantly higher rate of abstinence in heroin addicts within the first two years of follow-up, a greater and longer-lasting reduction in craving for heroin, as well as greater positive change in nonverbal unconscious emotional attitudes [91].

Until now, on the other hand, hallucinogens have not yet found full acceptance as a therapeutic technique [92], probably for ethical reasons.

Ketamine as a club drug

Club drugs are chemical substances used recreationally in social settings. Ketamine use is increasingly frequent among young people, especially during all-night dance parties, the so-called "rave parties". Ketamine, a phencyclidine derivative interacting with the N-methyl-D-aspartate channel, produces analgesic and amnestic effects at higher doses, often in association with vivid hallucinations and confusion, hostility, and delirium [93]. These are the mental and physical adverse effects searched by occasional and frequent users of club drugs, in particular ketamine [94]. It is widely reported that ketamine produces psychedelic effects in healthy volunteers [95] and there are common reports of hallucinations occurred in patients undergoing ketamine-based general anaesthesia.

Ketamine seems to produce acute and severe impairments of working, and of the episodic and semantic memory as well as psychotogenic and dissociative effects. Even some days after drug ingestion, recreational users present semantic memory impairment and dissociative and schizotypal symptomatology. On some cognitive measures there were no differences. All this can be interpreted as an enduring action of the drug [96].

In case of long-term, high-dose ketamine use, the user may present impaired recall and attention, and persisting visual anomaly [97]. It must also be remarked that the uncertain sources of these substances, acquired from pushers in a clandestine way, sometimes conveying contaminants or other drugs, make it difficult to evaluate the separate toxicity of ketamine [98]. Usually, a typical dose of ketamine is 1/8 g, usually taken intranasally, orally and intramusculary [99, 100], often mixed with other drugs and vitamins.

Ketamine dependence is often linked to the effects of other co-administered drugs, like cocaine, amphetamine, opioids, alcohol and cannabis, as well as to the psychological attractions towards its psychedelic properties consisting in psychedelic dreams (often forgotten afterward) accompanied by hallucinations, floating sensation, feeling of dissociation of the mind from the body, and near death sensation [101]. In long-term exposure tolerance, dependence, withdrawal signs, and flash back are described [102, 103].

Ketamine effects on surgical patients as well as on habitual and recreational users suggest its use with the aim of reproducing a condition similar to schizophrenia [104]. Schizophrenic patients suffer from positive and negative signs as well as emotional disturbance (blunted affect and discordance of emotional level). In healthy subjects its administration induces some positive symptoms (perceptual distortions), negative symptoms (emotional deficit, apathy, social withdrawal) and cognitive changes (memory impairment and preservation) similar to some aspects of schizophrenia. Ketamine psychotomimetic effects allow to draw several hypotheses related to neurotransmitter systems like glutamate, dopamine and serotonin in different cerebral areas [105]. Indeed, the use of ketamine in healthy volunteers may create some ethical problems, often related to possible memories of adverse effects, horrific hallucination or strange sensations. A recent study by Carpenter dispelled fears recognising high values to these studies [106].

References

1. Adam F, Libier M, Oszustowicz T et al (1999) Preoperative small-dose ketamine has no preemptive analgesic effect in patients undergoing total mastectomy. Anesth Analg 89:444-447
2. Reich DL, Silvay G (1989) Ketamine: an update on the first twenty-five years of clinical experience. Can J Anaesth 36:186-197
3. Maurset A, Oye I (1990) Ketamine: clinically useful - pharmacologically interesting. Nord Med 105:182-183
4. Ivani G, Vercellino C, Tonetti F (2003) Ketamine: a new look to an old drug. Minerva Anestesiologica 69:468-471
5. White PF, Way WL, Trevor AJ (1982) Ketamine - its pharmacology and therapeutic uses. Anesthesiology 56:119-136
6. Reves JG, Flezzani P, Kissin I (1987) Intravenous anesthetic induction drugs. In: Kaplan JA (ed) Cardiac Anesthesia. Grune and Stratton, New York, pp 466-469
7. Domino EF, Chodoff P, Corssen G (1965) Pharmacologic effects of CI-581, a new dissociative anesthetic in man. Clin Pharmacol Ther 6:279-291
8. David L, Reich MD, Silvay G (1989) Ketamine: an update on the first twenty-five years of clinical experience. Can J Anaesth 36:186-197
9. Restall J, Tully PJ, Ward PJ et al (1988) Total intravenous anaesthesia for military surgery. A technique using ketamine, midazolam and vecuronium. Anaesthesia 43:46-49
10. Bailie R, Craig G, Restall J (1989) Total intravenous anaesthesia for laparoscopy. Anaesthesia 44:60-63
11. Takrouri MS (1999) Anesthesia for laparoscopic general surgery. A special review. Middle East J Anesthesiol 15:39-62
12. Matsuki A (1991) A review of recent advances in total intravenous anesthesia. Masui 40:684-691
13. Parker MJ, Handoll HH, Griffiths R (2001) Anaesthesia for hip fracture surgery in adults. Cochrane Database Syst Rev CD000521
14. Aye T, Milne B (2002) Ketamine anesthesia for pericardial window in a patient with pericardial tamponade and severe COPD. Can J Anaesth 49:283-286
15. Roytblat L, Korotkoruchko A, Katz J et al (1993) Postoperative pain: the effect of a low-dose ketamine in addition to general anesthesia. Anesth Analg 77:1161-1165
16. Fu ES, Miguel R, Scharf JE (1997) Preemptive ketamine decreases postoperative narcotic requirements in patients undergoing abdominal surgery. Anesth Analg 84:1086-1090
17. Wilder-Smith OHG, Arendt-Nielsen L, Gäumann D et al (1998) Sensory changes and pain after abdominal hysterectomy: a comparison of anesthetic supplementation with fentanyl versus magnesium or ketamine. Anesth Analg 86:95-101
18. Suzuki M, Tsueda K, Lansing PS et al (1999) Small-dose ketamine enhances morphine-induced analgesia after outpatient surgery. Anesth Analg 89:98-103
19. Menigaux C, Fletcher D, Dupont X et al (2000) The benefits of intraoperative small-dose ketamine on postoperative pain after anterior cruciate ligament repair. Anesth Analg 90:129-135
20. Wilder-Smith OH (1995) Pre-emptive analgesia. Anaesthesist 44 Suppl 3:S529-S534
21. Sandler AN (1999) Post-thoracotomy analgesia and perioperative outcome. Minerva Anestesiol 65:267-274
22. Conacher ID (2001) Post-thoracotomy analgesia. Anesthesiol Clin North America 19:611-625
23. Taura P, Fuster J, Blasi A et al (2003) Postoperative pain relief after hepatic resection in cirrhotic patients: the efficacy of a single small dose of ketamine plus morphine epidurally. Anesth Analg 96:475-480
24. Astuto M, Disma N, Crimi E (2002) Two doses of oral ketamine, given with midazolam, for premedication in children. Minerva Anestesiol 68:593-598
25. Turhanoglu S, Kararmaz A, Ozyilmaz MA et al (2003) Effects of different doses of oral ketamine for premedication of children. Eur J Anaesthesiol 20:56-60

26. Bergman SA (1999) Ketamine: review of its pharmacology and its use in pediatric anesthesia. Anesth Prog 46:10-20
27. Pun MS, Thakur J, Poudyal G et al (2003) Ketamine anaesthesia for paediatric ophthalmology surgery. Br J Ophthalmol 87:535-537
28. Law AK, Ng DK, Chan KK (2003) Use of intramuscular ketamine for endoscopy sedation in children. Pediatr Int 45:180-185
29. Marhofer P, Koinig H, Kapral S (2003) The choice of drugs for caudal anaesthesia in children. An overview. Anaesthesist 52:55-67
30. Ozbek H, Bilen A, Ozcengiz D et al (2002) The comparison of caudal ketamine, alfentanil and ketamine plus alfentanil administration for postoperative analgesia in children. Paediatr Anaesth 12:610-616
31. Kruger AD (1998) Current aspects of using ketamine in childhood. Anaesthesiol Reanim 23:64-71
32. Baraka AS, Sayyd SS, Assaf BA (1997) Thiopental-rocuronium versus ketamine-rocuronium rapid-sequence intubation in parturients undergoing cesarean section. Anesth Analg 84:1104-1107
33. Yaubihi N, Oberoi GS (1994) Comparison of conventional anaesthesia, total intravenous ketamine and epidural block for abdominal hysterectomy. P N G Med J 37:209-213
34. Adams HA, Meyer P, Stoppa A et al (2003) Anaesthesia for caesarean section. Comparison of two general anaesthetic regimens and spinal anesthesia. Anaesthesist 52:23-32
35. Kee WD, Khaw KS, Ma ML et al (1997) Postoperative analgesic requirement after cesarean section: a comparison of anesthetic induction with ketamine or thiopental. Anesth Analg 85:1294-1298
36. Hee WC, Metias VF (2001) Intramuscular Ketamine in a parturient in whom pre-operative intravenous access was not possible. Br J Anaesth 86:891-893
37. Bonanno FG (2002) Ketamine in war/tropical surgery (a final tribute to the racemic mixture). Injury 33:323-327
38. Ezri T, Szmuk P, Stein A et al (2000) Peripartum general anaesthesia without tracheal intubation. Anaesthesia 55:421-426
39. Altissimi C (1979) Ketamine and analgesia during labor. Minerva Anestesiol 45:907-914
40. Adams HA, Hemelmann G (1990) 20 years of ketamine- a backward look. Anaesthesist 39:71-76
41. Friedberg BL (2003) Propofol ketamine anesthesia for cosmetic surgery in the office suite. Int Anesthesiol Clin 41:39-5012-5013
42. White PF (2002) The role of non-opioid analgesic techniques in the management of pain after ambulatory surgery. Anesth Analg 94:577-585
43. Darvas K, Janecsko M, Vimlati L et al (1999) Anesthesia ambulatory one-day surgery. Orv Hetil 140:2035-2040
44. Vinnik CA (1981) An intravenous dissociation technique for outpatient plastic surgery: tranquillity in the office surgical facility. Plast Reconstr Surg 67:799-805
45. Liang HS, Liang HG (1975) Minimizing emergence phenomena: subdissociative dosage of ketamine in balanced surgical anesthesia. Anesth Analg 54:312-316
46. Roytblat L, Levy J, Goldstein J et al (1986) Balanced anesthesia: low-dose ketamine/neuroleptoanalgesia. Curr Ther Res 40:646-652
47. Menigaux C, Fletcher D, Dupont X et al (2000) The benefits of intraoperative small-dose ketamine on postoperative pain after anterior cruciate ligament repair. Anesth Analg 90:129-135
48. Mathisen LC, Aasbø V, Ræder J (1999) Lack of pre-emptive analgesic effect of (R)-ketamine in laparoscopic cholecystectomy. Acta Anaesthesiol Scand 43:220-224
49. Doak GJ, Duke PC (1993) Oral clonidine premedication attenuates the haemodinamic effects associated with ketamine anaesthetic induction in humans. Can J Anaesth 40:612-618
50. Tanaka M, Nishikawa T (1994) Oral clonidine premedication attenuates the hypertensive response to ketamine. Br J Anaesth 73:758-762
51. Taittonen MT, Kirvelä OA, Aantaa R et al (1998) The effect of clonidine or midazolam

premedicationonperioperativeresponsesduringketamineanesthesia.AnesthAnalg87:161-167
52. Handa F, Tanaka M, Nishikawa T et al (2000) Effect of oral clonidine premedication on side effects of intravenous ketamine anesthesia: a randomized, double-blind, placebo-controlled study. J Clin Anesth 12:19-24
53. Cartwright PD, Pingel SM (1984) Midazolam and diazepam in ketamine anaesthesia. Anaesthesia 39:439-442
54. White PF (1983) Use of continuous infusion versus intermittent bolus administration of fentanyl or ketamine during outpatient anesthesia. Anesthesiology 59:294-300
55. Mankowitz E, Brock-Utne JG, Cosnett JE et al (1982) Epidural ketamine. A preliminary report: S Afr Med J 61:441-442
56. Rawal N (1995) Spinal antinociception: clinical aspects. Ann Med 27:263-268
57. Brock-Utne JG, Kallichurum S, Mankowitz E et al (1982) Intrathecal ketamine with preservative- histological effects on spinal nerve roots of baboons. S Afr Med J 61:440-441
58. Gebhardt B (1994) Pharmacology and clinical results with peridural and intrathecal administration of ketamine. Anaesthesist 43 Suppl 2:S34-S40
59. Bion JF (1984) Intrathecal ketamine for war surgery. A preliminary Study under field conditions. Anaesthesia 39:1023-1028
60. McDonnell FJ, Sloan JW, Hamann SR (2000) Advances in cancer pain management. Curr Oncol Rep 2:351-357
61. Bell R, Eccleston C, Kalso E (2003) Ketamine as an adjuvant to opioids for cancer pain. Cochrane Database Syst Rev 2003: CD003351
62. McQueen AL, Baroletti SA (2002) Adjuvant ketamine analgesia for the management of cancer pain. Ann Pharmacother 36(10):1614-1619
63. Kannan TR, Saxena A, Bhatnagar S et al (2002) Oral ketamine as an adjuvant to oral morphine for neuropathic pain in cancer patients. J Pain Symptom Manage 23:60-65
64. Fitzgibbon EJ, Hall P, Schroder C et al (2002) Low dose ketamine as an analgesic adjuvant in difficult pain syndromes: a strategy for conversion from parenteral to oral ketamine. Pain Symptom Manage 23:165-170
65. Vick PG, Lamer TJ (2001) Treatment of central post-stroke pain with oral ketamine. Pain 92:311-313
66. Mizuno J, Sugimoto S, Ikeda M et al (2001) Usefulness of epidural administration of ketamine for relief of postherpetic neuralgia. Masui 50:904-907
67. Jago RH, Thompson MC (1984) Ketamine and military anaesthesia. The effect of heavy papaverum premedication and althesin induction on the incidence of emergence phenomena. Anaesthesia 39:925-927
68. Restall J, Tully AM, Ward PJ et al (1988) Total intravenous anaesthesia for military surgery. A technique using ketamine, midazolam, and vecuronium. Anaesthesia 43:46-49
69. Bishop RA, Litch JA, Stanton JM (2000) Ketamine anesthesia at high altitude. High Alt Med Biol. 1:111-114
70. White PF (1988) Ketamine update: its clinical uses in anesthesia. Seminars in Anesthesia 7:113-126
71. Hennenberger A, Partecke BD (1995) Therapy of the severely burned child from the intensive care viewpoint. Unfallchirurg 98:193-197
72. Byer DE, Gould AB (1981) Development of tolerance to ketamine in an infant undergoing repeated anesthesia. Anesthesiology 54:255-256
73. Garcia Martinez JM (1999) Round table: Severe asthma in pediatrics: treatment of acute crises. Allergol Immunopathol (Madr) 27:53-62
74. Beveridge RC, Grunfeld AF, Hodder RV et al (1996) Guidelines for the emergency management of asthma in adults. CAEP/CTS Asthma Advisory Committee. Canadian Association of Emergency Physicians and The Canadian Society. CMAJ 155:25-37
75. Lau TT, Zed PJ (2001) Does ketamine have a role in managing severe exacerbation of asthma in adults? Pharmacotherapy 21:1100-1106

76. Howton JC, Rose J, Duffy S, et al (1996) Randomized, double-blind, placebo-controlled trial of intravenous ketamine in acute asthma. Ann Emerg Med 27:170-175
77. Sarma VJ (1992) Use of ketamine in acute severe asthma. Acta Anaesthesiol Scand 36:106-107
78. Jorgensen BG (1992) Ketamine as a broncholytic agent in status asthmaticus and as an anesthetic for patients with bronchial asthma. Ugeskr Laeger 154:2132-2135
79. Strube PJ, Hallam PL (1986) Ketamine by continuous infusion in status asthmaticus. Anesthesia 41:1017-1019
80. Hemmingsen C, Nielsen PK, Odorico J (1994) Ketamine in the treatment of bronchospasm during mechanical ventilation. Am J Emerg Med 12:417-420
81. Rock MJ, Reyes de la Rocha S, L'Hommedieu CS et al (1986) Use of ketamine in asthmatic children to treat respiratory failure refractory to conventional therapy. Crit Care Med 14:514-516
82. Nehama J, Pass R, Bechtler-Karsch A (1996) Continuous ketamine infusion for the treatment of refractory asthma in a mechanically ventilated infant: case report and review of the pediatric literature. Pediatr Emerg Care 12:294-297
83. Petrillo TM, Fortenberry JD, Linzer JF (2001) Emergency department use of ketamine in pediatric status asthmaticus. J Asthma 38:657-664
84. Youssef-Ahmed MZ, Silver P, Nimkoff L et al (1996) Continuous infusion of ketamine in mechanically ventilated children with refractory bronchospasm. Intensive Care Med 22:972-976
85.Gremmelt A, Braun U (1995) Analgesia and sedation in patients with head-brain trauma. Anaesthesist 44 Suppl 3:S559-S665
86.Fitzal S (1997) Ketamine and neuroprotection. Clinical outlook. Anaesthesist 46 Suppl 1:S65-S70
87.Mangini M (1998) Treatment of alcoholism using psychedelic drugs: a review of the program of research. J Psychoactive Drugs 30:381-418
88.Krupitsky EM, Grinenko AY (1997) Ketamine psychedelic therapy (KPT): a review of the results of ten years of research. J Psychoactive Drugs 29:165-183
89. Grinenko AIa, Krupitskii EM, Palei AI et al (1989) Treatment of alcoholism by affective counterattribution. Zh Nevropatol Psikhiatr Im S S Korsakova. 89:101-105
90. Sivolap IuP, Savchenkov VA (1994) Experience in using ketamine preparations in the psychotherapy of alcoholism. Zh Nevropatol Psikhiatr Im S S Korsakova 94:76-79
91. Krupitsky E, Burakov A, Romanova T et al (2002) Ketamine psychotherapy for heroin addiction: immediate effects and two-year follow-up. Subst Abuse Treat 23:273-283
92. Grieco A, Bloom R (1981) Psychotherapy with hallucinogenic adjuncts from a learning perspective. Int J Addict 16:801-827
93. Smith KM, Larive LL, Romanelli F (2002) Club drugs: methylenedioxymethamphetamine, flunitrazepam, ketamine hydrochloride, and gamma-hydroxybutyrate. Am J Health Syst Pharm 59:1067-1076
94. Jansen KL (2000) A review of the nonmedical use of ketamine: use, users and consequences. J Psychoactive Drugs 32:419-433
95. Bowdle TA, Radant AD, Cowley DS et al (1998) Psychedelic effects of ketamine in healthy volunteers: relationship to steady-state plasma concentrations. Anesthesiology 88:82-88
96. Curran HV, Morgan C (2000) Cognitive, dissociative and psychotogenic effects of ketamine in recreational users on the night of drug use and 3 days later. Addiction 95:575-590
97. Jansen KL (1990) Ketamine - can chronic use impair memory? Int J Addict 25:133-139
98. Gaulier JM, Canal M, Pradeille JL et al (2002) New drugs at "rave parties": ketamine and prolintane. Acta Clin Belg Suppl (1):41-46
99. Dalgarno PJ, Shewan D (1996) Illicit use of ketamine in Scotland. Psychoactive Drugs 28:191-199
100. Lim DK (2003) Ketamine associated psychedelic effects and dependence. Singapore Med J 44:31-34
101. Jansen KL, Darracot-Cankovic R (2001) The nonmedical use of ketamine, part two: A review of problem use and dependence. Psychoactive Drugs 33:151-158

102. Arditti J, Spadari M, de Haro L et al (2002) Ketamine - dreams and realities. Acta Clin Belg Suppl (1):31-33
103. Pal HR, Berry N, Kumar R et al (2002) Ketamine dependence. Anaesth Intensive Care 30:382-384
104. Kapur S, Seeman P (2002) NMDA receptor antagonists ketamine and PCP have direct effects on the dopamine D_2 and serotonin 5-HT_2 receptors-implications for models of schizophrenia. Mol Psychiatry 7:837-844
105. Micallef J, Tardieu S, Gentile S (2003) Effects of a subanaesthetic dose of ketamine on emotional and behavioral state in healthy subjects. Neurophysiol Clin 33:138-147
106. Carpenter WT Jr (1999) The schizophrenia ketamine challenge study debate. Biol Psychiatry 46:1081-1091

Neuroimaging studies on ketamine

U. FREO, C. ORI

Among anaesthetics, ketamine has the distinction of being the only antagonist of *N*-methyl-D-aspartate (NMDA) receptors approved for clinical use and a potent analgesic with only mild cardiovascular and respiratory depressant properties [1]. Ketamine, however, also has disadvantageous psychomimetic activity, which has been the major factor in limiting ketamine clinical use but also in modelling psychoses in animal and humans [1]. For all these reasons, ketamine has been extensively investigated with neuroimaging techniques.

Ketamine has been used as a tracer to image central nervous system pharmacokinetics, but in relatively few receptor studies, because of ketamine's lack of binding specificity for neuroreceptors and short half-life; development ketamine analogues for radiotracer synthesis and competition studies with neurotrasmitters tracers are currently on going. Inducibile c-Fos protein is a metabolic marker that is sensitive to a variety of pathophysiological conditions and serves also to evaluate ketamine neuroprotective and neurotoxic activities [2]. Finally, determination of regional cerebral metabolic rates for glucose (rCMRglc) and regional blood flow (rCBF) provide two surrogate indices of neuronal functional activities [3]. rCMRglc and rCBF are measured autoradiographically in animals with the [^{14}C] 2-deoxy-D-glucose [4] and [^{14}C]iodoantipyrine [5] techniques. rCMRglc and rCBF are determined in humans with positron emission tomography (PET) and ^{18}F-deoxy-D-glucose and ^{15}O- water ($H_2{}^{15}O$) [3, 6]. In the last 10 years techniques of magnetic resonance imaging have proven able to provide measures of rCBF and have been named functional magnetic resonance imaging (fMRI) [7].

The paper will review the contribution of neuroimaging techniques to the understanding of pharmacology of ketamine.

Receptor studies

Ketamine enantiomer analogues have been developed as PET radiotracers *S*(+) and *R*(-)[*N*-methyl-^{11}C] ketamine) to investigate ketamine pharmacokinetics and receptor binding in primate brain. In monkeys *S*(+)[*N*-methyl-^{11}C] ketamine binding affinity was in the micromolar range and half to a third that of *R*(-) enantiomer [8]. In healthy humans *S*(+)[*N*-methyl-^{11}C] ketamine radioactivity was short lasting (e.g. peak values by 6–9 min), highly concentrated (e.g. 5- to 7-fold that in body fluids) in thalamus, basal ganglia and cortices and displaceable by therapeutic doses of *S*(+)ketamine (e.g. 0.1–0.2 mg/kg) [9]. Radioactivity uptake of *S*(+)[*N*-methyl-^{11}C] ketamine is reduced in the temporal lobes of patients suffering from temporal lobe epilepsy suggesting that NMDA-receptor function is decreased in this clinical entity [10].

SPECT and PET dopaminergic ligands have been used to investigate ketamine dopaminergic targets. In monkeys, subanaesthetic ketamine (5 mg/kg, i.v. bolus) induced nystagmus and stereotyped movements and increased binding of *N*-[^{11}C]methylspiperone, a dopaminergic D_2 receptor ligand, in the striatum (e.g. specific binding) but not in cerebral cortex and cerebellum (e.g. aspecific binding) [11]; at the opposite and of the range, pentobarbital (25 mg/kg) produced deeper anaesthesia without psychotic symptoms and decreased the accumulation of *N*-[^{11}C]methylspiperone in the striatum [11]. In another monkey study striatal binding of dopaminergic D_2 receptor ligands was slightly decreased (e.g. *N*-[^{11}C]methylspiperone and [^{11}C]raclopride) [12] or unchanged (e.g. [^{18}F]fluoroclebopride) [13] during anaesthesia with isoflurane or ketamine, indicating that modifications in striatal D_2 receptors do not depend solely on changes in endogenous dopamine. In a series of monkey PET studies, Tsukada showed that ketamine anaesthesia (3 or 10 mg kg^{-1} h^{-1}, i.v. continuous infusion) in the striatum dose-dependently decreased labelling of [^{11}C]raclopride and increased striatal labelling by *L*-[beta-^{11}C]DOPA and [^{11}C]beta-CFT [2beta-carbomethoxy-3beta-(4-fluorophenyl)tropane] and [^{11}C]beta-CIT-FE [*N*-(2-fluoroethyl)-2beta-carbomethoxy-3beta-(4-iodophenyl)tropane] which are markers of dopamine synthesis and reuptake [14, 15]. Concurrent microdyalitic determinations showed that striatal dopamine concentrations were unaltered by ketamine [11, 14]. Hence, NMDA blockade by ketamine modulates dopamine turnover in the striatum by simultaneous enhancement of dopamine synthesis and transport and results in no overall change of dopamine striatal levels [14, 15].

In human PET studies ketamine at high subanaesthetic and anaesthetic doses did not change [^{11}C]raclopride binding [16, 17]. Other authors, however, used a different paradigm [18] and reported that ketamine [18, 19] and S(+)ketamine [20] decreased PET striatal [^{11}C]raclopride binding [18-20]. In addition, [^{11}C]raclopride binding was decreased by ketamine in a fashion similar to the way amphetamine decreased it [18] and was regionally correlated (e.g. in the ventral striatum) with heightened mood [18, 20]. In a SPECT study in normal human subjects, ketamine significantly enhanced the amphetamine-induced decrease in binding of [^{123}I]IBZM, a dopaminergic D_2 receptor ligand; such an effect was comparable in magnitude to the exaggerated response observed in schizophrenic patients [21]. Altogether the findings indicate that ketamine may, via NMDA receptors, modulate different dopaminergic functions and produce psychotic symptomatology [20]. Recently, a double PET study of D_2 receptor density and rCBF has been conducted in cats by means of [^{11}C]raclopride binding and $H_2{}^{15}O$. Ketamine anaesthesia did not alter or increased slightly striatally [^{11}C]raclopride binding and rCBF; in contrast halothane anaesthesia drastically increased both [^{11}C]raclopride binding and rCBF, suggesting that [^{11}C]raclopride binding may be heavily dependent on rCBF [22].

c-Fos studies

NMDA receptors have been implicated in neuronal damage from different pathological processes, and NMDA antagonists such as ketamine could have 'neuroprotective' activities. Ketamine blocked c-Fos induction by traumatic brain injury in mouse [2, 23] and rat [24] cerebral cortex, by devascularisation [25] and 4-aminopyridine seizures in rat cerebral cortex [26], by cocaine in rat basal ganglia [27], and by photic stimulation in the suprachiasmatic nucleus of hamsters [28].

NMDA receptors are implicated, however, in physiological brain processes including plasticity and NMDA receptor blockade by ketamine, and NMDA receptor antagonists may actually lead to 'toxic' neuronal changes. c Fos was found to be unaffected in earlier studies [2, 23] but was strongly induced in later studies [29, 30]. c-fos expression occurred in the posterior cingulate and retrosplenial cortices [29] in a stereospecific fashion (e.g. higher potency of *S*(+) vs *R*(-)ketamine) and was correlated with abnormal motor behaviour. For this reason, c-fos expression has been proposed as a possible marker of behavioural and neuronal toxic effects of ketamine [29]. The findings are consistent with higher anaesthetic potency but not with lesser postanaesthetic activation of *S*(+)ketamine [31, 32]; in addition, they suggest that only sedation/anaesthesia occurring at high doses, and not behavioural/psychomimetic activation occurring at low doses or during recovery from high doses of ketamine is related to c-fos expression.

Ketamine and NMDA antagonists are thought to induce abnormal motor behaviour by increasing dopaminergic release and neurotransmission in the ventral tegmental area, nucleus accumbens and medioprefrontal cortex [33]. Following ketamine, however, c-Fos expression has been observed in the posterior cingulate and retrosplenial cortices but not in dopaminergic areas [29].

c-Fos expression during ketamine anaesthesia (50 mg/kg) was enhanced by N_2O [34] and, consistently much reduced greatly in NMDA receptor knockout mice [35]. c-Fos expression was also blocked, however, by different gaseous (e.g. halothane, isoflurane and xenon) [36] and intravenous (e.g. propofol and diazepam) anaesthetics, all of which may have $GABA_A$ receptor antagonistic properties [34, 36, 37]. Consistently, bicuculline and flumazenil, two $GABA_A$ receptor antagonists, reversed propofol inhibition of c-fos expression by ketamine, further strengthening the idea that propofol blockade of ketamine activities involves or may be affected by $GABA_A$ receptor activation [30]. Gabazine, a $GABA_A$ antagonist, counteracted sedation and c-fos expression by $GABA_A$ agonists in specific sleep-promoting brain areas; gabazine, however, failed to affect sedation (c-Fos expression not determined) by intracerebroventricular ketamine (0.75–1.75 icv) [38]. Finally, ketamine-induced fos-like immunoreactivity was reduced by the sigma2 receptor antagonist rimcazole [35] and was unaffected [35] or decreased by the nonselective sigma antagonist haloperidol [39].

Overall, c-fos studies indicate that ketamine anaesthesia is mediated by NMDA receptors; changes in $GABA_A$, dopaminergic and sigma receptor functions are probably modulated by NMDA receptors. Further, c-fos studies indicate that $GABA_A$ antagonist sedatives and anaesthetics, such as propofol, are probably preferable to NMDA receptor agents, such as N_2O, in preventing and reducing psychomimetic and addictive properties of ketamine.

Cerebral metabolism and blood flow studies

Given its complex behavioural pharmacology, ketamine has been studied extensively in animals and humans with techniques of functional cerebral metabolism and blood flow. The aims of these studies have been to investigate the mechanisms of action of ketamine psychomimetic and anaesthetic activities.

In rodents, in a fashion similar to other NMDA antagonists, such as MK801 and phencyclidine, ketamine induces a biphasic dose-dependent behavioural continuum that consists in agitation, hyperlocomotion, ataxia and anaesthesia [31, 32]. Ketamine also has a very similar biphasic dose-dependent effect on rCMRglc. Low-dose ketamine (5 mg/kg) at steady state induces a subhypnotic condition and rCMRglc increases in most brain regions [33]. In mice and rats, after subanaesthetic ketamine (30 mg/kg i.p.) rCMRglc and 2-DG uptake, a nonquantitative index of glucose consumption, increases in medial prefrontal, cingulate and retrosplenial cortices, anterior ventral thalamic nucleus, basolateral amygdala and hippocampal formation and decreases in the lateral habenula and auditory system [40-44]. In rats but not in mice, subanaesthetic ketamine reduces rCMRglc in the auditory and sensory cortices, inferior colliculus, cerebellar dentate and vestibular nucleus, indicating that there are species differences in the rCMRglc response to ketamine [40, 44, 45].

Ketamine anaesthesia with larger doses (10-30 mg/kg i.v.; 30 mg/kg i.v. plus continuous infusion; 50 mg i.v.; 25-75 mg i.m.) [40, 44-46] leads to both rCMRglc increases in limbic, extrapyramidal and cortical areas and decreases in somatosensory and auditory regions. Ketamine anaesthesia with high doses (100-200 mg/kg i.p.) cause rCMRglc reductions almost exclusively [3, 46]. Postanaesthetic recovery from ketamine leads to sharp rCMRglc increases, especially in the limbic system [3, 40] that are similar to those observed after low subanaesthetic doses [3, 40]. rCMRglc effects of ketamine are stereospecific: after racemic and (*R*-) ketamine anaesthesia rats exhibited agitation and increased spontaneous motor activity; rCMRglc rose in several and decreased in few brain regions; in contrast, after *S*(+) ketamine rats did not present abnormal behaviour and appeared more heavily sedated; rCMRglc was increased in fewer regions and decreased in more regions than after racemic or *R*(-)ketamine [3].

The effects of ketamine on rCBF have been studied in animals and humans but these studies have yielded conflicting reports. Ketamine induces no change in rCBF in ventilated goats [47], rabbits [48] and rats [49]; Cavazzuti, however, with iodoantipyrine technique found that ketamine anaesthesia (e.g. 100 mg/kg) led to rCBF decreases in limbic regions of rats and that these were closely correlated with rCMRglc decreases [50]. In rats, ketamine anaesthesia alone does not alter absolute rCBF as measured with fMRI [51]; when added to fentanyl/fluanisone/midazolam, however, ketamine anaesthesia increases fMRI measured rCBF by 10-14% in the hippocampus, olfactory bulb and cortex [52]. In humans, added to isoflurane anaesthesia, ketamine causes no change or increase in rCBF of patients undergoing craniotomy [53, 54]. In ketamine-anaesthetized monkeys ketamine does not eliminate cortical processing of the motion stimulus and rCBF response to visual patterns is preserved [55]. These relevant discrepancies about ketamine effects on brain haemodyamics have been ascribed to differences in species, methods of ventilation and rCBF determination, ketamine dosage and background anaesthesia.

A number of studies have been conducted to investigate the involvement of NMDA and aminergic neurotransmitter systems in rCMRglc effects of ketamine. In parallel and independent studies, subanaesthetic doses of NMDA antagonists such as MK-801 (0.3-0.5 mg/kg i.p.) or phencyclidine have led to patterns of marked rCMRglc increases in limbic cortical regions, hippocampal formation, nucleus accumbens, and basolateral amygdala which are indistinguishable from subanaesthetic ketamine [3, 41] and suggest that NMDA receptor blockade is critical in ketamine rCMRglc effects [41]. In contrast, amphetamine leads to a different pattern of relative 2-DG uptake with increases in the ventral orbital cortex, medial septal, subthalamic, anterior pretectal and several thalamic nuclei, but not in the limbic and cortical regions [41]. As NMDA antagonists, such as ketamine and MK801, and amphetamine all increase dopaminergically mediated motor behaviours, the findings were interpreted as evidence that 2-DG uptake increases caused by subanaesthetic doses of ketamine depend on NMDA receptor antagonism and not on motor behaviour activation per se [41]; the findings also imply that dopaminergic activation is not sufficient to increase metabolic activity in limbic regions and, therefore, to induce psychomimetic changes [41].

Benzodiazepines are highly, and neuroleptics variably, effective in reducing agitation and c-fos expression induced by ketamine. The $GABA_A$ agent diazepam and neuroleptic droperidol, but not the acetylcholinesterase inhibitor physostigmine, prolongs the time of recovery of the righting reflex and tail flick responses and reduced agitation; none of these drugs alters rCMRglc activation by subanaesthetic ketamine [56]. Behavioural and cerebral metabolic activation in response to ketamine (30 mg/kg) were instead reduced in D_1 receptor knock out mice by pretreatment with the D_1 dopamine receptor antagonist SCH23390 (0.3 mg/kg) in wild mice [57] and by high doses of the 'atypical' antipsychotics clozapine and olanzapine in rats [58, 59]. The ability of high but not of low doses of olanzapine to block ketamine rCMRglc effects may be due to olanzapine and clozapine activities at other unknown target sites [41]. In rats, chronic, but not acute, pretreatment with the D_2 dopamine receptor antagonists haloperidol and risperidone attenuates rCMRglc increases induced by ketamine [60]; following chronic treatment olanzapine but not haloperidol further attenuates ketamine-induced cerebral metabolic increases. Hence, typical and atypical antipsychotics, although differing in their pharmacology can lead to plastic changes of NMDA receptors.

In humans most rCMRglc and rCBF studies have focused on ketamine subanaesthetic doses that determine and model psychotic symptoms. Specifically, subanaesthetic ketamine (0.3 mg/kg) induces psychotic symptoms, increases rCMRglc in the prefrontal [61] and anterior cingulate cortices [62] and rCBF in the anterior cingulate and medial prefrontal regions and inferior frontal cortices, and decreases rCBF in the cerebellum [63]. Scores for psychopathological symptoms correlated with rCMRglc and rCBF increases in different cortical and subcortical regions, suggesting that distribution networks rather than single regions may produce psychotic manifestations [62, 63]. rCBF changes had a monophasic time-course with a peak effect at 6-16 min [63]. In healthy humans, psychotomimetic doses (e.g. 15 mg and more in continuous infusion) of *S*(+)ketamine cause marked rCMRglc increases in frontal, anterior cingulate, parietal and left sensorimotor cortices and thalamus that are regionally (e.g. frontal and temporal lobes) correlated with psychotic symptoms [62]. *R*(-)Ketamine does not produce psychotic symptoms but a state of relaxation and significant rCMRglc decreases in the temporomedial cortex and left insula [62].

In the last few years fMRI technique have made it possible to image rCBF changes during emotional and cognitive stimulation/challenge in normal subjects and patients. In healthy subjects subanaesthetic ketamine (bolus 0.2-0.5 mg/kg) increases significantly dissociative phenomena and negative symptoms and alters emotional responses, but has variable effects on cognition. After ketamine, rCBF shown by fMRI, much like PET-measured rCBF, is increased in frontal, anterior cingulate, temporal and amygdalar regions and decreased in motor, somatosensory, occipital, posterior cingulate, cerebellar and thalamic regions [65]. Following ketamine (bolus 0.2-0.5 mg/kg) performance is unchanged in a gender discrimination task but is impaired in encoding/ retrieval and verbal fluency tasks [65-69]. During encoding and retrieval, ketamine enhances rCBF activation in the left inferior frontal gyrus, bilateral hippocampus, anterior cingulate gyrus and lateral temporal cortex [67] and in bilateral prefrontal cortex, respectively [68]. During a verbal fluency task, ketamine [69] causes greater rCBF activation in the prefrontal cortices and basal ganglia. During a continuous performance task ketamine prevents temporal rCBF deactivation [70]. Nicotine reverses memory impairment and rCBF changes brought about by ketamine during encoding/retrieval tasks [65]. Ketamine almost completely abolishes the normal rCBF pattern occurring in limbic and visual cortex to emotionally significant (e.g. fear) but not to 'neutral' face expression [71]. The findings are interpreted as evidence that in psychotic patients emotional blunting may be associated with reduced limbic responses to emotional stimuli and a relative increase in the visual cortical response to neutral stimuli [71].

rCBF is higher in the hippocampus of schizophrenic patients than in normal controls at rest and during a auditory discriminatory task but decreases, or "normalises", after neuroleptic medication [72]. In comparison to baseline, subanesthetic ketamine (0.3 mg/kg) reactivates psychotic symptoms, increases PET rCBF in the anterior cingulate cortex and decreases rCBF in the hippocampus and the primary visual cortex (lingual and fusiform gyri) [73]; ketamine reduces rCBF more markedly in schizophrenic patients than in healthy control subjects, suggesting that NMDA receptor function is abnormal in schizophrenia [72].

References

1. Reich DL, Silvay G (1989) Ketamine: an update on the first twenty-five years of clinical experience. Can J Anaesth 36:186-197
2. Dragunow M, Faull R (1989) The use of c-Fos as a metabolic marker in neuronal pathway tracing. J Neurosci Methods 29:261-265
3. Freo U, Ori C (2002) Mapping cerebral metabolic and blood flow effects of general anaesthetics. In: Gullo A (Ed) Anaesthesia Pain Intensive Care Emergency Medicine Vol 17. Springer-Verlag Italia, Milan pp 877-891
4. Sokoloff l, Reivich M, Kennedy C et al (1977) The [^{14}C]deoxyglucose method for the measurement of local cerebral glucose utilization. Theory, procedure, and normal values in the conscious and anesthetized albino rat. J Neurochem 28:897-916
5. Sakurada O, Kennedy C, Jehle J et al (1978) Measurements of local cerebral blood flow with iodo[^{14}C]antipyrine. Am J Physiol 234:H59-66
6. Herscovitch P, Markham J, Raichle ME (1983) Brain blood flow measured with intravenous $H^2{}_{15}O$. I. Theory and error analysis. J Nucl Med 24:782-789
7. Ogawa S, Lee TM, Kay AR et al (1990) Brain magnetic resonance imaging with contrast dependent on blood oxigenation. Proc Natl Acad Sci USA 87:9868-9872
8. Hartvig P, Valtysson J, Antoni G et al (1994) Brain kinetics of (*R*)- and (*S*)-[*N*-methyl-11C]ketamine in the rhesus monkey studied by positron emission tomography (PET). Nucl Med Biol 21:927-934
9. Hartvig P, Valtysson J, Lindner KJ et al (1995) Central nervous system effects of subdissociative doses of (*S*)-ketamine are related to plasma and brain concentrations measured with positron emission tomography in healthy volunteers. Clin Pharmacol Ther 58:165-173
10. Kumlien E, Hartvig P, Valind S et al (1999) NMDA-receptor activity visualized with (*S*)-[*N*-methyl-11C]ketamine and positron emission tomography in patients with medial temporal lobe epilepsy. Epilepsia 40:30-37
11. Onoe H, Inoue O, Suzuki K et al (1994) Ketamine increases the striatal *N*-[11C]methylspiperone binding in vivo: positron emission tomography study using conscious rhesus monkey. Brain Res 663:191-198
12. Kobayashi K, Inoue O, Watanabe Y et al (1995).Difference in response of D_2 receptor binding between ^{11}C-*N*-methylspiperone and ^{11}C-raclopride against anesthetics in rhesus monkey brain. J Neural Transm Gen Sect 100:147-151
13. Nader MA, Grant KA, Gage HD et al (1999) PET imaging of dopamine D_2 receptors with [18F]fluoroclebopride in monkeys: effects of isoflurane- and ketamine-induced anesthesia. Neuropsychopharmacology 21:589-596
14. Tsukada H, Harada N, Nishiyama S et al (2000) Ketamine decreased striatal [$^{(11)}$C]raclopride binding with no alterations in static dopamine concentrations in the striatal extracellular fluid in the monkey brain: multiparametric PET studies combined with microdialysis analysis. Synapse 37:95-103
15. Tsukada H, Nishiyama S, Kakiuchi T et al (2001) Ketamine alters the availability of striatal dopamine transporter as measured by [$^{(11)}$C]beta-CFT and [$^{(11)}$C]beta-CIT-FE in the monkey brain. Synapse 42:273-280
16. Aalto S, Hirvonen J, Kajander J et al (2002) Ketamine does not decrease striatal dopamine D(2) receptor binding in man. Psychopharmacology 164:401-406
17. Kegeles LS, Martinez D, Kochan LD et al (2002) NMDA antagonist effects on striatal dopamine release: positron emission tomography studies in humans. Synapse 43:19-29
18. Breier A, Adler CM, Weisenfeld N et al (1998) Effects of NMDA antagonism on striatal dopamine release in healthy subjects: application of a novel PET approach. Synapse 29:142-147
19. Smith GS, Schloesser R, Brodie JD et al (1998) Glutamate modulation of dopamine measured in vivo with positron emission tomography (PET) and ^{11}C-raclopride in normal human subjects. Neuropsychopharmacology 18:18-25

20. Vollenweider FX, Vontobel P, Oye I et al (2000) Effects of (*S*)-ketamine on striatal dopamine: a [^{11}C]raclopride PET study of a model psychosis in humans. J Psychiatr Res 34:35-43
21. Kegeles LS, Abi-Dargham A, Zea-Ponce Y et al (2000) Modulation of amphetamine-induced striatal dopamine release by ketamine in humans: implications for schizophrenia. Biol Psychiatry 48:627-640
22. Hassoun W, Le Cavorsin M, Ginovart N et al (2003) PET study of the [$^{(11)}$C]raclopride binding in the striatum of the awake cat: effects of anaesthetics and role of cerebral blood flow. Eur J Nucl Med Mol Imaging 30:141-148
23. Dragunow M, Goulding M, Faull RL et al (1990) Induction of c-fos mRNA and protein in neurons and glia after traumatic brain injury: pharmacological characterization. Exp Neurol 107:236-248
24. Herrera DG, Robertson HA (1990) N-methyl-D-aspartate receptors mediate activation of the c-fos proto-oncogene in a model of brain injury. Neuroscience 35:273-281
25. Herrera DG, Robertson HA (1989) Unilateral induction of c-fos protein in cortex following cortical devascularization. Brain Res 503:205-213
26. Szakacs R, Weiczner R, Mihaly A et al (2003) Non-competitive NMDA receptor antagonists moderate seizure-induced c-fos expression in the rat cerebral cortex. Brain Res Bull 59:485-493
27. Torres G, Rivier C (1993) Cocaine-induced expression of striatal c-fos in the rat is inhibited by NMDA receptor antagonists. Brain Res Bull 30:173-176
28. Abe H, Rusak B, Robertson HA (1992) NMDA and non-NMDA receptor antagonists inhibit photic induction of fos protein in the hamster suprachiasmatic nucleus. Brain Res Bull 28:831-835
29. Nishizawa N, Nakao S, Nagata A et al (2000) The effect of ketamine isomers on both mice behavioral responses and c-fos expression in the posterior cingulate and retrosplenial cortices. Brain Res 857:188-192
30. Nakao S, Nagata A, Miyamoto E (2003) Inhibitory effect of propofol on ketamine-induced c-fos expression in the rat posterior cingulate and retrosplenial cortices is mediated by GABAA receptor activation. Acta Anaesthesiol Scand 47:284-290
31. Benthuysen JL, Hance AJ, Quam DD et al (1989) Comparison of isomers of ketamine on catalepsy in the rat and electrical activity of the brain and behaviour in the cat. Neuropharmacology 28:1003-1009
32. Marietta MP, Way WL, Castagnoli N Jr et al (1977) On the pharmacology of the ketamine enantiomorphs in the rat. J Pharmacol Exp Ther 202:157-165
33. Bowers MB Jr, Hoffman FJ Jr (1984) Homovanillic acid in rat caudate and prefrontal cortex following phencyclidine and amphetamine. Psychopharmacology 84:136-137
34. Nagata A, Nakao Si S, Nishizawa N et al (2001) Xenon inhibits but $N_{(2)}O$ enhances ketamine-induced c-fos expression in the rat posterior cingulate and retrosplenial cortices. Anesth Analg 92:362-368
35. Nakao S, Miyamoto E, Masuzawa M et al (2002) Ketamine-induced c-fos expression in the mouse posterior cingulate and retrosplenial cortices is mediated not only via NMDA receptors but also via sigma receptors. Brain Res 926:191-196
36. Nakao S, Adachi T, Murakawa M et al (1996) Halothane and diazepam inhibit ketamine-induced c-fos expression in the rat cingulate cortex. Anesthesiology 85:874-882
37. Nagata A, Nakao S, Miyamoto E et al (1998) Propofol inhibits ketamine-induced c-fos expression in the rat posterior cingulate cortex. Anesth Analg 87:1416-1420
38. Nelson LE, Guo TZ, Lu J et al (2002) The sedative component of anesthesia is mediated by GABA(A) receptors in an endogenous sleep pathway. Nat Neurosci 5:979-984
39. Ma D, Wilhelm S, Maze M, Franks NP (2002) Neuroprotective and neurotoxic properties of the 'inert' gas, xenon. Br J Anaesth 89:739-746
40. Davis DW, Mans AM, Biebuyck JF, Hawkins RA (1988) The influence of ketamine on regional brain glucose use. Anesthesiology 69:199-205
41. Duncan GE, Miyamoto S, Leipzig JN, Lieberman JA (1999) Comparison of brain metabolic

activity patterns induced by ketamine, MK-801 and amphetamine in rats: support for NMDA receptor involvement in responses to subanesthetic dose of ketamine. Brain Res 843:171-183
42. Eintrei C, Sokoloff L, Smith CB (1999) Effects of diazepam and ketamine administered individually or in combination on regional rates of glucose utilization in rat brain. Br J Anaesth 82:596-602
43. Miyamoto S, Leipzig JN, Lieberman JA, Duncan GE (2000) Effects of ketamine, MK-801, and amphetamine on regional brain 2-deoxyglucose uptake in freely moving mice. Neuropsychopharmacology 22:400-412
44. Nelson SR, Howard RB, Cross RS, Samson F (1980) Ketamine-induced changes in regional glucose utilization in the rat brain. Anesthesiology 52:330-334
45. Crosby G, Crane AM, Sokoloff L (1982) Local changes in cerebral glucose utilization during ketamine anesthesia. Anesthesiology 56:437-443
46. Hammer RP Jr, Herkenham M (1983) Altered metabolic activity in the cerebral cortex of rats exposed to ketamine. J Comp Neurol 220:396-404
47. Schwedler M, Miletich DJ, Albrecht RF (1982) Cerebral blood flow and metabolism following ketamine administration. Can Anaesth Soc J 29:222-226
48. Oren RE, Rasool NA, Rubinstein EH (1982) Effect of ketamine on cerebral cortical blood flow and metabolism in rabbits. Stroke 18:441-444
49. Chi OZ, Wei HM, Klein SL, Weiss HR (1994) Effect of ketamine on heterogeneity of cerebral microregional venous O_2 saturation in the rat. Anesth Analg 79:860-866
50. Cavazzuti M, Porro CA, Biral GP et al (1987) Ketamine effects on local cerebral blood flow and metabolism in the rat. J Cereb Blood Flow Metab 7:806-811
51. Lei H, Grinberg O, Nwaigwe CI et al (2001) The effects of ketamine-xylazine anesthesia on cerebral blood flow and oxygenation observed using nuclear magnetic resonance perfusion imaging and electron paramagnetic resonance oximetry. Brain Res 913:174-179
52. Burdett NG, Menon DK, Carpenter TA et al (1995) Visualisation of changes in regional cerebral blood flow (rCBF) produced by ketamine using long TE gradient-echo sequences: preliminary results. Magn Reson Imaging 13:549-553
53. Mayberg TS, Lam AM, Matta BF et al (1995) Ketamine does not increase cerebral blood flow velocity or intracranial pressure during isoflurane/nitrous oxide anesthesia in patients undergoing craniotomy. Anesth Analg 81:84-89
54. Strebel S, Kaufmann M, Maitre L, Schaefer HG (1995) Effects of ketamine on cerebral blood flow velocity in humans. Influence of pretreatment with midazolam or esmolol. Anaesthesia 50:223-228
55. Leopold DA, Plettenberg HK, Logothetis NK (2002) Visual processing in the ketamine-anesthetized monkey. Optokinetic and blood oxygenation level-dependent responses. Exp Brain Res 143:359-372
56. Oguchi K, Arakawa K, Nelson SR, Samson F (1982) The influence of droperidol, diazepam, and physostigmine on ketamine-induced behavior and brain regional glucose utilization in rat. Anesthesiology 57:353-358
57. Miyamoto S, Mailman RB, Lieberman JA, Duncan GE (2001) Blunted brain metabolic response to ketamine in mice lacking D(1A) dopamine receptors. Brain Res 894:167-180
58. Duncan GE, Leipzig JN, Mailman RB, Lieberman JA (1998) Differential effects of clozapine and haloperidol on ketamine-induced brain metabolic activation. Brain Res 812:65-75
59. Duncan GE, Miyamoto S, Leipzig JN, Lieberman JA (2000) Comparison of the effects of clozapine, risperidone, and olanzapine on ketamine-induced alterations in regional brain metabolism. J Pharmacol Exp Ther 293:8-14
60. Duncan GE, Miyamoto S, Lieberman JA (2003) Chronic administration of haloperidol and olanzapine attenuates ketamine-induced brain metabolic activation. J Pharmacol Exp Ther 305:999-1005
61. Breier A, Malhotra AK, Pinals DA et al (1997) Association of ketamine-induced psychosis with focal activation of the prefrontal cortex in healthy volunteers. Am J Psychiatry 154:805-811

62. Vollenweider FX, Leenders KL, Oye I et al (1997) Differential psychopathology and patterns of cerebral glucose utilisation produced by (*S*)- and (*R*)-ketamine in healthy volunteers using positron emission tomography (PET). Eur Neuropsychopharmacol 7:25-38
63. Holcomb HH, Lahti AC, Medoff DR et al (2001) Sequential regional cerebral blood flow brain scans using PET with H2(15)O demonstrate ketamine actions in CNS dynamically. Neuropsychopharmacology 25:165-172
64. Vollenweider FX, Leenders KL, Scharfetter C et al (1997) Metabolic hyperfrontality and psychopathology in the ketamine model of psychosis using positron emission tomography (PET) and [^{18}F]fluorodeoxyglucose (FDG). Eur Neuropsychopharmacol 7:9-24
65. Beason-Held L, Holcomb H, Tamminga C (2003) Cognition and brain function: the effects of ketamine and nicotine in healthy subjects (abstract). Neuroimage, Human Brain Mapping 2003 Meeting, abstract 140
66. Abel KM, Allin MP, Kucharska-Pietura K et al (2203) Ketamine and fMRI BOLD signal: distinguishing between effects mediated by change in blood flow versus change in cognitive state. Hum Brain Mapp 18:135-145
67. Honey G, Honey R, Sharar S et al (2003) Investigation of the effects of low dose ketamine on episodic memory encoding using fMRI (abstract). Neuroimage, Human Brain Mapping 2003 Meeting, abstract 242
68. Honey G, Honey R, Sharar S et al (2003) Investigation on the effects of low dose ketamine on episodic memory retrieval using fMRI (abstract). Neuroimage, Human Brain Mapping 2003 Meeting, abstract 170
69. Fu C, Abel K, Alen M, Vythelingum G et al (2003) 'K' is for ketamine or knot, neural correlates of a ketamine-induced psychotic state on verbal fluency (abstract). Neuroimage, Human Brain Mapping 2003 Meeting, abstract 1286
70. O'Loughlin CJ, Sharar RS, Honey G et al (2003) Investigating the effects of ketamine in a continuous performance task using fMRI (abstract). Neuroimage, Human Brain Mapping 2003 Meeting, abstract 494
71. Abel KM, Allin MP, Kucharska-Pietura K et al (2003) Ketamine alters neural processing of facial emotion recognition in healthy men: an fMRI study. Neuroreport 14:387-391
72. Medoff DR, Holcomb HH, Lahti AC, Tamminga CA (2001) Probing the human hippocampus using rCBF: contrasts in schizophrenia. Hippocampus 11:543 550
73. Lahti AC, Holcomb HH, Medoff DR, Tamminga CA (1995) Ketamine activates psychosis and alters limbic blood flow in schizophrenia. Neuroreport 6:869-872

Neuroprotection by ketamine

S. Himmelseher, E. Kochs

The fundamental clinical obstacle to the use of ketamine for neuroprotection is the historical textbook dogma that ketamine is contraindicated in patients at risk of increases in intracranial pressure (ICP) [1, 2]. Early studies in animals and man revealed an increase in cerebral oxygen consumption ($CMRO_2$), cerebral blood flow (CBF) and ICP after ketamine [3-5]. However, various experimental and clinical data show that these findings lack consistency, which seems to be attributable to different study designs [6, 7], the absence or presence of controlled ventilation [8-11] and background anaesthetics or other medication [12-15]. Apart from practical use in haemorrhagic shock based on stimulatory effects on the cardiovascular system [16, 17], the well-known experimental neuroprotective efficacy of ketamine [18-20] has long remained clinically unexploited, with apparently having few if any implications for use in patients with intracranial lesions. When the classic concept of suppression of brain metabolism as the mainstay of cerebral protection by anaesthetics was questioned in recent years, interest in ketamine increasingly started to revive. The new pathophysiological thinking focused on a key role of glutamate signalling in the injury cascade, suggesting that neuronal death results from toxic concentrations of glutamate in the extracellular space and metabolic imbalances leading to apoptosis or delayed degeneration [21, 22]. Ketamine blocks the activation of excitatory glutamate receptors of the *N*-methyl-D-aspartate (NMDA) subtype by binding non-competitively to the phencyclidine site in the receptor channel in humans [23] and may have further effects of unknown clinical relevance [24, 25]. Two recent developments currently appear to demand a re-evaluation of ketamine for use in neurosurgical patients: first, *S*(+)-ketamine, the stereoisomer of racemic ketamine with the better therapeutic profile [25, 26], has demonstrated not only increased neuroprotective, but also neuroregenerative efficacy in experimental injury [27-29]; and secondly, drug preparations of *S*(+)-ketamine have been approved for clinical use in European countries.

The reality: cerebral pharmacology of ketamine

Effects on cerebral haemodynamics and metabolism

The net balance of a variety of brain and systemic effects of ketamine determines the drug's global action on cerebral haemodynamic variables. Ketamine's effects at cerebrovascular sites relate to the preexisting cerebrovascular tone induced by background anaesthetics [12, 30-32]. In spontaneously breathing patients, an increased arterial $PaCO_2$ after racemic ketamine appears to responsible for an increase in CBF or ICP [4]. In the case of impaired CBF autoregulation and after higher doses of racemic ketamine, ICP may be especially enhanced. Under controlled ventilation or with anaesthetics depressing brain metabolism, the ICP does not change [9, 11, 14, 15, 31-33]. In the presence of the cerebral vasodilator N_2O, racemic ketamine increases CBF and mean arterial pressure (MAP) even in ventilated animals [4, 34]. This may be caused by metabolic stimulation, impaired autoregulation or direct vasodilatation [35, 36]. Importantly, *S*(+)-ketamine does not impair the dynamic cerebrovascular autoregulation when combined with propofol in humans [37]. Racemic ketamine and its isomers heterogeneously inhibit brain metabolism in certain areas and simultaneously stimulate others, which is reflected in decreased CBF in regions with reduced metabolism and vice versa [6, 7, 38].

Irrespective of the current discussion on the optimal cerebral perfusion pressure (CPP) level [39, 40], ketamine's stimulatory action on the cardiovascular system may prevent systemic hypotension [16] and, with it, associated adverse outcomes after brain injury [41, 42] In addition to equivalent cardiovascular stimulatory effects at about half the dose [43], *S*(+)-ketamine offers further potential advantages over racemic ketamine: it caused less depression of the heart [44] and less vasorelaxation of the aorta [45]. Unlike the racemate, it did not reverse late cardiac preconditioning [46] and maintained muscle sympathetic activity during hypotensive challenge in volunteers [47]. In an approach to assessment of sedative regimens without haemodynamically depressive effects for intensive care patients, combinations of racemic or *S*(+)-ketamine and midazolam were also found to exert cardiovascular stimulation, but to a lesser degree than ketamine alone [43, 48, 49]. Combinations of *S*(+)-ketamine and propofol were reported to show almost balanced effects upon the systemic circulation [49-51]. To evaluate the key safety issue of possible rises of the ICP after ketamine in the setting of brain trauma, the agent was administered to head-injured patients under controlled ventilation and sedation with propofol or midazolam [14, 51]: no increases in ICP were observed, but rather slight decreases in ICP or CBF.

Taken together, these data imply that ketamine's stimulatory action on cerebral haemodynamic variables was probably overrated in the earlier days. When ketamine is used with an appropriate anaesthetic under controlled ventilation the contraindications based on concerns about prometabolic effects on the brain are no longer valid.

Effects in cells and animal models

A large body of evidence from numerous in vitro and animal investigations reveals that ketamine has important protective effects against injury from brain hypoxia, ischaemia, head trauma, reperfusion or seizure [18, 19, 52-61]. Most investigators related the neuroprotective effects observed to NMDA receptor blockade and associated reduction of glutamate excitotoxicity and necrotic cell death. Recent data also show less activation of proteins involved in neuronal apoptosis after ketamine and *S*(+)-ketamine [61-64]. Although the findings on this subject are hardly comparable in view of the tremendous differences in study methods and models, the preferred time of administration of racemic ketamine in simulated cerebral ischaemia appears to be before and during the insult. In contrast, when *S*(+)-ketamine was injected after global forebrain ischaemia [65], better neuroprotection was found in rat cerebral cortex than with *R*(-)-ketamine, which had no effect. The improved outcome in a rat model of incomplete cerebral ischaemia after use of *S*(+)-ketamine was probably based on NMDA receptor blockade and decreased sympathetic discharge [66]. When the stereoisomers of ketamine were studied for differences in neuroprotective effects in our hippocampal cell culture model and in brain slices [27-29], *S*(+)-ketamine preserved better metabolism and showed greater neuroprotective potential than racemic and *R*(-)-ketamine. Unexpectedly, *S*(+)-ketamine increased axonal re-outgrowth after axonal transection and enhanced expression of growth- and synaptosomal-associated proteins related to plasticity and repair in the adult brain [29]. Because nuclear transcription factors were involved in the phenomena observed, our interpretation of the data favours use of *S*(+)-ketamine over racemic ketamine in an approach to patient therapy.

NMDA antagonists themselves may be neurotoxic [67, 68]. However, a difference must be made between toxicity reported after higher than clinically usual doses in experimental work and toxicity observed in hypofunctional NMDA receptor states after profound blockade of NMDA receptors. Neurons have endogenous programmes to produce essential neuroprotective molecules (such as growth factors) which are regulated by synaptic activity [69, 70]. Not surprisingly, the brain seems to be particularly susceptible to NMDA receptor-mediated damage during developmental stages of synaptogenesis [67, 68]. The clinical implications of these experimental observations remain to be clarified.

Clinical uses

Sedation and analgesia in the intensive care unit

Only a small number of reports have so far been published on the effects of ketamine use in neurosurgical or brain-injured patients, the majority of studies having been performed in the intensive care unit. Advantages of using ketamine for sedation and analgesia in combined drug regimens have been shown in the non-neurosurgical patient population and include maintenance of haemodynamic stability and potentially catecholamine-sparing effects [49, 50, 71], a better tolerance of enteral nutrition due to greater gastrointestinal motility than with opioid use [72, 73] and little tachyphylaxis and few withdrawal phenomena [74, 75]. Two studies assessed these criteria in head-injured patients, one comparing a combination of midazolam and ketamine vs midazolam and fentanyl [76] and the other evaluating a continuous infusion regimen of midazolam and ketamine vs midazolam and sufentanil [77]. The main findings of the first study were comparable sedation and adverse effects after both drugs. The patients treated with ketamine, however, showed less need for exogenous vasopressors, higher average CPP values, and a better food intake [76]. Nevertheless, the 6-month outcome was similar for both groups. The second, more recent, study [77] revealed sufficient and comparable sedation and enteral nutrition after ketamine or sufentanil. No differences in ICP or CPP levels were observed. However, heart rate values were higher during 2 days of the 4-day study period with ketamine. In contrast, sufentanil-treated patients required more fluids on the first study day and showed a trend to greater need for vasopressors. Ketamine use was additionally associated with a slower recovery, but no extension of length of stay in the intensive care unit. To assess potential pharmacokinetic changes in intensive care patients with brain injury, one study determined the pharmacokinetics of ketamine and its active metabolites [78]. The results showed a greater increase in the volume of distribution than in total clearance, which caused a longer than estimated ketamine half-life. Based on the little clinical information available, it is most probably correct to conclude that ketamine can be safely administered in head-injured patients for sedation and analgesia. The reported study data are compatible with all of the pharmacological effects described above – except for readily observable neuroprotective actions of racemic ketamine. This should not discourage future investigators from starting the clinical trials needed, because none of the studies so far has been designed to assess neurological outcome parameters or surrogate variables.

Concluding remarks and outlook: need for proof of clinical efficacy

1. Optimised pharmacological strategies for neurosurgical patients demand the use of drugs that do not elevate the ICP or depress the systemic circulation, that maintain the cerebrovascular autoregulation as well as a coupling between CBF and metabolism, that allow for rapid drug recovery for neurological patient assessment, and that additionally show neuroprotective properties. Conceptually and based on the experimental evidence, *S*(+)-ketamine faithfully fulfils almost all the above criteria when used in an appropriate regimen with controlled ventilation.
2. From a pathophysiological point of view, the importance of the principle of glutamate neurotoxicity as a final common pathway for neurodegenerative processes remains unaltered. Cerebral microdialysis studies have confirmed increased glutamate concentrations in the extracellular space of patient brains during and after critical periods of injury cascades [22,79]. Expert opinion therefore advocates treatment approaches with noncompetitive NMDA-receptor antagonists to match periods of underlying secondary injury processes in patients with intracranial lesions [80].
3. The fact that previous clinical trials with NMDA-receptor antagonists in cardiopulmonary bypass [81] found only minor beneficial effects on neurological outcome or were stopped in the setting of head trauma [82] and after stroke [83] must not discourage future investigators from conducting research with ketamine in brain-injured patient populations. Up to now, all clinical trials that have evaluated NMDA-receptor antagonists have studied the effects of competitive blockers of the NMDA receptor channel. However, these compounds may have severe potential side effects for neurons due to complete and undifferentiated blockade of all neuronal NMDA receptors.

References

1. Madson JB, Cold GE (1990) The effects of anaesthetics upon cerebral circulation and metabolism. Experimental and clinical studies. Springer, Vienna New York
2. Hickey R (1999) Effects of anesthesia on cerebral and spinal cord physiology. In: Newfield P, Cottrell J (eds) Handbook of neuroanesthesia. Lippincott Williams & Wilkins, Philadelphia, pp 20-33
3. Gardner AE, Olson BE, Lichtiger M (1971) Cerebrospinal-fluid pressure during dissociative anesthesia with ketamine. Anesthesiology 35:226-228
4. Takeshita H, Okuda Y, Sari A (1972) The effects of ketamine on cerebral circulation and metabolism in man. Anesthesiology 36:69-75
5. Shapiro HM, Wyte SR, Harris AB (1972) Ketamine anesthesia in patients with intracranial pathology. Br J Anaesth 44:1200-1204
6. Cavazutti M, Porro CA, Biral GP et al (1987) Ketamine effects on local cerebral blood flow and metabolism in the rat. J Cereb Blood Flow Metabol 7:806-811
7. Chi O, Wei HM, Klein SL et al (1994) Effect of ketamine on heterogeneity of cerebral microregional venous O_2 saturation in the rat. Anesth Analg 79:860-866
8. Sari A, Okuda Y, Takeshita H (1972) The effect of ketamine on cerebrospinal fluid pressure. Anesth Analg 51:560-565
9. Schwedler M, Miletich DJ, Albrecht RF (1982) Cerebral blood flow and metabolism following ketamine administration. Can Anaesth Soc J 29:222-225
10. Akeson J, Björkman S, Messeter K et al (1993) Cerebral pharmcodynamics of anaesthetic and subanaesthetic doses of ketamine in the normoventilated pig. Acta Anaesthesiol Scand 37:211--218
11. Pfenninger E, Grünert A, Bowdler I et al (1985) The effect of ketamine on intracranial pressure during hemorrhagic shock under the conditions of spontaneous breathing and controlled ventilation. Acta Neurochir (Wien) 78:113-118
12. Dawson B, Michenfelder J, Theye R (1971) Effects of ketamine on canine cerebral blood flow and metabolism: modification by prior administration of thiopental. Anesth Analg 50:443-447
13. Nimkoff L, Quinn C, Silver P et al (1997) The effects of intravenous anesthetics on intracranial pressure and cerebral perfusion pressure in two feline models of brain edema. J Crit Care 12:132-136
14. Belopavlovic M, Buchthal A (1982) Modification of ketamine-induced intracranial hypertension in neurosurgical patients by pre-treatment with midazolam. Acta Anaesthesiol Scand 26:458-462
15. Mayberg TS, Lam AM, Matta BF et al (1995) Ketamine does not increase blood flow velocity or intracranial pressure during isoflurane / nitrous oxide anesthesia in patients undergoing craniotomy. Anesth Analg 81:84-89
16. White PF, Way WL, Trevor AJ (1982) Ketamine - its pharmacology and therapeutic uses. Anesthesiology 56:119-136
17. Himmelseher S, Pfenninger E (2000) Anaesthetic techniques and agents in neuroanesthesia – a comparison of German surveys in 1991 and 1997. Anaesthesiol Intensivmed 41:126-136
18. Choi DW (1990) Ketamine reduces NMDA receptor mediated neurotoxicity in cortical cultures. In: Domino EF (ed) Status of ketamine in anaesthesiology. NPP Books, Ann Arbor, Mich, pp 549-555
19. Hoffman WE, Pelligrino D, Werner C et al (1992) Ketamine decreases plasma catecholamines and improves outcome from incomplete cerebral ischemia in rats. Anesthesiology 76:755-762
20. Shapira Y, Lam AM, Eng CC et al (1994) Therapeutic time window and dose response of the beneficial effects of ketamine in experimental head injury. Stroke 25:1637-1643
21. Sattler R, Tymianski M (2001) Molecular mechanisms of glutamate receptor-mediated excitotoxic neuronal cell death. Mol Neurobiol 24:107-129
22. Sahuquillo J, Poca MA, Amoros S (2001) Current aspects of pathophysiology and cell dysfunction after severe head injury. Curr Pharm Des 15:1475-1483

23. Øye I, Paulsen O, Maurset A (1992) Effects of ketamine on sensory perception: evidence for a role of *N*-methyl-D-aspartate receptors. J Pharmacol Exp Ther 260:1209-1213
24. Orser BA, Pennefather PS, MacDonald JF (1997) Multiple mechanisms of ketamine blockade of *N*-methyl-D-aspartate receptors. Anesthesiology 86:903-917
25. Kohrs R, Durieux ME (1998) Ketamine: teaching an old drug new tricks. Anesth Analg 87:1186-1193
26. Schüttler J, Zsigmond E, White PF (1997) Ketamine and its isomers. In: White PF (ed) Textbook of intravenous anesthesia. Williams & Wilkins, Baltimore, pp 171-188
27. Mathews KS, Toner CC, McLaughlin DP et al (2001) Comparison of ketamine stereoisomers on tissue metabolic activity in an vitro model of global cerebral ischaemia. Neurochemistry Int 38: 367-372
28. Himmelseher S, Pfenninger E, Georgieff M (1996) The effects of ketamine-isomers on neuronal injury and regeneration in rat hippocampal neurons. Anesth Analg 83:505-512
29. Himmelseher S, Pfenninger E, Kochs E et al (2000) *S*(+)-Ketamine up-regulates neuronal regeneration associated proteins following glutamate injury in cultured rat hippocampal neurons. J Neurosurg Anesthesiol 12:84-94
30. Akeson J, Björkman S, Messeter K et al (1993) Low-dose midazolam antagonizes cerebral metabolic stimulation by ketamine in the pig. Acta Anaesthesiol Scand 37:525-531
31. Sakai K, Cho S, Fukusaki M et al (2000) The effects of propofol with and without ketamine on human cerebral blood flow velocity and response. Anesth Analg 90:377-382
32. Nagase K, Ida H, Dohi S (2002) *L*-Arginine and nitroglycerin restore hypercapnia-induced cerebral vasodilation in rabbits after its attenuation by ketamine. Anesth Analg 94:954-958
33. Friesen RH, Honda At (1987) Changes in anterior fontanel pressure in preterm neonates receiving isoflurane, halothane, fentanyl or ketamine. Anesth Analg 66:431-434
34. Oren RE, Rasool NA, Rubinstein EH (1987) Effect of ketamine on cerebral cortical blood flow and metabolism in rabbits. Stroke 1987:441-444
35. Wendling WW, Daniels FB, Chen D et al (1994) Ketamine directly dilates bovine cerebral arteries by acting as a calcium entry blocker. J Neurosurg 6:186-192
36. Shakunaga K, Kojima S, Jomura K et al (1998) Ketamine suppresses the production and release of endothelin 1 from cultured bovine endothelial cells. Anesth Analg 86:1098-1102
37. Engelhard K, Werner C, Möllenberg O et al (2001) *S*(+)-ketamine / propofol maintain dynamic cerebrovascular autoregulation in humans. Can J Anaesth 48:1034-1039
38. Vollenweider FX, Leenders KL, Oye I et al (1997) Differential psychopathology and patterns of cerebral glucose utilisation produced by (*S*)- and (*R*)-ketamine in healthy volunteers using positron emission tomography. Eur Neuropsychopharmacol 7:25-38
39. Brain Trauma Foundation, American Association of Neurological Surgeons, Joint Section on Neurotrauma and Critical Care (2000) Management and prognosis of severe traumatic brain injury. Brain Trauma Foundation, New York
40. Robertson CS (2001) Management of cerebral perfusion pressure after traumatic brain injury. Anesthesiology 95:2086-2095
41. Chesnut RM (1997) Avoidance of hypotension: condition sine qua non of successful severe head-injury management. J Trauma 42 (5 Suppl):S4-S9
42. Jeremitsky E, Omert L, Dunham CM et al (2003) Harbingers of poor outcome the day after severe head injury: hypothermia, hypoxia, and hypoperfusion. J Trauma 54:312-319
43. Doenicke A, Angster R, Mayer M et al (1992) The action of *S*-(+)-ketamine on serum catecholamine and cortisol. A comparison with ketamine racemate. Anaesthesist 41:585-587
44. Kunst G, Martin E, Graf BM et al (1999) Actions of ketamine and its isomers on contractility and calcium transients in human myocardium. Anesthesiology 90:1363-1371
45. Kanellopoulos A, Lenz G, Mühlbauer B (1998) Stereoselective differences in the vasorelaxing effects of *S*(+) and *R*(-) ketamine on rat isolated aorta. Anesthesiology 88:718-724
46. Müllenheim J, Rulands R, Wietschorke T et al (2001) Late preconditioning is blocked by racemic ketamine, but not by *S*(+)-ketamine. Anesth Analg 93:265-270

47. Kienbaum P, Heuter T, Pavlakovic G et al (2001) *S*(+)-Ketamine increases muscle sympathetic activity and maintains the neural response to hypotensive challenges in humans. Anesthesiology 94:252-256
48. Strebel S, Kaufman M, Maitre L et al (1995) Effects of ketamine on cerebral blood flow velocity in humans. Influence of pre-treatment with midazolam or esmolol. Anaesthesia 50:223-228
49. Adams HA (1997) *S*(+)-Ketamine. Circulatory interactions during total intravenous anesthesia and analgo-sedation Anaesthesist 46:1081-1087
50. Adams HA, Brausch M, Schmitz CS et al (2001) Analgosedation with (*S*)-ketamine / propofol vs. (S)-ketamine / midazolam: control and quality of sedation, stress response and haemodynamic reactions. Anaesthesiol Intensivmed Notfallmed Schmerzther 36:417-424
51. Albanese J, Arnaud S, Rey M, Thomachot L et al (1997) Ketamine decreases intracranial pressure and electroencephalographic activity in traumatic brain injury patients during propofol sedation. Anesthesiology 87:1328-1334
52. Weiss J, Goldberg MP, Choi DW (1986) Ketamine protects cultured neurons from hypoxic injury. Brain Res 380:186-190
53. Chan PH, Chu L (1989) Ketamine protects cultured astrocytes from glutamate-induced swelling. Brain Res 487:380-383
54. Lucas JH, Wolf A (1991) In vitro studies of multiple impact injury to mammalian CNS neurons: prevention of perikaryal damage and death by ketamine. Brain Res 543:181-193
55. Gonzalez JM, Loeb AL, Reichard PS, et al (1995) Ketamine inhibits glutamate-, *N*-methlyl-D-aspartate-, and quisqualate-stimulated cGMP production in cultured cerebral neurons. Anesthesiology 82:205-213
56. Church J, Zeman S, Lodge D (1988) The neuroprotective action of ketamine and MK-801 after transient cerebral ischaemia in rats. Anesthesiology 69:702-709
57. Smith DH, Okiyama TA, Gennarelli TA et al (1993) Magnesium and ketamine attenuate cognitive dysfunction following experimental head injury. Neurosci Lett 157:211-214
58. Fujikawa DG (1995) Neuroprotective effect of ketamine administered after status epilepticus onset. Epilepsia 36:186-195
59. Lin SZ, Chiou AL, Wang Y (1996) Ketamine antagonizes nitric oxide release from cerebral cortex after middle cerebral artery ligation in rats. Stroke 27:747-752
60. Spandou E, Karkavelas G, Soubasi V et al (1999) Effect of ketamine on hypoxic-ischemic brain damage in newborn rats. Brain Res 819:1-7
61. Chang ML, Yang J, Kem S et al (2002) Nicotinamide and ketamine reduce infarct volume and DNA fragmentation in rats after brain ischemia and reperfusion. Neurosci Lett 322:137-140
62. Zhang C, Shen W, Zhang G (2002) *N*-Methyl-D-aspartate receptor and L-type voltage-gated Ca channel antagonists suppress the release of cytochrome c and the expression of procaspase-3 in rat hippocampus after global brain ischemia. Neurosci Lett 328:265-268
63. Shen WH, Zhang CY, Zhang GY (2003) Modulation of I*k*B kinase autophosphorylation and activity following brain ischemia. Acta Pharmacol Sin 24:311-315
64. Engelhard K, Werner C, Eberspächer E et al (2003) The effect of the α_2-agonist dexmedetomidine and the *N*-methyl-D-aspartate antagonist *S*(+)-ketamine on the expression of apoptosis-regulating proteins after incomplete cerebral ischemia and reperfusion in rats. Anesth Analg 96:524--531
65. Proescholdt M, Heimann A, Kempski O (2001) Neuroprotection of *S*(+) ketamine isomer in global forebrain ischemia. Brain Res 904:245-251
66. Reeker W, Werner C, Möllenberg O et al (2000) High-dose *S*(+)-ketamine improves neurological outcome following incomplete cerebral ischemia. Can J Anaesth 47:572-578
67. Ikonomidou C, Bosch F, Miksa M et al (1999) Blockade of NMDA receptors and apoptotic neurodegeneration in the developing brain. Science 283:70-74
68. Pohl D, Bittigau P, Ishimaru MJ et al (1999) *N*-Methyl-D-aspartate antagonists and apoptotic cell death triggered by head trauma in developing rat brain. Proc Natl Acad Sci 96:2508-2513
69. Zafra F, Hengerer B, Leibrock (1990) Activity dependent regulation of BDNF and NGF mRNAs

in the rat hippocampus is mediated by non-NMDA glutamta receptors. EMBO J 9:3545-3550
70. Hardingham GE, Fukunaga Y, Bading H (2002) Extrasynaptic NMDARs oppose synaptic NMDARs by triggering CREB shut-off and cell death pathways. Nat Neurosci 5:405-414
71. Adams HA, Claussen E, Gebhardt B et al (1991) The use of ketamine and midazolam for analgesia and sedation in ventilated patients subject to obligatory treatment with catecholamines. Anaesthesist 40:238-244
72. Kolbel CB, Rippel K, Klar H et al (2000) Esophageal motility disorders in critically ill patients: a 24-hour manometric study. Intensive Care Med 26:1421-1427
73. Ostermann ME, Keenan SP, Seiferling RA et al (2000) Sedation in the intensive care unit. JAMA 283:1451-1459
74. Köppel C, Arndt I, Ibe K (1990) Effects of enzyme induction, renal and cardiac function on ketamine plasma kinetics in patients with ketamine long-term analgosedation. Eur J Drug Metab Pharmacokinet 15:259-263
75. Tsubo T, Sakai I, Okawa H et al (2001) Ketamine and midazolam kinetics during continuous hemodiafiltration in patients with multiple organ dysfunction syndrome. Intensive Care Med 27:1087-1090
76. Kolenda H, Gremmelt A, Rading S et al (1996) Ketamine for analgosedative therapy in intensive care treatment of head-injured patients. Acta Neurochir (Wien) 138:1193-1199
77. Bourgin A, Albanese J, Wereszczynski N et al (2003) Safety of sedation with ketamine in severe head injury patients: comparison with sufentanil. Crit Care Med 31:711-717
78. Hijazi Y, Bodonian C, Bolon M et al (2003) Pharmacokinetics and haemodynamics of ketamine in intensive care patients with brain or spinal cord injury. Br J Anaesth 90:155-160
79. Bullock R, Zauner A, Woodward JJ et al (1998) Factors affecting excitatory amino acid release following severe head injury. J Neurosurg 89:507-518
80. Narayan RK, Michel ME, and the Clinical Trials in Head Injury Study Group (2002) Clinical Trials in Head Injury. J Neurotrauma 19:503-518
81. Arrowsmith JE, Harrison MJ, Newman SP et al (1998) Neuroprotection of the brain during cardiopulmonary bypass: randomized trial of remacemide during coronary artery bypass in 171 patients. Stroke 29:2357-2362
82. Morris GF, Bullock R, Marshall SB et al (1999) Failure of the competitive *N*-methyl-D-aspartate antagonist selfotel (CGS 19755) in the treatment of severe head inury: results of two phase III clinical trials. The selfotel investigators. J Neurosurg 91:737-743
83. Albers GW, Goldstein LB, Hall D et al (2001) Aptiganel hydrochloride in acute ischemic stroke: a randomized controlled trial. JAMA 286:2673-2682

Pain relief by ketamine

S. Himmelseher, E. Kochs

Although advances in techniques for anaesthesia, surgery, and the protection of organs have resulted in reductions in age- and risk-adjusted mortality and morbidity, the incidence of perioperative pain has changed little over the past years. Given the increasing numbers of elderly people with age-related painful conditions and the improvements in the management of cancer with increased life expectancy, there is a large clinical need for successful perioperative pain treatment [1]. Because clinical efforts for pain therapy are currently being re-directed from empirical strategies to more targeted mechanistic approaches [2], ketamine has increasingly been used for treatment of acute and chronic pain in the perioperative setting [3, 4]. This development has been caused partly by enhanced knowledge of pathophysiological mechanisms that operate in pain pathways, where the importance of the activation of excitatory glutamate receptors of the *N*-methyl-D-aspartate (NMDA) subtype in nociceptive transmission, synaptic plasticity and pain sensitisation has been established for humans [5]. Ketamine binds non-competitively to the phencyclidine-binding site of the NMDA receptor channel [6]. When clinically used at subanaesthetic doses, the drug's analgesic efficacy correlates well with its inhibiting action on NMDA receptor-mediated pain facilitation [7, 8]. The clinical relevance of ketamine effects on other potential pain control mechanisms is not yet apparent.

The S(+)-stereoisomer of ketamine

Traditionally ketamine has been marketed as racemate, containing equimolar amounts of two enantiomers as a 1:1 mixture. The molecular structure of ketamine shows a chiral centre at the asymmetric carbon-2 atom of the cyclohexanone ring [6], which is responsible for two optical stereoisomers. *S*(+)-ketamine, the left-handed isomer of racemic ketamine, has an affinity for NMDA receptors that is fourfold that of right-handed R(-)-ketamine [7, 9]. Volunteer and investigational trials have shown that this difference results in a clinical analgesic potency of *S*(+)-ketamine that is about twice that of racemic and four times that of *R*(-)-ketamine [10-12]. *S*(+)-Ketamine has now been available for a few years in some European countries, and its clinical use at analgesic doses has confirmed its significant advantages over racemic ketamine, mainly reported in comparisons between the two drugs at anaesthetic doses [13]. According to our experience with regard to relevance for pain therapy, the use of *S*(+)-ketamine especially avoids unnecessary drug-load, thus reducing unwanted side effects while allowing for sufficient dosing combined with a faster recovery. From a pharmacokinetic point of view, the elimination clearance of *S*(+)-ketamine is significantly greater than that of racemic ketamine [13], most probably because of enantiomeric selectivity in hepatic metabolism by microsomal enzymes [14]. For equivalent drug effects, practical experience and a recent report [15] show that S(+)-ketamine has to be applied at about 75% of the former dose of racemic ketamine when used at a repeated dose or as a continuous infusion.

Clinical uses in the perioperative period

Intravenous low-dose ketamine as an analgesic adjunct to general anaesthesia

Over recent years, it has become increasingly evident that intravenous low-dose ketamine has beneficial effects on postoperative pain and opioid requirements when added as an analgesic adjunct to general anaesthesia. Ketamine decreased postoperative pain in a variety of settings, ranging from outpatient surgery to major abdominal procedures [16-23]. Nevertheless, several studies revealed failure of intravenous ketamine to enhance postoperative analgesia when applied intraoperatively [24-28]. This phenomenon can now be readily explained: first, in line with the discussion on the clinical utility of 'preemptive analgesia' [29], a single intravenous injection of racemic ketamine either before or after surgical incision [24-27] may not be sufficient to cause analgesic effects that last far into the postoperative period. Second, in view of the long-lasting injury process caused by surgical trauma and the subsequent inflammatory response, the low doses of ketamine used [24-27] are absolutely justifiable to achieve the targeted pain reduction. Third, when ketamine is used at a relatively low intravenous dose in combination with a multimodal regimen of several analgesics [24] or epidural anaesthesia [28], pain-inhibitory effects of low-dose ketamine are clinically likely to be masked. As a conclusion, the adequacy of the ketamine administration schedule is a crucial component in successful postoperative pain prevention. This has recently been confirmed in patients undergoing major abdominal surgery with a management strategy of combined general and epidural anaesthesia: optimised postoperative pain relief was found in gastrectomy patients who received an intraoperative ketamine infusion at a dose of 0.5 mg kg^{-1} h^{-1} preceded by a preincisional bolus of 1 mg/kg ketamine [29]; it was also reported in a long-term outcome trial which showed reduced incidence of residual pain until the sixth postoperative month in patients with adenocarcinoma surgery who were treated with a preincisional bolus of 0.5 mg/kg ketamine followed by a continuous infusion of 0.25 mg kg^{-1} h^{-1} ketamine [20]; and it is described in our recent study, where 0.2 mg/kg repeated intraoperative injections subsequent to an injection of 0.5 mg/kg *S*(+)-ketamine before surgical incision for major pelvic visceral procedures yielded better postoperative pain relief than single preincisional *S*(+)-ketamine use [30].

Low-dose ketamine and acute opioid tolerance

Ketamine and intraoperative opioid tolerance

The development of rapid tolerance and delayed hyperalgesia after the use of opioid analgesics has been demonstrated in volunteers [31-33] and in trials on acute intraoperative and postoperative opioid exposures in surgical patients [34, 35]. Because pronociceptive systems related to pain sensitisation have been associated with increased synaptic activity at the NMDA receptor level [36] and ketamine was reported to modulate remifentanil-induced analgesia in humans [31, 32], an inhibitory effect of ketamine on opioid-related phenomena may have contributed to the above aforementioned reductions in postoperative opioid requirements. In addition, supplementing a remifentanil-based anaesthesia with low-dose ketamine decreased the need for both intraoperative remifentanil and postoperative opioid analgesics after abdominal surgery [37]. Nevertheless, *S*(+)-ketamine given at a preincisional bolus of 0.5 mg/kg followed by an infusion of 0.12 mg kg^{-1} h^{-1} until 2 h after emergence from anaesthesia did not decrease intense somatic pain after remifentanil use [38]. Because this lack of effect probably relates to inappropriately low drug dose, the evaluation of adequate ketamine administration schedules in the setting of possible acute intraoperative opioid-induced phenomena could become of special clinical relevance.

Ketamine–opioid combinations in patient-controlled analgesia

Several clinical trials tested the combined use of ketamine and an opioid analgesic for intravenous patient-controlled analgesia (PCA). While the earlier studies reported better pain relief, decreased analgesic needs and fewer side effects with the drug combinations [39, 40], later trials did not find beneficial effects after ketamine addition [41-43]. Two main issues complicate the interpretation of these findings: on one hand, the drug combinations applied were chosen purely empirically with little clinical experience or expert knowledge of ketamine-opioid interactions in terms of clinical effects on postoperative pain states in this setting. Sometimes dose reductions of opioids or ketamine below analgesic effects of their own were suggested [3]. On the other hand, patients were studied with rather global assessment tools, such as pain rating scales or analgesic requirements in the immediate postoperative period. However, to identify long-term effects of analgesic treatment, more profound examinations of pain-related entities, such as long-lasting hyperalgesia, or outcome variables such as length of hospital stay, are necessary. The first problem has recently been approached with the use of optimisation models restricted by side effects for combinations of morphine with ketamine [44]. The procedure converged on a morphine-to-ketamine ratio of 1:1 and a lockout interval of 8 min for postoperative PCA after lumbar spine and hip surgery.

Low-dose ketamine as an analgesic adjunct to regional anaesthesia and analgesia

The reported advantages of combining low-dose ketamine with a local anaesthetic or other analgesics in peripheral or neuraxial regional analgesia and anaesthesia regimens consist in better pain relief and fewer side effects, resulting from reduced drug doses of local anaesthetics or analgesics [45-54]. This may easily be explained by blockade of NMDA receptors within in the spinal cord and a potential complementary antinociceptive action of the drug classes used. However, although ketamine shows local-anaesthetic-like properties [55], its peripheral effects do not suffice for profound local analgesia in volunteers when used as a single agent [56, 57]. At neuraxial site, sole ketamine induces analgesic effects at higher doses, but exerts central side effects that limit its clinical utility at least in awake patients [58]. The resorption and plasma uptake of peripheral or neuraxial ketamine has not yet been systematically analysed. Based on our experience and two studies on epidural and caudal use, ketamine gains rapid access to the systemic circulation with high bioavailability [59, 60]. Despite comparable plasma values during most of the postoperative observation period, the study in children showed more effective analgesia after caudal than after intramuscular *S*(+)-ketamine, suggesting supraspinal and local analgesic effects after caudal use. Because spinal neurotoxicity has been described in case reports after repeated intrathecal doses of ketamine prepared with preservatives (benzethonium chloride or chlorobutanol) [61, 62], only preservative-free drug preparations must be used for neuraxial administration. Nevertheless, although there is no evidence for spinal toxicity of preservative-free ketamine in man [63], we currently suggest its use only for the epidural site and in the lower dose range.

Ketamine and intraoperative regional blocks

Most trials investigating intraoperative ketamine as an analgesic additive to epidural regimens show improved analgesia, more rapid onset of epidural blockade and a local anaesthetic or opioid-sparing effect that lasts into the postoperative period [46-50, 64]. When low-dose *S*(+)-ketamine was used as one preincisional epidural injection, benefits over 48 h after orthopaedic surgery were observed [49, 50]. In contrast, single use of epidural low-dose racemic ketamine before surgical incision often resulted in a clinically insignificant effect until after surgery [65-67]. This was also reported, for example, when racemic ketamine was added preincisionally to an interscalene brachial plexus block [68]. The concept that beneficial outcomes from intraoperative low-dose ketamine can only be achieved after repeated or continuous administration during surgery thus appears also to be valid for regional anaesthesia. The critical element in treatment success or failure with ketamine is the provision of suppression of afferent nociceptive input with sufficient duration. Because enhanced inflammatory peripheral and spinal activity may extend into rehabilitative periods [69], research should be intensified to evaluate prolonged administration schedules using *S*(+)-ketamine.

Ketamine and caudal blockades in children

Caudal analgesia added to general anaesthesia is an effective anaesthetic regimen for paediatric surgery, but may be associated with such complications as prolonged motor blockade, systemic toxicity after accidental intravascular injection of local anaesthetics or respiratory depression after opioid use. Studies assessing caudal ketamine have shown efficient analgesia for both the intra- and the postoperative period [51, 60, 70-75]. Racemic ketamine provided better analgesic effects of prolonged duration when added to local anaesthetics [51, 70, 72], and 1 mg/kg *S*(+)-ketamine produced effective analgesia when applied as sole agent or in combination with other analgesics [60,71,73-75]. In the postoperative period, no increased incidence of psychic or other side effects after caudal ketamine was reported. This is supposedly related to the fact that the children were under general anaesthesia during the time when systemic drug concentrations were present at concentrations high enough to cause unwanted psychic side effects. In conclusion, although the regimen of caudal anaesthesia with *S*(+)-ketamine suggests clinical advantages over traditionally used local anaesthetics, accumulated clinical experience is required to confirm the safety of caudal use of the drug in children at these young ages.

Side effects and concerns

The most often encountered reservations about the use of ketamine as an analgesic agent are concerns about unacceptable mind-altering effects and protracted psychosis even after low-dose intraoperative use. However, psychic side effects are clearly dose dependent [76-78] and without relevance when patients receive a balanced general anaesthesia. In the recovery period, quiet surroundings and a confident atmosphere contribute to their reduced incidence. When ketamine is used alone in awake patients for analgesic therapy, the prophylactic administration of a sedative agent has mostly proved beneficial, because trials and clinical experience note a decline in mood, conscious perception, memory, and intellectual performance after about 0.2-0.5 mg/kg intravenous racemic or 0.25 *S*(+)-ketamine [76-79]. Interestingly, studies on low-dose ketamine-opioid combinations in postoperative pain therapy revealed fewer side effects after drug combinations than after either drug alone [39, 44]. Although the incidence of side effects after *S*(+)-ketamine appears to be similar to those after racemic ketamine [6, 79], volunteers who received *S*(+)-ketamine at equianalgesic doses of racemic ketamine demonstrated less tiredness and impairment in cognitive capacities [79, 80]. However, the greatest advantage of *S*(+)-ketamine for clinical pain therapy is its better analgesic potency compared with racemic ketamine, because it allows for efficient use at lower doses and correspondingly markedly reduced side effects.

Commentary on studies in the perioperative period: options and optimised pain therapy with low-dose ketamine

The currently available clinical trials on low-dose ketamine for pain therapy in the perioperative setting differ in design, protocols, and methods of analgesic strategy and treatment assessments. To allow for statements of general validity and applicability, new studies must be based on comparable control and treatment groups with regard to patients and acute and long-term medical management. Dose-response regimens of various low-dose ketamine administration schedules must be examined in comparison with other novel approaches to pain treatment strategies. The evaluation of optimised treatment protocols for use of low-dose intravenous *S*(+)-ketamine as an analgesic adjunct to general anaesthesia appears to be a high priority, given the promising results available and the ease with which such a regimen could be implemented.

1. As an optional recommendation and starting point for an administration schedule, pain therapy with intravenous *S*(+)-ketamine should be performed as a 0.5-mg/kg slow bolus injection before surgical incision; this should be followed by repeated injections of 0.25-0.5 mg/kg *S*(+)-ketamine spaced at 25-min intervals or by a continuous ketamine infusion of 0.15-0.35 µg kg^{-1} min^{-1}. The last drug injection or the infusion should be stopped at approximately 30 min before the end of the operation to prevent a prolonged period of patient awakening. If racemic ketamine is used, drug doses must be adapted and the last drug administration should be at least 50 min before surgical wound closure.
2. Because it may be possible that no fixed administration schedule is applicable for successful or optimised pain therapy with ketamine in an individual patient, it is advisable to administer the first two bolus doses or the preincisional bolus and an infusion of 20-min duration under careful patient monitoring. Further doses should then be titrated according to the patient's reaction to anaesthesia and the surgical stimuli in the course of the procedure. Apart from the analgesic effects, patients under general anaesthesia do need less of the intraoperative anaesthetics when ketamine is used in addition. Upon slow administration of low-dose ketamine only marginal or no side effects such as haemodynamic stimulation will occur. With this background, beneficial effects may even be observed in settings that have traditionally been regarded as contraindications to ketamine use, such as cardiovascular disease.
3. Nevertheless, the lack of long-term outcome data and our current state of knowledge mean we cannot yet set up treatment standards, let alone therapeutic guidelines, for pain therapy with analgesic doses of ketamine.

References

1. Raj PP (ed) (2000) Practical management of pain 3rd edn. Mosby, St Louis
2. Scholz J, Woolf CJ (2002) Can we conquer pain. Nat Neurosci Suppl 5:1062-1067
3. Schmid RL, Sandler AN, Katz J (1999) Use and efficacy of low-dose ketamine in the management of acute postoperative pain: a review of current techniques and outcomes. Pain 82:111-125
4. Bell R, Eccleston C, Kalso E (2003) Ketamine as an adjuvant to opioids for cancer pain (Cochrane review). Cochrane Database Syst Rev 1: CD003351
5. Michaelis EK (1998) Molecular biology of glutamate receptors in the central nervous system and their role in excitotoxicity, oxidative stress and aging. Prog Neurobiol 54:369-415
6. White PF, Way WL, Trevor AJ (1982) Ketamine - its pharmacology and therapeutic uses. Anesthesiology 56:119-136

7. Øye I, Paulsen O, Maurset A (1992) Effects of ketamine on sensory perception: evidence for a role of *N*-methyl-D-aspartate receptors. J Pharmacol Exp Ther 260:1209-1213
8. Hartvig P, Valtysson J, Lindner KH et al (1995) Central nervous system effects of subdissociative doses of (*S*)-ketamine are related to plasma and brain concentrations measured with positron emission tomography in healthy volunteers. Clin Pharmacol Ther 58:165-173
9. Zeilhofer HU, Swandulla D, Geisslinger G et al (1992) Differential effects of ketamine enantiomers on NMDA receptor currents in cultured neurons. Eur J Pharmacol 213:155-158
10. Arendt-Nielsen L, Nielsen J, Petersen-Felix S et al (1996) Effect of racemic mixture and the (*S*+)-isomer of ketamine on temporal and spatial summation of pain. Br J Anaesth 77:625-631
11. White PF, Schüttler J, Shafer A et al (1985) Comparative pharmacology of the ketamine isomers. Br J Anaesth 57:197-203
12. Mathisen LC, Skjelbred P, Skoglund LA et al (1995) Effect of ketamine, an NMDA receptor inhibitor, in acute and chronic orofacial pain. Pain 61:215-20
13. Schüttler J, Zsigmond E, White PF (1997) Ketamine and its isomers. In: White PF (ed) Textbook of intravenous anesthesia. Williams & Wilkins, Baltimore, pp 171-188
14. Kharasch ED, Labroo R (1992) Metabolism of ketamine stereoisomers by human liver microsomes. Anesthesiology 77:1201-1207
15. Ihmsen H, Geisslinger G, Schüttler J (2001) Stereoselective pharmacokinetics of ketamine: *R*(-)-ketamine inhibits the elimination of *S*(+)-ketamine. Clin Pharmacol Ther 70:431-438
16. Fu ES, Miguel R, Scharf JE (1997) Preemptive ketamine decreases postoperative narcotic requirements in patients undergoing abdominal surgery. Anesth Analg 84:1086-1090
17. Stubhaug A, Breivik H, Eide PK et al (1997) Mapping of punctuate hyperalgesia around a surgical incision demonstrates that ketamine is a powerful suppressor of central sensitization to pain following surgery. Acta Anaesthesiol Scand 41:1124-1132
18. Suzuki M, Tsueda K, Lansing PS et al (1999) Small-dose ketamine enhances morphine-induced analgesia after outpatient surgery. Anesth Analg 89:98-103
19. Menigaux C, Fletcher D, Dupont X et al (2000) The benefit of intraoperative small-dose ketamine on postoperative pain after anterior cruciate ligament repair. Anesth Analg 90:129-135
20. Aida S, Yamakura T, Baba H et al (2000) Preemptive analgesia by intravenous low-dose ketamine and epidural morphine in gastrectomy: a randomized double-blind study. Anesthesiology 92: 1624-1630
21. de Kock M, Lavand'homme P, Waterloos H (2001) Balanced analgesia in the perioperative period: is there a place for ketamine. Pain 92:373-380
22. Menigaux C, Guignard B, Fletcher D et al (2001) Intraoperative small-dose ketamine enhances analgesia after outpatient knee arthroscopy. Anesth Analg 93:606-612
23. Guignard B, Coste C, Costes H et al (2002) Supplementing desflurane-remifentanil anesthesia with small-dose ketamine reduces perioperative analgesic requirements. Anesth Analg 95:103-108
24. Mathisen LC, Aasbo V, Raeder J (1999) Lack of pre-emptive analgesic effect of (R)-ketamine in laparoscopic cholecystectomy. Acta Anaesthesiol Scand 43:220-224
25. Adam F, Libier M, Oszustowicz T et al (1999) Preoperative small-dose ketamine has no preemptive analgesic effect in patients undergoing total mastectomy. Anesth Analg 89:444-447
26. Dahl V, Ernoe PE, Steen T et al (2000) Does ketamine have preemptive effects in women undergoing abdominal hysterectomy procedures. Anesth Analg 90:1419-1422
27. Holthusen H, Backhaus P, Boeminghaus F et al (2002) Preemptive analgesia: no relevant advantage of preoperative compared with postoperative intravenous administration of morphine, ketamine, and clonidine in patients undergoing transperitoneal tumor nephrectomy. Reg Anesth Pain Med 27:249-253
28. Ilkjaer S, Nikolajsen L, Hansen TM et al (1998) Effect of i.v. ketamine in combination with epidural bupivacaine or epidural morphine on postoperative pain and wound tenderness after renal surgery. Br J Anaesth 81:707-712
29. Moinche S, Kehlet H, Dahl JB (2002) A qualitative and quantitative systematic review of preemptive analgesia for postoperative pain relief. Anesthesiology 96:725-741

30. Argiriadou H, Himmelseher S, Papagiannopoulou P et al (2003) Improvement of pain treatment after major abdominal surgery by intravenous S(+)-ketamine. Anesth Analg (in press)
31. Vinik HR, Kissin I (1998) Rapid development of tolerance to analgesia during remifentanil infusion in humans. Anesth Analg 86:1307-1311
32. Luginbuhl M, Geber A, Schnider TW et al (2003) Modulation of remifentanil-induced analgesia, hyperalgesia, and tolerance by small-dose ketamine in humans. Anesth Analg 96:726-732
33. Koppert W, Sittl R, Scheuber K et al (2003) Differential modulation of remifentanil-induced analgesia and postinfusion hyperalgesia by *S*-ketamine and clonidine in humans. Anesthesiology 99:152-159
34. Chia YT, Liu K, Wang JJ et al (1999) Intraoperative high dose fentanyl induces postoperative fentanyl tolerance. Can J Anaesth 46:872-877
35. Guignard B, Bossard AE, Coste C et al (2000) Acute opioid tolerance: intraoperative remifentanil increases postoperative pain and morphine requirement. Anesthesiology 93:409-417
36. Mao J (1999) NMDA and opioid receptors: their interactions in antinociception, tolerance and neuroplasticity. Brain Res Rev 30:289-304
37. Guignard B, Coste C, Costes H et al (2002) Supplementing desflurane-remifentanil anesthesia with small-dose ketamine reduced perioperative opioid analgesic requirements. Anesth Analg 95:103-108
38. Jaksch W, Lang S, Reichhalter R et al (2002) Perioperative small-dose *S*(+)-ketamine has no incremental beneficial effects on postoperative pain when standard-practice opioid infusions are used. Anesth Analg 94:981-986
39. Javery KB, Usssery TW, Steger HG et al (1996) Comparison of morphine and morphine with ketamine for postoperative analgesia. Can J Anaesth 43:212-215
40. Adrianssens G, Vermeyen KM, Hoffmann VL et al (1999) Postoperative analgesia with i.v. patient-controlled morphine: effect of adding ketamine. Br J Anaesth 83:393-396
41. Burstal R, Danjoux G, Hayes C et al (2001) PCA ketamine and morphine after abdominal hysterectomy. Anaesth Intensive Care 29:246-251
42. Reeves M, Lindholm DE, Myles PS et al (2001) Adding ketamine to morphine for patient-controlled analgesia after major abdominal surgery: a double-blinded, randomized controlled trial. Anesth Analg 93:116-120
43. Murdoch CJ, Crooks BA, Miller CD (2002) Effect of the addition of ketamine to morphine in patient-controlled analgesia. Anaesthesia 57:484-488
44. Sveticic G, Gentilini A, Eichenberger U et al (2003) Combinations of morphine with ketamine for patient-controlled analgesia: a new optimization method. Anesthesiology 98:1195-1205
45. Tverskoy M, Oren M, Vaskovich M et al (1996) Ketamine enhances local anesthetic and analgesic effect of bupivacaine by peripheral mechanism: a study in postoperative patients. Neurosci Lett 215:5-8
46. Wong CS, Lu CC, Cheng CH et al (1997) Pre-emptive analgesia with ketamine, morphine and epidural lidocaine prior to total knee replacement. Can J Anaesth 44:31-37
47. Abdel-Ghaffar ME, Abdulatif M, Al-Ghandi A et al (1998) Epidural ketamine reduces postoperative epidural PCA consumption of fentanyl / bupivacaine. Can J Anaesth 45:103-109
48. Wu CT, Yeh CC, Yu JC et al (2000) Pre-incisional epidural ketamine, morphine and bupivacaine combined with epidural and general anaesthesia provides pre-emptive analgesia for upper abdominal sugery. Acta Anaesthesiol Scand 44:63-68
49. Himmelseher S, Argiriadou H, Ziegler-Pithamitsis D et al (2001) Small-dose S(+)-ketamine reduces postoperative pain when applied with ropivacaine in epidural anesthesia for total knee arthroplasty. Anesth Analg 92:1290-1295
50. Lauretti GR, Oliveira AP, Rodrigues AM et al (2001) The effect of transdermal nitroglycerin on spinal S(+)-ketamine antinociception following orthopedic surgery. J Clin Anesth 13:576-581
51. Naguib M, Sharif AM, Seraj M et al (1991) Ketamine for caudal analgesia in children: comparison with caudal bupivacaine. Br J Anaesth 67:559-564
52. Chia YY, Liu K, Liu YC et al (1998) Adding ketamine in a multimodal patient-controlled epidural

regimen reduces postoperative pain and analgesic consumption. Anesth Analg 86:1245-1249
53. Tan PH, Kuo MC, Kao PF et al (1999) Patient-controlled epidural analgesia with morphine or morphine plus ketamine for postoperative pain relief. Eur J Anesthesiol 16:820-825
54. Subramaniam K, Subramaniam B, Pawar DK et al (2001) Evaluation of the safety and efficacy of epidural ketamine combined with morphine for postoperative analgesia after major upper abdominal surgery. J Clin Anaesth 13:339-344
55. Wagner LE, Gingrich KJ, Kulli JC et al (2001) Ketamine blockade of voltage-gated sodium channels. Evidence for a shared receptor site with local anesthetics. Anesthesiology 95:1406-1413
56. Warncke T, Jorum E, Stubhaug A (1997) Local treatment with the *N*-methyl-D-aspartate receptor antagonist ketamine inhibits development of secondary hyperalgesia in man by a peripheral action. Neurosci Lett 227:1-4
57. Pedersen JL, Galle TS, Kehlet H (1998) Peripheral analgesic effects of ketamine in acute inflammatory pain. Anesthesiology 89:58-66
58. Hawksworth C, Serpell M (1998) Intrathecal anesthesia with ketamine. Reg Anesth Pain Med 23:283-288
59. Pedraz JL, Lanao JM, Calvo MB et al (1987) Pharmacokinetic and clinical evaluation of ketamine administered by IV and epidural routes. Int J Clin Pharmacol Ther Tox 25:77-80
60. Koinig H, Marhofer P, Krenn CG et al (2000) Analgesic effects of caudal and intramuscular S(+)-ketamine in children. Anesthesiology 93:976-980
61. Karpinsky N, Dunn J, Hansen L et al (1997) Subpial vacuolar myelopathy after intrathecal ketamine: report of a case. Pain 73:103-105
62. Stotz M, Oehen HP, Gerber H (1999) Histological findings after long-term infusion of intrathecal ketamine for chronic pain: a case report. J Pain Symptom Manage 18: 223-228
63. Yang CY, Wong CS, Chang JY et al (1996) Intrathecal ketamine reduces morphine requirements in patients with terminal cancer pain. Can J Anaesth 43:379-83
64. Yanli Y, Eren A (1996) The effect of extradural ketamine on onset time and sensory block in extradural anaesthesia with bupivacaine. Anaesthesia 51:84-86
65. Kucuk N, Kizilkaya M, Tokdemir M (1998) Preoperative epidural ketamine does not have a postoperative opioid sparing effect. Anesth Analg 87:103-106
66. Weir PS, Fee JPH (1998) Double-blind comparison of extradural block with three bupivacaine-ketamine mixtures in knee arthroplasty. Br J Anaesth 80:299-301
67. Subramaniam K, Subramaniam B, Pawar DK et al (2001) Preoperative epidural ketamine in combination with morphine does not have a clinically relevant intra- and postoperative opioid-sparing effect. Anesth Analg 93:1321-1326
68. Lee IO, Kim WK, Kong MH et al (2002) No enhancement of sensory and motor blockade by ketamine added to ropivacaine interscalene brachial plexus blockade. Acta Anaesthesiol Scand 46: 821-826
69. Yaksh TL, Hua XY, Kalcheva I et al (1999) The spinal biology in humans and animals of pain states generated by persistent afferent input. Proc Natl Acad Sci 96:7680-7686
70. Johnston P, Findlow D, Aldrige LM et al (1999) The effect of ketamine on 0.25% and 0.125% bupivacaine for caudal epidural blockade in children. Paediatr Anaesth 9:31-34
71. Marhofer P, Krenn CG, Plochl W et al (2000) *S*(+)-Ketamine for caudal block in paediatric anaesthesia. Br J Anaesth 84:341-345
72. Lee HM, Sanders GM (2000) Caudal ropivacaine and ketamine for postoperative analgesia in children. Anaesthesia 55:806-810
73. De Negri P, Ivani G, Visconti C et al (2001) How to prolong postoperative analgesia after caudal anaesthesia with ropivacaine in children: *S*-ketamine versus clonidine. Paediatr Anaesth 11: 679-683
74. Ozbek H, Bilen A, Ozcengiz D et al (2002) The comparison of caudal ketamine, alfentanil and ketamine or alfentanil administration for postoperative analgesia in children. Paediatr Anaesth 12:610-616
75. Hager H, Marhofer P, Sitzwohl C et al (2002) Caudal clonidine prolongs analgesia from caudal *S*(+)-ketamine in children. Anesth Analg 94:1169-1172

76. Bowdle TA, Radant AD, Cowley DS et al (1998) Psychedelic effects of ketamine in healthy volunteers. Relationship to plasma concentrations. Anesthesiology 88:82-88
77. Krystal JH, Karper LP, Seibyl JP et al (1994) Subanesthetic effects of the noncompetitive NMDA antagonist, ketamine, in humans. Arch Gen Psychiatry 51:199-214
78. Vollenweider FX, Leenders KL, Oye I et al (1997) Differential psychopathology and patterns of cerebral glucose utilisation produced by (*S*)- and (R)-ketamine in healthy volunteers using positron emission tomography. Eur Neuropsychopharmacol 7:25-38
79. Pfenninger EG, Durieux ME, Himmelseher S (2002) Cognitive impairment after small-dose ketamine isomers in comparison to equianalgesic racemic ketamine in human volunteers. Anesthesiology 96:357-366
80. White PF, Schüttler J, Shafer A et al (1985) Comparative pharmacology of the ketamine isomers. Br J Anaesth 57:197-203

Neurotoxicity of ketamine and nitrous oxide

V. JEVTOVIC-TODOROVIC

Since its first clinical administration in 1965 by Corssen and Domino [1], the dissociative anaesthetic ketamine, a derivative of phencyclidine (PCP), has been used in many clinical settings. Unlike other intravenous anaesthetics (e.g. barbiturates, benzodiazepines, propofol), ketamine provides significant analgesia without depressing cardiovascular and respiratory functions. Therefore it is frequently used for sedation of paediatric and critically ill patients.

Nitrous oxide (N_2O), although introduced more than 150 years ago, is the most commonly used inhalational anaesthetic in human medicine. It is a colourless and tasteless gas with low anaesthetic potency: the minimum alveolar concentration that prevents purposeful movements in response to supramaximal noxious stimulation in 50% of subjects (MAC) for N_2O is about 155-180 vol% in rats [2] and 104-110 vol% in humans [3]. Thus, in order to administer an effective concentration of N_2O without compromising oxygenation, hyperbaric conditions are required. Since normobaric conditions are used in daily anaesthesia practice, N_2O is commonly combined with more potent inhalational and intravenous anaesthetics.

Mechanism of anaesthetic action of ketamine and N_2O

Modern medicine has not achieved a clear understanding of how general anaesthetics render patients unconscious and confer analgesia. However, research over the past 30 years suggests two main mechanisms: (1) increased inhibitory neurotransmission through $GABA_A$ (γ-amino-butyric acid) receptors, and (2) decreased excitatory transmission through NMDA (*N*-methyl-D-aspartate) glutamate receptors [4]. Agents that increase GABAergic transmission ($GABA_A$ agonists) are found among both intravenous anaesthetics (benzodiazepines, barbiturates, propofol, etomidate) [4] and inhalational anaesthetics (isoflurane, enflurane, sevoflurane, desflurane) [5]. Agents that decrease excitatory transmission, known traditionally as dissociative anaesthetics, were only recently recognized to be noncompetitive antagonists of NMDA glutamate receptors. Ketamine and PCP powerfully block ion conductance through NMDA glutamate receptors by acting at a "PCP" site within the NMDA receptor-ion channel [6].

Until recently, ketamine was the only clinically used anaesthetic known to be an NMDA antagonist. However, in 1998 we reported [7] that N_2O is an NMDA antagonist, having the same basic properties as ketamine, i.e. it protects neurons of the young adult brain in vivo against the excitotoxic action of NMDA. This excitotoxicity results from hyperactivation of NMDA receptors and is prevented by drugs that block NMDA receptors. N_2O also inhibits inward currents elicited by NMDA in vitro in a dose-dependent and noncompetitive manner (as demonstrated using whole-cell patch-clamp recording from cultured hippocampal neurons) (Fig. 1) [7]. In contrast, N_2O had no significant effect on GABA-induced chloride currents. We have recently demonstrated that the synaptic targets of N_2O, as an NMDA antagonist, are confined to postsynaptic sites in cultured hippocampal neurons [8]. These results suggest that N_2O interacts postsynaptically with NMDA receptor-gated ion channels and does not affect presynaptic glutamate release.

Ketamine and N_2O share not only their mechanism of anaesthetic action but many clinical characteristics as well [9, 10]. Both agents are sympathomimetics that increase blood levels of circulating norepinephrine, leading to increases in peripheral vascular resistance, cardiac output and blood pressure. Both are good analgesics and amnestics that do not interfere with hypoxic or hypercarbic stimulation of respiration, and both maintain a high level of skeletal muscle tone. In addition, both agents increase cerebral blood flow, causing elevated intracranial pressure, and both cause postoperative nausea and vomiting.

Neurotoxic effects of ketamine and nitrous oxide

Psychotomimetic effects

The dissociative anaesthetics PCP and its derivative ketamine have psychotomimetic properties. Shortly after PCP was introduced as a general anaesthetic in the late 1950s, it was withdrawn because of its prominent and sometimes prolonged psychotomimetic actions. Because the psychotomimetic reactions associated with ketamine anaesthesia – hallucinations, delusions, agitation and disturbance in affect [11-13] – were less pronounced and less prolonged, and could be attenuated by co-administration of benzodiazepines or barbiturates [14, 15], this adverse side effect of ketamine has since been regarded as undesirable but manageable.

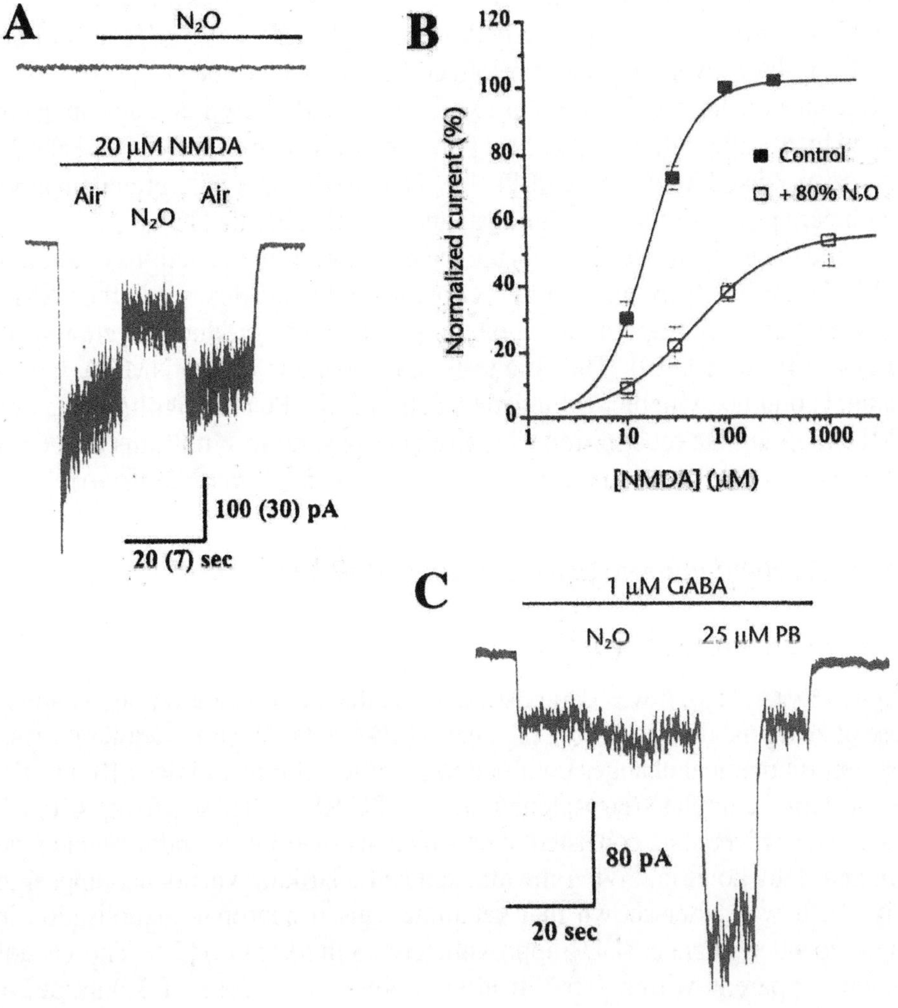

Fig. 1 N_2O inhibits neuronal NMDA- but not GABA-gated currents. In all experiments depicted, 80% N_2O was used. **(A)** *Upper trace:* N_2O has no effects on the holding current. *Lower trace:* the steady-state inward current in the presence of NMDA +air is inhibited with sharp onset and offset by N_2O. *Horizontal bars* indicate time of application and *numbers in parentheses* indicate calibration for upper trace. **(B)** N_2O causes a rightward and downward shift of the NMDA concentration-response curve indicating a mixed competitive-noncompetitive antagonism. All *points* are the average of 5-8 cells and are normalized to the current evoked by 100 μM NMDA, with *vertical bars* indicating ±SE and *solid line* representing best fit using the equation described in Methods. **(C)** The same concentration of N_2O that profoundly blocks NMDA currents has very little effect upon GABA-mediated currents, while an equipotent anaesthetic concentration of pentobarbital potentiated the GABA current by 38%

N_2O causes psychotomimetic disturbances manifested as pleasant (joyful) sensations, body image distortions, hallucinations and the disturbance in affect which led to the name "laughing gas". Due to its short duration of action (N_2O is rapidly eliminated from the body through the lungs), these psychotomimetic effects are less severe and less prolonged than for ketamine.

Because of these sensations of exhilaration and altered perception accompanied by the alleviation of physical pain, ketamine ("special K") [16] and N_2O have been abused for many years [17]. N_2O abuse is especially prevalent among health care professionals and medical and dental students [18].

While the mechanisms underlying the psychotomimetic actions of ketamine and N_2O are not fully understood, clinically relevant doses of other NMDA antagonist drugs (competitive or noncompetitive) also produce psychotomimetic side effects [19, 20]. This suggests that blockade of the NMDA receptor channel complex, whether achieved by action at the PCP recognition site or the NMDA/Glutamate recognition site, produces psychotic symptoms (see *Correlation between psychotomimetic effects and cerebrocortical neurotoxicity*).

Cerebrocortical neurotoxicity in young adult brain

Reversible neurotoxic reaction

About 15 years ago, it was demonstrated [21] that administration of a single low dose of ketamine (or one of several other NMDA antagonists) to adult rats caused pathomorphological changes confined to specific neurons in layers III and IV of the posterior cingulate/retrosplenial cortex (PC/RSC). These changes, initially described as reversible, consisted of conspicuous swelling of endoplasmic reticulum and mitochondria, giving the affected cell a striking vacuolated appearance (Fig. 2). It was latter shown that ketamine caused neuronal vacuolisation in a dose-dependent manner (ED_{50} approximately 48 mg/kg, s.c.) [22]. The vacuoles became apparent within 0.5-1 h after a single low dose of ketamine, and gradually disappeared approximately 4-5 h posttreatment. Similarly, a N_2O dose-response study revealed that at concentrations only moderately higher that those used in humans, this agent triggered a robust vacuole reaction in the PC/RSC of the adult rat brain (EC_{50} was approximately 120 vol%) [7, 22].

This reaction was also reversible: at 150-vol% (approximately MAC for N_2O) it took about 3 h of continuous N_2O anaesthesia to achieve maximal vacuolisation, but vacuoles gradually disappeared approximately 3 h after N_2O was terminated [23].

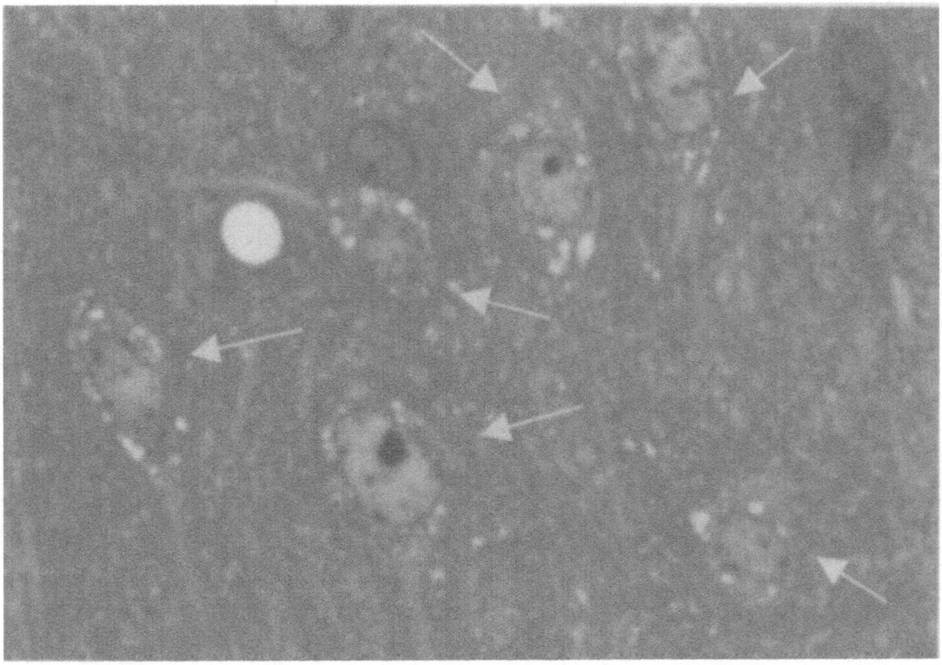

Fig. 2 Light microscopic section showing vacuolisation of all neurons in the field *(multiple arrows)* depicted in layers III and IV of the PC/RSC after 3 h of exposure to 150 vol% (magnification x480)

Sex and age dependency

Early studies showed that sex influenced sensitivity to the neurotoxic effects of MK801 and PCP, with female rats more sensitive than males [21]. Recently we demonstrated that male and female adult rats exposed to a range of doses of ketamine (from 20 to 80 mg/kg, s.c.) show different response patterns (Fig. 3A) [22]. A significant neurotoxic reaction occurred at a lower dose in females, and the neurotoxic response across the entire range of doses of ketamine revealed a greater degree of sensitivity in female rats than in males. However, the profile of N2O sensitivity was identical for male and female rats (Fig. 3B).

Experiments using low concentrations of N_2O (50 and 75 vol%) provided no evidence of a PC/RSC neurotoxic reaction in either male or female adult rats. At higher concentrations of N_2O, a concentration-dependent neurotoxic reaction occurred in both sexes. The EC_{50} values revealed no significant differences in sensitivity between males and females (calculated EC_{50} was 104±15 vol % and 117±1 vol% for males and females, respectively). Hence, susceptibility to ketamine, but not to N_2O, is gender related, with females being

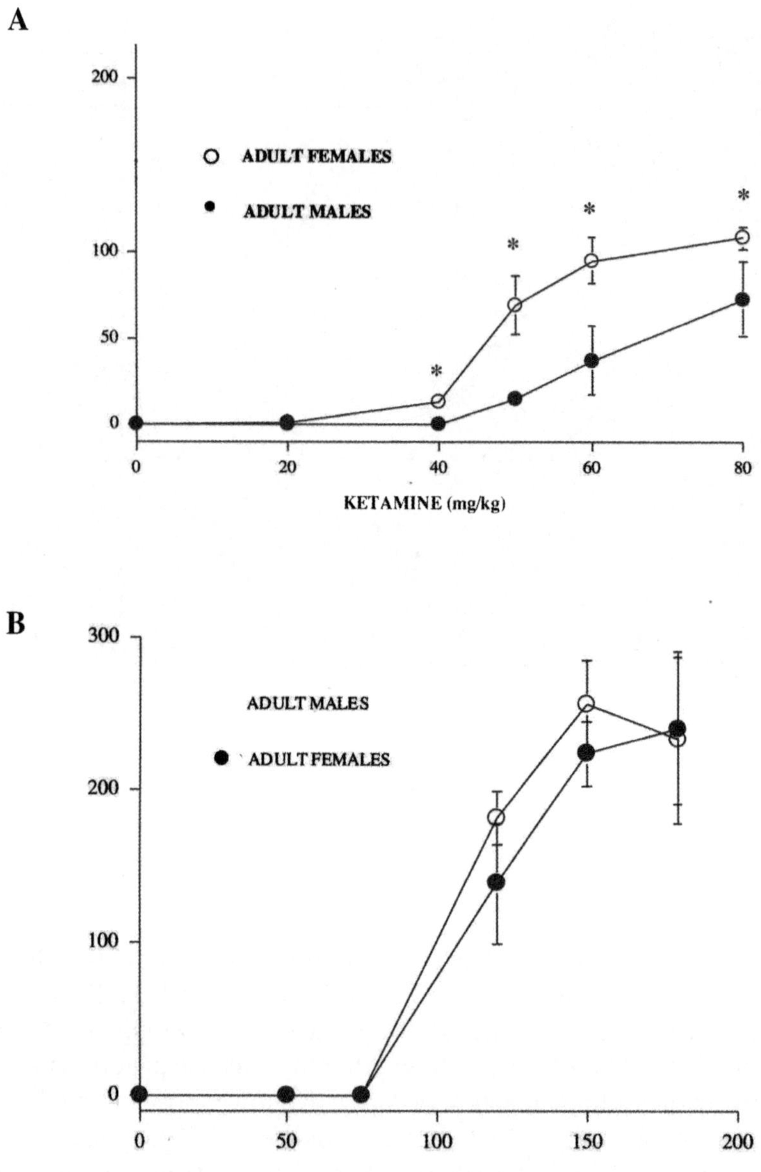

Fig. 3 (A) Neurotoxicity in PC/RSC neurons caused by exposure of adult male rats *(closed circles)* and adult female rats *(open circles)* for 3 h to ketamine is dose-dependent. Adult female rats were more sensitive to ketamine neurotoxicity compared to adult males. * Significantly different compared with males given the same dose of ketamine, $P<0.05$; n=7-10 per treatment group. **(B)** Neurotoxicity in PC/RSC neurons caused by exposure of adult male rats *(open circles)* and adult female rats *(closed circles)* for 3 h to N_2O is dose-dependent. Dose-response curves are steep (n=7-10 per treatment group)

more sensitive than males. Lack of gender differences in N_2O sensitivity may help explain the gender differences in the response to ketamine (and certain other NMDA antagonists). Ketamine is metabolised more efficiently by the male than by the female rat liver [23], while N_2O undergoes almost no metabolic conversion [24] but is rapidly eliminated via the lungs. Thus, ketamine is substantially biotransformed by hepatic mechanisms that are less efficient in females than males, whereas N_2O is not subject to this or any other sex-influenced biotransformation process. This seems the most likely explanation for the sex differential observed with ketamine (and certain other NMDA antagonists: MK801, PCP), but not N_2O neurotoxicity.

Since N_2O and ketamine are commonly used in paediatric patients, we conducted several studies to examine the age dependency profile of the acute vacuolar reaction in PC/RSC neurons of rats [22]. We found that male and female rats exposed to MAC for N_2O (150 vol%) at several ages from infancy to adulthood displayed an age-dependent neurotoxic reaction which was absent at 8 days of age, barely detectable at 1 month, and increasingly more severe at 2, 3 and 8 months of age (Fig. 4A).

The age-dependency profiles were virtually identical for males and females, with no gender differences in the severity of the neurotoxic reaction at any age. Thus age, but not sex, influences sensitivity to N_2O neurotoxicity. When male and female rats of several ages were exposed to a fixed dose of ketamine (60 mg/kg, i.p.), they displayed strikingly different response patterns (Fig. 4B). Females began displaying a significant neurotoxic reaction at 2 months, which became more severe at 3 months and strikingly severe at 8 months. Males showed almost no reaction at any developmental age (8 days, 1, 2 or 3 months). Thus, vulnerability to ketamine neurotoxicity is age dependent in both male and female rats, although male rats are less sensitive than female rats, having a later onset of sensitivity and displaying a less robust neurotoxic reaction in adulthood after full sensitivity develops. Hence, sensitivity to both ketamine and N_2O neurotoxicity are age dependent, with sensitivity to either agent greater in adulthood than at any pre-adult age.

Combined N2O and ketamine neurotoxicity

Because both N_2O and ketamine have neurotoxic potential and are sometimes administered in combination to human patients, we recently addressed the issue of whether they potentiate each other's neurotoxicity [25]. When N_2O and ketamine were combined, the neurotoxic response was markedly augmented compared with the response to either drug alone. Figure 5A illustrates the degree of neurotoxicity obtained with various doses of ketamine when administered with a fixed concentration of N_2O. For example, if the concentration of

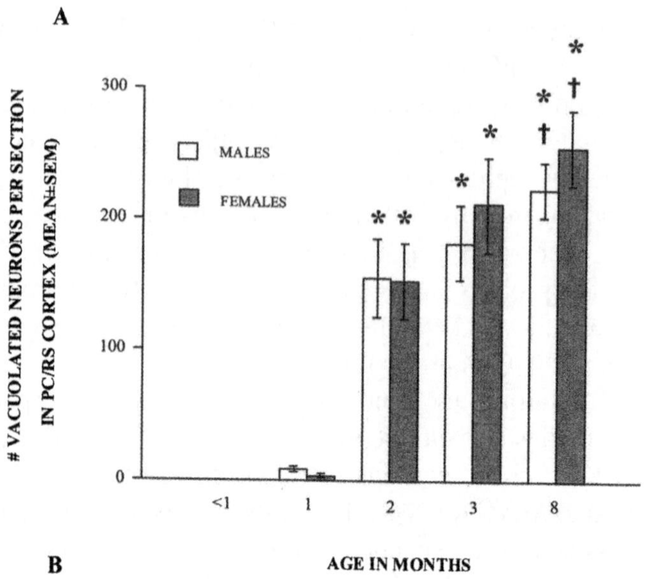

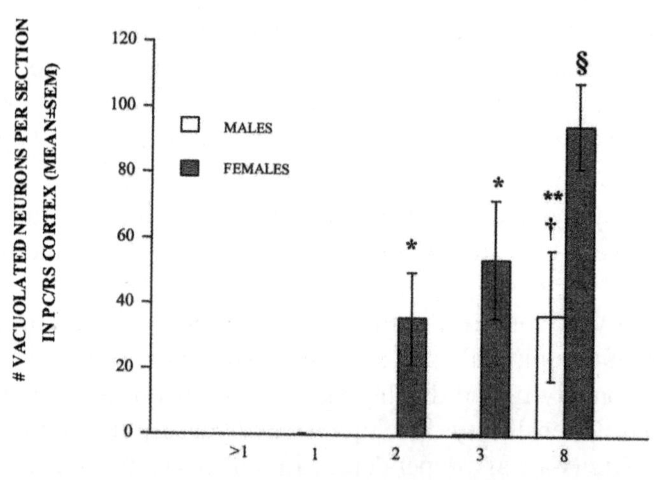

Fig. 4 (A) Neurotoxicity in PC/RSC neurons caused by N_2O (150 vol%) is age dependent in males and females. At 8 days of age, rats of both sexes are totally insensitive, and they become gradually more sensitive as they pass through adolescence into full adulthood. * Significantly different compared with 8-day-old and 1-month-old rats ($P < 0.0005$, males and females). † Significantly different compared with 2-month-old rats ($P < 0.0005$ and $P=0.022$ for males and females, respectively) (n=9-12 per treatment group). **(B)** Neurotoxicity in PC/RSC caused by ketamine (60 mg/kg, s.c.) is age-dependent in males and females. At 8 days of age, rats of both sexes were totally insensitive. Female rats become gradually more sensitive as they pass through adolescence into adulthood. *Significantly different compared with 8-day-old and 1-month-old female rats, $P=0.005$. § Significantly different compared with 2-month-old female rats, $P<0.005$. Male rats remain insensitive to ketamine-induced neurotoxicity until they reach full adulthood. † Significantly different compared with 8-day-old, 1- and 2-month-old male rats, $P<0.005$; n=7-10 per treatment group. In adulthood, male rats are significantly less sensitive than female to ketamine-induced neurotoxicity (** $P=0.02$)

N_2O was 75 vol% (ineffective concentration), adding an ineffective dose of ketamine (20 mg/kg) produced a robust vacuolar reaction approximately equal to the most severe reaction elicited by any dose of ketamine alone. If the concentration of N_2O was at its EC_{50} (approximately 120 vol%), adding various doses of ketamine resulted in a reaction several-fold what would be expected from a given dose of ketamine alone. The ED_{50} of ketamine when combined with N_2O at 120 vol% was 8.8 mg/kg. This is less than one-fifth of the ED_{50} for ketamine when given alone (ED_{50} 47.5 mg/kg).

Because the effect at low doses was greater than could be explained by simple additivity, we performed an isobolographic analysis and found that the fractional value (the sum of the ratios of the ED_{50} values for ketamine and N_2O determined alone and jointly) was less than 1, supporting the interpretation that the N_2O-ketamine interaction is synergistic (Fig. 5B).

Because neither N_2O nor ketamine depresses cardiorespiratory functions, their combined use is considered appropriate for situations (e.g. trauma, elderly and obstetric patients) in which respiratory and haemodynamic depression must be avoided [10]. Yet, the fact that low concentrations of N_2O and ketamine, administered in combination, can cause a severe neurotoxic reaction in the rat cerebral cortex raises a question about the safety of this practice. For example, when a nontoxic dose (20 mg/kg, i.p.) of ketamine (equivalent to 3 mg/kg, i.m. in humans) [10] was supplemented with a nontoxic concentration (50 vol%) of N_2O (equivalent to 35 vol% N_2O in humans) [3], the neurotoxic reaction was more severe than that produced by any dose of ketamine alone (Fig. 5A). While interspecies comparisons do not provide a precise risk evaluation, it is significant that the doses used in our rats, when converted to human dose equivalents, fall within the ranges often used in human anaesthesia (ketamine doses of 5-10 mg/kg, i.m., and N_2O concentrations up to 75 vol%) [9, 10].

Irreversible neurotoxic reaction

Although single low doses of NMDA antagonists cause acute reversible vacuolar changes in PC/RSC, high doses or repeated lower doses over several days cause irreversible degeneration of neurons in several cortico-limbic brain regions in addition to PC/RSC [26, 27]. While ketamine is known to cause a reversible vacuole reaction in PC/RSC neurons, it remains to be shown whether it may cause neuronal death. A recent series of studies on neuronal death found that if one MAC of N_2O (150-vol%) is administered continuously for 12-16 h to young adult rats, neuronal degeneration occurs in PC/RSC and other cortical brain regions (e.g. perirhinal cortex) [28].

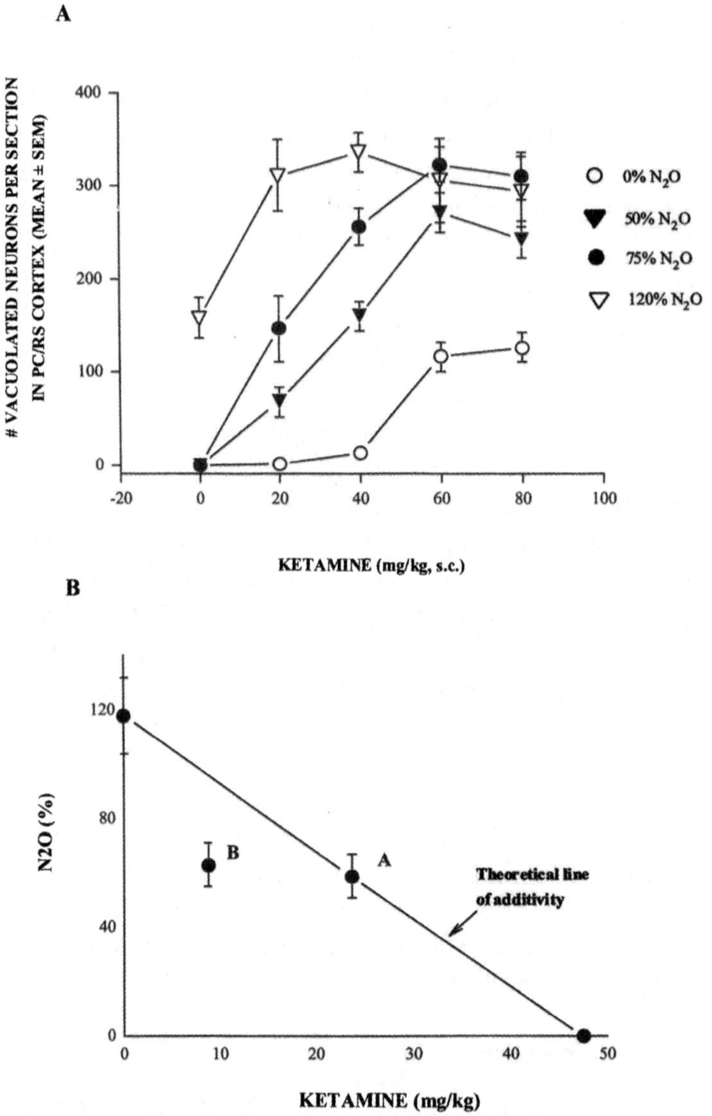

Fig. 5 (A) N_2O significantly potentiates the neurotoxicity caused by ketamine. Adult female rats were exposed to ketamine either alone or in combination with various concentrations of N_2O (as indicated) for 3 h. The ketamine neurotoxicity curve is shifted markedly upward and to the left by combination with concentrations of N_2O (50 or 75 vol%) which by themselves are not neurotoxic. The number of vacuolated neurons in PC/RSC in the presence of N_2O+ketamine is significantly higher than in the presence of the corresponding dose of ketamine alone ($P<0.05$). The control condition for N_2O experiments is normobaric or hyperbaric air and for ketamine is saline i.p. and is depicted as 0 vol% and 0 mg/kg, respectively (n=10-12 per treatment group). **(B)** Isobolographic curve for the interaction between N_2O and ketamine. The EC_{50} for N_2O is plotted on the y-axis and the ED_{50} for ketamine on the x-axis. The line connecting these two points is the theoretical line of additivity. *Point A* is the theoretical additive ED_{50} point. The experimental ED_{50} *point B* for the combination falls bellow the theoretical line of additivity suggesting a synergistic (supra-additive) interaction

Mechanism of ketamine and N_2O neurotoxicity

An evaluation of the neurotoxicity of ketamine, N_2O (also PCP and MK801), has revealed that these agents create a network disturbance featuring disinhibition as the primary operative mechanism [29, 30]. Glutamate is a major regulator of inhibitory tone; it performs this function primarily by tonically stimulating NMDA receptors on GABAergic inhibitory neurons, neurons which normally restrain major cholinergic and glutamatergic excitatory pathways that innervate certain cerebrocortical neurons. Thus, blockade of NMDA receptors in this network abolishes GABAergic inhibition, releasing excitatory pathways from inhibition. These disinhibited excitatory pathways excessively stimulate cerebrocortical neurons, causing excitotoxic injury. The longer the NMDA receptor blockade is maintained, the greater the chance that excitotoxic damage will convert from reversible to irreversible. We have demonstrated that various classes of drugs, if co-administered with ketamine and/or N_2O (also MK801), prevent both reversible and irreversible neurotoxic reactions induced by ketamine and/or N_2O (and MK801). Agents exhibiting this neuroprotective property include $GABA_A$ agonists (benzodiazepines, barbiturates, propofol, halothane, isoflurane), $\alpha 2$ adrenergic agonists, $5HT_{2A}$ serotonergic agonists, cholinergic muscarinic antagonists and non-NMDA glutamate antagonists [7, 26-35]. Each of these seemingly diverse agents acts at receptors that modulate either the glutamatergic or cholinaergic (or both) pathways which mediate the neurotoxic reaction. Evidence suggests that blockade of either pathway confers effective protection, suggesting that simultaneous hyperactivity in both pathways is required for the neurotoxic reaction to occur.

The effectiveness of GABAergic anaesthetics (e.g. benzodiazepines, barbiturates, propofol, halothane, isoflurane) in preventing the pathomorphological reaction triggered in rat brain by ketamine and N_2O, individually or combined [7, 25, 28], is noteworthy because in clinical anaesthesia GABAergic agents are commonly included in the drug cocktail used to induce and maintain general anaesthesia. Therefore, although the practice of combining N_2O or/and ketamine with GABAergic anaesthetics was not conceived for safety purposes, it appears that increased safety has been achieved.

Correlation between psychotomimetic effects and cerebrocortical neurotoxicity

It is not established whether the human brain is vulnerable to these neurotoxic phenomena (i.e. vacuolar reaction and/or neuronal degeneration). However, N_2O and ketamine (and most if not all other NMDA antagonists) do trigger psychotic reactions in adult humans [11-15, 19, 20] (see *Psychotomimetic effects*). A growing body of evidence suggests that the two phenomena are mediated by a common mechanism involving similar neuronal circuitry [36]. If this is correct, the psychotomimetic symptoms induced by N_2O and/or ketamine may be clinical manifestations of the psycho-toxic process that causes occult pathomorphological changes in cerebrocortical neurons. Indeed, the psychotomimetic reaction in humans can be suppressed or prevented by the same drugs (e.g. benzodiazepines, barbiturates, α_2 adrenergic agonists) that block the neurotoxic manifestations in rodent brains [21, 31-35]. In addition, the neurotoxic reactions in rats and psychotomimetic reactions in humans have the same age dependency profile, both phenomena occurring in adulthood but not at pre-adult ages [30]. The invulnerability of pre-adult humans to the psychotogenic effects of ketamine explains its frequent use in paediatric anaesthesia [10].

Cerebrocortical neurotoxicity in the aged brain

An impressive decline in NMDA receptor-binding sites and/or NMDA receptor function has been shown in the aged brain of several species (mice, rats, monkeys) [37-39]. This age-related deficit of NMDA receptors has been demonstrated in several brain regions, including the cerebral cortex, hippocampus, and striatum. Thus, an age-related loss of NMDA receptors and the functional capacity of this receptor system may explain, in part, the memory deficits of the elderly and their increased susceptibility to psychological disturbances (e.g. confusion, delusions). By blocking NMDA receptors, NMDA antagonists render the NMDA receptor system acutely hypofunctional. We proposed that the aged brain with hypofunctional NMDA receptors might be acutely sensitive to the effects of ketamine and N_2O (individually or in combination). Our recent study supports this hypothesis. When female rats (6 or 18 months old) were subjected to N_2O or ketamine individually, the neurotoxicity of N_2O alone was similar in young and aged animals. In contrast, aged animals were substantially more sensitive than young animals to ketamine neurotoxicity: doses of ketamine which were nontoxic in young animals induced significant neurotoxic reactions in the PC/RSC of aged animals. When combined, the potentiation of N_2O neurotoxicity by ketamine (or vice versa) resulted in a neurotoxic reaction 2-3 times as severe (with respect to the number of neurons exhibiting vacuoles) in aged as in young adult animals [40]. This age-dependent effect of ketamine may also reflect diminished hepatic metabolism of ketamine in aged animals. Because N_2O undergoes minimal metabolism [24], hepatic efficacy plays little part in its neurotoxicity; thus, no age differential was observed.

Cerebrocortical neurotoxicity in immature (developing) brain

Although the research presented thus far indicates that the immature brain (up to 2 weeks of age) [7, 29, 41] is completely insensitive to the mechanism by which ketamine and N_2O injure the adult brain, this does not signify that these agents are innocuous for the developing brain. On the contrary, during synaptogenesis the immature brain is exquisitely sensitive to a different mechanism of damage by NMDA antagonist drugs. During synaptogenesis, which in humans lasts from 6 months of gestation to 3 years after birth, two classes of drugs – NMDA antagonists and $GABA_A$ agonists – can trigger widespread apoptotic neurodegeneration in the developing brain. Ikonomidou and colleagues demonstrated that when ketamine was repeatedly administered to 7-day-old rat pups (to maintain a steady blockade of NMDA receptors for at least 8 h) widespread apoptotic neurodegeneration was detected in several brain regions [42]. This sensitivity to ketamine was high on postnatal days 0 and 3, increased between postnatal days 3 and 7, and then decreased sharply between 7 and 14 days postnatally. Knowing that prolonged administration of ketamine results in severe neuroapoptosis, we investigated the effects of a single dose of ketamine. A single dose of ketamine is often administered for sedation or induction of paediatric or obstetric anaesthesia. Given ketamine's short duration of action, it was assumed that such use posed no risk of apoptosis in the developing brain. However, in our study, a single dose of ketamine (40 mg/kg, s.c.) to infant mice caused significantly higher apoptosis in the striatum and cortex than was observed in saline-treated controls [43].

We have also studied the effect of N_2O on the developing brain. N_2O, much like ketamine, can induce apoptotic degeneration. Our recently published study shows that, although N_2O alone did not cause apoptosis in the immature brain, it significantly potentiated the neurotoxic damage caused by midazolam (a benzodiazepine commonly used for sedation in paediatric patients) and isoflurane [44]. A clinically relevant combination of anaesthetics (9 mg/kg midazolam, followed by 6 h of 75 vol% N_2O and 1 vol% isoflurane anaesthesia) was administered to 7-day-old rats, resulting in robust apoptotic neurodegeneration affecting several major regions of the brain (thalamus, hypothalamus, amygdala, caudate nucleus, frontal, parietal, temporal, occipital, cingulate cortices, hippocampus and subiculum) (Fig. 6).

Anaesthesia-treated animals showed significant and persistent learning/memory deficits (confirmed by radial arm maze and Morris water maze tests) compared with controls up to 160 days (young adulthood) (Fig. 7). Well-designed clinical studies are needed to assess the relevance of these animal findings to obstetric or paediatric anaesthesia.

In conclusion, N_2O and ketamine are valuable general anaesthetics that have

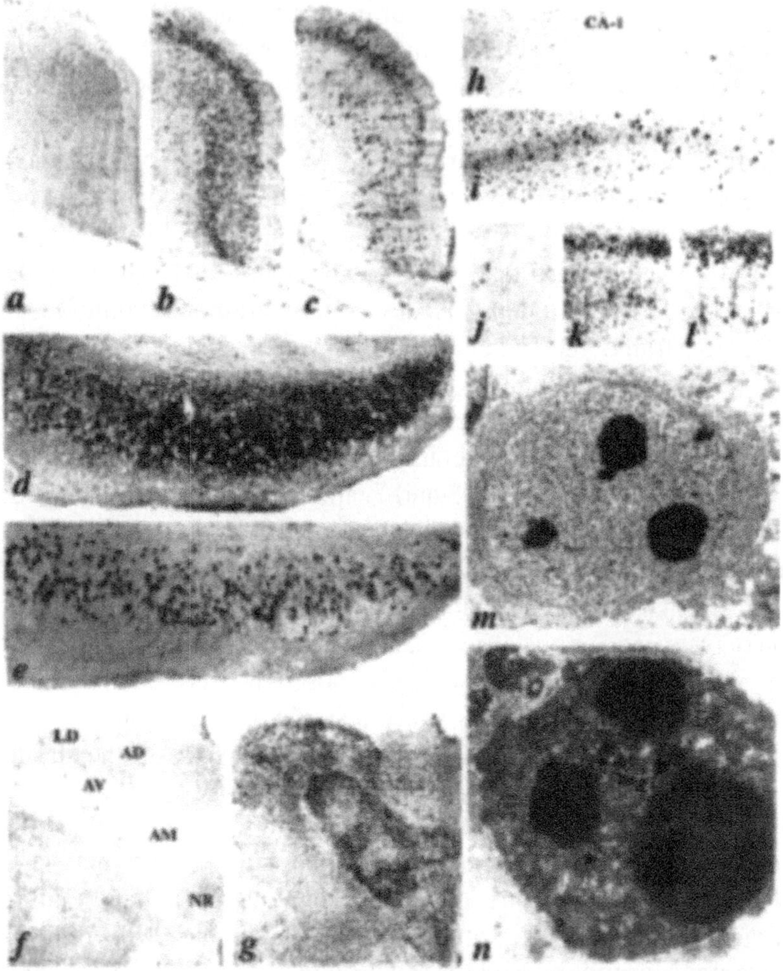

Fig. 6 Triple anaesthetic cocktail induces apoptotic neurodegeneration. ***a*** - ***l*** Light micrographic scenes from various brain regions of either a control rat (***a***, ***f***, ***h***, ***j***) or a rat exposed to the triple anaesthetic cocktail (***b*** – ***e***, ***g***, ***i***, ***k***, ***l***). Some sections are stained by the DeOlmos silver method (***a***, ***b***, ***d***, ***f***, ***g***, ***k***) and the remainder are immunocytochemically stained to reveal caspase-3 activation (***c***, ***e***, ***h***, ***i***, ***j***, ***l***). The regions illustrated are: posterior cingulate/retrosplenial cortex (***a***, ***b***, ***c***); subiculum (***d***, ***e***); anterior thalamus (***f***, ***g***); rostral CA-1 hippocampus (***h***, ***i***) and parietal cortex (***j***, ***k***, ***l***). The individual nuclei shown in the anterior thalamus (***f***, ***g***) are laterodorsal (LD), anterodorsal (AD), anteroventral (AV), anteromedial (AM) and nucleus reuniens (NR). ***m***, ***n*** Electron micrographic scenes depicting the ultrastructural appearance of neurons undergoing apoptosis. The cell in ***m*** displays a very early stage of apoptosis, in which dense spherical chromatin balls are forming in the nucleus at a time when the nuclear membrane remains intact and very few changes are evident in the cytoplasm. The cell in ***n*** exhibits a much later stage of apoptosis, in which the entire cell is condensed, the nuclear membrane is absent and there is intermixing of nuclear and cytoplasmic constituents. These are hallmark characteristics of neuronal apoptosis as it occurs in the in vivo mammalian brain

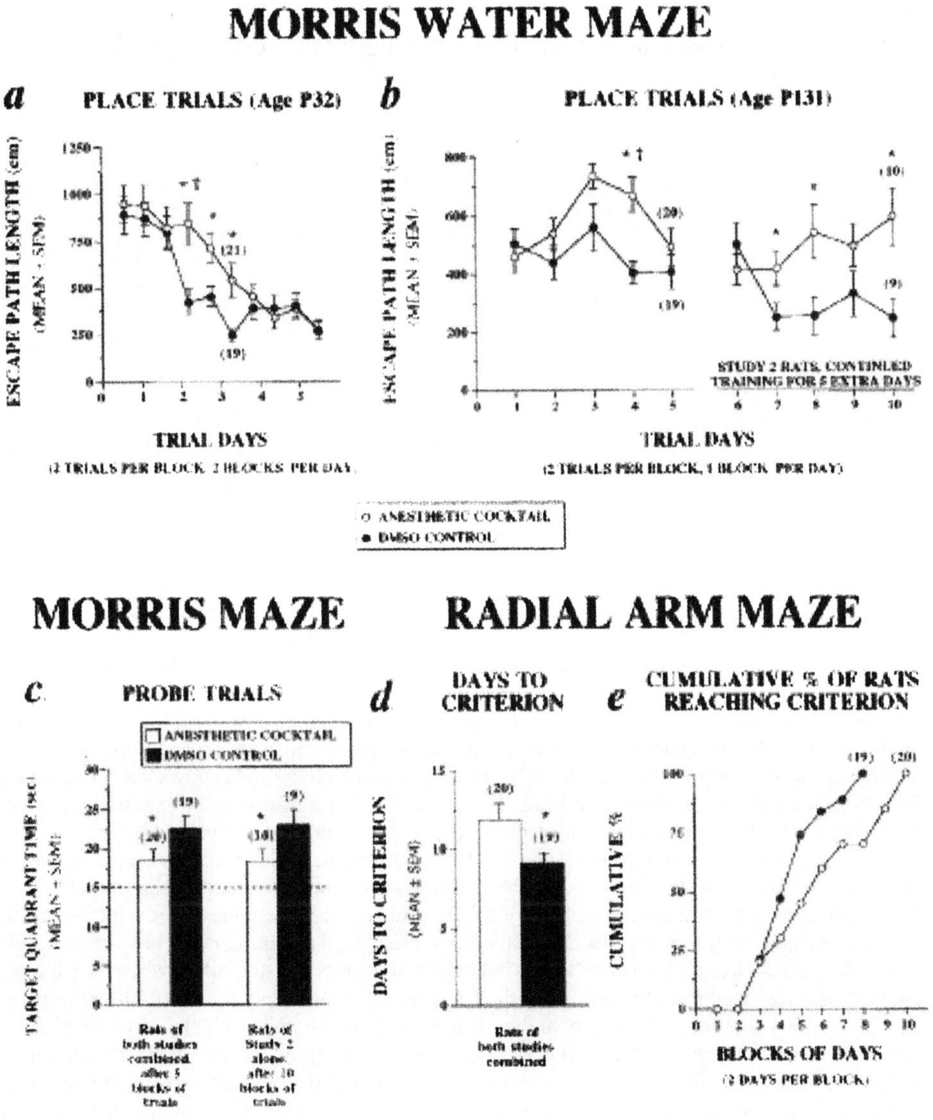

Fig. 7 Effects of neonatal triple anaesthetic cocktail treatment on spatial learning. ***a*** Rats were tested at P32 for their ability to learn the location of a submerged (not visible) platform. An ANOVA of the escape path length data yielded a significant main effect of treatment (*P*= 0.032), and a significant treatment by blocks of trials interaction (*P*= 0.024) indicating that the performance of the anaesthetic cocktail rats was significantly inferior to that of control rats during place training. Subsequent pairwise comparisons indicated that differences were greatest during blocks 4, 5 and 6 (*p* = 0.003, 0.012, and 0.019, respectively). However, the anaesthetic-cocktail rats improved their performance to control-like levels during the last 4 blocks of trials. ***b*** Rats were retested as adults (P131) for their ability to learn a different location of the submerged platform *cont.* →

an important role in clinical anaesthesia. However, a growing body of evidence suggests that their neurotoxic potential cannot be ignored and should be continuously assessed and systematically studied in well-designed animal and clinical studies.

The graph on the *left* represents the path length data from the first 5 place trials, when all rats were tested. An ANOVA of these data yielded a significant main effect of treatment ($P = 0.013$), indicating that the control rats, in general, exhibited significantly shorter path lengths in swimming to the platform compared to anaesthetic cocktail rats. Subsequent pairwise comparisons showed that differences were greatest during block 4 ($P=0.001$). The graph on the *right* shows the data from study 2 rats which received 5 additional training days as adults. During these additional trials the control group improved their performance and appeared to reach asymptotic levels, while the anaesthetic cocktail rats showed no improvement. An ANOVA of these data yielded a significant main effect of treatment ($P= 0.045$) as well as a significant treatment by blocks of trials interaction ($P =0.001$). Additional pairwise comparisons showed that group differences were greatest during blocks 7, 8, and 10 ($P= 0.032$, 0.013, and 0.017, respectively). ***c*** Probe trial performance of anaesthetic cocktail and control rats during adult testing. Search behaviour of the rats was quantified when the submerged platform was removed from the pool after the last place trials in blocks 5 and 10. The *histogram* on the *left* presents data for rats in both studies 1 and 2 combined after 5 blocks of place trials were completed. The *histogram* on the *right* presents data for rats in study 2 alone, after 10 blocks of place trials were completed. The *dotted line* represents the amount of time that animals would be expected to spend in the target quadrant based on chance alone. Both *histograms* show that the control rats spent significantly more time in the target quadrant than the anaesthesia-exposed rats, regardless of whether the probe tests were performed on both study groups after 5 blocks or only on the study 2 rats after 10 trials. ***d*** and ***e*** Data from the radial arm maze test performed on P53 to evaluate spatial working memory capabilities are shown. ***d*** A *histogram* showing that the anaesthetic cocktail rats required significantly more days to reach a criterion demonstrating learning (8 correct responses out of the first 9 responses for 4 consecutive days) than did controls. ***e*** Plotting the days to criterion data as the cumulative percent of rats reaching criterion in each group as a function of blocks of training days shows that the acquisition rate of the anaesthetic cocktail rats began to slow around the 4th block of trials and remained slower throughout the rest of the experiment.
Numbers in *parentheses* in each *graph* indicate sample sizes. $^{*}P < 0.05$; $^{\dagger}P <$ Bonferroni corrected level: 0.005 in ***a***; 0.01 in ***b***

References

1. Corssen G, Domino EF (1966) Dissociative anesthesia: further pharmacologic studies and first clinical experiences with the phencyclidine derivative CI-581. Anesth Analg 45:29
2. Gonsowski CT, Eger II EI (1994) Nitrous oxide minimum alveolar anesthetic concentration in rats is greater than previously reported. Anesth Analg 79:710-712
3. Hornbein TF, Eger EI II, Winter PM et al (1982) The minimum alveolar concentration of nitrous oxide in man. Anesth Analg 61:553-556
4. Franks NP, Lieb WR (1994) Molecular and cellular mechanism of general anesthesia. Nature 367:607-614
5. Nishikawa K, MacIver MB (2001) Agent-selective effects of volatile anesthetics on GABAA receptor-mediated synaptic inhibition in hippocampal interneurons. Anesthesiology 94:340-347
6. Lodge D, Anis NA (1982) Effects of phencyclidine on excitatory amino acid activation of spinal interneurons in the cat. Eur J Pharmacol 77:203-204
7. Jevtovic-Todorovic V, Todorovic SM, Mennerick S et al (1998) Nitrous oxide (laughing gas) is an NMDA antagonist, neuroprotectant and neurotoxin. Nat Med 4:460-463
8. Mennerick S, Jevtovic-Todorovic V, Todorovic SM et al (1998) Effect of nitrous oxide on excitatory and inhibitory synaptic transmission in hippocampal cultures. J Neurosci 18:9716-9726
9. Stevens WC, Kingston HGG (1992) Inhalation anesthesia. In: Barash PG et al (eds) Clinical anesthesia. Lippincott, Philadelphia, pp 439-465
10. Fragren RJ and Avram MJ (1992) Nonopioid intravenous anesthetesia. In: Barash PG et al (eds) Clinical anesthesia. Lippincott, Philadelphia, pp 385-412
11. Luby ED, Gottlieb JS, Cohen BD et al (1962) Model psychosis and schizophrenia. Am J Psychiatry 119:61
12. Krystal JH, Karper LP, Seibyl JP et al (1993) Dose-related effects of the NMDA antagonist, ketamine, in healthy humans. Schizophr Res 9:240-241
13. Newcomer JW, Farber NB, Jevtovic-Todorovic V et al (1999) Ketamine-induced NMDA receptor hypofunction as a model of memory impairment in schizophrenia. Neuropsychopharmacology 20:106-118
14. Magbagbeola JAO, Thomas NA (1974) Effect of thiopentone on emergence reactions to ketamine anaesthesia. Can Anaesth Soc J 21:321
15. White PF, Way WL, Trevor AJ (1982) Ketamine – its pharmacology and therapeutic uses. Anesthesiology 56:119
16. Bovill JG, Coppell, L, Dundee JW et al (1971) Current status of ketamine anesthesia. Lancet I:1285
17. Dohrn CS, Lichtor JL, Coalson DW et al (1993) Related articles, links reinforcing effects of extended inhalation of nitrous oxide in humans. Drug Alcohol Depend 31:265-280
18. Gillman MA (1992) Nitrous oxide abuse in perspective. Clinical Neuropharmacol 15:297-306
19. Herrling PL (1994) D-CPPene (SDZ EAA 494), a competitive NMDA antagonist: results from animal models and first results in humans. Neuropsychopharmacology 10: (Part 1):591S
20. Grotta J (1995) Why do all drugs work in animals but none in stroke patients? 2. Neuroprotective therapy. J Intern Med 237:89
21. Olney JW, Labruyere J, Price MT (1989) Pathological changes induced in cerebrocortical neurons by phencyclidine and related drugs. Science 244:1360
22. Jevtovic-Todorovic V, Wozniak DW, Benshoff ND et al (2001) Comparative evaluation of the neurotoxic properties of ketamine and nitrous oxide. Brain Res 895:264-267
23. Jevtovic-Todorovic V, Benshoff N, Olney JW (1998) Prolonged nitrous oxide anesthesia kills neurons in the adult rat brain. J Neurosurg Anesthesiol 10:257
24. Livingston A, Waterman AE (1977) Influence of age and sex on the duration of action of ketamine in rats. Br J Pharmacol 59:491
25. Hong K, Trudell JR, O'Neil JR et al (1980) Metabolism of nitrous oxide by human and rat intestinal contents. Anesthesiology 52:16-19

26. Jevtovic-Todorovic V, Benshoff N, Olney JW (2000) Ketamine potentiates cerebrocortical damage induced by the common anesthetic agent nitrous oxide in adult rats. Br J Pharmacol 130:1692-1698
27. Wozniak DF, Dikranian K, Ishimaru MJ et al (1998) Disseminated corticolimbic neuronal degeneration induced in rat brain by MK-801: potential relevance to Alzheimer's disease. Neurobiol Dis 5:305-322
28. Corso TD, Sesma MA, Tenkova TI et al (1997) Multifocal brain damage induced by phencyclidine is augmented by pilocarpine. Brain Res 752:1-14
29. Olney JW, Labruyere J, Wang G et al (1991) NMDA antagonist neurotoxicity: mechanism and protection. Science 254:1515-1518
30. Olney JW, Farber NB (1995) NMDA antagonists as neurotherapeutic drugs, psychotogens, neurotoxins, and research tools for studying schizophrenia. Neuropsychopharmacology 13:335--345
31. Jevtovic-Todorovic V, Kirby CO, Olney JW (1997) Isoflurane and propofol block neurotoxicity caused by MK-801 in the rat posterior cingulate/retrosplenial cortex. Cereb Blood Flow Metab 17:168-174
32. Ishimaru M, Fukamauchi F, Olney JW (1995) Halothane prevents MK-801 neurotoxicity in the rat cingulate cortex. Neurosci Lett 193:1-4
33. Farber NB, Foster J, Duhan NL et al (1995) Alpha 2 adrenergic agonists prevent MK-801 neurotoxicity. Neuropsychopharmacology 12:347-349
34. Farber NB, Foster J, Duhan NL et al (1996) Olanzapine and fluperlapine mimic clozapine in preventing MK-801 neurotoxicity. Schizophr Res 21:33-37
35. Farber NB, Hanslick J, Kirby C et al (1998) Serotonergic agents that activate 5HT2A receptors prevent NMDA antagonist neurotoxicity. Neuropsychopharmacology 18:57-62
36. Farber NB, Kim SH, Dikranian K et al (2002) Receptor mechanisms and circuitry underlying NMDA antagonist neurotoxicity. Mol Psychiatry 7:32-43
37. Gonzales RA, Brown LM, Jones TW et al (1991) *N*-Methyl-D-aspartate mediated responses decrease with age in Fischer 344 rat brain. Neurobiol Aging 12:219-225
38. Magnusson KR, Cotman CW (1993) Age-related changes in excitatory amino acid receptors in two mouse strains. Neurobiol Aging 14:197-206
39. Wenk GL, Walker LC, Price DL et al (1991) Loss of NMDA, but not GABA-A, binding in the brains of aged rats and monkeys. Neurobiol Aging 12:93-98
40. Beals JK, Carter LB, Jevtovic-Todorovic V (2003) Neurotoxicity of nitrous oxide and ketamine is more severe in aged than in young rat brain. Ann NY Acad Sci 993:1
41. Farber NB, Wozniak DF, Price MT et al (1995) Age-specific neurotoxicity in the rat associated with NMDA receptor blockade: potential relevance to schizophrenia? Biol Psychiatry 38:788--796
42. Ikonomidou C, Bosch F, Miksa M et al (1999) Blockade of NMDA receptors and apoptotic neurodegeneration in the developing brain. Science 283:70-74
43. Young C, Tenkova T, Wang H et al (2003) A single sedating dose of ketamine causes neuronal apoptosis in developing mouse brain (abstract). Soc Neurosci (in press)
44. Jevtovic-Todorovic V, Hartman RE, Izumi Y et al (2003) Early exposure to common anesthetic agents causes widespread neurodegeneration in the developing rat brain and persistent learning deficits. J Neurosci 23:876-882

Models of acute pain service

G. GALIMBERTI, M. PIVA, A. GULLO

Postoperative acute pain is a syndrome, whose physiopathologic mechanisms are now well known: all of them result from surgical operations, which are invasive acts. Postoperative acute pain is semeiologically meaningless and physiologically useless; however, it is responsible for a range of nervous, hormonal and metabolic responses, which are unhealthy for patients and jeopardise their prognoses, since they entail longer hospital stays and, therefore, increased social costs. Nowadays, patients still regard this kind of pain as an inevitable part of the price to be paid for surgical treatments; moreover, medical and paramedical staff members often believe that pain is an inherent part of surgery and apply unsuitable approaches and treatments. Therefore, postoperative acute pain control units should be established in surgical departments, not only to treat such pain, but mainly to provide information, education and training.

In fact, national epidemiological surveys show a significant prevalence of pain in hospitals, as well as heterogeneous use of techniques and drugs to control postoperative acute pain, which are applied in different ways even on different wards. Recently, in Italy, the importance of postoperative acute pain control has been recognised by relevant legislation, stressing both the urgency of this issue at the national level, and the need to make its treatment and management consistent throughout the country [1]. The guidelines laid down in the said legislation are aimed specifically at increasing the attention paid by the staff involved in care processes to pain, so that they will implement all possible measures to fight pain, but they also contain recommendations for provision of permanent training and education to medical and paramedical staff and for the dissemination of information and raising of public awareness. They also advise that a person responsible for the implementation of these guidelines should be appointed to each health unit, as should a painless hospital board (PHB), including health management representatives, pain treatment experts, postoperative acute pain treatment specialists, and the operators usually dealing with pain control treatments, especially nurses.

Postoperative acute pain control unit

Evidence for shorter stays in hospital and of lower morbidity and mortality rates has been reported whenever effective postoperative analgesia has been applied. Therefore, the establishment of "acute pain services" (APS), as they referred to in the literature, is increasingly frequent. An APS is a heterogeneous organisation, including medical (anaesthesiologists, surgeons, specialists) and paramedical (professional nurses specialised in postoperative acute pain treatment, nurses on surgical wards) staff, which reports to the anaesthesia and resuscitation service and supports the various wards. Many models of APS have been described in the literature; however, the main ones are the model described by Ready and applied in the United States [2], and that proposed in Sweden by Rawal [3], which interestingly spread to other parts of Europe. The former, which is focused on anaesthesiologists, is undoubtedly effective and technically advanced, but it is also very expensive and too selective; the latter, which is based on nurses and supervised by anaesthesiologists, cuts operating costs and increases the number of patients followed up postoperatively, since instead of establishing a new service it optimises the work of a range of in-house professionals, thus enabling them to follow up almost all patients who have undergone surgery.

Postoperative acute pain

Usually, acute pain is associated with a precise disease or trauma and has a predictable length that is generally limited to the time required to repair the injury. The most typical acute pain is postoperative pain, which is usually characterised by abrupt onset and variable intensity, and which is limited in time (the patient usually recovers in less than 7 days). Postoperative pain varies in different patients and even in the same patient over time: this variability depends not only on the pre-existing disease, its location, and the type of surgery, but also, and sometimes mainly, on the factors resulting from the pain/tissue injury ratio, which is associated with many cultural, religious, socio-economic and racial aspects and depends on the patients' histories, and especially on their previous experience of pain [4].

Pain physiopathology

Pain appears as a consequence of an injury to the intertegumentary organ or to system structures; a tissue injury leads to the release of neuro-mediators such as bradykinin (BK), serotonin (5-HT), and potassium ions. 5-HT is responsible for vasodilatatory reactions, oedema, and the triple reaction described by Lewis; BK entails the activation of (mechanothermal) C-amyelinated fibre receptors and the A2-cycloxygenase phospholipase cascade, which is responsible for the synthesis of many eicosanoids (prostaglandins, prostacyclins, leukotrienes) [5]. Therefore, BK and potassium ions are responsible for the activation of receptors, whereas prostaglandins prolong sensitisation and lead to a decreased pain stimulation threshold. These recruitment and sensitisation processes of both nociceptors and primary afferences are called peripheral hyperalgesia, which is described as an alteration of sensitivity leading to a remarkable increase in the intensity of the stimulus-induced painful sensation [6, 7]. Primary hyperalgesia is provoked by the release of vasoactive algogenic peptides from injured cells, and it is a response that appears in only a few minutes; conversely, secondary hyperalgesia is a delayed response, whose origin is complex and not yet completely clear and which involves both peripheral sensitisation and CNS modifications. Hardy et al. were the first to suggest that secondary hyperalgesia was a consequence of medullary modifications: the nociceptive information transmission from the injured area to posterior horns would also lead to "sensitisation" (central hyperalgesia) of medullary neurons receiving afferences from the areas that are not directly injured. Sensitisation could be mediated by a decrease in tonic inhibition and the establishment of new synaptic contacts [5]. The synapses of nerve endings at primary afferences in posterior horns are formed according to a precise anatomical pattern, which maintains the spatial localisation of peripherally applied stimuli. Second-order nociceptive nerve cells with their cell bodies in dorsal horns and their axon endings in the thalamus are divided into two types: some respond to a light stimulus and increase the response when the stimulus becomes more intense (harmful), and some only respond to harmful stimuli. These nerve cells are called WDR (wide dynamic ranger) and NS (nociceptive specific) nerve cells, respectively [7]. The synapses of second-order nociceptors and WDR nerve cells are somatotopically organised, but recent findings have shown that these synapses can be changed. The response of WDR nerve cells gradually increases as a consequence of repeated stimuli. This phenomenon is called "wind-up" of nerve cells; some spontaneous modifications have been found as a consequence of nociceptive stimuli (plastic modifications) [8].

They result in the extension of a nerve cell reception field, and also in sensitisation to stimuli other than nociceptive ones; therefore, this phenomenon, which is called "central sensitisation", is characterised by a facilitated activation of nerve cells in the spinothalamic section by nonpainful stimuli induced by slow-conducting fibres (C-amyelinated fibres). As a matter of fact, the wind-up mechanism can modify the anatomo-physiological characteristics of nerve cells through a range of biochemical and morphostructural events, which are not yet perfectly known and are universally called "neuroplasticity". This extremely complex phenomenon, which involves the release of chemical mediators, activation of secondary intracellular messengers, appearance of specific previously latent oncogenes, and modification of cyto-skeletal elements, is likely to create and represent a sort of neurochemical "memory" of previously suffered pains. Although the physiology of this phenomenon is not yet well known, a key event could be the intracellular transduction of extracellular signals leading to a cascade of phosphorylation–dephosphorylation events, which play an important role in the modulation of the activity of many molecules. In fact, repeated nociceptive stimulation entails the release of a range of excitatory neurotransmitters such as glutamate and aspartate amino acids, which activate the *N*-methyl-D-aspartate (NMDA) and alpha-amino-3-hydroxy-5-methyl-4-isoxazolepropionate (AMPA) receptors located in the nerve cells of dorsal horns [9]. In particular, NMDA receptors induce the release of substance P and neurokinin A, thus maintaining spinal hypersensitisation and reinforcing the transmission of nociceptive stimuli [10]. Following this activation of receptors, calcium rapidly increases in nerve cells and proto-oncogenes are transcribed; after repeated sensorial stimuli there is an increase in the expression of genes by some postsynaptic nerve cells. For instance, *c-fos* and *c-jun* proto-oncogenes fall within this cellular programme that ensures such aspects of synaptic plasticity as the ability of nerve cells to modify their synapses on the basis of previous, repeated, and intense events [11]. Therefore, the appearance of new antigens in spinal cord nerve cells, which is a phenotypic expression of the aforementioned proto-oncogenes, could be the first signal of a structural and chronic modification of the synthesis of proteins, which entails a persisting trail of pain.

When passing from acute pain to chronic pain, at the roots of dorsal ganglions other factors, such as the nitric oxide level, local blood flow regulation and glutaminergic mechanisms [12, 13], are likely to play an important part. Recently, efforts to relieve postoperative pain have focused on preventive treatments aimed at reducing the activation of the NMDA subtype of excitatory glutamate receptors. Although AMPA receptors are involved in the nociceptive mechanisms of the spinal cord, the effects of the antagonists of AMPA receptors are controversial: it was reported that they inhibit the first acute stage, but not the second, tonic, stage. These phenomena are very significant from a clinical point of view [8-14]; in fact, clinical manifestations associated with central sensitisation and secondary hyperalgesia lead to increased pain intensity, as well as to the appearance of allodynia and alterations in regional sympathetic tone [8]. Central sensitisation can persist for a long time after trauma because biochemical structural modifications can occur at dorsal horns, e.g. the expression of *c-fos* proto-oncogene, which is likely to be a marker of prolonged functional changes such as central sensitisation and "wind-up" [15].

Systemic effects of acute pain

Treatment is also necessary because acute pain is associated with modifications to organs and systems, whose involvement can be harmful to the patient. Tissue injury entails deep neuroendocrine changes owing to stimulation of the hypothalamus, which is directly linked to pain paths. These "stress reactions" are characterised by the incretion of catabolic hormones and inhibition of anabolic substances, such as testosterone and insulin. They lead to mobilisation of substrata, and also to hyperglycaemia and negative nitrogen balance. Although, at the beginning, hypermetabolism, which is associated with stress reactions, increases the energy available to the body, the said modifications, when persisting over time, can adversely affect the patient's outcome. Two mechanisms are involved. The first one, i.e. excessive loss of proteins, can lead to muscular mass reduction and, consequently, delayed functional recovery; the second, i.e. immunosuppression resulting from the decrease in immunoglobulins and white cell activity, can lead to increased sensitivity to infections. Together with the response of the hypothalamus, a sympathetic nervous system reaction appears, which directly affects the cardiovascular system. This increases hydrosaline retention and therefore the heart burden; angiotensin causes diffused vasoconstriction; catecholamines increase heart rate, myocardial contractility, and systemic vascular resistance. All these events lead to hypertension, tachycardia, and arrhythmia, which can lead to myocardial ischaemia in patients with reduced coronary reserve. Moreover, low hydrosaline retention, when associated with the aforementioned effects, can irreparably worsen situations of low haemodynamic compensation. From the respiratory point of view, neuroendocrine modifications increase extracellular water in the lungs, thus altering the ventilation/perfusion ratio. After surgery to chest and abdomen, pain induces reflexes that increase intercostal musculoskeletal tension, reduce the patient's residual functional capacity (RFC), and reduce the cough reflex, thus leading to hypoventilation and decreased overall pulmonary capacity. These modifications favour the appearance of atelectatic areas, which worsen the ventilation/perfusion ratio abnormality and lead to hypoxaemia. In the event of major surgery, these effects can reduce RFC by 25–50% from the preoperative values [16]. At first, hypoxaemia increases the ventilation/minute ratio, thus leading to hypocapnia; thereafter, owing to persisting respiratory hyperactivity, it can lead to respiratory insufficiency and hypercapnia in predisposed patients. The aforementioned neuroendocrine modifications are responsible for reflex inhibition of gastrointestinal functionality and subsequent postoperative ileus, which entails nausea, vomit, patient discomfort, and possibly worsened hyperventilation [17]. The consequences in terms of stress on the immune system are particularly interesting. Lymphocytopenia, leucocytosis, and reticular system depression can occur [18]. These effects lower the resistance to pathogens and could be a key factor in the development of perioperative infectious complications. The main stress-mediated effects on coagulation are alterations in blood viscosity, platelet functionality and fibrinolysis [19, 20]. All these effects entail hypercoagulation, which significantly increases the risk of deep vein thrombosis (DVT) and pulmonary embolism (PE) in compulsorily immobilised patients. Therefore, treatment of postoperative acute pain is essential not merely from the ethical and humane point of view, but also to considerably improve the patient's outcome, thus significantly reducing morbidity and mortality.

Recommendations for postoperative pain treatment

It is widely recognised that proper postoperative pain treatment considerably helps to improve perioperative morbidity, which is reflected in fewer postoperative complications, shorter hospital stay, and lower costs, especially in high-risk patients (ASA III-V) who have undergone major surgical operations [21]. Similarly, the risk/benefit ratio should be taken into account, given that complications of analgesic treatment techniques can never be excluded. All hospitals should implement postoperative acute pain treatment protocols for all patients who undergo surgery. At the same time, suitable pain measurement tools should be used for proper assessment of treatment effectiveness. Pain measurement should be added to the so-called vital parameters, such as heart rate, arterial pressure, temperature and diuresis, to be regularly monitored over the 24-hour period. Proper planning of postoperative pain treatment should take account of a range of factors:

- Expected incidence of postoperative pain intensity and length;
- Implementation of quickly available tools to "measure" and to "assess" pain at rest and in motion (verbal scales, numbered scales, relevant visual linear patterns);
- Organisation of existing resources;
- Identification of the staff involved in these procedures.

The determinants of postoperative pain [22]

1. Surgery:
   - Surgery location and nature of the injury that leads to surgery;
   - Characteristics of intraoperative trauma and type of anaesthesia, premedication, preparation;
   - Postoperative conditions: drains, tubes and catheters, feeding autonomy, canalisation.
2. Patient:
   - Age, sex, individual pain threshold;
   - Sociocultural factors, religious beliefs, personality, anxiety, depression, locus of control, cognitive and behavioural learning patterns, previous experiences;
   - Fear of drug addiction, overdose, side effects of drugs.
3. Environment:
   - Preoperative information and preparation;
   - Medical and paramedical staff, and their relationships with the patient;
   - Supporting staff (physiotherapists, psychologists, etc.) and supporting treatments for functional recovery (rehabilitation and early mobilisation);
   - Presence of elements supporting the patient's autonomy (enabling the patient to regain control over the situation).

Materials and methods

In the light of international experiences, and taking into account Rawal's Swedish model, we have tried to organise our assistance to patients who have undergone surgery by working, from September 1998, within the complex Anaesthesia, Reanimation and Analgesic Treatment organisation at the University of Trieste, which serves the Cattinara Hospital, a Postoperative Acute Pain Service (APS). This APS is focused on professional nurses, on the one hand, and practitioners specialising in anaesthesiology and reanimation, on the other, who work under the anaesthesiologist's supervision and have a key role, since they perform direct postoperative clinical monitoring of patients, especially with reference to regular recording of postoperative acute pain intensity on clinical records. Within this model, it is up to the operating theatre anaesthesiologist to decide whether the patient is to be admitted to APS or not, on the basis of the following inclusion criteria: (1) Patient with ASA = 2; (2) surgery length ≥ 3 h. Thereafter, the anaesthesiologist fills in the postoperative analgesic treatment record, which is collected by the APS professional nurse, who then monitors postoperative acute pain by means of a visual analogue scale (VAS).

A VAS value ≤ 3, corresponding to mild pain on an ordinal scale of adjectives, is acceptable. During the postoperative period pain intensity is measured and recorded, together with the other vital parameters, every hour in the waking-up room until the patient becomes stable and a VAS ≤ 3 is obtained. Thereafter, it is measured and recorded every 3 h in surgical wards for the first 48–72 h.

Moreover, we usefully tried to identify, for each type of surgery, some groups of surgical operations that are postoperatively associated with mild, moderate and severe pain, and to identify for each group the drug or mixture of drugs that is the most effective. For instance, with reference to mild pain, FANS or paracetamol (p.o. or i.v.) is enough. With reference to moderate pain, combinations of FANS-meperidine or FANS-tramadol (i.v.) are recommended. Alternatively, in the event of peridural administration, local anaesthetics or opioids, alone or combined, can be used. Finally, with reference to severe pain the pattern used for moderate pain can be applied but with the relevant doses increased. In this case, morphine-FANS (i.v.) or morphine-local anaesthetic (peridurally administered) combinations should be preferred.

Results

From 1 January to 31 December, 2002 the APS at the Cattinara Hospital holistically followed up 1,170 patients (694 males [60%], 462 females [39%] and 14 transsexuals [1%]), with a mean age of 61.6±16.4 years (m±SD) and a range comprised between 5 and 97 years. The said patients had undergone various types of surgery. The breakdown of patients by type of surgery and by type of surgical operation showed a marked prevalence of general surgical operations (*n*=638; 54.53%) and major surgical operations (*n*=565, 48.29%). With reference to primary analgesic methods, the most popular technique was intravenous administration (*n*=1008; 86.15%), followed by peridural administration (*n*=149; 12.74%), mixed intravenous/peridural administration (*n*=3; 0.26%), rectal administration (*n*=3; 0.26%), subcutaneous administration (*n*=1; 0.09%), subarachnoid administration (*n*=1; 0.09%), and oral administration (*n*=1; 0.09%); with reference to administration devices, the most popular device was the elastomeric pump (*n*=961; 82.14%), followed by phleboclysis (*n*=187;15.98%), boluses (*n*=11; 0.94%), phleboclysis/boluses (*n*=1; 0.09%), and microjet (*n*=1; 0.09%). In 182 patients (15.56%), skin infiltration was performed; moreover, 688 patients (58.80%) required postoperative recharges, whereas the analgesic treatment administered during the first 48 h was sufficient for the rest of patients. Furthermore, 82.73% of patients (*n*=968) received intraoperative analgesic boluses, i.v.-administered FANS in 38.84% of cases

(n=376), i.v.-administered opioid in 53% (n=513), and peridurally administered opioid in 8.16% (n=79). The i.v.-administered analgesic mixture (n=1008) was made up of FANS in 6 cases (0.6%), opioids in 289 cases (28.67%) and a combination of both in 713 cases (70.73%). The FANS administered was ketorolac in 100% of cases, with an average dose over 48 h of 129.01±48.23 mg (m±SD); the opioids administered were meperidine in 757 cases (75.55%), with an average dose over 48 h of 319.42±105.56 mg (m±SD) and an average dose (mg kg^{-1} h^{-1}) over 48 h of 0.105±0.038 mg (m±SD); morphine in 87 cases (8.68%) with an average dose over 48 h of 41.32±14.29 mg (m±SD), and an average dose (mg kg^{-1} h^{-1}) over 48 h of 0.012±0.0033 (m±SD); tramadol in 156 cases (15.57%) with an average dose over 48 h of 235.26±186.68 mg (m±SD), and an average dose (mg kg^{-1} h^{-1}) over 48 h of 0.55±3.22 (m±SD).
The peridurally administered analgesic mixture (n=149) was morphine in 4 cases (2.68%), local anaesthetic in 42 cases (28.19%), morphine and local anaesthetic in 101 cases (67.78%), and other drugs in 2 cases (1.34%). The average dose of morphine over 24 h was 3.031±2.049 mg (m±SD) with an average dose (mg kg^{-1} h^{-1}) over 24 h of 0.00084±0.00041 (m±SD); the local anaesthetics administered were bupivacaine in 27 cases (18.88%) with an average dose over 24 h of 70.50±33.70 mg (m±SD) and an average percentage concentration of 0.14±0.13 (m±SD); ropivacaine in 110 cases (76.92%) with an average dose over 24 hours of 167.83±52.72 mg (m±SD) and an average percentage concentration of 0.138±0.044 (m±SD); levobupivacaine in 4 cases (2.80%), with an average dose over 24 h of 91.66±26.02 mg (m±SD), and an average percentage concentration of 0.47±0.25 (m±SD). With reference to 328 treated patients (28.03%), the analgesic treatment was not enough; they therefore required a "rescue dose" during the first 24 h after surgery. The rescue medication was FANS in 142 cases (44.24%). It was administered to 126 patients (88.76%), by the i.v. primary analgesic technique, with an average dose of 34.56±16.72 mg (m±SD) and to 17 patients (11.97%), by peridural primary analgesic technique, with an average dose of 30.00±0.00 mg (m±SD). The rescue medication consisted of opioids in 188 cases (58.56%). It was administered to 180 patients (95.74%) by the intravenous primary analgesic technique; the opioids administered were morphine in 21 cases (11.67%), with an average dose of 7.22±8.08 mg (m±SD), meperidine in 151 cases (83.89%) with an average dose of 66.33±53.12 mg (m±SD), and tramadol in 8 cases (4.44%), with an average dose of 87.5±23.14 mg (m±SD).

Opiate rescue doses were also administered to 8 patients (4.25%) by the peridural primary analgesic technique; the opioids administered were morphine in 6 cases (75%), with an average dose of 3.33±1.37 mg (m±SD), and meperidine in 2 cases (25%) with an average dose of 20.00±0.00 mg (m±SD). Finally, the rescue medication was a local anaesthetic in 49 patients (15.26%) treated by the peridural primary analgesic technique; the local anaesthetic administered were ropivacaine in 42 cases (87.50%), with an average percentage concentration of 0.186±0.035 (m±SD) and an average amount of 6.84±2.36 ml (m±SD); bupivacaine in 6 cases (12.50%), with an average percentage concentration of 0.073±0.043 (m±SD) and an average amount of 9.83±6.21 ml (m±SD); and levobupivacaine in 1 case (2.00%), with an average percentage concentration of 0.125, and an average amount of 6 ml. With reference to postoperative monitoring, the overall trend of VAS in followed-up patients was consistently ≤3 both at rest and during movement; the same held true for the patients who had undergone general surgical, orthopaedic, otolaryngological, plastic, and urological operations.

Conversely, the patients who had undergone neurosurgical and chest surgical operations recorded values ≥3 at the first measurements, especially in motion, but never values in excess of 4, i.e. the upper threshold accepted by many hospitals and in line with the said type of surgery, which is particularly stressful for the patient. With reference to the type of surgery, the trend of VAS for operations of minor, medium, and major severity was always acceptable (the values were always ≤3). Moreover, during the postoperative period, the following elements were analysed: (a) stages of sedation during the first, second, and third hours, which were 0.97±0.82 (m±SD), 0.69±0.70 (m±SD), and 0.38±0.58 (m±SD), respectively; (b) breathing frequencies during the first, second, and third hours, which were 18.86±3.33 breaths per minute (m±SD), 18.94± 3.07 breaths per minute (m±SD), and 19.79± 2.86 breaths per minute (m±SD), respectively; (c) stages of motor block after peridural analgesia, according to the simplified Bromage scale, which were, at the first hour, stage 1 for 103 patients (69.13%), stage 2 for 7 patients (4.70%), and stage 3 for 1 patient (0.67%); at the second hour, stage 1 for 98 patients (65.77%), stage 2 for 2 patients (1.34%), and stage 3 for 1 patient (0.67%); at the third hour, stage 1 for 103 patients (69.13%), stage 2 for 1 patient (0.67%), and stage 3 for 1 patient (0.67%); (d) incidence of hypotension (AP≤100), which was recorded in 80 patients only (6.84%). Other side effects appeared in 154 patients (13.16%), namely: nausea/vomiting in 51 cases (4.36%), mental confusion in 43 cases (3.68%), headache in 14 cases (1.20%), dysphoria/hallucinations in 13 cases (1.11%), itching in 8 cases (0.68%), restlessness/anxiety in 7 cases (0.60%), paraesthesia in lower limbs in 6 cases (0.51%), raised temperature in 4 cases (0.34%), shivering in 1 case (0.09%), vasodepressor syncope in 1 case (0.09%), erythema in 1 case (0.09%), respiratory standstill in 1 case (0.09%), and phlebitis in 1 case (0.09%). The average length of primary analgesia was 75.21±35.66 h (m±SD), with a range of 0–216 hours; in 2002, total paramedical checks were 12,209, with an average per patient of 10.53±5.17 (m±SD), whereas total medical checks were 2,607, with an average per patient of 2.27±1.50 (m±SD), and a range of 0–10.

Discussion and conclusions

The APS at the Cattinara Hospital, as presently organised, has been repeatedly changed from September 1998. At first, in addition to operating theatre anaesthesiologists, the project envisaged pain treatment nurses and practitioners specialising in anaesthesiology, the identification of paramedical and surgical "representative staff members" within the various wards, and of a co-ordinating anaesthesiologist to be responsible for the APS, who were intented to interact with the paramedical and medical staff on the various wards and with the out-patient department anaesthesiologist. In practice, owing to difficulties in identifying "pain representatives" within the various wards, as well as an anaesthesiologist responsible for the APS, the service, which has been in operation since 1998, has been relying essentially on operating theatre anaesthesiologists, pain nurses, practitioners specialising in anaesthesiology, ward nurses and surgeons, supported by the anaesthesiologist on duty, who interact between themselves and with the out-patient department anaesthesiologist, thus covering all working days from 7:30 a.m. to 7:30 p.m. In the light of several qualitative and quantitative data analyses, some changes to the original organisation were recommended. The first development of the APS at the Cattinara Hospital occurred between 1998 and 2001, and was the suppression of the operating theatre anaesthesiologist's function; in this model, all patients who undergo surgery are dealt with according to the standard protocols and orders for their type of surgery, which are prescribed by the operating theatre anaesthesiologist, who also decides whether or not to admit the patient to the APS, according to the aforementioned inclusion criteria. In this case too, the key elements are pain nurses and practitioners specialising in anaesthesiology, who interact with the anaesthesiologist and with surgical wards and are supported by the chronic pain team. The limit of this model is coverage, since the service is provided from Monday to Friday, and from 7:30 a.m. to 7:30 p.m. Therefore, nights and non-working days are not covered. The second development took place in 2002: the problem of coverage provided during the day and on working days only was overcome by training, educating and raising the awareness of practitioners specialising in anaesthesiology, who, thanks to beepers for emergencies, can cover nights and non-working days, thus supporting the action of the anaesthesiologist on duty, and ensuring a 24-h coverage to patients. In 2002, the APS at the Cattinara Hospital provided full follow-up for 1,170 patients, i.e. 20.34% of patients that had undergone surgery (*n*=5752); although this rate can be regarded as relatively low in absolute terms, it includes the patients who are worst affected from a psychophysical point of view, who required a special assistance during their postoperative period and were directly followed up by the APS team. The rest of the patients were followed up by the staff of their own surgical wards, according to standard analgesic protocols and prescriptions entered by the operating theatre anaesthesiologist in their anaesthesiology records. The analyses performed on the data obtained in our study confirm the effectiveness of the APS, which is undoubtedly an effective organisational approach to the control of postoperative acute pain. Moreover, the low incidence of side effects, the overall VAS value both at rest and during movement and for the various types of surgery, which was consistently ≤3 during the first 4 days of postoperative hospitalisation, demonstrate that our postoperative analgesic protocols, which use relatively low drug doses (close to, although higher than, the effective dose of 50), are safe. The evolution of patients' perioperative management, and in particular, of postoperative acute pain treatment, presupposes a sort of "resumption" of the original APS Trieste project in line with the act dated May 24, 2001, which adopted the "Painless Hospital" project. Finally, we would like to suggest and recommend the following priorities to guarantee an increasingly well-qualified health service meeting the population's needs and expectations: preference of patient safety and simple techniques in all circumstances; progression to regular pain measurement and recording; choice of operations on the basis of evidence; whenever possible, tailoring treatments to individual patients' needs; choice of the most suitable drugs, types, and modes of administration; initiation of a permanent training and education process for the staff working in health facilities; provision of information to raise public awareness.

References

1. Italian Republic (2001) Act dated May 24, 2001. Agreement entered into by the Ministry of Health, the Regions, and the Autonomous Provinces on the guidelines relative to the project "Painless Hospital". Official Journal of the Italian Republic; general series no. 149 (29/06/2001)
2. Ready LB, Oden R, Chadwich HS et al (1988) Development of an anesthesiology-based postoperative pain management service. Anesthesiology 68:100-106
3. Rawal N, Berggren L (1994) Organization of acute pain service: a low cost model. Pain 57:117-123
4. Cronin M, Redfern PA, Utting JE (1973) Psychiatry and postoperative complaints in surgical patients. Br J Anaesth 45:879-884
5. Raja SN, Meyer RA, Campbell JN (1988) Peripheral mechanism of somatic pain. Anesthesiology 68:571-580

6. Raja SN, Campbell JN, Meyer RA (1984) Evidence for different mechanism of primary and secondary hyperalgesia. Brain 107:1179-1188
7. Besson JM, Chaouch A (1987) Peripheral and spinal mechanism of nociception. Physiol Rev 67:67
8. Woolf CJ (1983) Evidence for a central component of post-injury pain hypersensitivity. Nature 306:686-688
9. Liu H, Mantyh PW, Basbaum AI (1997) NMDA-receptor regulation of substance P release from primary afferent nociceptors. Nature 386:721-724
10. Harris JA, Corsi M, Quartaroli M et al (1996) Upregulation of spinal glutamate receptor in chronic pain. Neuroscience 74:7-12
11. Schaible HG, Jarrott B, Hope PJ, Duggan AW (1990) Release of immunoreactive substance P in the spinal cord during development of acute arthritis in the knee joint of the cat: a study with antibody microprobes. Brain Res 529:214-223
12. Meller ST, Gebhart GF (1993) Nitric oxide (NO) and nociceptive processing in the spinal cord. Pain 52:127-136
13. Coderre TJ (1993) The role of excitatory aminoacid receptors and intracellular messengers in persistent nociception after tissue injury in rats. Mol Neurobiol 7:229-246
14. Woolf CJ (1989) Recent advances in the pathophysiology of acute pain. Br J Anaesth 63:139-146
15. Hunt SP, Pini A, Evan G (1987) Induction of c-fos-like protein in spinal cord neurons following sensory stimulation. Nature 328:632-634
16. Rawal N, Sjostrand U, Christofferson E et al (1984) Comparison of intramuscolar and epidural morphine for post-operative analgesia in grossly obese. Influence on post-operative ambulation and pulmonary function. Anesth Analg 63:583-592
17. Donovan I, Alexander-Williams J (1976) Postoperative gastric retention and delayed gastric emptying. Surg Clin North Am 56:1413
18. Pollock RE, Lotzova E, Stanford SD (1991) Mechanism of surgical stress impairment of human perioperative natural killer cell cytotoxicity. Arch Surg 126:338-342
19. Tuman KJ, Spiess BD, McCarthy RJ, Ivankovich AD (1987) Effects of progressive blood loss on coagulation as measured by thromboelastography. Anesth Analg 66:856-863
20. Garcia-Frade LJ, Landin L, Avello AG et al (1987) Changes in fibrinolysis in the intensive care patient. Thromb Res 47:593 599
21. Ballantyne JC, Carr DB, De Ferranti S et al (1998) The comparative effects of post operative analgesic therapies on pulmonary outcome: cumulative meta-analyses of randomized, controlled trials. Anesth Analg 86:598-612
22. Nolli M, Nicosia F (2000) Postoperative pain management. Aims and organization of a strategy for postoperative acute pain therapy. Minerva Anestesiol 66:585-601

BLOOD TRANSFUSION

Platelet transfusion: when, how and how much?

V. De Angelis

The use of platelets in therapy has become widespread in recent decades. The treatment of haematological and nonhaematological malignancies, bone marrow transplantation procedures and cardiac surgery are responsible for the vast majority of platelet transfusions. However, transfusion of platelets is associated with different post-transfusion reactions: infections due to bacterial contamination are the most frequent side effects of platelet transfusion, but, although less frequent, alloimmunisation, febrile nonhaemolytic reactions, viral infections and transfusion-associated lung injury (TRALI) are also detected by the network of haemovigilance [1]. Finally, platelet concentrates are very costly blood components, and blood and blood components are becoming increasingly scarce in Europe.

This paper will deal with the elements that help clinicians to identify patients who will benefit from platelet transfusion ("When"), how to transfuse platelets properly and to perform the post-transfusion surveillance ("How") and what is the correct amount of platelets to be transfused ("How much") in order to maximise benefits and to minimise risks of transfusion and to allow proper utilisation of this scarce and costly resource.

Platelet products

Platelets for transfusion can be prepared either by separation from units of whole blood or by apheresis from a single donor [2]. In the first case, four to six platelet concentrates from whole blood (PCs-WB), each containing from $0.55\text{-}0.75 \times 10^{11}$ platelets, represent a standard "therapeutic dose"; commonly, in Europe the concentrates are pooled in a single bag and resuspended either in plasma or in protein-free additive solution, to reduce the amount of plasma and/or to allow reinfusion in plasma-incompatible recipients. The single-donor platelets are produced by apheresis technologies (SD-PA), and current standards require that a SD-PA will contain at least 2×10^{11} platelets but usually a content of 3×10^{11} platelets per bag is standard in the European blood establishments [3].

Different studies [4, 5] have shown that the two preparations are comparable in post-transfusion recovery, platelet survival and haemostatic effects. Thus, the main differences are related to costs (which are higher for SD-PA than for PCs-WB) and to the availability of the product; clearly, when requiring platelets matched by HLA or platelet-specific antigens for alloimmunised recipients, the SD-PA product is the only possibility. Also, there can be concern about the pool origin of the PCs-WB, which exposes the recipient to a greater number of donors, thus increasing the likelihood of infection transmission; however, current techniques used in blood banks to test blood units for different infectious agents have greatly reduced this risk and there is no evidence of any difference in transfusion-transmitted infection rates between oncology patients receiving SD-PA and PCs-WB preparations. Moreover, although beyond the scope of this review, methods for inactivation of pathogens in platelet preparations are currently under investigation in blood establishments and in a few years products meeting higher safety standards will become available [6].

When

In clinical practice, it is commonly recognised that with a platelet count higher than 50,000/mL bleeding due to thrombocytopenia is highly improbable, while, with a platelet count between 10,000 and 50,000/μL, it becomes possible only following trauma, invasive procedures, ulceration etc.; the probability of spontaneous bleeding with platelet counts between 5,000 and 10,000/mL and less than 5,000/μL is high and very high, respectively.

The decision to transfuse a patient with thrombocytopenia must be taken with due consideration for:

1. Origin of thrombocytopenia
2. Platelet count
3. Coexisting diseases and/or medications
4. Platelet function
5. Surgery

Thrombocytopenia resulting from decreased production

Most commonly, severe thrombocytopenia starts after chemotherapy for the treatment of haematological and nonhaematological malignancies. However, bone marrow aplasia, myelodysplasia and bone marrow (or stem cell) transplantation show similar patterns of decreased production of platelets.

Although there are no randomised studies comparing the incidence of serious bleeding and survival in patients transfused prophylactically vs therapeutically, prophylactic transfusion of platelets in severe thrombocytopenic patients is a commonly accepted clinical practice, and the ASCO guidelines for platelet transfusion [7] recommend that "prophylactic platelet transfusion be administered to patients with thrombocytopenia resulting from impaired bone marrow function." The number of 10,000 platelets/μL as threshold for prophylactic transfusion in adult leukaemia is generally accepted, since it is based on level I evidence and is scored as a grade A recommendation; moreover, the same threshold seems to be acceptable in paediatric leukaemia patients. However, higher thresholds may be accepted in newborns or in the presence of comorbidities, such as haemorrhage, hyperthermia, hyperleukocytosis, rapidly decreasing platelet count, coexisting coagulation abnormalities or use of antiplatelet drugs. Platelet transfusion is also indicated at higher levels when patients undergo invasive procedures (see below).

A similar practical approach also seems to be useful for patients with solid tumours [7].

Thrombocytopenia resulting from increased consumption

Patients with immune thrombocytopenia (ITP) and patients with spleen enlargement (e.g. cirrhotic patients) usually do not benefit from platelet transfusion; in ITP, platelets transfused are immediately destroyed by the antibodies of the recipient, while in the second case they are trapped in the enlarged spleen and are not available for the haemostatic function. In thrombotic thrombocytopenic purpura, transfusion of platelets is not indicated or even contraindicated, owing to the possible thrombogenic effect of the transfusion. The same appears to be true for disseminated intravascular coagulation (DIC), unless a contextual appropriate therapy for the underlying cause of DIC is effective [8].

Platelet dysfunction

Platelet dysfunction may originate in congenital or acquired conditions that impair a normal adhesive or aggregating platelet function. In Glanzmann and in Bernard-Soulier syndromes, two inherited platelet defects, the absence or the alteration of membrane glycoproteins that mediate the interaction of platelet with adhesion molecules leads to impaired platelet capability for interactation with injured vessels, thus leading to a bleeding tendency [9]. However, the most common causes of impaired platelet function are related to the use antiplatelet drugs (e.g. ASA or monoclonal antibodies against platelet membrane glycoproteins) or to underlying diseases, such as myeloma and uraemia. In all these conditions platelet transfusion must be considered only in the case of active bleeding or if surgery is needed.

For patients treated with monoclonal antibodies inhibiting the function of platelet membrane receptorial glycoproteins, a recent report by Lemmer [10] suggests that transfusion of one standard platelet concentrate allows a successful cardiac operation in a patient receiving antibodies until a few hours before operation.

Surgery

Thrombocytopenic patients may need invasive diagnostic or therapeutic procedures. There are several lines of evidence to show that with a platelet count higher than 40,000-50,000/μL patients do not require platelet transfusion during major surgery [11]; however, some procedures (e.g. bone marrow aspiration and lumbar puncture) can also be safely performed at a count of 20,000/μL [12], while in neurosurgery, cardiac surgery or surgery in some anatomical districts, e.g. the eye, where even modest bleeding can be very harmful, a platelet count as high as 100,000/μL may be needed [13]. Regardless of the platelet count, platelet transfusion may be necessary if a patient treated with inhibitors of platelet membrane glycoproteins mediating the interaction of platelets with adhesion molecules is undergoing surgery [10].

If platelets are administered before surgery a platelet count must be performed to ensure that the target increase in platelet count has been reached.

Conditions in which platelet transfusion is indicated and those in which it must be avoided [14] are summarized in Table 1:

Table 1 Indications and contraindications for platelet transfusion

Common indications	
1.	Congenital or acquired platelet defects in patients undergoing surgery or actively bleeding
Surgical indications:	
1.	Platelet count > 50,000/μL is accepted in patients undergoing most surgical interventions and vaginal delivery
2.	Platelet count between 50,000 and 100,000/μL may be required for neurological, cardiac, ocular and some ORL interventions
Medical indications:	
1.	< 10,000/μL in patients with thrombocytopenia due to bone marrow aplasia (e.g. after chemotherapy for haematological and nonhaematological malignancies) when stable and without signs of bleeding
2.	< 20,000/μL patients with thrombocytopenia due to bone marrow aplasia and one of more of the following conditions: bleeding, rapidly decreasing platelet count, fever, infections, spleen enlargement, use of antiplatelet or anticoagulant drugs

Platelet transfusion should not be performed	
1.	In patients with thrombocytopenia due to increased consumption (immune thrombocytopenia, thrombotic thrombocytopenic purpura, DIC)
2.	As a prophylaxis for extracorporeal circulation
3.	As a prophylaxis for bleeding if platelet count is 10,000/μL, the patient is stable and no complications are recorded

How

Platelets express ABO antigens on their membrane, and therefore ABO compatibility should be respected when transfusing platelets; however, transfusion of ABO-incompatible platelets is associated with a lower, but not absent, platelet recovery; therefore, in critical conditions of platelet availability, an ABO-mismatched transfusion can be safely performed, provided that the patient's life is at risk [8]. The amount of plasma in which platelets are suspended (normally about 250 mL) makes any haemolytic reaction in the recipient due to plasma incompatibility or to fluid overload unlikely, except in paediatric patients: in this case, the suspension of platelets in a small-volume, protein-free additive solution will avoid unfavourable reactions [15].

Platelets do not express Rh(D) antigens on their membrane; nevertheless, red cells contaminating platelet concentrates may cause anti-D immunization in the recipient. There is a wide consensus that at least RhD negative children and women of childbearing age should receive anti-D immunoprophylaxis when transfused with platelets from Rh(D) positive donors. A dose of 25 μg of anti-D immunoglobulin will protect against 1 ml of Rh(D) positive red cells and should be given as soon as possible and within 72 hrs from the exposure [16].

Platelet concentrate are stored in the blood bank at a controlled temperature (22±2°C) and with gentle agitation to prevent aggregation, which would make the transfusion ineffective. Therefore, platelet concentrate, once issued by the blood bank to the clinical ward, must be immediately transfused, since different conditions of temperature or storage allow rapid and irreversible impairment of platelet function. Platelets must never be kept at a temperature below 20°C.

It must be also outlined that, due to the limited shelf-life of stored platelets, platelets for patients scheduled for surgery must not be transfused on the day before the intervention, but not until immediately before surgery, to obtain the maximum haemostatic efficacy.

Finally, the time required for platelet transfusion must not exceed 20-30 min.

Patients receiving a platelet transfusion must be observed, in the subsequent period, for the possible appearance of post-transfusion complications, such as allergic reactions, hyperthermia, sepsis (due to bacterial contamination of the concentrate) and TRALI. In any case of undesired side effects, the blood bank must be immediately notified and a consultant from the blood bank medical staff must evaluate the case.

How much

The coexistence of thrombocytopenia and bleeding (or highly probable bleeding risk) defines the need for platelet transfusion. The amount of platelets to be transfused must take into consideration the actual condition of the patient and the increment necessary to reach a platelet count sufficient to stop bleeding and to prevent re-bleeding. Therefore, the amount of platelets to be transfused can be defined by the platelet count to be reached in the patient, starting from the recorded count, bearing in mind that the platelet splenic pool accounts for about 30% of the total platelet number:

Dose: desired increment (platelets/μL) × patient's blood volume × 1.5:

Clearly, different factors may influence the increment of platelet count following transfusion and, therefore, the dose of platelets to be transfused. For instance, in cases of platelet functional defect (whether congenital or acquired) the quantitative criteria cannot be utilised and platelet transfusion will be required only in patients at very high risk of bleeding (e.g. before surgery) or actually bleeding, regardless of the platelet count or the "desired increment". Moreover, although the expected post-transfusion platelet recovery in mathematical models is about 60%, the coexistence of comorbidities may lower the recovery to 40% or 20% and also frustrate the effort to increase platelet count following allogeneic platelet transfusion. Fever, sepsis, bleeding, consumption coagulopathy, antiplatelet and/or anticoagulant drugs, antibiotics and antimycotics progressively lower the post-transfusion increment, while the presence of antiplatelet alloantibodies causes a true refractory state. Thus, platelet counts performed 1 h and 24 h after the end of platelet transfusion can help in differentiating a refractory state due to antiplatelet alloantibodies (with lack of response 1 h after the transfusion) from an accelerated consumption of the transfused platelets (which appears as a platelet increment after 1 h but a fall of the platelet count to baseline after 24 h). Therefore, this simple approach can help in monitoring the efficacy of transfusion and the need for more platelet transfusion.

Many guidelines and consensus conferences have focused attention on protocols for the optimal dose in platelet transfusion and the more recent published data are summarised below:

1) NIH Consensus Conference on platelet transfusion [17]: 5 U of platelet concentrate in adult patients
2) British Committee for Standards in Haematology [18]: dose: desired increment × estimated blood volume of patient / 0.67.
3) Council and Scientific Advisory board of the German Medical Association [19]: dose: desired increment × blood volume × 1.5
4) American Society of Anesthesiologists Task Force on Blood Component Therapy [6]: therapeutic dose: 1 platelet concentrate/10 kg body weight.

Some recently published trials performed in patients with haematological malignancies [20-22] seem to suggest that higher amounts of transfused platelets are associated with higher post-transfusion increment, longer transfusion-free intervals and, as a result, with lower costs of platelet transfusion; thus, the recommended transfusion dose in thrombocytopenic patients with haematological malignancies is 0.7×10^{11} platelets/kg body weight, corresponding to 1.5 W/10 kg body weight or a SD-PA containing $5\text{-}6 \times 10^{11}$ platelets. Clearly, although very suggestive, these data must be confirmed.

Finally, the ultimate decision on transfusion must be taken with due consideration for the clinical circumstances of the patient and the policy of the local blood establishment on production and use of blood components. To emphasise this conclusion, the Consensus Conference on Platelet Transfusion held by the Royal College of Physicians of Edinburgh recommend the use of a "single therapeutic dose" and a "unit-by-unit" practice with monitoring of patient response to transfusion [23].

Essential indicators that must be taken into account when evaluating patient response to platelet transfusion are [24]:

1. Clinical efficacy (cessation of bleeding).
2. Platelet recovery (R):
   R = (Platelet count after transfusion – Platelet count before transfusion)/Number of transfused platelets × 100.
3. Post-transfusion corrected count increment (CCI):

CCI = (Platelet count/ml after transfusion – Platelet count before transfusion)/ Number of transfused platelets (× 10^{11} platelets) × Body surface area.

4. Post-transfusion survival of platelets: the corrected increment (CCI) is evaluated 1 h and 24 h after transfusion; CCI of at least 7.5×10^9 platelets/L at 1 h and of at least 4.5×10^9 platelets/L at 24 h after transfusion are considered acceptable, while lower values indicate a refractory state, either immunological or nonimmunological.

Conclusions

Blood establishments must maintain a fully implemented quality system in the preparation and storage of platelet concentrates to guarantee high standards of the products and thus ensure a controlled and effective platelet transfusion with viable thrombocytes. On the other hand, clinicians must control, as far as possible, all events that may negatively influence the effectiveness of platelet transfusion. Moreover, a multidisciplinary approach is highly recommended, in which clinicians and transfusion medicine specialists define a policy aimed at selecting both platelet preparation and conditions of use which optimise transfusion efficacy and increase the duration of transfusion-free intervals in patients. Finally, research must develop indicators aimed at predicting transfusion need and monitoring the effectiveness of platelet transfusion.

References

1. Wilkinson J, Wilkinson C (2001) Administration of blood transfusions to adults in general hospital settings: a review of the literature. J Clin Nurs 10:161-170
2. Murphy S, Heaton WA, Rebulla P (1996) Platelet production in the Old World – and the New. Transfusion 36:751-754
3. Council of Europe (1988) Guide to the preparation, use and quality assurance of blood components, 4th edn.
4. Patel IP, Ambinder E, Holland JF et al (1978) In vivo and in vitro comparison of single donor platelets and multiple-donor pooled platelets transfusions in leukemic patients. Transfusion 18:116-119
5. Turner VS, Hawker RJ, Mitchell SG et al (1994) Paired in vivo and in vitro comparison of apheresis and recovered platelet concentrates stored for five days. J Clin Apheresis 9:189-194
6. Corbin F (2002) Pathogen inactivation of blood colmponents: current status and introduction of an approach using riboflavin as a photosensitizer. Int J Hematol 76 (Suppl 2):253-257
7. Schiffer CA, Anderson KC, Bennet CL (2001) Platelet transfusion for patients with cancer: clinical practice guidelines of the American Society for Clinical Oncology. J Clin Oncol 19:1519-1538
8. Mollison PL, Engelfriet CP, Contreras M (1993) Blood transfusion in clinical medicine, 9th edn. Blackwell Scientific Publications, Oxford
9. LoScalzo J, Scheffer AI (1998) Thrombosis and hemorrhage. Williams Wilkins, Baltimore
10. Lemmer JH Jr, Metzdorff MT, Krause AH Jr et al (2000) Emergency coronary artery bypass graft surgery in abciximab-treated patients. Ann Thorac Surg 69:90-95
11. National Institutes of Health (1987) Consensus Conference: Platelet transfusion therapy.Transfus Med Rev 1:195-200
12. Howard SC, Gajjr A, Ribeiro RC et al (2000) Safety of lumbar puncture in children with acute lymphoblastic leukemia and thrombocytopenia. JAMA 284:2222-2224
13. Practice guidelines for blood component therapy. A report by the American Society of Anesthesiologists Task Force on Blood Component Therapy (1996) Anesthesiology 84:732-745
14. Norfolk DR, Ancliffe PJ, Contreras M et al (1998) Consensus Conference on platelet transfusion. Royal College of Physicians of Edinburgh. Br J Haematol 101:609-617
15. Heatn WAL, Rebulla P, Pappalettera M et al (1997) A comparative analysis of different methods for routine blood components preparation. Transfus Med Rev 11:116-129

16. Lee D, Contreras M, Robson SC et al (1999) Recommendations for the use of anti-D immunoglobin for Rh prophylaxis. Transfus Med Rev 9:93-97
17. NIH Consensus Conference on platelet transfusion (1987) Transfus Med Rev 3:195-217
18. Murphy MF, Brozovic B, Murphy W et al (1992) Guidelines for platelet transfusions. British Committee for Standards in Haematology, Working Party of the Blood Transfusion Task Force. Transfus Med 2:311-318
19. Council and Scientific Advisory Board of the German Medical Association (1995) Guidelines for therapy with blood components and plasma derivatives. Deutscher Ärtze-Verlag
20. Roy AJ, Jaffe N, Djerassi I (1973) Prophylactic platelet transfusions in children with acute leukemia: a dose response study. Transfusion 13:283-290
21. Norol F, Bierling P, Roudot-Thoraval F et al (1998) Platelet transfusion: a dose-response study. Blood 92:1448-1453
22. Ackerman SJ, Klumpp TR, Guzman GI et al (2000) Economic consequences of alterations in platelet transfusion dose: analysis of a prospective, randomized, double-blind trial. Transfusion 40:1457-1462
23. Royal College of Physicians of Edinburgh (1998) Consensus Conference on Platelet Transfusion. Transfus Med 8:149-151
24. Davis KB, Slichter SJ, Corash L (1999) Corrected count increment and percent platelet recovery as measures of posttransfusion platelet response: problems and a solution. Transfusion 39:586-592

Erythropoietin in the critically ill

H.L. Corwin

The issues surrounding red blood cell (RBC) transfusion are important in the critically ill. Anaemia is very common in the critically ill; almost 95% of patients admitted to the intensive care unit (ICU) have a haemoglobin level below normal by ICU day 3 [1]. As a result, critically ill patients receive a significant number of RBC transfusions during their ICU stay. Studies almost a decade ago found that over 50% of all patients admitted to the ICU were transfused during their ICU stay [2]. Among patients with a prolonged ICU stay (greater than 1 week), 85% received a transfusion [3]. On average, these latter patients were each transfused with over 9 units of RBCs during their ICU admission. These transfusions were not restricted to the early ICU course, but rather were transfused at a rate of 2 to 3 units per week. In a descriptive study of critical care units in the United States [4], on a single day almost 14% of patients in critical care units are transfused (ranging from 4% in CCUs to 27% in SICUs).

Transfusion practice in response to this anaemia has changed little over the last decade. In a recent survey of 4,892 ICU patients, approximately 50% of patients admitted to ICUs across the United States had received transfusions on average of almost 5 RBC units [5]. There were also ongoing RBC transfusions given to these patients throughout their ICU stay. These observations are virtually identical to those made in earlier studies [2-4]. Similarly, the mean pre-transfusion haemoglobin observed, i.e. the "transfusion trigger", was 8.6 g/dL, also comparable to that described in earlier reports [2, 3]. RBC transfusions were not restricted to the ICU. Thirteen percent of patients discharged from the ICU received almost three RBC units following ICU discharge. Post-ICU RBC transfusions increased the total number of RBC units transfused by almost 15%, and therefore had a significant impact on the total number of RBC units administered to critically ill patients.

A similar observational study of transfusion practice in ICUs across Western Europe has also been reported [6]. Data were collected on 3,534 patients admitted to ICUs during a 2-week period in late 1999. A total of 42% of patients were transfused with approximately 5 RBC units during the 28-day study period. The mean pre-transfusion haemoglobin level was 8.4 g/dL. The similarity of the results of this study, of the US study and of our study is striking and suggests a remarkable consistency in current transfusion practice within the critical care community.

A major factor contributing to anaemia and the need for blood transfusions in the critically ill patient is phlebotomy. Smoller and Kruskall [7] found that almost half of their ICU patients receiving blood transfusions were phlebotomised with withdrawal of more than the equivalent of 1 unit of blood. The ICU patients reported in this study, on average, had 65 cc per day taken by phlebotomy. Phlebotomy blood losses in this range are consistent with those in other reports on critically ill patients and are often associated with the development of anaemia [2].

However, the view of anaemia in the critically ill as simply the result of excess phlebotomy is not completely accurate [8]. Red cell production in critically ill patients is not normal, and decreased levels of RBC production are also involved in the development and maintenance of the anaemia observed in the critically ill. There is a growing literature suggesting that the anaemia observed in the critically ill is an underproduction anaemia consistent with what is commonly referred to as the anaemia of chronic inflammatory disease.

Over 90% of ICU patients have low serum iron (Fe), total iron binding capacity (TIBC), and Fe/TIBC ratio, but have a normal or, more usually, an elevated serum ferritin level [1, 9]. At a time when the iron levels are abnormal, serum EPO levels are only mildly elevated, with little evidence of reticulocyte response to endogenous EPO [1]. Rogiers et al. [10] compared EPO levels in critically ill patients and those in patients with iron deficiency anaemia. Although EPO levels were somewhat higher than in adults without anaemia, they were significantly lower than in patients with iron deficiency anaemia despite similar levels of haematocrit. A comparably blunted EPO response to physiological stimuli has also been reported in critically ill children [11].

This blunted EPO response observed in the critically ill appears to result from inhibition of the *EPO* gene by inflammatory mediators [12, 13]. It has also been shown that these same inflammatory cytokines directly inhibit red cell production by the bone marrow and may produce the distinct abnormalities of iron metabolism [14, 15]. Levels of interleukin-1 (IL-2) are elevated in patients with rheumatoid arthritis and are proportional to the degree of anaemia. IL-1 activates T lymphocytes, which increase the production of interferon gamma, which in turn directly inhibits red cell production in vitro. Similarly, levels of tumour necrosis factor (TNF) are elevated in patients with inflammatory and infectious diseases and with cancer. TNF also inhibits erythropoiesis, both in vitro and when administered to human beings [16]. Thus, the anaemia of chronic disease is an anaemia of immune activation in reaction to new foreign antigens (bacteria, parasites, viruses, neoplasms), with the production of cytokines that inhibit the action of EPO on bone marrow cells and the production of EPO by the kidney, thereby producing an underproduction anaemia. As such, the bone marrow in many of these patients may respond to the administration of exogenous EPO, in spite of their critical illness. This may present a therapeutic option for the treatment of the anaemia of critical illness.

The effectiveness of rHuEPO has been firmly established in patients undergoing a variety of orthopaedic procedures [17-20]. Patients with haemoglobin levels of $10 \leq 13$ g/dL benefited most from rHuEPO therapy. Several controlled trials using rHuEPO for general surgery have also been reported. Heiss et al. performed a randomised controlled double-blind trial in patients undergoing colorectal surgery [21]. They observed a significant increase in erythropoietic activity associated with rHuEPO therapy, although no significant difference in the frequency of allogeneic transfusions was noted between the two groups. Poulsen et al. also completed a randomised controlled double-blind study on colorectal surgery patients. The rHuEPO group demonstrated a significantly greater reticulocyte count and smaller intraoperative blood loss, and received no blood transfusions [22]. Similarly, a randomised controlled double-blind study of colorectal surgical patients receiving the same dose range demonstrated that the rHuEPO group had a significantly higher mean haemoglobin concentration throughout the perioperative period. In addition, the rHuEPO group had a significantly lower mean number of units transfused [23]. The efficacy of r-HuEPO has also been studied in patients undergoing cardiac surgery [24-25]. However, the safety of using r-HuEPO in this population remains unresolved. At this time, r-HuEPO is not approved for use among cardiac surgery patients, but may be considered in special circumstances, such as in patients who refuse blood products for religious reasons.

Erythropoietin therapy may also have a role in the critically ill patient, particularly those with longer ICU stays (e.g. greater than 1 week). In patients with multiple organ failure, rHuEPO therapy (600 units/kg) has been shown to stimulate erythropoiesis [26]. In a small randomised placebo-controlled trial (160 patients), therapy with rHuEPO resulted in an almost 50% reduction in RBC transfusions compared with placebo [27]. Erythropoietin was given at a dose of 300 units/kg daily for 5 days followed by every-other-day dosing until ICU discharge. Despite receiving fewer RBC transfusions, patients in the rHuEPO group had a significantly greater increase in haematocrit.

The efficacy of rHuEPO demonstrated in the small trial was the basis for a recently completed randomised controlled trial of 1,302 patients [28]. In this trial, rHuEPO was given weekly at a dose of 40,000 units. All patients received three weekly doses, and patients who remained in the ICU on study day 21 received a fourth dose. Treatment with rHuEPO resulted in a 10% reduction in the number of patients receiving any RBC transfusion (60.4% placebo vs 50.5% rHuEPO, $P < 0.0004$) and a 20% reduction in the total number of RBC units transfused (1,963 units placebo vs 1,590 units rHuEPO, $P < 0.001$). Similar to the initial study, the increase in haemoglobin from baseline to final was greater in the rHuEPO group. Clinical outcomes were similar in the rHuEPO and placebo groups.

The effects of critical illness persist well after discharge from the ICU. Therefore, the "chronically" critically ill constitute a large and important population of patients. In a small randomised controlled trial (86 patients) of patients admitted to a long-term acute care facility, a weekly dose of 40,000 units for up to 12 weeks was shown to decrease the exposure to allogeneic blood [29]. There was a reduction in the total units of RBCs transfused in the rHuEPO group (113 units placebo vs 73 units rHuEPO). In addition, patients receiving rHuEPO were also less likely to be transfused (61% placebo vs 31% rHuEPO, $P < 0.006$). Increase in haemoglobin from baseline to final was greater in the rHuEPO group. Mortality (19% rHuEPO, 29.5% placebo) and adverse clinical events were not significantly different.

Taken together, these studies [27-29] demonstrate that EPO therapy in both "acute" and "chronic" critically ill patients will result in a decrease in RBC transfusion and a rise in haemoglobin level. This supports the hypothesis that the critically ill patient has an anaemia that is consistent with anaemia of critical illness and characterised in part by a relative erythropoietin deficiency.

Erythropoietin therapy is generally safe and well tolerated. The incidence of thrombosis in particular has been closely monitored in patients who receive EPO. A review of four prospective studies including a total of 869 orthopaedic surgery patients demonstrated a similar incidence of thrombotic/vascular events in 619 patients treated with EPO and in 250 patients receiving placebo [30]. In the trials in the critically ill there was no increase in the number of adverse clinical events reported with rHuEPO therapy [27-29]. In particular, there was no increased risk of thromboembolic complications. However, the power of these studies may have been too low to identify less common adverse events. Recently, the occurrence of pure red-cell aplasia associated with the presence of anti-erythropoietin antibodies was reported in a small number of chronic renal failure patients treated with rHuEPO administered subcutaneously [31]. This complication was not observed in the trials in the critically ill; however, treatment duration and follow-up were relatively short.

In view of questions that have been raised regarding the safety and efficacy of RBC transfusions [32], does a reduction in RBC transfusions with rHuEPO therapy lead to better clinical outcomes ? The studies in critically ill patients have not demonstrated differences in clinical outcome associated with RBC transfusion reduction. Further study is necessary to determine whether there are clinical outcome benefits in critically ill patients admitted to either the ICU and/or long-term acute care facilities associated with the reduction in the exposure to RBC transfusion with epoetin administration.

References

1. Rodriguez RM, Corwin HL, Gettinger A et al (2001) Nutritional deficiencies and blunted erythropoietin response as causes of the anemia of critical illness. J Crit Care 16:36–41
2. Corwin L, Parsonnet KC, Gettinger A (1995) RBC transfusion in the ICU: is there a reason? Chest 108:767–771
3. Littenberg B, Corwin H, Gettinger A et al (1995) A practice guideline and decision aide for blood transfusion. Immunohematology 11:88-92
4. Groeger JS, Guntupalli KK, Strosberg M et al (1993) Descriptive analysis of critical care units in the United States: Patient characteristics and intensive care unit utilization. Crit Care Med 21:279-291
5. Corwin HL, Abraham E, Fink MP et al (2001) Anemia and blood transfusion in the critically ill: current clinical practice in the US—The CRIT Study (abstract). Crit Care Med 29 (Suppl):A2
6. Vincent JL, Baron JF, Gattinoni L et al (2002) Anemia and blood transfusions in the critically ill: An epidemiological, observational study. JAMA 288:1499-1507
7. Smoller BR, Kruskall MS (1986) Phlebotomy for diagnostic laboratory tests in adults: pattern of use and effect on transfusion requirements. N Engl J Med 314:1233-1235
8. Burnum JF (1986) Medical vampires. N Engl J Med 314:1250-1251
9. Van Iperen CE, Gaillard CAJM, Kraaijenhagen RJ et al (2000) Response of erythropoiesis and iron metabolism to recombinant human erythropoietin in intensive care unt patients. Crit Care Med 28:2773-2778
10. Rogiers P, Zhang H, Leeman M et al (1997) Erythropoietin response is blunted in critically ill patients. Intensive Care Med 23:159-162
11. Krafte-Jacobs B, Levetown ML, Bray GL et al (1994) Erythropoietin response to critical illness. Crit Care Med 22:821-826
12. Frede S, Fandrey J, Pagel H et al (1997) Erythropoieitn gene expression is suppressed after lipopolysaccharide or interluekin-1B injections in rats. Am J Physiol 272:R1067-1071
13. Jelkmann W (1998) Proinflammatory cytokines lowering erythropoieitn production. J Interferon Cytokine Res 18:555-559
14. Means RT, Krantz SB (1992) Progress in understanding the pathogenesis of the anemia of chronic disease. Blood 80:1639-1647
15. Krantz SB (1994) Pathogenesis and treatment of the anemia of chronic disease. Am J Med Sci 307:353:353-359
16. Blick M Sherwin SA, Rosenblum M, Guttterman J (1987) Phase I study of recombinant tumor necrosis factor in cancer patients. Cancer Res 47:2986-2989
17. Keating EM (1998) Current options and approaches for blood management in orthopedic surgery. J Bone Joint Surg Am 80:750-762
18. Canadian Orthopedic Perioperative Erythropoietin Study Group (1993) Effectiveness of perioperative recombinant human erythropoietin in elective hip replacement. Lancet 341:1227-1232
19. Faris PM, MA Ritter, RI Abels (1996) The effects of recombinant human erythropoietin on

perioperative transfusion requirements in patients having a major orthopedic operation. J Bone Joint Surg Am 78:62-72
20. De Andrade JR, Jove M, Landon G et al (1997) Baseline hemoglobin as a predictor of risk of transfusion and response to epoetin alfa in orthopedic surgery patients. Am J Orthop 25:533-542
21. Heiss MM, Tarabichi A, Delanoff C et al (1996) Perisurgical erythropoietin application in anemic patients with colorectal cancer: A double-blind randomized study. Surgery 119:523-527
22. Poulsen KA, Qvist N, Winther K, Boesby S (1998) Haemostatic aspects of recombinant erythropoietin in colorectal surgery. Eur J Surg 164:211-215
23. Qvist N, Boesby S, Wolff B, Hansen CP (1999) Recombinant human erythropoietin and hemoglobin concentration at operation and during the postoperative period: reduced need for blood transfusions in patients undergoing colorectal surgery. World J Surg 23:30-35
24. Sowade O, Ziemer S, Sowade B et al (1997) The effect of preoperative recombinant erythropoietin therapy on platlets and hemostasis in patients undergoing cardiac surgery. J Lab Clin Med 129, 376-383
25. D'Ambria MN, Gray RJ, Hillman R et al (1997) Effect of recombinant human erythropoietin on transfusion risk in coronary bypass patients. Ann Thorac Surg 64:1686-1693
26. Gabriel A, Kozek S, Chiari A et al (1998) High-dose recombinant human erythropoietin stimulates reticulocyte production in patients with multiple organ dysfuction syndrome. J Trauma 44:361--366
27. Corwin HL, Gettinger A, Rodriguez RM et al (1999) Efficacy of recombinant human erythropoietin in the critically ill patient: a randomized double blind placebo controlled trial. Crit Care Med 27:2346-2350
28. Corwin HL, Gettinger A, Rodriguez RM et al (2002) Efficacy of recombinant human erythropoietin in the critically ill patient: a randomized double blind placebo controlled trial. JAMA 288:2827-2835
29. Silver M, Bazan A, Corwin HL et al (2003) A randomized double blind placebo controlled trial of recombinant human erythropoietin in long term acute care patients. Crit Care Med 31 (Suppl):A167
30. De Andrade JR, Frei D, Guilfoyle M (1999) Integrated analysis of thrombotic/vascular event occurrence in epoetin alfa treated patients undergoing major, elective orthopedic surgery. Orthopedics 22:S113-118
31. Eckardt K-U, Casadevall N (2003) Pure red-cell aplasia due to anti-erythropoietin antibodies. Nephrol Dial Transplant 18:865-869
32. Hebert PC, Wells G, Blajchman MA et al (1993) A multicenter, randomized, controlled clinical trial of transfusion requirements in critical care. Transfusion Requirements in Critical Care Investigators, Canadian Critical Care Trials Group. N Engl J Med 340:409-417

Acute normovolaemic haemodilution

C. Bandeira Margarido, D. Aya Otsuki, J.O.C. Auler

The potential risk of transmission of infectious diseases and of other adverse effects, including transfusion reaction, immunosuppression, transfusion-related acute lung injury, has reinforced a general reappraisal of transfusion and a critical analysis of its benefits, risks and costs in the clinical and surgical settings. At the same time, research into alternatives to allogeneic red blood cell transfusion and physiological effects of lower haemoglobin levels has been developed. Critically ill patients in intensive care units usually require red cell transfusion to compensate anaemia caused by bleeding or the need to augment oxygen delivery. Unfortunately, these critically ill patients may be more susceptible than others to the immunosuppressive complications of transfusion.

Compensatory mechanisms in anaemia

The major physiological consequence of lowered haemoglobin levels is a reduced oxygen-carrying capacity of the blood. There are compensatory mechanisms for avoiding tissue hypoxia, such as peripheral vascular dilatation, increased blood flow, increased extraction of oxygen from the blood and increased cardiac output [1]. Among the various changes that occur during anaemia and haemodilution the decrease in blood viscosity is extremely important [2]. The blood viscosity reduction causes changes in blood flow of the venous territory, causing a significant increase in venous return and preload and also of the arterial vascular bed leading to a decrease in afterload. These modifications promote an increase in systolic volume by the Starling mechanism and consequently increase cardiac output with maintenance of arterial pressure [3, 4]. At the same time, systemic vascular resistance decreases as a result of nitric oxide liberation [5].

The cardiac output response to anaemia is the most important compensatory mechanism that contributes to the maintenance of oxygen delivery. Nevertheless, when cardiac output does not increase, oxygen delivery can still be maintained to some degree owing to the augmentation of the oxygen extraction rate [4]. During haemodilution, a redistribution of cardiac output and oxygen transport occurs in favour of organs with a lower capacity to increase oxygen extraction, i.e. heart and brain.

It is important to note that anaesthesia can influence and even blunt the cardiovascular response associated with acute normovolaemic haemodilution (ANH). Most anaesthetic agents decrease myocardial contractility and venous return, so that they may blunt the compensatory increase in cardiac output observed during ANH. Ickx et al. [6] studied forty patients undergoing major abdominal surgery who were randomised to undergo ANH either awake (awake group, n=20) or with fentanil-nitrous oxide-isoflurane anaesthesia (anaesthetised group, n=20). Anaesthesia significantly reduced the cardiac output response associated with ANH. In this group, the increase in cardiac index was smaller (Fig. 1) and related solely to an increase in stroke index. Oxygen delivery decreased, but oxygen consumption was maintained as oxygen extraction increased.

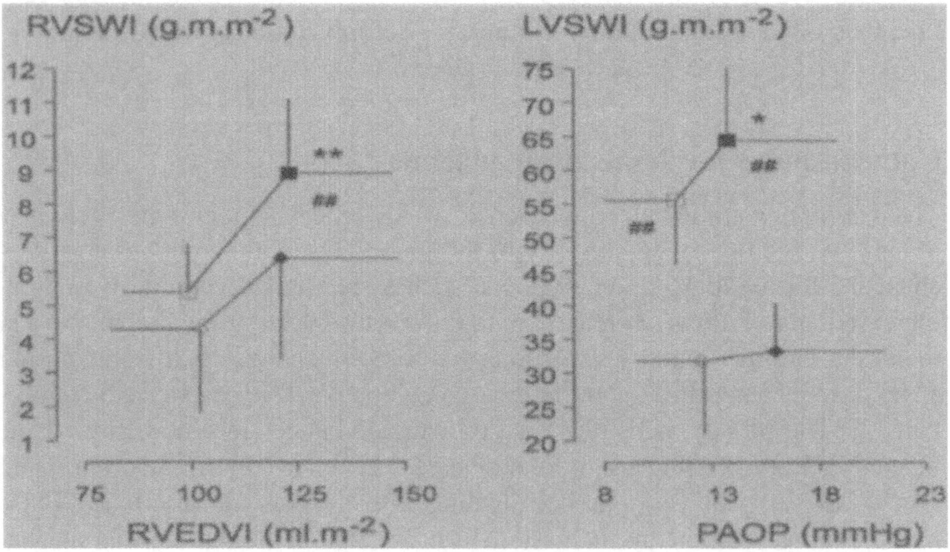

Fig. 1 *Left*: Evolution of right ventricular stroke work index (RVSWI) as a function of right ventricular end-diastolic volume index (RVEDVI) during acute normovolaemic haemodilution. *Right*: Evolution of left ventricular stroke work index (LVSWI) as a function of pulmonary artery occluded pressure (PAOP) during acute normovolaemic haemodilution. *Squares* = awake patients; *diamonds* = anaesthetised patients; *open symbols* = before ANH; *closed symbols* = after ANH. *P <0.05; **P <0.01 after versus before acute normovolaemic haemodilution. ## P <0.01 in awake versus anaesthetised group [6]

Alternatives to allogeneic red blood cell transfusion

Intraoperative restrictive and preoperative red cell transfusion strategies may be used individually or in combination [7]:

a. Preoperative autologous blood donation
b. Preoperative use of erythropoietin
c. Acute normovolaemic haemodilution
d. Intraoperative cell salvage and retransfusion
e. Pharmacological treatment (aprotinin, ε-aminocaproic acid, tranexamic acid)
f. Anaesthesia technique (normothermia, fluid replacement, hyperoxic ventilation, hypotensive anaesthesia)
g. Minimal haemoglobin levels
h. Transfusion algorithms based on coagulation monitoring
i. Artificial O_2 carriers

Preoperative autologous donation is a safe procedure for patients scheduled to undergo elective surgery. This technique requires that patients donate blood on several preoperative visits in the weeks preceding surgery.

ANH was described as a blood conservation strategy more than 30 years ago. In this technique whole blood is removed from a patient while the circulating blood volume is maintained with simultaneous infusion of acellular fluid, crystalloid or colloid [8]. The blood is stored at room temperature and is reinfused into the patient in the operating room after major blood loss has ceased, or sooner if indicated. Comparison of ANH with preoperative autologous blood donation and intraoperative blood salvage shows that haemodilution is less costly, technically simple and needs minimal preoperative preparations. Although ANH seems to be a clinically useful blood-saving technique [9-11], a meta-analysis published in 1998 showed that its efficacy was not well established at that time [12]. However, in 2002 Matot demonstrated in a clinical prospective trial (n=78) that in a significant number of patients with ASA status I and II undergoing major liver resection ANH may make exposure to allogeneic blood transfusion unnecessary (Table 1) [13].

All of these techniques have been used efficaciously in certain situations and have to be implemented in general clinical practice. It is important to point out that many of them can be combined to improve overall efficacy [7]. Combinations of ANH with preoperative erythropoietin, antifbrinolytic drugs, cell salvage, haemodilution performed with artificial oxygen carriers and all together have been proposed [14].

Table 1 Transfusion of packed erythrocytes and outcome variables

	ANH	Control
Transfusion of packed erythrocytes		
No. of patients transfused* (%)	4† (10)	14 (36)
Median units tranfused (range)	0 (0–13)	0 (0–16)
Postoperative complications (%)		
Intraabdominal infection	1 (2.5)	3 (7.7)
Wound infection	1 (2.5)	4 (10.3)
Biliary leak	3 (7.7)	2 (5.1)
Small bowel obstruction	1 (2.5)	0
Intraabdominal bleeding	2 (5.1)	0
Pneumonia	1 (2.5)	1 (2.5)
Others	3 (7.7)	2 (5.1)
Total	9 (23)	8 (20)

* All blood obtained by acute normovolemic haemodilution (ANH) was returned and is not included in this analysis. † $P < 0.05$ compared with control group

Intensive care unit setting

Blood restrictive strategies imply acceptance of minimal haemoglobin levels and knowledge of oxygen delivery and cell utilisation physiology and of the importance of underlying diseases. The historical "hemoglobin of 10g/dl and hematocrit of 30%" transfusion trigger have been discussed, and recent guidelines for blood transfusion recommend haemoglobin levels of 6.0 to 8.0g/dl, except for critically ill patients with known risk factors, such as impaired cardiovascular function and increased metabolic demands [15].

In a recent multicentre study a total of 838 intensive care unit patients were randomised to receive transfusions according to liberal (Hb <7 g/dl) or conservative criteria (Hb <10 g/dl). The restrictive arm received significantly fewer transfusions with no increase in mortality, with the possible exceptions of patients with acute myocardial infarction and unstable angina [16].

Studies in patients with ischaemic heart disease provide evidence that conservative transfusion strategies are associated with lower mortality [17, 18]. Patients with impaired cardiovascular function have lower limits in terms of physiological reserve, and less ability to increase cardiac output. These conditions limit the tolerance of anaemia in elderly patients with acute myocardial infarction.

Haemodilution in clinical settings

The indications can be divided into groups, mainly based on the purposes, target haematocrits and whether blood is removed or not.

1. ANH to decrease exposure to allogeneic transfusions in patients subjected to elective surgery and to avoid transfusing blood products to Jehovah's witnesses.
2. Haemodilution without removal of blood from the patient, to maintain and even improve the blood flow to organs and tissues. This technique can be used in microvascular surgery and in vasospasm following subarachnoid haemorrhage, and it has been studied as a treatment for acute ischaemic stroke.
3. Haemodilution established in CEC due to prime solution.

Haemodilution to avoid allogeneic transfusion

Major surgical procedures

The use of ANH to conserve erythrocytes and avoid allogeneic transfusions has been advocated by several organisations and transfusion experts. However, its use has remained controversial because of its uncertain efficacy and safety. In addition to the potential risks of not maintaining normovolaemia, theoretically, ANH could cause an increase in surgical blood loss because of increased blood flow (increased cardiac output and lower blood viscosity); decreased concentrations of clotting factors, since these are removed together with erythrocytes, and the effects of the fluid, such as hetastarch, on clotting factors and platelet function [19]. ANH requires expertise, takes time and can divert the attention of the anaesthesiologist from other patient care issues.

ANH is one of the few procedures in medicine that lend themselves to mathematical modelling. Analyses have shown that efficacy of haemodilution requires [19]:

1. High initial haematocrits.
2. Low haematocrits after ANH ("target").
3. Significant blood loss (a recent analysis by Weiskopf suggests that surgical blood loss should be 0.7 or more of the patient's blood volume for ANH to result in a saving of at least one unit of blood).
4. Blood loss within specific range.

Matot et al. have published evidence showing that ANH can be efficacious if used correctly in the appropriate patient population. These authors conclude that in patients with ASA status I – II undergoing major liver resection ANH may allow a significant number of patients to avoid exposure to allogeneic blood. Unfortunately, until now, its safety remains unknown [13].

Jehovah's witnesses

In general, Jehovah's witnesses will accept neither the administration of homologous blood products nor the readministration of autologous products that have left the circulation. However, their faith allows significant personal discretion, so that the wishes of each patient must be clarified. Few will permit the administration of the common whole blood components, and the majority will decline preoperative autodonation, but many will accept procedures that maintain extracorporeal blood in continuity with the circulation. The acceptability of cardiopulmonary bypass, acute normovolaemic haemodilution, and perioperative cell salvage must be clarified with each patient individually. Most will permit administration of erythropoietin [20].

Haemodilution to improve blood flow to organs and tissues

Microvascular surgery

Microvascular surgery includes both replantation – the reattachment of a completely severed body part, and revascularisation – the reestablishment of blood flow through a severed body part. Most replantation surgery involves the upper extremity. Anaesthetic management in microvascular surgery includes maintenance of blood flow through microvascular anastomoses, positioning considerations associated with a long surgical procedure during which the patient must lie completely still, and replacement of blood and fluid losses, which may be extensive.

Maintenance of blood flow through microvascular anastomoses is paramount for limb or graft viability. Blood flow may be improved by increasing the perfusion pressure, preventing hypothermia, and using vasodilators and sympathetic blockade. Microvascular perfusion pressure depends on both adequate intravascular volume and oncotic pressure. Blood loss during microvascular surgery is typically continual and insidious. Unrecognised bleeding and migration of intravascular fluid into the third space reduce microvascular perfusion pressure and must be corrected. However, overzealous use of a crystalloid results in generalised oedema, also of the replanted body part, whereas excessive transfusion of blood products increases the blood viscosity and therefore decreases flow. Evidence suggests that the use of phenylephrine to support blood pressure does not jeopardise blood flow to the tissue being replanted. Rheologically, the oxygen-carrying capacity of blood is optimised with a haematocrit of 30%. Normovolaemic haemodilution can be used to improve tissue blood flow and decrease transfusion requirements in patients without significant cardiovascular, cerebrovascular and renal disease. Preoperative autologous blood donation and intraoperative use of a cell saver also significantly reduce the number of homologous units that need to be transfused. Arterial cannulation allows frequent assessment of haemoglobin levels and acid–base status, as well as direct blood pressure measurement.

There are other measures that can be used for the purpose of improving blood flow:

– To avoid hypothermia resulting in vasoconstriction, sympathetic activation, with shivering, increased oxygen demand, a leftward shift of the oxygen–haemoglobin dissociation curve, and altered coagulation, can be induced.
– The use of vasodilators has also been studied in the treatment of perioperative vasospasm: local anaesthetics and papaverine, applied *topically;* volatile anaesthetics, direct-acting vasodilating agents; regional anaesthesia; antithrombotics (heparin) and fibrinolytics (streptokinase, urokinase, low–molecular-weight dextran) are used to preserve blood flow in microvascular anastomoses [20].

Vasospasm after subarachnoid haemorrhage

The treatment of subarachnoid haemorrhage has been revolutionised since the introduction of the "triple H" therapy more than 20 years ago. Hypervolaemia, hypertension and haemodilution serve to improve cerebral blood flow in patients with vasospasm and abnormal autoregulation. In most centres triple H therapy is used only when vasospasm is recognised, whereas some clinicians use triple H prophylactically. This treatment involves the use of crystalloid and colloid solutions, and often the intravenous administration of vasopressors, such as phenylephrine or dopamine. Because of the risk of myocardial ischaemia, congestive heart failure, pulmonary oedema, intracranial haemorrhage, hypertensive encephalopathy, or increased brain oedema, this treatment regimen requires close observation and cardiovascular monitoring. Along with other routine clinical parameters followed in ICUs, central venous pressure is augmented with crystalloid and colloid infusion to maintain normal or slightly elevated hydratation and intravascular volume status. This has the additional effect of diluting the circulating blood constituents (haemodilution). An ideal haematocrit of 30-40% is thought to provide the optimal level of reduced blood viscosity, thereby improving the cerebral blood flow. Although improved outcomes are attributed to triple H therapy, its usefulness has been studied in few well-controlled randomised studies. Small randomised trials do not show a clear benefit; 60-70% show an early clinical response in controlled series [21].

Acute ischaaemic stroke

Studies of the triple H therapy in the setting of acute ischaemic stroke have given inconclusive, but generally negative, results. At present, strategies to improve blood flow by changing the rheological characteristics of the blood or by increasing perfusion pressure are not established as useful. Haemodilution is not recommended outside the clinical trial setting for the treatment of most patients with acute ischaemic stroke [22].

Cardiopulmonary bypass (CPB)

CPB is a technique that diverts venous blood from the heart, adds oxygen, removes CO_2, and returns the blood to a large artery. The CPB machine has five basic components: a venous reservoir, an oxygenator, a heat exchanger, a main pump and an arterial filter. Prior to use, the CPB circuit must be primed with fluid (1200-1800ml for adults). A crystalloid solution is generally used, but other components are frequently added, including colloid (albumin or heta-starch), mannitol, heparin, bicarbonate, and potassium. At the onset of bypass, haemodilution usually decreases the haematocrit to about 22-25% in most patients. Blood is used as a priming solution for small paediatric and severely anaemic adult patients to prevent severe haemodilution.

The advantages of haemodilution during the CPB are:

- An increase in microcirculation due to a decreasing blood viscosity
- Decreased metabolic acidosis
- Increased urine output
- Reduced amount blood needed

The disadvantages are:

- Decreased oxygen carrying capacity
- Postoperative extracellular fluid overload
- Possible pulmonary oedema
- Hypotension resulting from decreased viscosity and peripheral resistance
- Decreased concentrations of calcium, magnesium, phosphate and zinc

As hypothermia and a nonpulsatile flow are used during CPB, the compensatory mechanisms in anaemia, previously described, cannot be seen during CPB. For example, while haemodilution increases blood flow and causes vasodilatation, hypothermia decreases it and causes vasoconstriction. In view of this, it is important to point out that haemodilution is only one of the components of CPB and its physiological effects are complex and beyond the scope of this chapter [23].

Contraindications to ANH are [6]:

- Unstable angina
- Congestive heart failure (New York Heart Association III/IV)
- Valvular disease
- Eletrocardiographic rhythms other than regular sinus
- Uncontrolled hypertension
- Significant respiratory disease (arterial oxygen partial pressure less than 60 mmHg at room air)
- Uncontrolled diabetes mellitus
- Acute infection
- Coagulopathy
- Hepatic disease
- Renal disease
- Hydroxyethyl starch allergy

Experimental settings current in our laboratory

As cited before, there are many controversies about such aspects of ANH as its real benefits, selection of target haematocrit, kind of fluid to maintain normovolaemia, anaesthetic as well as the haemodynamic responses [24]. Haemodiluition is, then, still under evaluation and requires experimental studies to answer all these questions. Our group have been studying haemodilution in experimental settings to address some of these points:

Fraga [25] studied 25 dogs subjected to mechanical ventilation during anaesthesia: 5 in the control group and the other animals, were subjected to ANH with Ringer's lactate (n=10) or hydroxyethyl starch (6% HES, n=10). The Swan Ganz catheter was used to evaluate echocardiography and electronic microscopy, haemodynamic data, cardiac function and histological modifications. Final haemoglobin concentration was 3.2 mg/dl in the RL group and 3.6 mg/dl with HES. Cardiac index was increased in both groups during haemodilution; nevertheless it had significantly decreased in the RL group at the end of investigation (80 minutes). A significant decrease in pulmonary and systemic vascular resistance was noted as well as a significant increase in both pulmonary wedge and central venous pressures in the RL group. Both groups exhibited a significant decrease in the index of subendocardial perfusion during haemodilution. A linear modification of haemodynamic parameterswas noted throughout the experiment, followed by a haemoglobin reduction that was more pronounced in the RL group. Parameters of tissue oxygenation were longer preserved in the HES group, while plasma osmolarity was significantly decreased in the RL group. Echocardiographic evaluation demonstrated a decline in cardiac function at the end of experiment, while it was maintained stable in the HES group. Histopathological analysis revealed minor to moderate lesions in cardiac cells in the HES group and moderate to serious lesions in the RL group. Based on results achieved in these experiments it can be assumed that ANH with 6% HES is better able to yield haemodynamic stability and cardiac cell preservation than RL even in the presence of critical haemoglobin levels.

In another study, ANH was performed with two different solutions (lactated Ringer's and hydroxyethyl starch) to evaluate its pulmonary effects and the haemodynamic changes by means of echocardiography and tonometric parameters. The target haematocrit was established as around 15%. Values obtained by the transoesophageal echography showed no difference after ANH. There is a tendency for a decrease in gastric pH in both groups, which is more evident with lactated Ringer's, but not significantly so.

Regarding the pulmonary effects, in the RL group there is a tendency for a time-dependent decrease in compliance and in PaO_2/FiO_2.

New horizons

Because of the potential adverse effects of ANH, combined methods have been studied and recommended in order to minimise risks [7, 14].

Haemoglobin-based oxygen carriers and perfluorocarbon emulsions are artificial oxygen carriers. These drugs have been extensively studied and can be used in association with ANH; so that a greater volume of normal blood can be removed. Using human polymerised haemoglobin as a blood substitute in acute trauma and emergency surgery, the frequency of allogeneic RBC transfusion could be reduced. The clinical benefits of artificial carriers of oxygen still needs confirmation.

References

1. Varat MA, Adolph RJ, Fowler NO (1972) Cardiovascular effects of anemia. Am Heart J 83:415-426
2. Martin E, Hansen E, Peter K (1987) Acute limited normovolemic hemodilution: a method for avoiding homologous transfusion. World J Surg 11:53-59
3. Fahmy NR, Chandler HP, Patel DJ et al (1980) Hemodynamics and oxygen availability during acute hemodilution in conscious man (abstract). Anesthesiology 53(Suppl):584
4. Gallagher JD (1995) Hemodilution: physiology and limits of anemia. In: Lake CL, Moore RA (eds) Blood hemostasis, transfusion and alternatives in the perioperative period. Raven Press, New York, pp 345-380
5. Doss DN, Estafanous FG, Ferrario CM et al (1995) Mechanism of systemic vasodilation during normovolemic hemodilution. Anesth Analg 81:30-34

6. Ickx BE, Rigolet M, Van der Linden PJ (2000) Cardiovascular and metabolic response to acute normovolemic anemia. Effects of anesthesia. Anesthesiology 93:1011-1016
7. Spahn DR, Casutt M (2000) Eliminating blood transfusions. Anesthesiology 93:242-255
8. Monk TG, Goodnough LT (1998) Acute normovolemic hemodilution. Clin Orthop 357:74-81
9. Helm RE, Klemperer JD, Rosengart TK et al (1996) Intraoperative autologous blood donation preserves red cell mass but does not decrease postoperative bleeding. Ann Thorac Surg 62:1431-1441
10. Kochamba GS, Pfeffer TA, Sintek CF et al (1996) Intraoperative autotransfusion reduces blood loss after cardiopulmonary bypass. Ann Thorac Surg 61:900-903
11. Kahraman S, Altunkaya H, Celebioglu B et al (1997) The effect of acute normovolemic hemodilution on homologous blood requirements and total estimated red blood cell volume lost. Acta Anaesthesiol Scand 41:614-617
12. Bryson GL, Laupacis A, Wells GA (1998) Does acute normovolemic hemodilution reduce perioperative allogenic transfusion? A meta-analysis. Anesth Analg 86:9-15
13. Matot I, Scheinin O, Jurim O et al (2002) Effectiveness of acute normovolemic hemodilution to minimize allogenic blood transfusion in major liver resections. Anesthesiology 97:794-800
14. Auler JOC (2001) Haemodilution in clinical anesthesia. Minerva Anestesiol 67:355-357
15. American college of physicians (1992) Practice strategies for elective red blood cell transfusion. Ann Intern Med 116:403-406
16. Hebert PC, Wells G, Blajchman MA et al (1999) A multicenter, randomized, controlled clinical trial of transfusion requirements in critical care. N Engl J Med 340:409-417
17. Hebert PC, Yetisir E, Martin C et al (2001) Is a low transfusion threshold safe in critically ill patients with cardiovascular diseases? Crit Care Med 29:227-234
18. Wu WC, Rathore SS, Wang Y et al (2001) Blood transfusion in elderly patients with acute myocardial infarction. N Engl J Med 345:1230-1236
19. Weiskopf RB (2002) Hemodilution and candles. Anesthesiology 97:773-775
20. Petrovitch CT, Drumond JC (2001) Hemotherapy and hemostasis. In: Barash PJ, Cullen BF, Stoelting RK (eds) Clinical anesthesia, 4th edn Lippincott/Williams and Wilkins, Philadelphia, pp 201-236
21. Janjua N, Mayer AS (2003) Cerebral vasoespasm after subarachnoid hemorrhage. Curr Opin Crit Care 9:113-119
22. Adams PH, Adams RJ, Brott T et al (2003) Guidelines for the early management of patients with ischemic stroke. A scientific statement from the Stroke Council of the American Stroke Association. Stroke 34:1056-1083
23. Morgan GE, Mikhail MS, Murray MJ (2001) Clinical anesthesiology, 3th edn McGraw-Hill/Appleton & Lange, Philadelphia 433-471
24. Fantoni DT (2001) Hemodilution in experimental setting. Minerva Anestesiol 67:351-354
25. Fraga AO (2002) Acute Normovolemic Hemodilution with Ringer's lactate or hydroxyethyl starch 6% in dogs: cardiovascular, metabolic, respiratory and histopathological evaluation. Thesis, University of São Paulo Medical School

NEUROLOGICAL ILLNESS

Acute neuropathies in sepsis

N. LATRONICO, B. GUARNERI, A. CANDIANI

Several infections can cause acute neuropathies. Leprosy is the commonest cause of peripheral neuropathy and is still important in developing countries where the disease is endemic, the *Mycobacterium leprae* selectively affecting the skin and nerves [1]. Peripheral neuropathies may be found in up to 50% of patients infected with HIV [2]. Neuropathies may be related to the immunological reactions against viral antigens, immunodepression, opportunistic infections, and iatrogenic complications of anti-viral drugs [3]. Hepatitis C virus infection has been found in cryoglobulinaemic neuropathies [4]. Poliomyelitis, diphtheria and Lyme disease are other rare causes of neuropathy [3].

These diseases seldom cause acute life-threatening organ failure requiring intensive care unit (ICU) admission. A more common ICU situation is that of acute neuropathies developing after ICU admission and complicating the clinical course of critically ill patients. Sepsis is a well recognised clinical syndrome promoting organ dysfunction and failure. Brain, lungs, kidneys, muscles, heart and peripheral circulation are commonly affected. In this chapter we examine whether the peripheral nervous system is also liable to sepsis.

Definition of sepsis

Bone et al. defined sepsis as the systemic host response to infection, severe sepsis as sepsis associated with organ dysfunction, hypoperfusion or hypotension, and septic shock as sepsis with arterial hypotension despite adequate fluid resuscitation [5]. These definitions were confirmed at the 2001 International Sepsis Definitions Conference, where a staging system for sepsis was also proposed [6]. Mechanisms through which sepsis causes organ failure are incompletely understood. They are briefly reviewed, with special attention to the peripheral nervous system.

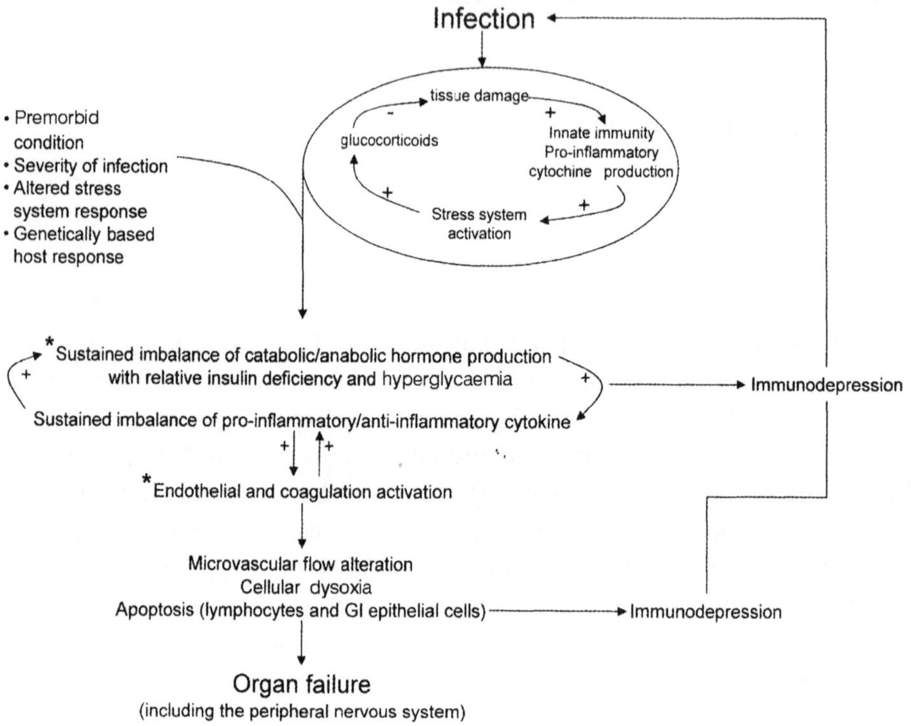

Fig. 1 Pathogenesis of organ failure in sepsis: a complex interplay between the innate immunity, the stress system (hypothalamic–pituitary–adrenal axis), the inflammatory and coagulation system is at the base of organ failure. * Pathogenetic mechanisms which have been specifically demonstrated for peripheral nervous system failure

Cellular dysoxia and hibernation

Microvascular changes limiting nutrient blood flow undoubtedly occur [7]; however, massive ischaemic tissue necrosis is rarely observed in patients dying from sepsis and multiorgan failure (MOF). Indeed, increased tissue oxygen tension has been demonstrated [8, 9], suggesting that the predominant defect might lie in cellular oxygen use (tissue dysoxia or cytopathic hypoxia) rather than in oxygen delivery. Hotchkiss et al. in a seminal paper in patients dying from MOF, showed that organs had a normal macroscopic and microscopic appearance [10]. Apoptosis – programmed cell death – was the only relevant histological finding. Apoptosis was not, however, widespread, but involved only two types of cells: the lymphocytes and the gastrointestinal epithelial cells.

This net divergence between in vivo evidence of organ failure and absence of histological evidence of substantial organ damage is not easily explained, but again points to cellular dysoxia as a leading pathogenetic mechanism. "Cell hibernation" or "cell stunning", a situation in which the cell shifts to fetal gene expression and a lower energy-using state, has been proposed as an explanation for the cell's avoiding necrosis [11]. An analogy is found in the setting of myocardial infarction and "stunned" myocardium.

The stunned peripheral nerve

It is interesting that these same events seem to operate in the neuromuscular system. In our study of 24 critically ill neurological sepsis patients [12], all had reduced amplitudes of the action potential (a powerful energy-consuming process) or nerves were inexcitable, indicating an axonal neuropathy. However, at nerve biopsy, 14 of the 22 patients examined had a normal nerve and only 8, an axonal neuropathy. The divergence between electrophysiological and histological findings was observed in patients with early biopsies, while findings were congruent in late biopsies. We speculated that in the sepsis-related low-energy state, the nerves were trying to maintain their structure and thus to survive by reducing or abolishing (hopefully temporarily) the function, a phenomenon easily documented by electrophysiological testing [12, 13]. With persisting sepsis, the energy supply and/or use is not restored and histological alterations ensue. A recent study confirms our hypothesis, showing mitochondrial dysfunction and decreased ATP concentrations to be strongly related to organ dysfunction and outcome in patients with sepsis [14]. The authors' conclusion was that bioenergetic failure is an important pathophysiological mechanism underlying multiorgan dysfunction. Initially, sepsis may be characterised by increases in inflammatory mediators, but as sepsis persists there is a shift toward an anti-inflammatory immunosuppressive state. It is uncertain whether this sequential response to sepsis does always take place, and individual variation exists. In fact, host genetic factors have been shown to determine the concentrations of inflammatory and anti-inflammatory cytokines produced, thus influencing whether persons have marked hyper-inflammatory or hypo-inflammatory responses to infection. Sepsis-induced immunosuppression is, however, a well-demonstrated phenomenon.

Cytokines, adhesion molecules and coagulation

Innate immunity is the first line of defence against infection and is activated by invading pathogens [15]. Innate immune responses must be tightly regulated, as unbalanced inflammatory reactions can result in devastating inflammatory responses with tissue injury, vascular collapse and MOF [16]. Recognition of bacterial products activates several intracellular signalling pathways with activation of transcription factors (NF-kB, AP-1, Fos, Jun), expression of immune response genes and release of several effector molecules, such as cytokines [17]. Cytokines have an essential role in orchestrating the immune responses to an invading pathogen, but these cytokines can directly affect organ function and may also act indirectly through secondary mediators (thromboxanes, leukotrienes, platelet-activating factor, prostaglandins, complement). Cytokines, as well as endotoxin, also boost the expression of adhesion molecules on endothelial cells and neutrophils [17, 18]. The endothelial adherence of activated neutrophils and their transmigration into the extravascular space result in microvascular (reduced capillary flow) and tissue injury. Recent research has provided the first evidence of the endothelial cells' activation of the microvessels in the endoneurium of human peripheral nerve in patients with critical illness polyneuropathy (CIP) [19]. Inflammatory molecules and bacterial products also amplify the tissue-factor expression on endothelial cells with activation of the extrinsic pathway of the coagulation [11]. This is a key event, coupling activation of inflammation with activation of coagulation, leading to the development of disseminated intravascular coagulation. Activated protein C, a protein with antithrombotic, profibrinolytic, and anti-inflammatory effects, has been shown to reduce the mortality in patients with severe sepsis at the cost of increases in the frequency of bleeding events [20].

What happens into the cell?

Energy metabolism can be deranged on the basis of either decreased delivery of oxygen to cells or an alteration in the functioning of mitochondria [17]. Microcirculatory blood flow maldistribution, and hence decreased delivery of nutrients to cells, is well demonstrated [7], although the extent to which changes in microvascular perfusion lead directly to organ system failure is still debated. How can the extravasation of activated neutrophils cause mitochondrial dysfunction and cytopathic hypoxia?

Neutrophils are a potent source of proinflammatory cytokines, principally tumour necrosis factor (TNF) and interleukin 1, and TNF has been shown to depolarise mitochondria, thus disrupting ATP synthesis through opening of the mitochondrial permeability transition pore and dissipation of the mitochondrial protonic gradient [21]. Another potential cause of cellular dysoxia is the activation of the enzyme poly(ADP-ribose) polymerase (PARP) [22, 23]. Under normal conditions PARP is relatively inactive in cells. However, PARP is activated by the presence of single-strand breaks in nuclear DNA, which can be induced by various endogenously generated oxidants, such as peroxynitrite and hydrogen peroxide. Depletion of cellular levels of NAD can thereby cause the energy crisis in cells. Generation of free radicals can be a consequence of mitochondrial hypoxia and these potent oxidants can also initiate proinflammatory signal transduction pathway, including activation of the transcription factor nuclear factor-κB, important in the regulation of tumour necrosis factor expression [24]. In synthesis, pro-inflammatory cytokines can disrupt mitochondrial energy production with mitochondrial leakage of free radicals further enhancing the transcription of pro-inflammatory cytokines. DNA damage with activation of PARP and consequent NAD depletion closes the vicious circle.

Insulin deficiency and hyperglycaemia

Witt et al. showed that elevated serum glucose, together with reduced serum albumin and prolonged ICU stay, is an independent predictor for the development of CIP [25]. The authors hypothesised the hyperglycaemia-related increase in endovascular resistance with reduced nerve blood flow and endoneurial hypoxia might be the mechanism. More recently, Van den Berghe et al. [26] showed that intensive insulin therapy reduced the number of deaths from MOF in patients with sepsis; concurrently, the incidence of CIP was also reduced by 44%. There was a positive linear correlation between the risk of polyneuropathy and the mean blood glucose level both with conventional and with intensive insulin treatment. The risk of CIP with conventional insulin treatment was, however, more than double that with intensive insulin treatment.

The anti-apoptotic effects of insulin and its trophic effects on mucosal and skin barriers, as well as the deleterious effects of hyperglycaemia on macrophage or neutrophil function and endovascular resistance are the purported explanations [26-29]. Van den Berghe's results are consistent with CIP being due to the same mechanisms that are currently postulated to cause dysfunction of other organ systems during sepsis and MOF. Relative insulin deficiency and/or hyperglycaemia must have a pivotal role.

Definition of CIP

CIP is a relatively new entity, whose description goes back to the early 1980s by different groups in France, Canada and the United States. However, Bolton and coworkers must be given the credit for the systematic appraisal of its clinical and electrophysiological aspects [30, 31]. CIP is an acute axonal sensory-motor polyneuropathy, mainly affecting the peripheral nerves of the lower limbs. On histological investigation the affected nerve shows a reduced number of fibres with maintained myelin sheaths [32], which makes sense of the electrophysiological findings: the amplitude of the nerve action potential is reduced, while the nerve conduction velocity is preserved.

The exact incidence of CIP is unknown owing to wide variation in diagnostic criteria and patients studied [33], but certainly CIP is not a rare complication, being described in 58% of patients with prolonged ICU stay [34], 68.5% of patients with sepsis [35], 70% of patients with MOF [25], 76% of patients with septic shock [36], 82% of patients with sepsis and MOF [37] and 100% of acutely ill neurologic patients with severe sepsis [12]. A recent multicentre French study showed that 16.9-35.2% of patients who undergo mechanical ventilation for 7 or more days and achieve satisfactory recovery of consciousness actually develop *clinically detectable* paresis [38].

Clinical signs and evolution of CIP

Involvement of motor nerves explains the acute flaccid muscle weakness and paralysis. Involvement of peripheral motor nerves is usually generalised, but can be more pronounced for the inferior limbs [39]. Cranial nerves are usually, but not invariably, spared. The authors have seen cases of patients completely paralysed, but conscious ("locked-in") because of CIP or critical illness myopathy (CIM) or both. Deep tendon reflexes are usually absent, but their presence does not exclude this diagnosis. Sensory symptoms are often overlooked due to the difficulty of properly evaluating patients in their acute phase. Limb paralysis usually becomes clinically evident over the first 2-3 ICU weeks; however, it is possible that the onset is earlier and remains unnoticed, because the patient's consciousness is often altered (sedation, primary disease) and the physicians' attention is polarised towards life-threatening problems. Cases have been described in which there was a sudden onset of paralysis in the first 2-3 ICU days [40, 41]. Patients with severe sepsis or septic shock seem to be particularly at risk, but it is uncertain whether some patients have had CIP or rather CIM.

In one case, a patient with post-traumatic coma became acutely quadriplegic only a few hours after the onset of high fever and hypotension [41]. A missed traumatic lesion of the cervical spine was suspected, but an MRI was normal. Neurophysiological investigations (electroneurography and electromyography) led to the diagnosis of CIP.

In comatose patients, an acute flaccid paralysis due to CIP can lead to an unreasonably pessimistic prognosis [12]. In fact, an absent reflex motor response to pain suggests profound central nervous system deterioration and poor outcome. If CIP is suspected as the cause of paralysis, a careful neurological and neurophysiological investigation should be done and CIP excluded before an opinion is given on prognosis.

Involvement of the phrenic nerve and diaphragm is not uncommon [42, 43] and may cause acute neuromuscular respiratory failure. Failed weaning of patients from the ventilator was the initial clinical problem alerting physicians to the possible involvement of the neuromuscular respiratory system in critically ill patients [30-32] and is still the commonest clinical presentation in today's ICU practice. Patients with CIP require the ventilator for a longer period of time, but not always because of difficult weaning [44], reflecting the complexity of factors explaining prolonged ventilation (pre-existing diseases, malnutrition, cardiac and respiratory dysfunction, infections). In a small case series [45], CIP and CIM were responsible for acute neuromuscular respiratory failure after resolution of the respiratory and cardiac dysfunctions, successful weaning from the ventilator, and ICU discharge. In such cases CIP might be responsible for unplanned ICU readmission or even unexpected death.

The available data on long-term outcome suggest that patients with CIP usually recover in a matter of months after ICU discharge, although motor disturbances may persist for years [46]. In one series, clinical motor and sensory neurological deficits in patients with protracted critical illness were found up to 5 years after ICU discharge [47]. In other series, the evolution was more benign, recovery being complete within 3-6 months of ICU discharge [38]. Since CIP and CIM often coexist [12] it is possible that patients with a prevalent myopathic component recover earlier than patients with CIP alone.

Septic or critical illness polyneuropathy?

Several authors have reported CIP in patients suffering from SIRS and sepsis [12, 48, 49]. Recently, bacteraemia and vasopressor support for more than 3 days were found to be independent risk factors for CIP [26]. However, De Jonghe et al. have demonstrated in their systematic review of risk factors for CIP that only in one study was sepsis associated with the occurrence of CIP (and/or CIM). Indeed, in their prospective cohort study, sepsis was not an independent risk factor for the development of clinically relevant CIP, while female sex, number of days with dysfunction in two organs, duration of mechanical ventilation, and corticosteroid administration were [38]. At present, there is no unequivocal evidence from clinical studies to support a causal relation between sepsis and CIP.

Do you not have an EMG machine?

CIP is an easy diagnosis to make. EMG is the diagnostic gold standard, and a reduced amplitude of the compound muscle action potential and sensory nerve action potential, or peripheral nerve inexcitability in a critically ill patients with MOF is virtually diagnostic [31]. Usually both sensory and motor nerves are involved [30], but pure motor and pure sensory forms have also been described [12, 50]. It must be emphasised that, if the patient fails to activate his/her muscles voluntarily, *the diagnosis will invariably be CIP*, even if an acute myopathy is ongoing [51]. For this reason, we prefer the term critical illness myopathy or neuropathy (CRI.MY.NE) [12] to the term CIP, at least until a complete clinical and neurophysiological investigation can be done.

Some authors suggest that the new onset of weakness in the critically ill patient is "such a characteristic entity that it may be diagnosed reliably on clinical grounds and that [this] adds little useful information" [52]. They propose easily applicable criteria to diagnose CIP without an EMG machine. Whether or not this method is as accurate as EMG, it offers a bright alternative wherever a specialist clinical neurophysiologist is not present or no portable EMG machine is available.

Conclusions

Several pathologic conditions, including sepsis, trauma, burns, acute central nervous system diseases and pancreatitis, can cause organ failure, including CIP. Sepsis is a leading cause, but the pathogenetic mechanisms are common to all critical conditions. Therefore, the term CIP is still appropriate. What is changing is the shift towards appreciating the involvement of peripheral nerves *and* muscles. The alarming acronym CRI.MY.NE. ("crimine" means crime in Italian) emphasises this concept.

References

1. Haimanot RT, Melaku Z (2000) Leprosy. Curr Opin Neurol 13:317-322
2. Simpson DM (2002) Selected peripheral neuropathies associated with human immunodeficiency virus infection and antiretroviral therapy. J Neurovirol 8 Suppl 2:33-41
3. Creange A (2000) [Infectious neuropathies]. Rev Prat 50:743-748
4. Mayo MJ (2003) Extrahepatic manifestations of hepatitis C infection. Am J Med Sci 325:135-148
5. Bone RC, Balk RA, Cerra FB et al (1992) Definitions for sepsis and organ failure and guidelines for the use of innovative therapies in sepsis. The ACCP/SCCM Consensus Conference Committee. American College of Chest Physicians/Society of Critical Care Medicine. Chest 101:1644-1655
6. Levy MM, Fink MP, Marshall JC et al (2003) 2001 SCCM/ESICM/ACCP/ATS/SIS International Sepsis Definitions Conference. Intensive Care Med 29:530-538
7. Ince C, Sinaasappel M (1999) Microcirculatory oxygenation and shunting in sepsis and shock. Crit Care Med 27:1369-1377
8. Rosser DM, Stidwill RP, Jacobson D, Singer M (1995) Oxygen tension in the bladder epithelium rises in both high and low cardiac output endotoxemic sepsis. J Appl Physiol 79:1878-1882
9. Boekstegers P, Weidenhofer S, Pilz G, Werdan K (1991) Peripheral oxygen availability within skeletal muscle in sepsis and septic shock: comparison to limited infection and cardiogenic shock. Infection 19:317-323
10. Hotchkiss RS, Swanson PE, Freeman BD et al (1999) Apoptotic cell death in patients with sepsis, shock, and multiple organ dysfunction. Crit Care Med 27:1230-1251
11. Hotchkiss RS, Karl IE (2003) The pathophysiology and treatment of sepsis. N Engl J Med 348:138-150
12. Latronico N, Fenzi F, Recupero D et al (1996) Critical illness myopathy and neuropathy. Lancet 347:1579-1582
13. Latronico N (2000) Monitoring of peripheral nerves and muscle function in patients with multiple organ dysfunction syndrome. Crit Care Med 28:3375
14. Brealey D, Brand M, Hargreaves I et al (2002) Association between mitochondrial dysfunction and severity and outcome of septic shock. Lancet 360:219-223
15. Astiz ME, Rackow EC (1998) Septic shock. Lancet 351:1501-1505
16. Bochud PY, Calandra T (2003) Pathogenesis of sepsis: new concepts and implications for future treatment. BMJ 326:262-266
17. Fink MP, Evans TW (2002) Mechanisms of organ dysfunction in critical illness: report from a Round Table Conference held in Brussels. Intensive Care Med 28:369-375
18. Adrie C, Pinsky MR (2000) The inflammatory balance in human sepsis. Intensive Care Med 26:364-375
19. Fenzi F, Latronico N, Refatti N, Rizzuto N (2003) Enhanced expression of E-selectin on the vascular endothelium of peripheral nerve in critically ill patients with neuromuscular disorders. Acta Neuropathol (Berl) 106:75-82
20. Bernard GR, Vincent JL, Laterre PF et al (2001) Efficacy and safety of recombinant human activated protein C for severe sepsis. N Engl J Med 344:699-709
21. Pastorino JG, Simbula G, Yamamoto K et al (1996) The cytotoxicity of tumor necrosis factor depends on induction of the mitochondrial permeability transition. J Biol Chem 271:29792-29798
22. Cuzzocrea S, Costantino G, Mazzon E, Caputi AP (1999) Protective effect of N-acetylcysteine on multiple organ failure induced by zymosan in the rat. Crit Care Med 27:1524-1532
23. Cuzzocrea S, Zingarelli B, Costantino G et al (1999) Protective effect of poly(ADP-ribose) synthetase inhibition on multiple organ failure after zymosan-induced peritonitis in the rat. Crit Care Med 27:1517-1523
24. Chandel NS, Trzyna WC, McClintock DS, Schumacker PT (2000) Role of oxidants in NF-kappa

B activation and TNF-alpha gene transcription induced by hypoxia and endotoxin. J Immunol 165:1013-1021
25. Witt NJ, Zochodne DW, Bolton CF et al (1991) Peripheral nerve function in sepsis and multiple organ failure. Chest 99:176-184
26. van den Berghe G, Wouters P, Weekers F et al (2001) Intensive insulin therapy in the critically ill patients. N Engl J Med 345:1359-1367
27. Gao F, Gao E, Yue TL et al (2002) Nitric oxide mediates the antiapoptotic effect of insulin in myocardial ischemia-reperfusion: the roles of PI3-kinase, Akt, and endothelial nitric oxide synthase phosphorylation. Circulation 105:1497-1502
28. Singleton JR, Baker BL, Thorburn A (2000) Dexamethasone inhibits insulin-like growth factor signaling and potentiates myoblast apoptosis. Endocrinology 141:2945-2950
29. Van den Berghe G, Wouters PJ, Bouillon R et al (2003) Outcome benefit of intensive insulin therapy in the critically ill: insulin dose versus glycemic control. Crit Care Med 31:359-366
30. Bolton CF, Gilbert JJ, Hahn AF, Sibbald WJ (1984) Polyneuropathy in critically ill patients. J Neurol Neurosurg Psychiatry 47:1223-1231
31. Bolton CF, Laverty DA, Brown JD et al (1986) Critically ill polyneuropathy: electrophysiological studies and differentiation from Guillain-Barré syndrome. J Neurol Neurosurg Psychiatry 49:563-573
32. Zochodne DW, Bolton CF, Wells GA et al (1987) Critical illness polyneuropathy. A complication of sepsis and multiple organ failure. Brain 110 (Pt 4):819-841
33. Latronico N, Candiani A (1999) Neuromuscular disorders acquired in the ICU. Intensive Care Med 25:645
34. Leijten FS, Harinck-de Weerd JE, Poortvliet DC, de Weerd AW (1995) The role of polyneuropathy in motor convalescence after prolonged mechanical ventilation. JAMA 274:1221-1225
35. Garnacho-Montero J, Madrazo-Osuna J, Garcia-Garmendia JL et al (2001) Critical illness polyneuropathy: risk factors and clinical consequences. A cohort study in septic patients. Intensive Care Med 27:1288-1296
36. Tepper M, Rakic S, Haas JA, Woittiez AJ (2000) Incidence and onset of critical illness polyneuropathy in patients with septic shock. Neth J Med 56:211-214
37. Berek K, Margreiter J, Willeit J et al (1996) Polyneuropathies in critically ill patients: a prospective evaluation. Intensive Care Med 22:849-855
38. De Jonghe B, Sharshar T, Lefaucheur JP et al (2002) Paresis acquired in the intensive care unit: a prospective multicenter study. JAMA 288:2859-2867
39. Zochodne DW, Bolton CF (1996) Neuromuscular disorders in critical illness. Baillieres Clin Neurol 5:645-671
40. Tennila A, Salmi T, Pettila V et al (2000) Early signs of critical illness polyneuropathy in ICU patients with systemic inflammatory response syndrome or sepsis. Intensive Care Med 26:1360--1363
41. Latronico N, Rasulo FA, Recupero D et al (1998) Acute quadriplegia with delayed onset and rapid recovery. Case report. J Neurosurg 88:769-772
42. Maher J, Rutledge F, Remtulla H et al (1995) Neuromuscular disorders associated with failure to wean from the ventilator. Intensive Care Med 21:737-743
43. Sander HW, Saadeh PB, Chandswang N et al (1999) Diaphragmatic denervation in intensive care unit patients. Electromyogr Clin Neurophysiol 39:3-5
44. van Mook WN, Hulsewe-Evers RP (2002) Critical illness polyneuropathy. Curr Opin Crit Care 8:302-310
45. Latronico N, Guarneri B, Alongi S et al (1999) Acute neuromuscular respiratory failure after ICU discharge. Report of five patients. Intensive Care Med 25:1302-1306
46. de Seze M, Petit H, Wiart L et al (2000) Critical illness polyneuropathy. A 2-year follow-up study in 19 severe cases. Eur Neurol 43:61-69
47. Herridge MS, Cheung AM, Tansey CM et al (2003) One-year outcomes in survivors of the acute respiratory distress syndrome. N Engl J Med 348:683-693

48. Bolton CF (1996) Sepsis and the systemic inflammatory response syndrome: neuromuscular manifestations. Crit Care Med 24:1408-1416
49. Bolton CF, Young GB (1997) Critical illness polyneuropathy due to parenteral nutrition. Intensive Care Med 23:924-925
50. Coakley JH, Nagendran K, Yarwood GD et al (1998) Patterns of neurophysiological abnormality in prolonged critical illness. Intensive Care Med 24:801-807
51. Latronico N, Fenzi F, Boniotti C et al (1993) Acute reversible paralysis in critically ill patients. Acta Anaestesiol Ital 44:157-171
52. Morris C, Trinder JT (2002) Electrophysiology adds little to clinical signs in critical illness polyneuropathy and myopathy. Crit Care Med 30:2612

Stroke management in the early phase

P.D. SCHELLINGER

Stroke is the third most common cause of death in the industrialised countries, after myocardial infarction and cancer, and the single most common reason for permanent disability [1]. Up to 85% of all strokes are of ischaemic origin, and mostly due to blockage of a cerebral artery by a blood clot [2]. Emergency brain resuscitation in acute cardiovascular disease (CVD) and the initial clinical and neurological evaluation in general take place in the emergency room setting. The definitive discrimination between ischaemic stroke, intracerebral haemorrhage (ICH) and subarachnoid haemorrhage (SAH) is made by neuroradiological examination. Once ICH has been ruled out, the aetiology of ischaemic stroke can be determined by several ancillary tests, which are described in detail elsewhere [3].

The therapeutic nihilism concerning ischaemic stroke is definitely not justified. Every acute stroke patient has to be recognised as severely ill, irrespective of severity of symptoms [4]. Of course, only a minority of patients are in a life-threatening condition, and these are more frequently patients with ICH. Nevertheless, there are often underlying conditions, such as cardiac disease (infarction, insufficiency, arrhythmias), hypo- or hypertension, renal disease, diabetes, electrolyte imbalances and dehydration, and in addition the possibility of impending intracranial hypertension and progression of infarct. Time is of the essence in brain resuscitation and diagnosis of ischaemic stroke, as the time window for causal treatment of patients with acute brain infarction, i.e. systemic/intravenous or local/intraarterial thrombolysis with rt-PA (rsp prourokinase or urokinase) is as narrow as 3-6 h, and only occasionally more in isolated patients [5-7]. Accordingly, a new urgency for immediate treatment has developed during recent years – the decade of the brain – so that all initial measures taken, including clinical examination, elicitation of patient history and the organisation of further diagnostic procedures and consequent specific treatment, should be done simultaneously rather than in sequence. The selection of special treatment strategies may already be ongoing before the final decision on therapy of the specific subtype of stroke has been made. Speed and rapid decision making are essential.

Initial evaluation in the emergency room

All of the following may also be implemented into the preclinical stage if feasible. The initial assessment of a patient with presumed stroke includes pulmonary function, heart rate (HR) and blood pressure (BP), pupillary reaction and vigilance. Minimum monitoring consists in pulse oxymetry, continuous recording of ECG (at least one lead) and repeated measurements of BP. Simultaneously, two peripheral venous lines are inserted. A central venous catheter (CVC) or the femoral vein route is only indicated when antebrachial veins are not accessible. Introduction of a CVC is time consuming and risky if applied in a hurry or by an inexperienced physician [8]. Moreover one has to take into account that in an emergency situation all drugs can be given via a large-bore cubital vein cannula. With a venous line in place, blood samples for an instant blood glucose test, clinical chemistry, coagulation assays and haematology studies are taken. Until the arrival of the laboratory results, standard electrolyte solutions (isotonic saline, Ringer lactate etc.) are given. For practical reasons several stopcocks should be applied to the venous cannulas to give direct access for not only infusions but also i.v. injections and "flush-in injections" with normotonic saline. If deemed necessary an arterial blood gas sample is taken. The easiest and therefore fastest access is the femoral artery.

After an approach to the stroke patient the ABC rule of closer evaluation of airways, breathing and pulmonary function may become necessary. Pulse oximetry is a useful and fast tool to detect ventilatory distress. In ischaemic stroke, however, unstable airways and breathing abnormalities are rare. Exceptions are large hemispheric infarctions (MCA or MCA/ACA), vertebrobasilar territory infarctions, sustained seizure activity and, of course, intracranial haemorrhage, which has not been ruled out at this point in patient management. Some patients with acute MCA or ICA infarction may have breathing abnormalities due to neurogenic ventilatory dysfunction, loss of protective reflexes with danger of aspiration or neurogenic pulmonary oedema [2, 9]. It must be taken into account that there may also be preexisting extracerebral conditions, such as chronic obstructive pulmonary disease (COPD), cardiac insufficiency and asthma, that predispose to ventilatory distress and may be exacerbated during acute stroke. Furthermore it is known that oxygen saturations slightly above 90%, which are in general considered to be sufficient, do not necessarily reflect the situation in the brain, where especially in the deep white matter there may be profound hypercarbia and hypoxaemia [10]. Therefore we recommend the application of a nasal tube with 4–6 l oxygen per minute, which generally suffices to keep oxygen saturation within the range of 95-100% and is an easy way to improve oxygenation without any side effects. With a pathological breathing pattern, severe hypoxaemia or hypercarbia, danger of aspiration or progressive loss of vigilance early endotracheal intubation is recommended. The decision on whether to intubate and ventilate a patient should take into consideration his or her age, medical condition before stroke, extent of brain injury, deficits to be expected in survival and of course the presumed wishes of the patient. Many neurologists have never considered stroke patients to be candidates for intubation and ventilation, except for those electively intubated for angiography or operation [11]; our own data show a 1-year survival rate of almost one third among intubated patients and an improved Barthel and Rankin score in the survivors [12].

Blood glucose levels must be measured in every patient with suspected stroke [13, 14]. Hyperglycaemia in stroke leads to increased formation of lactic acid, drop in pH and accumulation of other metabolites and worsens neuronal damage, though hypoglycaemia also seems to worsen stroke [15, 16]. The aim therefore should be to normalise blood glucose into a range of 100 mg/dl – 200 mg/dl, high-osmolarity glucose solutions (40%) should be avoided in acute stroke [17]. It should be borne in mind that glucocorticoids and catecholamines, whether endo- or exogeneous, also raise blood glucose levels via increased glucose formation and increased peripheral insulin resistance, respectively [18]. Fever is commonly present in acute stroke, resulting from infection, altered cerebral regulatory mechanisms in temperature, dehydration or other reasons. Both experimental [19] and clinical data show that temperature raised by even 0.5°C is associated with poor outcome in ischaemic stroke [20-22]. Azzimondi et al. found in 78 patients with stroke and fever that a rise in body temperature to 37.9°C or higher was an independent risk factor for a worse prognosis in stroke, with an odds ratio of 3.4 [23]. Patients who have fever in acute stroke should be treated with antipyretics such as acetaminophen or metamizole (beware of a drop in BP). Also, in the first few days after stroke body temperature should be kept within a normal range either by physical measures, e.g. cooling blankets, intravascular cooling devices, or causal therapy, e.g. antibiotics in the case of infection.

After the emergency assessment described above, a targeted neurological examination has to be done. Cardiovascular risk factors, prothrombotic premedications such as birth control pills, a history of trauma or migraine and antithrombotics such as warfarin, ASA, dipridamole or clopidogrel alone or in combination may give important clues. Rare causative factors such as drug use, multisystem disease (vasculitis) or postpartum state should also be considered. Auscultation and palpation of heart and peripheral pulses with special attention to subclavian and carotid bruits, an orienting check of all other organ systems and blood pressure in **both** arms when vertebrobasilar disease is suspected are assessed. Funduscopic examination may reveal signs of general vascular disease, such as hyaline plaques, cholesterol or other embolies. Pharmacological pupillary dilatation should never be used in acute stroke, as the early signs of brain stem compromise, such as loss of pupillary reaction or mydriasis, cannot be seen. The extent and nature of the neurological examination varies between patients. The unconscious patient may be assessed using the Glasgow Coma Scale (GCS), primitive reflexes (Babinski) and brain stem reflexes / cranial nerve function (pupillary light reaction, corneal reflex, deviation of gaze, oculocephalic reflex) [24]. Noxious stimuli such as pinching the skin of the proximal arm and vigorous pressure to the nailbeds and other verbal or tactile stimulation are used [24]. Careful attention to the patient's responses, the presence of a hemiparesis or hemisensory loss may be elicited. Abnormal posturing gives a clue to the extent of brain stem compromise. Meningism can be tested for in the same way as in the awake patient and an increase in neck muscle tone evaluated by placing a hand under the occiput and flexing the head forward. The National Institutes of Health Stroke Scale (NIHSS) is a useful tool for the neurological evaluation of the awake patient [25]. The examination can be done rapidly within 5-10 min, is easy to perform also for nonneurologists, and has good inter-rater reliability [26]. At this point it still has to be kept in mind that it is impossible to differentiate between ICH and ischaemic stroke. No treatment that might be a potential hazard in either disease, i.e. ICH and ischaemia, should be initiated before a CT scan or stroke MRI has been obtained.

Stroke imaging

In spite of discouraging reports that CT cannot demonstrate ischaemic tissue changes during the first 12 hours after symptom onset [27, 28], it has been generally accepted in the academic stroke community that CT can demonstrate early infarct signs within the first 2-6 hours after stroke. The reported sensitivity of early CT findings ranges from 12% to 92%, depending on the infarct signs, the exact time window of the investigated population, and the authors. The most common sign of early infarct is a frequently subtle grey matter and/or cortical hypodensity [29-32]. Other early infarct signs include the loss of the insular ribbon [33], sulcal effacement due to early oedema in 12-41% of stroke patients [29-31, 34], and the hyperdense middle cerebral artery sign (HMCAS) in 40-60% of patients with angiographically demonstrated MCA occlusion [26, 35-37]. More recent studies have reported incidences of early CT signs of infarction between 53% and 92% within the first 6 h for all acute stroke patients [29-31, 34, 35, 38]. There is an association between the size of early hypodensities and the risk of a secondary haemorrhage [39] and clinical outcome, as early parenchymal hypodensity of more than 50% of the MCA territory is associated with mortality of up to 85% [35]. ECASS I and II showed that in patients with a small area of hypoattenuation (< 33% of the MCA territory), treatment increased the chance of a good clinical outcome, while rt-PA in patients with a large area of hypoattenuation (> 33% of the MCA territory) had no benefit but increased the risk of a fatal brain haemorrhage [30]. While several studies have shown the usefulness of early CT findings in selecting patients for intravenous thrombolytic therapy, other studies have demonstrated that physicians, including general radiologists and neurologists, do not uniformly achieve a sufficient level of sensitivity for identifying CT contraindications for thrombolytic therapy [40]. However, radiologists can be trained to recognise early infarct signs on CT, and the positive effect of being trained to read the CT scans of hyperacute stroke patients has recently been demonstrated in a large trial [31]. CT angiography (CTA) can provide additional information on stenoses or occlusions in the basal arteries of the brain [41], as nonionic contrast material does not affect infarction volume or worsen the symptoms of cerebral ischaemia [42]. In addition to the assessment of a major vessel occlusion, CTA has the potential to deliver information about the quality of the collateral circulation; contrast enhancement in arterial branches beyond the occlusion occurs in those patients [41, 43]. Volume CT scanners may produce images which can be used to construct functional maps of cerebral blood volume, cerebral blood flow, or time to peak enhancement, utilising a first-pass curve of a contrast bolus [44]. However, at present only one to two slices, and not images of the whole brain, can be obtained.

The need for an all-round diagnostic tool with which all the important pathophysiologic aspects of hyperacute stroke can be investigated is evident. Such a method must answer five decisive questions: (1) Where and how large is the actual area of irreversible ischaemic brain damage? (2) How old is the infarction? (3) Is there tissue at risk, and if so how much? (4) Is there a vessel occlusion and if so where is it? (5) Is an ICH or another underlying, nonischaemic disease present? At present, the decision to initiate intravenous rt-PA treatment is based on clinical findings and CT scanning. The reported diagnostic yield of CT within 3 h after symptom onset does not adequately meet these criteria [45]. The advent of new MRI techniques such as perfusion- and diffusion- weighted imaging (PWI, DWI) has revolutionised diagnostic imaging in stroke [46, 47]. DWI may delineate infarcted brain tissue in less than 1 h after symptom onset, probably within minutes [48], although there is accumulating evidence to show that in the very early stage of stroke there may be reversible DWI changes [49, 50], while PWI defines the area of cerebral hypoperfusion. The absolute volume difference or the ratio of PWI and DWI reveals the ischaemic tissue potentially at risk of irreversible infarction [51, 52]. It must be clearly stated that the PWI/DWI mismatch concept is a simplified approach, as the DWI abnormality does not always define the core and the PWI abnormality includes oligogaemic tissue that is not doomed to die whether recanalisation ensues or not. However, the simple approach holds true for 90-95% of all acute stroke patients and therefore is practical and valid for most patients. MRA can reliably assess the cerebral vessel status [53]. Stroke MRI further allows a definitive diagnosis of ICH within the first hours of stroke [54-56] and possibly also that of subarachnoid haemorrhage [57]. Several studies have reported early findings of stroke MRI within the first 6-12 h, demonstrating the feasibility and practicality of this method in the setting of acute stroke and thrombolytic therapy [47, 51, 58-63]. In essence, the presence of a vessel occlusion according to MRA is associated with a PWI/DWI mismatch, the stroke MRI setting that defines the ideal candidate for thrombolysis [61, 64]. In addition, there are five studies that clearly demonstrate that early recanalisation achieved by thrombolysis results in significantly smaller infarcts and a significantly better clinical outcome [50, 51, 61, 63, 65]. Although presently limited by a low availability, the utility of stroke MRI is likely to lie in the early identification of those patients in whom outcome and final infarct size, ultimately the patient's fate, have not yet been determined. Furthermore, cost effectiveness is likely as there is no need for CT or Doppler ultrasound in the hyperacute stage of stroke. With an increasing distribution and round the-clock availability of stroke MRI, the identification of patients who are more suitable for thrombolytic therapy and of those who are not may lead to increased benefit and fewer complications in patients receiving thrombolytic therapy [61]. Furthermore, the rather strictly defined therapeutic window may be qualified and individualised according to the findings in each patient. Published data from Roether et al. and unpublished data from Kuelkens et al. suggest that stroke MRI-guided therapy within 3-6 h may be at least as effective as CT-guided therapy in the 3-h time window [66, 67].

Thrombolytic therapy

After introduction of thrombolytic therapy for the treatment of acute myocardial infarction in the early 1990s [68], major trials for the evaluation of this new therapeutic approach to ischaemic stroke were initiated. Occlusion of a brain vessel leads to a critical reduction in cerebral perfusion and, within minutes, to ischaemic infarction with a central infarct core of irreversibly damaged brain tissue and an area, which can be more or less large, of hypoperfused but still vital brain tissue (the ischaemic penumbra), which can be salvaged by rapid restoration of blood flow [16, 69]. Therefore, the underlying rationale for the introduction and application of thrombolytic agents is the lysis of an obliterating thrombus and subsequent reestablishment of cerebral blood flow by cerebrovascular recanalisation [70]. Proof of an occluded vessel by Doppler ultrasound, CT, MR or digital subtraction angiography should be established, at least when i.v. thrombolysis is performed later than 3 h after symptom onset; however, it is not yet required to decide whether thrombolytic therapy is indicated. Overall, the watchword "time is brain" holds true; therefore, a rapid workup of any patient who is a potential candidate for thrombolytic therapy is mandatory. The delivery of thrombolytic agents locally, at or within the occluding thrombus, has the advantage of providing a higher concentration of the particular thrombolytic agent where it is needed while minimising the concentration systemically. Hence, local intra-arterial thrombolysis has the potential for greater efficacy with regard to arterial recanalisation rates and greater safety with regard to lower risk of haemorrhage. The technique involves performing a cerebral arteriogram, localising the occluding clot, navigating a microcatheter to the site of the clot and administering the lytic agent at or inside the clot, with or without mechanical dissolution of the thrombus.

Meta-analyses of the ECASS I and II, NINDS, ATLANTIS trials [71, 72] assessed the benefit of rt-PA. In the first meta-analysis by Hacke et al., ICH, the most relevant complication of thrombolytic therapy, occurred significantly more often in patients receiving rt-PA (144 / 1,034 versus 43 / 1,010; OR 3.23, CI 2.39 – 4.37), and was increased slightly less in the 3-h time window and at the lower dosage (41 / 393 versus 15 / 389; OR 2.68, CI 1.56 – 4.62). There was no significant difference in mortality between rt-PA and placebo (OR 1.07, CI 0.84 – 1.36), but a slight trend towards a lower mortality was seen in the 0.9 mg/kg and 3-h group (OR 0.91, 0.63 – 1.32). Rt-PA, on the other hand, led to a 37% reduction in death and dependence regardless of dose and time window (OR 0.63, CI 0.53 – 0.76). If treated with the lower dose and within 3 h the chance of an unfavourable outcome was reduced by 45% (OR 0.55, CI 0.41 – 0.72). For every 1,000 patients treated with either dose there are 90 fewer patients who are dead or disabled but 96 haemorrhages more than expected with placebo. Conversely, for 1,000 patients treated with 0.9 mg/kg and within 3 h, there are 65 additional ICH and 140 fewer patients are dead or disabled. The NNT for all doses and time windows is 11; that for the 3-h and 0.9-mg/kg group is 7. These values are far better than the NNT for thrombolysis in myocardial infarctions, which is 30 – 40 [71]. Wardlaw et al. included in their Cochrane Library meta-analysis all 17 randomised trials of thrombolysis with a total of

5,216 patients (2,889 of whom were treated in rt-PA trials) regardless of time window, dosage, administration route and substance. The main objectives were to show that thrombolytic therapy reduces the risk of late death and increases the risk of early and fatal ICH, and that the benefit at outcome (reduction of death and dependence) offsets any early hazard. Symptomatic and fatal ICH were significantly more common as a result of thrombolytic therapy (symptomatic ICH: OR 3.53, CI 2.79 – 4.45, $P < 0.000001$; fatal ICH: OR 4.15, CI 2.96 – 5.84). This translates into 70 additional instances of symptomatic ICH for patients receiving thrombolysis and 29 / 1,000 (OR 3.2) additional instances of fatal ICH in rt-PA patients but 92 / 1,000 (OR 6.03) additional ICH in those patients receiving streptokinase as opposed to placebo. Despite this, thrombolytic therapy administered up to 6 h after ischaemic stroke significantly reduced death or dependence at the end of follow-up (55.2% versus 59.7%, OR 0.83, CI 0.73 to 0.94, P=0.0015), which is equivalent to 44 fewer patients being dead or dependent per 1,000 treated (CI 15 – 73). For patients treated with rt-PA only, the OR was 0.79 (CI 0.68 – 0.92, P = 0.001) or 57 deaths / dependence prevented per 1,000 patients treated (CI 20 – 93). An alternative end-point analysis yields similar results for favourable versus unfavourable outcome (OR 0.79 for all patients and 0.76 for rt-PA patients). When treatment was given within 3 h after stroke onset there was an even better risk reduction for dependency or death (55.2% versus 68.3%; OR 0.58, CI 0.46 to 0.74, P= 0.00001) or 126 fewer dead or dependent patients per 1,000 treated. The difference in benefit of rt-PA between the 0 – 3 h window and the 3 – 6 h window was nonsignificant but showed a trend towards better improvement with early therapy (OR 0.7 vs 0.76). The authors conclude that the significant increase in early death and fatal and nonfatal symptomatic ICH are offset by the significant reduction of disability in survivors. Therapy with rt-PA is associated with less risk and more benefit than are other substances.

Recently, Brott presented a new metaanalysis of the NINDS, ECASS I and II and ATLANTIS studies in San Antonio at the American Stroke Association meeting [73]. They quadrotomised the time interval to treatment in 90-min intervals (0-90; 91-180; 181-270; 271-360) and analysed the ratio of patients with an excellent outcome (mRS $\leq$ 1, NIHSS $\leq$ 1, BI $\geq$95) in 2,776 patients. They found a significant correlation of outcome with time from symptom onset. The odds ratios for favourable outcome were 2.83, 1.53, 1.4 and 1.16, respectively, with the last OR missing statistical significance. Within the first 3 h there were significant OR changes at 10-min increments. The lower confidence interval intersects with 1.0 at 285 min after symptom onset. Most interestingly, the significant effect in favour of rt-PA is mainly on the cost for patients in the mRS range from 2-5, but there is no difference in death (mRS 6). Thus, the negative correlation of time loss with outcome is again established (time is brain), but this is not directly comparable with the other meta-analyses as the chosen end-point is much more favourable in the latter analysis.

Intra-arterial thrombolytic therapy of acute M1 and M2 occlusion with 9 mg / 2 h significantly improves outcome if administered within 6 h after stroke onset. Seven patients need to be treated in order to protect 1 patient from death or dependence. The higher rate of symptomatic ICH (10.2% in PROACT II versus 8.8% in ECASS II, 6.4% in NINDS and 7.2% in ATLANTIS) is very well explained by the far larger baseline severity of stroke in PROACT II (NIHSS of 17 in PROACT II versus 11 in ECASS II and ATLANTIS, and 14 in NINDS). According to the Cochrane meta-analysis, combining PROACT I and II data (34), there is a 0.55 OR (CI 0.31-1.00) for death or disability, an OR of 2.39 (CI 0.88-6.47) for early symptomatic ICH (7-10 days), and an OR of 0.75 (CI 0.4-1.42) for death from all causes at follow-up. Although recanalisation rates may be superior with intra-arterial (66%) than with intravenous (»55%) thrombolysis, and may even be increased by careful mechanical disruption of a thrombus, in addition to the lytic effect of the drug, a limited availability of centres with a 24-h interventional neuroradiology service 7 days a week may restrict the use of this therapy. On the other hand, the clinically more severe strokes may benefit even more from an intra-arterial than from an intravenous approach. Furthermore, the time to eventual recanalisation may be substantially shorter with intra-arterial thrombolysis. Another intra-arterial rpro UK trial (PROACT III), which is partly stroke MRI based and aimed at reducing the rate of screening angiography and optimising patient selection is under way.

Overall, thrombolysis with 0.9 mg/kg rt-PA for acute ischaemic stroke within 6 h leads to an overall clinically significant effect in favour of treated patients but is associated with an excess rate of symptomatic ICH, which does not, however, have an effect on mortality. Intravenous rt-PA (0.9 mg/kg; maximum of 90 mg) is therefore the recommended treatment within 3 h after stroke symptom onset. Thrombolytic therapy should be performed in centres experienced in the use of the procedure. The benefit from the use of intravenous rt-PA for acute ischaemic stroke beyond 3 h from onset of symptoms is lower, but definitely present in selected patients. The adjunctive use (and also the optimal timepoint of use) of antithrombotic agents is still controversial, and at present no recommendations can be given about concomitant administration of heparin or antiplatelet agents during thrombolytic therapy. Intravenous rt-PA is not recommended when the time of onset of stroke cannot be ascertained reliably; this includes patients in whom strokes are recognised when they wake. Intravenous administration of streptokinase for acute ischaemic stroke is dangerous and not indicated. Data on the efficacy of any other intravenously administered thrombolytic drugs are not available to allow any recommendations. A stroke-MRI-based study on the efficacy of recombinant desmoteplase (DSPA, derived from saliva of the vampire bat *Desmodus rotundus*) for treatment of stroke in the 3- to 9-h time window is under way (DIAS=desmoplase in acute ischaemic stroke). Finally, the benefits of arterial recanalisation may be supplemented by neuronal protection (first protocol drafts under way), particularly when the two strategies are used simultaneously and if they can be used very soon after symptom onset. At present thrombolytic therapy is still underutilised. Among the major problems are that relatively few candidates meet the clinical and time criteria. Educating the general public to regard stroke as a treatable emergency and training emergency caregivers in the use of thrombolysis may decrease these problems. Healthcare institutions should be made aware of the potential for long-term cost savings, once stroke management is optimised and thrombolysis is more widely available. Patients and their relatives should be informed not only of the hazards of thrombolytic therapy, but also of its potential benefit and thus the risk inherent in **not** being treated.

Malignant or space-occupying middle cerebral artery infarction

Patients with acute, near-complete middle cerebral artery (MCA) or panhemispheric infarction may develop massive concomitant oedema with significant midline shift or compression of the basal cisterns, resulting in clinical signs of uncal herniation, a condition called "malignant" MCA infarction [74]. This syndrome is defined clinically and by means of CT scanning criteria. The patients are somewhat younger (about 10 years on average) than other stroke patients. Standard antioedema treatment often fails to prevent herniation and brain death, which may occur in up to 80% of the cases [74].

It is quite uncommon for a patient with acute ischaemic stroke to show signs of raised ICP within the first 24 h, as the maximum of oedema formation is reached around day 3-5 [17, 24, 75-77]. However, complete MCA infarctions in young patients with small outer CSF spaces, an acute carotid T-occlusion or extensive ICH can cause profound swelling and midline shift [2]. Initial clinical signs of elevated intracranial pressure are reduced vigilance, vomiting and hiccups and, in the further course, unilaterally or bilaterally dilated pupils with loss of pupillary response to light and loss of corneal reflex. If these signs are present acute actions taken are intubation, if possible with thiopental for induction of anaesthesia, hyperventilation (pCO_2 28-32 mmHg), i.v. boluses of mannitol 20% 125 ml or Hyper Haes (NaCl 10% plus hydroxyethyl starch), and if these are not successful, TRIS-buffer 10 ml and as a last effort 250-500 mg thiopental [78]. If those immediate measures do not lead to normalisation of pupillary reaction and corneal reflexes it is necessary proceed to to resuscitation and try to perform a CCT scan as soon as possible to obtain information on the aetiology of the stroke [2]. Usually these patients show a rapid decline in consciousness and develop signs of herniation 2-4 days after the onset of symptoms. Most patients require intubation and artificial ventilation. During the further clinical course failure of medical treatment for elevated intracranial pressure (ICP) occurs. Once the ICP has moved into critical values (20 mmHg or beyond), both clinical appearance and CT already show signs of herniation. Brain death usually occurs between days 2 and 5 after the onset of stroke.

Moderate hypothermia (33 - 36°C) has been shown to reduce secondary brain injury and infarction size and to improve neurological outcome in animal models with either focal or global ischaemia [79]. Most of the studies used a narrow time-window between 60 and 90 min. However, several clinical trials in head-injured patients have shown a significant reduction in ICP and cerebral blood flow, better neurological outcome and limited secondary brain injury, though the time window varied between 6 h and 16 h. The duration of hypothermia varied from 24 h to 48 h, while neither the optimal duration of hypothermia nor the optimal time after the trauma for therapy in these patients could be identified [80]. Recently the first clinical trial on the use of moderate hypothermia in severe MCA infarction was published [81]. Hypothermia was induced a mean of 14 h after the ischaemic injury. Hypothermia was maintained over 72 h to overcome the maximum brain swelling, which is known to occur between days 2 and 5 after ischaemia. All patients in this study fulfilled the criteria for diagnosis of a malignant MCA infarction. The mortality was only 44%, and the survivors reached a favourable outcome with Barthel indices ranging from 60 to 85. Hypothermia significantly reduced the ICP. However, rewarming the patients constantly led to a secondary rise of ICP, which required additional ICP therapy with mannitol. In some cases it even exaggerated the initial ICP levels. This rebound after rewarming might be due to a proposed hypermetabolic response after induced hypothermia, as described after cardiopulmonary bypass. A new series of patients indicates that modified rewarming protocol may well reduce the ICP elevation that occurs during and after rewarming [82]. Ventricular ectopy and fibrillation limit the extent of hypothermia, but this is known to occur only at temperatures below 30°C. In the above study, pneumonia was the only severe side effect of moderate hypothermia. Other side effects of hypothermia, which have been shown in animal studies, are clotting abnormalities and coagulopathy. In humans the enzymatic reactions of the coagulation cascade were shown to be strongly inhibited by hypothermia. Though an elevation of high serum amylase and lipase levels is frequently observed, the association between hypothermia and pancreatitis is poorly understood as yet.

Although case series impressively show a dramatic reduction in mortality in patients with both cerebellar and hemispheric space-occupying infarction if decompressive surgery is performed, there are no controlled data to support its superiority. The rationale of decompressive surgery is to allow expansion of the oedematous tissue away from the lateral ventricle, the diencephalon and the mesencephalon to reduce intracranial pressure, to increase perfusion pressure and to preserve cerebral blood flow by preventing further compression of the collateral vessels. These factors may help to increase cerebral blood flow in areas surrounding ischaemic regions, thereby preventing further brain tissue necrosis. The hypothesis is supported by a recent experimental stroke study on the value of decompressive surgery [83, 84]. In human space-occupying hemispheric infarction, surgical treatment has been reported to lower mortality and improve the unfavourable outcome [85, 86]. It has been shown in a spherical model that the diameter of the craniectomy needs to be at least 12 cm. The temporal bone should be resected to the skull base. The dura is opened and an adjusted, biconvex dural patch (lyophilised dura or homologous temporal fascia) is placed into the incision. In surviving patients an artificial bone flap is re-implanted 6-12 weeks after surgery. There is some controversy about whether infarcted tissue should be resected or not. There are some reports with positive results in outcome and neurological function [87]. However, since in acute stroke the margins of the infarction are poorly defined and differentiation between definitely damaged tissue and the ischaemic penumbra is not possible, we do not remove the ischaemic tissue. Surgical complications include infections, subdural or epidural haematoma, space-occupying subdural CSF hygroma, and paradoxical herniation after the swelling period. Close clinical follow-up, including palpation of the trepanation site, ICP monitoring, and daily B-mode scanning of the affected hemisphere for detection of epidural or subdural blood and its space-occupying effect on the lateral ventricle, may ensure that these events are found in time and prevent an unfavourable outcome in these patients.

In the first Heidelberg trial, space-occupying MCA infarction was defined as massive supratentorial infarction involving the territory of the MCA or both MCA and anterior cerebral artery (ACA). The definition also included the dynamic aspect of the syndrome by including reversible signs of herniation: increasing space-occupying oedema with a midline shift of more than 10 mm at the septum pellucidum level documented on serial CT. Thirty-two patients underwent surgery. The control group consisted of 21 patients who had left hemispheric malignant MCA infarcts and patients whose relatives did not give informed consent to performance of the operation. Without surgery, 76% patients (16/21) with space-occupying hemispheric infarction died from herniation despite maximal conservative treatment. Only 5 patients survived, and all of them were moderately disabled. Mortality in the surgically treated group was significantly lower (32%, 11/32), 21 patients surviving: 7 of the survivors were rated as severely disabled and dependent, while 14 were independent and only mildly or moderately disabled. More than 80% reached a Barthel index of 60 or above. Of the left-hemispheric patients, only a few were left with a complete global aphasia, while all others have severe Broca aphasia [85]. During the evaluation of the pilot study we realised that in some patients the intervention seemed to come too late. Furthermore, by looking at the CT scan, and the clinical course of the patients it seemed feasible to identify patients who are prone to develop malignant MCA infarct within the next 24-36 h. We therefore changed the protocol: we no longer wait for signs of reversible herniation. Surgery is performed as soon as the CT scan shows a complete MCA infarction leading to significant mass effect with displacement of the lateral ventricle and midline shift and when the patient's consciousness level is deteriorating. Using these entry criteria, the mean time from stroke onset to intervention dropped from 39 h to 21 h in the second part of the study. We included 31 patients in that trial. This approach lead to a further decrease in mortality to 16% (5/31). The number of independent or moderately disabled patients was 17 [86]. In both trials taken together, we observed 8 haemorrhages within the infarcted area which did not require surgical intervention. Eight epidural bleedings occurred. They were all detected by daily B-mode ultrasound monitoring and easily evacuated. We did not have any deaths related to surgery in decompression for MCA infarction. Decompressive surgery should be performed early enough to prevent irreversible damage to adjacent brain structures. On the other hand, the procedure should not be performed too early to avoid the inclusion of patients who probably would not need decompressive surgery for survival. Early CT signs of infarction, initial clinical presentation, and angiographical or other information (TCD, MRA) about arterial occlusion site and state of collateral blood flow should be obtained. In Heidelberg we increasingly use dynamic MRI studies for early patient selection. The next prospective case series started in late 1998. Eleven patients have now been enrolled. New results will be available after 25 patients have been included. In the US a NINDS-funded phase II trial (HEADDFIRST) will be launched in the near future. This trial will be a randomised controlled clinical trial.

References

1. WHO Task Force: Stroke (1989) Recommendations on stroke prevention, diagnosis, and therapy. Report of the WHO Task Force on Stroke and Other Cerebrovascular Disorders. Stroke 20:1407-1431
2. Hacke W, Steiner T, Schwab S (1996) Critical management of the acute stroke: medical and surgical therapy. In: Batjer HH, Caplan LR, Freiberg L, Greenlee RG Jr, Kopitnik TH Jr, Young WL eds. Cerebrovascular disease. Lippincott-Raven, Hagerstown, 523-533
3. Schellinger P, Steiner T (1998) Emergency and intensive-care treatment after a stroke. Recommendations of the European Consensus Group. Nervenarzt 69:530-539
4. Hacke W, Kaste M, Olsen TS et al (2000) European Stroke Initiative (EUSI) recommendations for stroke management. Cerebrovasc Dis (in press)
5. Albers GW, Amarenco P, Easton JD et al (2001) Anthithrombotic and thrombolytic therapy for ischemic strroke. Chest 119:300S-320S
6. Schellinger PD, Fiebach JB, Mohr A et al (2001) Thrombolytic therapy for ischemic stroke – a review. I. Intravenous thrombolysis. Crit Care Med 29:1812-1818
7. Schellinger PD, Fiebach JB, Mohr A et al (2001) Thrombolytic therapy for ischemic stroke – a review. II. Intra-arterial thrombolysis, vertebrobasilar stroke, phase IV trials, and stroke imaging. Crit Care Med 29:1819-1825
8. Mansfield PF, Hohn DC, Fornage BD et al (1994) Complications and failures of subclavian-vein catheterization. N Engl J Med 331:1735-1738
9. Schwarz S, Schwab S, Keller E et al (1997) Neurogenic impairment of cardiopulmonary function in acute cerebral lesions. Nervenarzt 68:956-962
10. Kennealy JA, McLennan JE, Loudon RG, McLaurin RL (1980) Hyperventilation induced cerebral hypoxia. Am Rev Respir Dis 122:407-412
11. Burtin P, Bollaert PE, Feldman L et al (1994) Prognosis of stroke patients undergoing mechanical ventilation. Intensive Care Med 20:32-36
12. Steiner T, Mendoza G, De Georgia M et al (1997) Prognosis of stroke patients requiring mechanical ventilation in a neurological critical care unit. Stroke 28:711-715
13. Pulsinelli WA, Waldman S, Sigsbee B (1980) Experimental hyperglycemia and diabetes mellitus worsen stroke outcome. Trans Am Neurol Assoc 105:21-24
14. Pulsinelli WA, Levy DE, Sigsbee B et al (1983) Increased damage after ischemic stroke in patients with hyperglycemia with or without established diabetes mellitus. Am J Med 74:540-544
15. Wagner KR, Kleinholz M, de Courten Myers GM, Myers RE (1992) Hyperglycemic versus normoglycemic stroke: Topography of brain metabolites, intracellular ph, and infarct size. J Cereb Blood Flow Metab 12:213-222
16. Hacke W, Stingele R, Steiner T et al (1995) Critical care of acute ischemic stroke. Intensive Care Med 21:856-862
17. Ringleb P, Dörfler A, Hacke W (1996) Intensivmedizinische Behandlung der akuten zerebralen Ischämie. Intensivmed Notfallmed 33:307-315
18. Toni D, De Michele M, Fiorelli M et al (1994) Influence of hyperglycaemia on infarct size and clinical outcome of acute ischemic stroke patients with intracranial arterial occlusion. J Neurol Sci 123:129-133
19. Busto R, Dietrich WD, Globus MY-T et al (1987) Small differences in intraischemic brain temperature critically determine the extent of ischemic injury. J Cereb Blood Flow Metab 7:729-738
20. Terent A, Andersson B (1981) The prognosis for patients with cerebrovascular stroke and transient ischemic attacks. Ups J Med Sci 86:63-74
21. Hindfelt B (1976) The prognostic significance of subfebrility and fever in ischaemic cerebral infarction. Acta Neurol Scand 53:72-79
22. Reith J, Jorgensen HS, Pedersen PM et al (1996) Body temperature in acute stroke: relation to stroke severity, infarct size, mortality, and outcome. Lancet 347:422-425

23. Azzimondi G, Bassein L, Nonino F et al (1995) Fever in acute stroke worsens prognosis. A prospective study. Stroke 26:2040-2043
24. Jannett B, Teasdale D, Braakmarz R (1979) Prognosis of patients with severe head injury. Neurosurgery 4:283-289
25. The National Institute of Neurological Disorders and Stroke rt-PA Stroke Study Group (1995) Tissue plasminogen activator for acute ischemic stroke. N Engl J Med 333:1581-1587
26. Tomsick T, Brott T, Barsan W et al (1996) Prognostic value of the hyperdense middle cerebral artery sign and stroke scale score before ultraearly thrombolytic therapy. AJNR Am J Neuroradiol 17:1-7
27. Gilman S (1998) Imaging the brain. First of two parts. N Engl J Med 338:812-820
28. Gilman S (1998) Imaging the brain. Second of two parts. N Engl J Med 338:889-896
29. von Kummer R, Nolte PN, Schnittger H et al (1996) Detectability of cerebral hemisphere ischaemic infarcts by ct within 6 h of stroke. Neuroradiology 38:31-33
30. von Kummer R, Allen KL, Holle R et al (1997) Acute stroke: usefulness of early CT findings before thrombolytic therapy. Radiology 205:327-333
31. von Kummer R (1998) Effect of training in reading CT scans on patient selection for ecass ii. Neurology 51:S50-S52
32. Bozzao L, Bastianello S, Fantozzi LM et al (1989) Correlation of angiographic and sequential ct findings in patients with evolving cerebral infarction. AJNR Am J Neuroradiol 10:1215-1222
33. Truwit CL, Barkovich AJ, Gean-Marton A et al (1990) Loss of the insular ribbon: another early CT sign of acute middle cerebral artery infarction. Radiology 176:801-806
34. Horowitz SH, Zito JL, Donnarumma R et al (1991) Computed tomographic-angiographic findings within the first five hours of cerebral infarction. Stroke 22:1245-1253
35. von Kummer R, Meyding-Lamade U, Forsting M et al (1994) Sensitivity and prognostic value of early ct in occlusion of the middle cerebral artery trunk. AJNR Am J Neuroradiol 15:9-15
36. Tomsick TA, Brott TG, Chambers AA et al (1990) Hyperdense middle cerebral artery sign on ct: Efficacy in detecting middle cerebral artery thrombosis. AJNR Am J Neuroradiol 11:473--477
37. Leys D, Pruvo JP, Godefroy O et al (1992) Prevalence and significance of hyperdense middle cerebral artery in acute stroke. Stroke 23:317-324
38. Tomura N, Uemura K, Inugami A et al (1988) Early CT finding in cerebral infarction: Obscuration of the lentiform nucleus. Radiology 168:463-467
39. Bozzao L, Angeloni U, Bastianello S et al (1991) Early angiographic and CT findings in patients with hemorrhagic infarction in the distribution of the middle cerebral artery. AJNR Am J Neuroradiol 12:1115-1121
40. Schriger DL, Kalafut M, Starkman S et al (1998) Cranial computed tomography interpretation in acute stroke: physician accuracy in determining eligibility for thrombolytic therapy. JAMA 279:1293-1297
41. Knauth M, Kummer Rv, Jansen O et al (1997) Potential of CT angiography in acute ischemic stroke. AJNR Am J Neuroradiol 18:1001-1010
42. Doerfler A, Engelhorn T, von Kummer R et al (1998) Are iodinated contrast agents detrimental in acute cerebral ischemia? An experimental study in rats. Radiology 206:211-217
43. Wildermuth S, Knauth M, Brandt T et al (1998) Role of CT angiography in patient selection for thrombolytic therapy in acute hemispheric stroke. Stroke 29:935-938
44. Hamberg LM, Hunter GJ, Halpern EF et al (1996) Quantitative high-resolution measurement of cerebrovascular physiology with slip-ring CT. AJNR Am J Neuroradiol 17:639-650
45. Hacke W, Kaste M, Fieschi C et al (1998) Randomised double-blind placebo-controlled trial of thrombolytic therapy with intravenous alteplase in acute ischaemic stroke (ecass II). Lancet 352:1245-1251
46. Warach S, Dashe JF, Edelman RR (1996) Clinical outcome in ischemic stroke predicted by early diffusion-weighted and perfusion magnetic resonance imaging: a preliminary analysis. J Cereb Blood Flow Metab 16:53-59

47. Barber PA, Darby DG, Desmond PM et al (1998) Prediction of stroke outcome with echoplanar perfusion- and diffusion-weighted MRI. Neurology 51:418-426
48. Conturo TE, McKinstry RC, Aronovitz JA, Neil JJ (1995) Diffusion MRI: precision, accuracy and flow effects. NMR Biomed 8:307-332
49. Kidwell CS, Alger JR, Di Salle F et al (1999) Diffusion MRI in patients with transient ischemic attacks. Stroke 30:1174-1180
50. Kidwell CS, Saver JL, Mattiello J et al (2000) Thrombolytic reversal of acute human cerebral ischemic injury shown by diffusion/perfusion magnetic resonance imaging. Ann Neurol 47:462-469
51. Jansen O, Schellinger PD, Fiebach JB et al (1999) Early recanalization in acute ischemic stroke saves tissue at risk defined by MRI. Lancet 353:2036-2037
52. Schlaug G, Benfield A, Baird AE et al (1999) The ischemic penumbra: operationally defined by diffusion and perfusion MRI. Neurology 53:1528-1537
53. Jansen O, Heiland S, Schellinger P (1998) Neuroradiological diagnosis in acute ischemic stroke. Value of modern techniques. Nervenarzt 69:465-471
54. Linfante I, Llinas RH, Caplan LR, Warach S (1999) MRI features of intracerebral hemorrhage within 2 hours from symptom onset. Stroke 30:2263-2267
55. Patel MR, Edelman RR, Warach S (1996) Detection of hyperacute primary intraparenchymal hemorrhage by magnetic resonance imaging. Stroke 27:2321-2324
56. Schellinger PD, Jansen O, Fiebach JB et al (1999) A standardized MRI stroke protocol: comparison with CT in hyperacute intracerebral hemorrhage. Stroke 30:765-768
57. Wiesmann M, Mayer T, Yousri I et al (1999) Comparison of FLAIR and fast spin-echo MR imaging at 1.5 T for detection of acute subarachnoid hemorrhage. Joint Annual Meeting of the American Society of Neuroradiology
58. Tong DC, Yenari MA, Albers GW et al (1998) Correlation of perfusion- and diffusion-weighted MRI with NIHSS score in acute (0.5 hour) ischemic stroke. Neurology 50:864-870
59. Baird AE, Warach S (1999) Imaging developing brain infarction. Curr Opin Neurol 12:65-71
60. Beaulieu C, de Crespigny A, Tong DC et al (1999) Longitudinal magnetic resonance imaging study of perfusion and diffusion in stroke: evolution of lesion volume and correlation with clinical outcome. Ann Neurol 46:568-578
61. Schellinger PD, Jansen O, Fiebach JB et al (2000) Monitoring intravenous recombinant tissue plasminogen activator thrombolysis for acute ischemic stroke with diffusion and perfusion MRI. Stroke 31:1318-1328
62. Schellinger PD, Jansen O, Fiebach JB et al (2000) Feasibility and practicality of MR imaging of stroke in the management of hyperacute cerebral ischemia. AJNR Am J Neuroradiol 21:1184-1189
63. Schellinger PD, Fiebach JB, Jansen O et al (2001) Stroke magnetic resonance imaging within 6 hours after onset of hyperacute cerebral ischemia. Ann Neurol 49:460-469
64. Rordorf G, Koroshetz WJ, Copen WA et al (1998) Regional ischemia and ischemic injury in patients with acute middle cerebral artery stroke as defined by early diffusion-weighted and perfusion-weighted MRI. Stroke 29:939-943
65. Marks MP, Tong D, Beaulieu C et al (1999) Evaluation of early reperfusion and iv rt-pa therapy using diffusion- and perfusion-weighted MRI. Neurology 52:1792-1798
66. Röther J, Schellinger PD, Gass A et al (2002) Effect of intravenous thrombolysis on MRI parameters and functional outcome in acute stroke. Stroke 33:2438-2445
67. Külkens S, Schwark C, Schellinger PD et al (2003) Thrombolysis in ischemic stroke 3 to 6 hours after symptom onset using a MR-based algorithm. International Stroke Conference, Phoenix, AZ, USA. February 13-15th, 2003
68. The GUSTO Angiographic Investigators (1993) The effects of tissue plasminogen activator, streptokinase or both on coronary artery patency, ventricular function, and survival after acute myocardial infarction. N Engl J Med 329:1615-1622
69. Astrup J, Siesjö B, Symon L (1981) Thresholds in cerebral ischemia - the ischemic penumbra. Stroke 12:723-725

70. Hacke W, Willig V, Steiner T (1997) Update on thrombolytic therapy in ischemic stroke. Fibrinolysis & Proteolysis 11:1-4
71. Hacke W, Brott T, Caplan L et al (1999) Thrombolysis in acute ischemic stroke: controlled trials and clinical experience. Neurology 53:S3-14
72. Wardlaw JM, del Zoppo G, Yamaguchi T (2002) Thrombolysis for acute ischaemic stroke (Cochrane review). The Cochrane Library
73. Brott TG (2002) A combined metaanalysis of NINDS, ECASS I and II, ATLANTIS. International Stroke Conference, San Antonio, Tex, 7-9 February 2002
74. Hacke W, Schwab S, Horn M et al (1996) 'Malignant' middle cerebral artery territory infarction: clinical course and prognostic signs. Arch Neurol 53:309-315
75. Schwab S, Aschoff A, Spranger M et al (1996) The value of intracranial pressure monitoring in acute hemispheric stroke. Neurology 47:393-398
76. Frank JI (1995) Large hemispheric infarction, deterioration, and intracranial pressure. Neurology 45:1286-1290
77. Raichle ME (1983) The pathophysiology of brain ischemia. Ann Neurol 13:2-10
78. Schwarz S, Schwab S, Bertram M et al (1998) Effects of hypertonic saline hydroxyethyl starch solution and mannitol in patients with increased intracranial pressure after stroke. Stroke 29:1550-1555
79. Karibe H, Chen J, Zarow GJ et al (1994) Delayed induction of mild hypothermia to reduce infarct volume after temporary middle cerebral artery occlusion in rats. Neurosurgery 80:112-119
80. Clifton GL, Miller ER, Choi SC et al (2001) Lack of effect of induction of hypothermia after acute brain injury. N Engl J Med 344:556-563
81. Schwab S, Schwarz S, Spranger M et al (1998) Moderate hypothermia in the treatment of patients with severe middle cerebral artery infarction. Stroke 29:2461-2466
82. Steiner T, Friede T, Aschoff A et al (2001) Effect and feasibility of controlled rewarming after moderate hypothermia in stroke patients with malignant infarction of the middle cerebral artery. Stroke 32(12):2833-2835
83. Doerfler A, Forsting M, Reith W et al (1996) Decompressive surgery in a rat model of "malignant" cerebral hemispherical stroke: experimental support for an aggressive therapeutic approach. J Neurosurg 85:853-859
84. Forsting M, Reith W, Schabitz WR et al (1995) Decompressive craniectomy for cerebral infarction. An experimental study in rats. Stroke 26:259-264
85. Rieke K, Schwab S, Krieger D et al (1995) Decompressive surgery in space-occupying hemispheric infarction: Results of an open, prospective trial. Crit Care Med 23:1576-1587
86. Schwab S, Steiner T, Aschoff A et al (1998) Early hemicraniectomy in patients with complete middle cerebral artery infarction. Stroke 29:1888-1893
87. Nussbaum E, Wolf A, Sebring L (1991) Complete temporal lobectomy for surgical resuscitation of patients with transtentorial herniation secondary to unilateral hemisperic swelling. Neurosurgery 29:62-66

Guillain-Barré syndrome

A. KRUGER, S. BHAGWANJEE

Background

In 1859, Landry documented a clinical profile of generalised weakness and distal paraesthesia. Almost 60 years later, in 1916, Georges Guillain and Jean Barré redefined the same clinical condition, but in addition identified an increase in proteins in the cerebrospinal fluid. Based on this description, the term Guillain-Barré syndrome was first coined.

Guillain-Barré syndrome (GBS) occurs in all ages and both sexes (male:female 1.5:1) and is not specific to any ethnic group. The incidence is 1-2 per 100 000 in the population. The subtypes appear to favour certain geographic regions. The form with acute inflammatory demyelinating polyneuropathy is predominant in the USA, Europe and Australia while that with acute motor axonal neuropathy occurs more frequently in China [1].

This paper will endeavour to deal with the relevant clinical aspects and the intensive care of the syndrome.

Pathophysiology

GBS is an acute, inflammatory, ascending, demyelinating polyneuropathy [2, 3]. It is autoimmune in nature, with humoral and cellular reactions to the gangliosides in peripheral nerves. It is rapidly progressive in nature and often has a sensory component [4].

It most commonly follows a viral infection, but often no clear precipitating factor can be identified. Several other triggers have been identified, including:

- Mycoplasma [5]
- Hodgkin's disease [5]
- Lupus [5]
- Campylobacter [1, 6]
- Malaria [7]
- Ebstein-Barr virus

- Cytomegalovirus
- Vaccinations (rabies, tetanus)
- Pregnancy
- Trauma
- HIV [2]

There are three recently described clinical subtypes [4, 6]:

- Acute inflammatory demyelinating polyneuropathy (AIDP) – 75%
- Acute motor axonal neuropathy (AMAN) – 10-20%
- Acute motor and sensory axonal neuropathy (AMSAN)

A variant of the GBS exists, the Miller Fisher syndrome [4, 6]. This syndrome consists of a combination of ophthalmoplegia, ataxia and areflexia without weakness.

Diagnostic criteria

The diagnostic criteria for GBS were first devised in 1978 and have since been modified [5]. These are defined by clinical, laboratory and electrodiagnostic criteria. Of all the criteria, the two most consistent are progressive motor weakness of more than one limb and areflexia. Often there is symmetrical involvement of the limbs. Typically the disease begins as bilateral lower limb weakness that ascends to involve the upper limbs.

Campylobacter jejuni is now regarded as a major precipitator of GBS [6]. The acute clinical picture of diarrhoea and positive stool cultures is usually absent by the time the neuropathy begins; however, antibodies to *C. jejuni* will be present [6].

The precise pathophysiology of this syndrome is not clear. It may be that both peripheral nerves and the *C. jejuni* share antigenic sites [6]. As a result, an immune response to the *C. jejuni* produces an equivalent antibody response to the peripheral nerves.

The histology is characterised by infiltration of the peripheral nerves by leucocytes. The prognosis is better when only the myelin of the nerves is affected. This pattern of involvement produces weakness without profound paralysis. Axonal involvement is associated with a worse prognosis, since paralysis is almost invariably present.

Clinical presentation

The clinical presentation ranges from mild weakness to severe paralysis requiring intubation and ICU admission. It usually follows a gastrointestinal or respiratory tract infection. By the time the neuropathy presents, the fever and malaise have subsided. As a result, any patient who presents with a neuropathy and signs of systemic illness, such as vomiting and abdominal pain should be screened for another illness especially toxic ingestion. These symptoms are most likely not to represent GBS.

There is loss of deep tendon reflexes as the ascending neuronal involvement develops. Occasionally, the autonomic nervous system is involved and the patient presents with profound autonomic instability.

The differential diagnosis should include:

- Central nervous system disorders
- Myelopathy
- Muscle and neuromuscular junction disorders, such as myasthenia gravis
- Other infections, such as botulism
- Toxin ingestion (thallium)
- Non-metastatic manifestation of malignancies

The diagnosis is based on the history and a careful neurological examination. Certain special investigations such as electrophysiology and cerebrospinal fluid (CSF) examination are important anciliary tests to confirm the diagnosis and to exclude the other possible causes. The CSF demonstrates 0.5–2.5g/l of protein and few or no cells.

The natural history of the disease starts with a deterioration in power followed by a plateau phase where no new weakness is observed. Recovery takes place over many months. Most patients recover without the need for intensive care. However, those patients who do require intensive care are particularly prone to morbidity and mortality. Overall, 90% of patients will recover with no disability, while 10% will have residual weakness.

Management

Equal attention must be paid to both supportive and specific therapy for the condition. The degree of supportive therapy will depend on the severity of the disease. It should include:

- Surveillance for respiratory paralysis, with intubation and ventilation where needed. Loss of airway control occurs before the inability to breathe. It can occur rapidly.

- Deep vein thrombosis prophylaxis. This includes elastic stockings and low- molecular-weight heparins.
- Monitoring for arrhythmias and managing any autonomic instability [4].
- Pain management. This would include one or more of the following interventions: steroids, narcotics, carbamazepine, epidural anaesthesia, gabapentin and nonsteroidal anti-inflammatories
- Infection control and management
- Nutrition. Ileus may occur but is usually transient. Total parenteral nutrition is rarely required. Given the chronicity of the disease and the benefits of enteral feeding, this is the preferred route for long-term feeding.
- Physiotherapy: passive (and where possible active physiotherapy) is essential to prevent contractures.
- Psychological support. The disease is chronic and very distressing to both the patient and the family. Simple and sophisticated psychological support must be considered. The use of antidepressants may be required in some patients.

The active management includes the following:

- Plasma exchange
- Intravenous immunoglobulin
- Steroids

Plasma exchange

The Cochrane review (2001) suggests that plasma exchange should be considered the gold standard for therapy in GBS [8]. Compared with supportive therapy alone, it definitely offers improvements in time to walking, percentage of patients ventilated, duration of ventilation and severe sequelae at 1 year. The recommended regimen is one of total plasma exchange: 50 ml/kg every alternate day for 4-5 sessions. The replacement solution is albumin.

Intravenous immunoglobulin

This intervention has been shown to improve the clinical outcome [4, 9]. The suggested dose regimen is 0.4 g kg^{-1} day^{-1} for 5 days.

Current practice varies depending on availability of these therapeutic modalities. Based on current data, it appears that the use of either plasma exchange and or immunoglobulin are equally efficacious in ameliorating the severity and duration of the disease [4]. The number of ventilated days and time to walking are decreased. Combination therapy is suggested only for severe motor paralysis. Some clinicians repeat either plasma exchange or intravenous immunoglobulins if the patient relapses.

Steroids

There have been many trials addressing the role of steroids in GBS. A recent literature review suggests that despite the inflammatory (immune-mediated) nature of this condition, no trial has conclusively shown an improvement in clinical picture or an improved outcome [4].

After one of these specific interventions, the next most important intervention is effective intensive care. A high mortality is seen in these patients where ICU facilities are unavailable [2].

Outcome

Early morbidity and mortality is related to delays in establishing airway control and institution of intermittent positive airway pressure (IPPV) in patients whose respiratory muscles are affected. Autonomic nervous system instability – though uncommon – is also an important cause of early fatalities. Delayed morbidity and mortality are related to the chronicity of the disease and the need for protracted intensive care. Sepsis and pulmonary embolus are common sequelae in these patients. Thirty percent of patients with GBS will require mechanical ventilation and, hence, admission to the ICU [2, 3, 10]. Mortality has decreased over the years (5-7% overall and 15-30% with ventilation) and is seen more frequently in severe forms of GBS, older patients and those with co-existing medical conditions [6]. Patients who stay less than 3 weeks in the ICU have lower morbidity rates.

The main reasons for admission to the ICU include:

- Intensive monitoring of the patient as the disease is rapidly progressing.
- Respiratory weakness/bulbar weakness.
- Autonomic dysfunction which manifests with cardiac arrhythmias, blood pressure swings, pupil abnormalities, sweating, urine retention, ileus/constipation.

Henderson et al. reviewed 114 patients admitted to the Mayo Medical Center. Their findings were similar to those in other studies [10]. The commonest causes of morbidity include:

- Respiratory: tracheobronchitis and pneumonia.
- Sepsis: from bacteraemia, invasive lines and ICU causes such as acalculous cholecystitis and bedsores.

- Other: gastrointestinal bleeds, deep vein thrombosis and pulmonary embolus, urinary tract infections and hyponatraemia.

Most of the above are non-specific. They include many of the usual morbidity factors seen in intensive care units. The longer the paralysis and the longer the period of mechanical ventilation, the higher the morbidity.

This same study found that a third of patients needed mechanical ventilation for less than 3 weeks [10]. Overall, 30% of GBS patients require mechanical ventilation. As a result, early monitoring and identification of respiratory failure are needed. In addition, the decision to ventilate depends on the rapidity of the disease progression in the particular patient and the site of the weakness.

Sharshar et al. followed up 722 patients and identified six predictors of the need for mechanical ventilation [3]:

- Time from onset to admission in the ICU 7 days
- Inability to cough
- Inability to stand
- Inability to lift the elbows
- Inability to lift the head
- Raised liver enzymes

They concluded that patients with at least one predictor should be admitted to the ICU. Most (85%) patients with 4 predictors will require mechanical ventilation. In addition, the authors agree with the findings in another study that bulbar dysfunction and a decrease in vital capacity are also early warning signs of the need for mechanical ventilation [11].

Other more specific recommendations for early intubation include:

- Vital capacity <20ml/kg
- Mean inspiratory pressure 30 cmH_2O
- Mean expiratory pressure 40 cm/H_2O

or a

- Reduction of >30% in any of the above parameters

Should the patient need intubation, the use of suxemethonium (scoline) is absolutely contraindicated. Postsynaptic acetylcholine (extrajunctional) receptors increase in number during the disease. The depolarising action of suxemethonium normally provokes potassium release. In this disease the severe hyperkalaemia associated with the use of scoline is very likely to lead to cardiac arrest. These patients do not respond to resuscitation from hyperkalaemia, so that scoline should be avoided.

HIV and GBS

Numerous reports have alluded to the occurrence of GBS in HIV-positive patients [2, 5, 12]. It manifests at the time of seroconversion, i.e. early in the disease process. Seropositive and -negative patients have the same clinical course as long as the CD4 count is greater than 200×10^6 cells/l [2].

A variant exists that includes cell counts in the CSF of 11-50 mononuclear leucocytes/mm^3. It appears that the lower the CD4 count in HIV-positive patients the more cells are present in the CSF. Hence, the variant form of CSF presentation is more common [5].

Conclusions

While GBS is a relatively uncommon condition in the general ICU population, it certainly poses unique challenges to the intensivist. An understanding of the pathophysiology and clinical course will allow for the early identification of high-risk patients. Early deaths can be prevented by adequate assessment of the airway, the need for ventilation and the identification of autonomic instability. Since these patients often spend many months in ICU, chronic complications of intensive care are frequently encountered. Meticulous attention to their prevention and early treatment will impact favourably on morbidity and mortality. Lastly, it is essential that appropriate attention be directed to psychological support – an often neglected consideration – for this protracted disease.

References

1. Ho TW, Mishu, B, Li CY et al (1995) Guillain-Barré syndrome in northern China. Relationship to *Campylobacter jejuni* infection and anti-glycolipid antibodies. Brain 118:597-605
2. Schleicher GK, Black A, Mochan A, Richards GA (2003) Effect of human immunodeficiency virus on intensive care unit outcome of patients with Guillain-Barré syndrome. Crit Care Med 6:1848-1850
3. Sharshar T, Chevret S, Bourdain F, Raphael JC (2003) Early predictors of mechanical ventilation in Guillain-Barré syndrome. Crit Care Med 1:278-283
4. Winer JB (2002) Treatment of Guillain-Barré syndrome. A review. Q J Med 95:717-721
5. Asbury AK, Cornblath DR (1990) Assessment of current diagnostic criteria for Guillain-Barré syndrome. Annals Neurol 27:S21-24
6. Bolton CF (1995) The changing concepts of Guillain-Barré syndrome. N Engl J Med 333:1415-1417
7. Sokrab TE, Eltahir A, Idris MN, Hamid M (2002) Guillain-Barré syndrome following acute falciparum malaria. Neurology 59:1281-1283
8. Raphael JC, Chevret S, Hughes RAC (2001) Plasma exchange for Guillain-Barré syndrome (Cochrane Review). Oxford Update Software, Oxford

9. Green DM (2002) Advances in the management of Guillain-Barré syndrome. Curr Neurol Neurosci Rep 2:541-548
10. Henderson RD, Lawn ND, Fletcher DD et al (2003) The morbidity of Guillain-Barré syndrome admitted to the intensive care unit. Neurology 60:17-21
11. Lawn ND, Fletcher DD, Henderson RD et al (2001) Anticipating mechanical ventilation in Guillain-Barré syndrome. Arch Neurol 58:893-898
12. Brannagan TH, Zhou Y (2003) HIV-associated Guillain-Barré syndrome. J Neurol Sci 208:39-42

TRAUMA OPERATIVE PROCEDURES

Pre-hospital care and triage in trauma

W. UMMENHOFER, R. ALBRECHT, D. SCHEIDEGGER

During the last three decades, the frequency of fatal motor vehicle accidents has been significantly reduced in most industrialised countries. Nevertheless, major trauma continues to be the most common cause of death between the ages of 1 to 44. Injury accounts for more lost years of life than either cancer or heart disease [1]. About 5 million people died worldwide in 1990 as a result of trauma [2]. Demographic projections suggest that deaths from trauma will probably increase to 8.4 million by 2020 [3], becoming a growing burden mainly on low-income countries [4].

Mortality has now become a recognised endpoint in statistical evaluation of health problems and medical strategies. Trauma, death and permanent disability are now used as one of the measures by which severity of injury and quality of medical care are determined. On the other hand, survival of major trauma and return to productivity might be a more important issue for injured people and for corporate policymakers, resulting in worthwhile economic investments in integrated trauma systems paying dividends in terms patients' quality of life [5, 6].

Pre-hospital care and triage are important parts of an integrated trauma system. Structure and quality of emergency medical systems (EMS) may significantly influence the long-term outcome of trauma victims and must therefore provide effective strategies for handling major trauma.

Advanced life support, basic life support or mere transportation?

The past century has witnessed dramatic improvements in the care of injured patients. Before World War I mortality associated with closed femur fractures was greater than 50% and gunshot wounds to the abdomen resulted in a 90% probability of death [1]. Most improvements in outcome are due to antibiotics, modern surgical techniques, and intensive care, but decreasing evacuation time of trauma victims from the scene and increasing knowledge of trauma resuscitation has also undoubtedly contributed to this success. Accordingly, during the last three decades, pre-hospital advanced life support (ALS) activities were estimated to have very positive advantages, although they were not unanimously accepted [7]. But with the era of evidence-based medicine (EBM), new standards of care have been defined. According to these standards, there is almost no evidence that pre-hospital care has had an impact on morbidity or mortality except for cases of nontraumatic and out-of-hospital cardiac arrest [8]. The recently published Cochrane review [9] suggests that the promotion of programmes teaching ALS techniques should be discontinued in view of the lack of evidence supporting their effectiveness.

Obviously, the increased possibilities for pre-hospital invasive therapeutic procedures at the emergency site are not always lifesaving, but include new risks that can potentially further harm the trauma patient in addition to being time consuming. Indeed, there is even evidence that pre-hospital care can be detrimental. One American outcome study found that trauma patients, even severely injured patients, who were transported by private transportation had a lower mortality than those transported by professional EMS [10]. A large database study done in the United States by Dula et al. also supported these findings [11].

Surprisingly, scepticism regarding ALS procedures for trauma patients is restricted to the pre-hospital area. For in-hospital management of major trauma, Advanced Trauma Life Support (ATLS™) algorithms have been widely accepted, with courses introduced worldwide under the auspices of the American College of Surgeons Subcommittee on Trauma. Therefore, it might be worthwhile to consider some aspects of the 'ABCDE' algorithms (Airway, Breathing, Circulation, Disability, Environment) for pre-hospital care. Within these algorithms, there are specific controversial issues regarding airway, circulation and disability, which are addressed below.

Pre-hospital airway management

If, as indicated by the ATLS™ in-hospital priorities, an obstructed airway is the quickest killer in the multiply injured patient [12], then there is no a priori reason for delaying treatment until the patient is in the emergency room (ER). But, as for in-hospital purposes, pre-hospital airway management requires accurate assessment of the patient's respiratory status in order to determine which series of skills and procedures need to be performed. Assessment methods include focused history, observation, auscultation and familiarity with monitoring procedures such as pulse oximetry, capnography and electrocardiography. The skills performed consist in basic airway management, i.e., head positioning, opening the airway, suctioning, placing oropharyngeal or nasopharyngeal airway adjuncts, administration of high-flow oxygen and bag-valve-mask ventilation. Advanced airway management skills include the technique of rapid sequence intubation (RSI) with rescue strategies for failed intubation scenarios, e.g. laryngeal mask airway or cricothyrotomy.

Until recently, advanced airway management skills performed by EMS personnel have been widely accepted and regarded as successful with low adverse event rates [13-15]. The euphhoria over airway management skills has vanished completely. Intubation performed by basic emergency technicians has been questioned as a result of detrimental complications [16]. Moreover, as Liberman et al. point out in a meta-analysis and critical review of the literature, there is no advantage for intubation at the accident scene with regard to the final outcome [17]. It was also reported that patients who received bag-valve-mask ventilation had an adjusted survival rate fivefold that of patients who had on-scene tracheal intubation [18].

Several potential risks, such as an increase in intracranial pressure [19, 20], vomiting and, most fatal, unrecognised oesophageal intubation, are also associated with laryngoscopy and attempted intubation without the use of drugs. Consequently, paramedics in some trauma systems in the United States have tried to use drugs to facilitate pre-hospital intubation; however, complications and failed intubation rates are still high [18, 19, 21]. Thus, the recently published Cochrane review [9] favours discontinuing the promotion of advanced techniques because of the lack of evidence about the effectiveness of ATLS training for ambulance crews.

Gausche-Hill reviewed current controlled studies available for pre-hospital airway management [22], and her data reveal that pre-hospital endotracheal intubation is associated with variable success, morbid complications, lack of clear effect on improving patient outcome, prolonged scene time, which might delay definitive care, and inequity of application in all patients. It is evident that reassessment of our present operating procedures is needed.

This reassessment should address the following three important questions: First, is endotracheal intubation necessary in the pre-hospital trauma patient? Second, if yes, what is the most effective way of efficiently performing the procedure? Third, if sedation and neuromuscular blockade are used, who should do it?

Endotracheal intubation in the field

The following two quotes are in the Advanced Trauma Life Support manual, "Prevention of hypoxemia requires a protected, unobstructed airway and adequate ventilation that must take priority over all other conditions," and "The unconscious head-injured patient, the patient obtunded from alcohol and/or other drugs, and the patient with thoracic injuries may have compromised ventilatory effort. In these patients, endotracheal intubation is intended to: (1) provide an airway, (2) deliver supplementary oxygen, (3) support ventilation, and (4) prevent aspiration. Maintaining oxygenation and preventing hypercarbia are critical in managing the trauma patient, especially if the patient has sustained a head injury" [12].

Airway problems have been cited as the main cause of mortality in otherwise survivable injuries [23]. When dealing with the importance of airway protection in severely head-injured patients (Glasgow Coma Score of 8 or less), most authors refer to the investigation of Winchell and Hoyt [24]. They showed that intubated patients had a significantly lower mortality (26%) than patients who remained unintubated until arrival at hospital (36%). Because it is not known whether attempted or failed intubation caused harm and contributed to mortality in the nonintubated group, interpreting the results of this nonrandomized, retrospective study is difficult. The paramedics did not use drugs to facilitate intubation attempts, and the ability to intubate a trauma patient without sedation or neuromuscular blockade is a strong predictor of poor outcome [25]. In contrast to Winchell and Hoyt's study, another retrospective study in patients with severe head injury found that pre-hospital intubation did not improve survival [26]. The weakness of all these studies was that they were retrospective. However, data from new prospective studies are now available. In a well-designed, randomised investigation, Gausche et al. compared survival and neurological outcomes of paediatric patients treated by bag-valve-mask ventilation and in patients treated by endotracheal intubation in a pre-hospital setting [27]. Their results did not reveal any significant difference between the two groups in survival or in neurological outcome. The results suggest that complications and undetected failures of invasive airway protection outweigh the potential benefits, and that bag-valve-mask ventilation is the superior technique for injured children in a paramedic-based system. For adult patients with severe but nonacutely lethal traumatic brain injury, paramedic RSI protocols were associated with an increase in mortality and a decrease in good outcome in two new prospective trials [28, 29].

Thus, the first question regarding the necessity of endotracheal intubation in the field has to be answered clearly in a philosophical manner; theoretically, it is yes (ATLS™); practically, it is no. And, if done at all, medical research has to more clearly define which patients would most benefit from either field or hospital intubation. Effective airway management implies that the procedure, based on sound scientific evidence, will be used only on the patients who will benefit most from the procedure [22].

Safe procedures for endotrachael pre-hospital intubation in trauma patients

Common hazards for successful invasive airway management are patient combativeness, lack of practice and the concomitant need for in-line cervical stabilisation [30-32]. Even in patients with a Glasgow Coma Score (GCS) of 3, there is airway reactivity (gag and cough reflexes) with a considerable potential to promote intubation failure [30-33]. Attempting intubation in trauma patients without support of a sedative and muscle-relaxant drugs is often impossible. Furthermore, laryngoscopy without drugs can lead to a rise in intracranial pressure [34, 35]. The 'gold standard' [36] for emergency intubation attempts is RSI with a sedative induction agent (such as thiopental, ketamine or etomidate), followed by administration of a rapidly acting neuromuscular blocking agent (such as succinylcholine) to induce unconsciousness and motor paralysis, which is associated with a decrease in intubation failures and complications [13, 37-45]. But sedative and neuromuscular agents facilitate intratracheal intubation only for professional providers. For personnel not accustomed to the effects and side effects of these drugs, new dangers and complications can arise. Therefore, knowledge and skills are the main determinants of successful RSI procedures, and thus the use of the technique should be restricted to professional providers.

Profile of personnel providing pre-hospital endotracheal intubation

The specialty of pre-hospital care, like emergency medicine, is marked by high stress, immediacy of patients' needs, incomplete data and an inability to control the volume of patients that must be treated [22]. Endotracheal intubation requires meticulous assessment of difficult intubation scenarios such as are common in the pre-hospital setting. Combative patients, laryngoscopy impaired by blood and external restricting factors, such as an unpredictable environment including poor lighting or sunlight, inclement weather, concomitant cervical immobilisation and interference or disruption from bystanders, make endotracheal intubation a challenge even for experienced providers. The technique requires knowledge and expertise in using RSI procedures with an awareness of drug dosage and side effects. Hypovolaemia will necessitate reduction of sedative drug dosage. In case of significant intra-abdominal haemorrhage, loss of wall tension following neuromuscular blockade will result in deep hypotension and, therefore, should be withheld initially for certain cases of abdominal trauma. For RSI, preoxygenation and only short attempts at laryngoscopy are part of the procedure. Rescue equipment such as laryngeal mask and surgical airways should be immediately available, and providers should be mentally prepared to apply them. Inline stabilisation of the cervical spine, cricoid pressure, awareness of drug kinetics and pharmacodynamics in hypovolaemic patients as well as reliable assessment of tube position are necessary; additional pharmacotherapy (ongoing sedation, continuous muscle relaxation with nondepolarising neuromuscular blockade) will be required. Paramedics have only limited experience and on-the-job skills for invasive airway management [46]. As Pepe pointed out, a given paramedic may perform endotracheal intubation only on one or two patients each year, or perform a paediatric intubation once every 15 to 20 years [47].

Therefore, only personnel who are involved in the daily clinical routine of airway management should perform endotracheal intubation in the hostile pre-hospital environment. Traditionally, airway management has been a skill that was perfected, taught and, to a certain degree, sequestered by anaesthetists. But it is the technique and experience, not the profession, that makes the difference. Meanwhile, RSI is a safe procedure if performed by emergency physicians, whether in an in-hospital setting [48] or in the field [49]. On the other hand, for paramedic-based systems, bag-valve-mask ventilation [21] or noninvasive airway devices such as the laryngeal mask airway or the new laryngeal tube [50, 51] may be advantageous.

Accordingly, EMS administrators must critically evaluate the quality of pre-hospital airway management that they are providing to patients within their system by collecting the data necessary to identify quality issues and developing strategies to implement change [22]. Although the utility of airway management at the accident scene is controversial, it is generally agreed that it is not the intervention per se (i.e. endotracheal intubation) but rather the conditions, skills, and performance that might be the possible variables which affect outcome [27, 52]. Davis has shown a high incidence of inadvertent hyperventilation and a substantially higher incidence of transient hypoxia for paramedic-based RSI procedures than has been reported for trauma intubations in the resuscitation suite [29]. On the other hand, for selected group of patients, pre-hospital invasive airway management may well have an influence on the later prognosis if performed by skilled individuals like anaesthetists [53, 54].

Spinal stabilisation

In the United States, the lifetime medical costs resulting from spinal cord injury (SCI) have been estimated at 9 billion dollars per year in 1994 [55]. SCI results in long-term disability, often with profound effects on the quality of life of the affected individuals and their careers [56]. Acute traumatic SCI is estimated to occur in only 3% of trauma admissions [57]. But, unfortunately, about half of these injuries involve the cervical spine with the threat of quadriplegia [58]. The aim of pre-hospital immobilisation is to stabilise the spine by restricting mobility, thus preventing secondary SCI during extrication, resuscitation, transport and evaluation of trauma patients with suspected spinal instability [56]. It is estimated that 5% of trauma patients with cervical spine injuries have a missed or delayed diagnosis [59]. In one study, the rescue team did not suspect SCI in 14% of the trauma patients despite clinical evidence [60]. Occult cervical SCI might be missed more likely in patients who are distracted by pain from other injuries or in patients with an obtunded or otherwise altered level of consciousness.

Pre-hospital spinal immobilisation has nevertheless been questioned despite its widespread use. Arguments have been made that spinal cord damage occurs at the time of the impact and that subsequent movement is generally not significant enough to cause further damage [61]. If this is true, then in-hospital immobilisation should also be discontinued. Presumably, in-hospital movement is much less than that of pre-hospital transfer procedures. On the other hand, Muckart et al. reported two cases of SCI as a possible result of endotracheal intubation in patients with undiagnosed cervical spine fractures; in both cases, intubation had been performed without protective measures like inline stabilisation, and neurological symptoms occurred after the procedure [62]. Indeed, many immobilisation procedures might be unnecessary. Most trauma patients do not have spinal instability and hence will not benefit from spinal immobilization. The incidence of SCI in the United States is estimated to be between 40 and 50 cases per million people per year [63]. If, as reported by Orledge and Pepe, approximately 5 million patients in the United States receive spinal immobilisation every year [64], 4.99 million patients are immobilised unnecessarily. But perhaps it is exactly the overly conservative use of immobilisation that prevents higher incidences of SCI. If these routine procedures are abandoned, proper assessment of patients and consideration of mechanisms of trauma will need to become necessary conditions for immobilisation. In doubt or in the case of unconscious patients, immobilisation should still be performed.

Of course, spinal immobilisation is not without adverse effects. Case series have shown that rigid collars might cause airway difficulties, increased intracranial pressure [65], increased risk of aspiration [66], restricted respiration [67], dysphagia [68] and skin ulceration [69]. The ATLS™ protocol for the in-hospital primary survey gives the highest priority to "airway and cervical spine control"[12]; there is no obvious reason that the same perspective should not also apply to the pre-hospital setting.

The WHO Pre-Hospital Trauma Care Steering Committee concluded that the effect of pre-hospital spinal immobilisation on mortality, neurological injury, spinal stability, and adverse effects in trauma patients remains uncertain. Because airway obstruction is a major cause of preventable death in trauma patients, and spinal immobilisation, particularly of the cervical spine, can contribute to airway compromise, the possibility that immobilisation may increase mortality and morbidity cannot be excluded [56]. Thus, if advanced airway management is abandoned, immobilisation procedures also might be challenged.

Trauma fluid resuscitation

On the one hand, "stop the bleeding" procedures are generally considered necessary for external bleeding in the pre-hospital setting. On the other hand, there exists little consensus regarding volume resuscitation, and much discussion has taken place during the last decade regarding this matter. The ongoing debate on "what to give?" (i.e. crystalloids, colloids, hypertonic solutions or oxygen-carrying blood substitutes) has been partly replaced by the controversy of "when to give?" and "how much to give?"

Most traditional strategies for fluid resuscitation focus on controlled haemorrhage shock models. But when considering early deaths from haemorrhage, uncontrolled bleeding scenarios leading to hypovolaemic shock are more realistic. Both penetrating and blunt trauma can lead to uncontrolled haemorrhage. Limited fluid resuscitation has been shown to have benefit in animal studies [70-73] and in a clinical trial [74].

What to give?

The main objective of fluid resuscitation from hypovolaemia is to increase oxygen delivery to vital organs to maintain viability yet not increase bleeding before surgical haemostasis. The optimal fluid for such a limited (i.e., hypotensive) fluid resuscitation should have certain characteristics, but this still needs to be determined. The fluid should rapidly restore plasma volume, microcirculatory flow and oxygen delivery and have no significant side effects, such as a deleterious immune response. It should be readily stored and transported, and it should be inexpensive. Standard plasma substitutes increase volume and flow, but may actually decrease oxygen delivery because of haemodilution [75]. Regarding the current pros and cons of crystalloids and colloids in trauma resuscitation, meta-analyses suggest that the choice of fluid used for resuscitation has little or no effect on mortality. In contrast, when only resuscitation of trauma patients is considered, the results suggest that resuscitation with colloids carries an increased mortality. Crystalloids should therefore, even when all limitations and nuances of interpretation are considered, continue to remain the fluids of choice for the resuscitation of trauma patients in haemorrhagic shock [76].

When to give and how much?

A recent Cochrane review [77] has concluded that there is no evidence from randomised controlled trials to support the pre-hospital use of early or large volume intravenous fluid administration in cases of uncontrolled haemorrhage. Results from most investigations indicate that efforts to return blood pressure to normal in bleeding patients can be counterproductive [78]. However, several questions remain, such as the optimal blood pressure and maximal safe duration of hypotension. There are a significant number of civilian (difficult extrication scenarios) and military (prolonged evacuation scenarios) trauma victims who, because of distance or tactical situations, must survive in a hypovolaemic state for a prolonged period of time between injury and surgical intervention. Prolonged limited fluid resuscitation has not been explored [75].

Triage in the field: assessment, evaluation and re-evaluation

As in the case of the obstructed airway, it is not only whether the right intervention has been selected or the technique has been performed safely that is crucial, but, most importantly, whether the assessment of injury, concomitant circumstances and patient's disorders are correctly determined that can make the difference. The common question of should we "scoop and run" or "stay and play" could be answered, as Pepe and Stewart pointed out, by another simple question, "For which patient?" [79]: "Under the uncontrolled circumstances of the pre-hospital environment, cookbook protocols are often difficult to follow and sound clinical judgement has become an essential ingredient in the decision-making process." You need the time course of stabilisation or deterioration of severely injured patients, which usually takes place within the initial time of the in-hospital treatment, to understand the core contents of the ATLS™ principle of assessment and re-assessment. The experience that comes with frequent management of unstable trauma victims is a necessary component for developing sound clinical judgement. This judgement might be essential to assess well-defined subgroups of patients who require volume resuscitation at the scene of injury, such as during prolonged extrication procedures or in elderly patients with coexisting cardiovascular compromise.

Pre-hospital scoring systems are widely used in the United States. They are typically employed to assist pre-hospital personnel in determining which patients require trauma centre care, but they are not recommended as the sole determinant of triage [80]. Pre-hospital scoring systems have been shown to lead to both under- and over-triage of trauma patients [81]. Under-triage denies the benefits of trauma centres to patients who need them most. Over-triage results in patients not requiring trauma centre care overburdening the system [82]. Protocols and scoring systems have been developed to assist pre-hospital personnel in correctly triaging trauma patients, but have not been able to achieve both high sensitivity and high specificity [83]. When obvious indicators, such as hypoxaemia, multiple injury, focal neurological deficits for choice of destination and in-hospital trauma team activation, are missing, the pre-hospital GCS score may be used to reduce over-triage and under-triage rates. Norwood et al. have demonstrated that a GCS score ≤ 14 accurately predicts the need for full trauma team activation and patient hospitalisation after motor vehicle collisions [84]. For a triage tool to be useful, it must be used. But despite the education of all pre-hospital personnel in the use of the GCS, an actual score was only reported in 72% of the patients before arrival in the emergency department [84]. Perhaps the presence of a trained physician can decrease the rate of over-triage by increasing the probability that the correct destination will be selected for an injured patient [85].

Responsibility in pre-hospital trauma care

Today, three primary forces drive health care policy in America and in most developed countries: efforts to control costs, to improve access and to produce and ensure delivery of high-quality care. Until recently, adverse outcomes were predicted primarily by patient factors, but results of inquiries, such as the United Kingdom's study on preventable deaths following trauma [86], indicate that complication rates alone are a poor measure of provider quality. A better measure of provider quality than mere complication rates might be the failure to rescue a patient [87]. For the field of anaesthesiology, the ability to rescue the patient from underlying disease is dependent on clinical skills. Both death rates and failure to rescue were inversely related to the proportion of board-certified anaesthetists on the anaesthesia-provider staff. Stated in positive terms the more board-certified anaesthetists are involved in the delivery of anaesthesia care, the better the outcomes as measured by survival rates and rescue from complications.

Pre-hospital procedures in trauma patients are often regarded as mere time-consuming efforts. Physicians tend to disregard time passed in the pre-hospital setting, but, although controversial, time has been shown to be the only valid predictor of outcome in the multiply injured patient [88-90]. Consistent with the efficacy of time reduction are results that support the use of private transportation by bystanders or police for trauma patients, thereby, saving the time that would have been required by professional EMS to reach the scene [10, 11].

However, Spaite et al. found no objective proof that the primary determinant of outcome for the trauma patient is the time interval from injury to the operating theatre [91]. For patients transported directly to a trauma centre time factors did not adversely affect outcome, providing they did not exceed the first hour after injury; this was true even for the most severely injured patients [92]. The time used for pre-hospital interventions, such as endotracheal intubation, venous access or immobilisation would save time in the ER and thus not necessarily increase the total injury-to-operating theatre interval. Perhaps the lack of designated emergency departments and less well-structured in-hospital performance in Europe accounts for the loss of time that is expected to be gained by these accident scene procedures. Furthermore, the ATLS™ -guided "golden hour of trauma", i.e. the time limit not to be exceeded for life-saving surgical definitive care, might nowadays only be applicable for a minority of multiply traumatised patients: the management of trauma patients has become increasingly nonoperative, especially for solid abdominal organ injuries. In a retrospective chart review of two trauma centres, only 15% of patients underwent operative interventions [93]. If this is so, ALS interventions in the field could partly replace ER-based procedures without time loss or harm for a majority of trauma victims.

As has been shown for helicopter emergency services with specially trained physicians, ALS only benefits a small number of patients. The most important target groups are patients with cardiovascular disease and severe trauma. The most important life-saving measure was airway control [94]. Therefore, not surprisingly, Lossius et al. demonstrated a benefit in terms of life-years gained in every 14th patient using an expert panel-based investigation of a pre-hospital anaesthetist-manned EMS [53]. The pre-hospital setting is a hazardous environment. Conditions for health care providers are usually much worse than the "safe" surroundings of an ER. Therefore, in the field, the quality of the caregiver engaged in essential life-saving procedures should not be inferior. This not only refers to airway management, but also includes assessment of patients, awareness of hazards and pitfalls and, of course, in the context of litigation, responsibility for a given mission. Who decides to terminate resuscitation or, often more difficult, not to start it? Even in the pre-hospital setting, the leader of a trauma team should be an experienced anaesthetist or emergency physician. Trauma education must involve manual skills accomplished elsewhere (i.e. administration of anaesthesia or regular performance of resuscitation in the emergency room) and focus on standard life-saving procedures and the peculiar challenges of the pre-hospital environment such as extrication procedures or triage principles in multiple casualty events [95].

Different systems have different problems. It is still questioned whether a physician's involvement in pre-hospital trauma care results in an improved outcome in severely injured patients. However, this is also true for paramedic-based systems. If airway management, volume replacement, and spinal immobilisation are discontinued because of their detrimental potential, there is not much left in the way of treatment to be performed in the field. The approaches that have been used to develop the current pre-hospital trauma literature do not permit the development of a consensus opinion on the impact of each system component on patient outcome. Perhaps, as Spaite et al. pointed out, and this may be a continuing paradigm even in the era of "evidence-based medicine", most pre-hospital trauma research is still "emphasizing the wrong issues, asking the wrong questions, and using the wrong methods" [96].

Finally, the benefit of EMS systems cannot be measured only in life-years gained and financial considerations. The service is expected by society for many other reasons. Most importantly, it gives a feeling of security and comfort, with helicopter availability valued particularly in remote rural areas [94].

References

1. Stewart RM, Myers JG, Dent DL et al (2003) Seven hundred fifty-three consecutive deaths in a level I trauma center: the argument for injury prevention. J Trauma 54:66-70
2. Murray CJL, Lopez AD (1996) Global health statistics: a compendium of incidence, prevalence and mortality estimates for over 200 conditions. Harvard University Press, Boston
3. Murray CJ, Lopez AD (1997) Alternative projections of mortality and disability by cause 1990-2020: Global Burden of Disease Study. Lancet 349:1498-1504
4. Murray CJ, Lopez AD (1997) Mortality by cause for eight regions of the world: Global Burden of Disease Study. Lancet 349:1269-1276
5. Morris JA, Jr., Sanchez AA, Bass SM et al (1991) Trauma patients return to productivity. J Trauma 31:827-833
6. Frutiger A, Ryf C, Bilat C et al (1991) Five years' follow-up of severely injured ICU patients. J Trauma 31:1216-1225
7. Bissell RA, Eslinger DG, Zimmerman L (1998) The efficacy of advanced life support: a review of the literature. Prehosp Disast Med 13:77-87
8. Spaite D, Benoit R, Brown D et al (1995) Uniform prehospital data elements and definitions: a report from the uniform prehospital emergency medical services data conference. Ann Emerg Med 25:525-534
9. Sethi D, Kwan I, Kelly AM et al (2002) Advance trauma life support training for trauma crews.

In The Cochrane Library, issue 2. WHO Pre-Hospital Trauma Care Steering Committee. Update Software, Oxford
10. Demetriades D, Chan L, Cornwell E et al (1996) Paramedic vs. private transportation of trauma patients. Effect on outcome. Arch Surg 131:133-138
11. Dula DJ, Moyer B, Skiendzielewski J et al (2000) Outcome associated with private vehicle and ambulance transport of motor vehicle crash victims to trauma centers. Ann Emerg Med 36 Suppl 77:297
12. American College of Surgeons Committee on Trauma (1993) Advanced Trauma Life Support (ATLS). Course for Physicians, 5th edn, Chicago, Ill
13. Hedges JR, Dronen SC, Feero S et al (1988) Succinylcholine-assisted intubations in prehospital care. Ann Emerg Med 17:469-472
14. Syverud SA, Borron SW, Storer DL et al (1988) Prehospital use of neuromuscular blocking agents in a helicopter ambulance program. Ann Emerg Med 17:236-242
15. Murphy-Macabobby M, Marshall WJ, Schneider C et al (1992) Neuromuscular blockade in aeromedical airway management. Ann Emerg Med 21:664-668
16. Spaite D (1998) Intubation by basic EMTs: lifesaving advance or catastrophic complication? Ann Emerg Med 31:276-277
17. Liberman M, Mulder D, Sampalis J (2000) Advanced or basic life support for trauma: meta-analysis and critical review of the literature. J Trauma 49:584-599
18. Eckstein M, Chan L, Schneir A et al (2000) Effect of prehospital advanced life support on outcomes of major trauma patients. J Trauma 48:643-648
19. Blostein PA, Koestner AJ, Hoak S (1998) Failed rapid sequence intubation in trauma patients: esophageal tracheal combitube is a useful adjunct. J Trauma 44:534-537
20. Pelucio M, Halligan L, Dhindsa H (1997) Out-of-hospital experience with the syringe esophageal detector device. Acad Emerg Med 4:563-568
21. Gausche M, Lewis RJ (2000) Out-of-hospital endotracheal intubation of children. JAMA 283:2790-2792
22. Gausche-Hill M (2003) Ensuring quality in prehospital airway management. Curr Opin Anesthesiol 16:173-181
23. Hussain LM, Redmond AD (1994) Are pre-hospital deaths from accidental injury preventable? BMJ 308:1077-1080
24. Winchell RJ, Hoyt DB (1997) Endotracheal intubation in the field improves survival in patients with severe head injury. Trauma Research and Education Foundation of San Diego. Arch Surg 132:592-597
25. Lockey D, Davies G, Coats T (2001) Survival of trauma patients who have prehospital tracheal intubation without anaesthesia or muscle relaxants: observational study. BMJ 323:141
26. Murray JA, Demetriades D, Berne TV et al (2000) Prehospital intubation in patients with severe head injury. J Trauma 49:1065-1070
27. Gausche M, Lewis RJ, Stratton SJ et al (2000) Effect of out-of-hospital pediatric endotracheal intubation on survival and neurological outcome: a controlled clinical trial. JAMA 283:783-790
28. Bochicchio GV, Ilahi O, Joshi M et al (2003) Endotracheal intubation in the field does not improve outcome in trauma patients who present without an acutely lethal traumatic brain injury. J Trauma 54:307-311
29. Davis DP, Hoyt DB, Ochs M et al (2003) The effect of paramedic rapid sequence intubation on outcome in patients with severe traumatic brain injury. J Trauma 54:444-453
30. Stewart RD, Paris PM, Winter PM et al (1984) Field endotracheal intubation by paramedical personnel. Success rates and complications. Chest 85:341-345
31. Krisanda TJ, Eitel DR, Hess D et al (1992) An analysis of invasive airway management in a suburban emergency medical services system. Prehosp Disast Med 7:121-126
32. Karch SB, Lewis T, Young S et al (1996) Field intubation of trauma patients: complications, indications, and outcomes. Am J Emerg Med 14:617-619
33. Moulton C, Pennycook AG (1994) Relation between Glasgow Coma Score and cough reflex. Lancet 343:1261-1262

34. Ampel L, Hott KA, Sielaff GW et al (1988) An approach to airway management in the acutely head-injured patient. J Emerg Med 6:1-7
35. Walls RM (1993) Rapid-sequence intubation in head trauma. Ann Emerg Med 22:1008-1013
36. Adnet F, Lapostolle F, Ricard-Hibon A et al (2001) Intubating trauma patients before reaching hospital: revisited. Crit Care 5:290-291
37. Li J, Murphy-Lavoie H, Bugas C et al (1999) Complications of emergency intubation with and without paralysis. Am J Emerg Med 17:141-143
38. Ma OJ, Atchley RB, Hatley T et al (1998) Intubation success rates improve for an air medical program after implementing the use of neuromuscular blocking agents. Am J Emerg Med 16:125-127
39. Vijayakumar E, Bosscher H, Renzi FP et al (1998) The use of neuromuscular blocking agents in the emergency department to facilitate tracheal intubation in the trauma patient: help or hindrance? J Crit Care 13:1-6
40. Wang HE, O'Connor RE, Domeier RM (2001) Prehospital rapid-sequence intubation. Prehosp Emerg Care 5:40-48
41. Wang HE, O'Connor RE, Megargel RE et al (2000) The utilization of midazolam as a pharmacologic adjunct to endotracheal intubation by paramedics. Prehosp Emerg Care 4:14-18
42. Wayne MA, Friedland E (1999) Prehospital use of succinylcholine: a 20-year review. Prehosp Emerg Care 3:107-109
43. Wayne MA, Slovis CM, Pirrallo RG (1999) Management of difficult airways in the field. Prehosp Emerg Care 3:290-296
44. Pace SA, Fuller FP (2000) Out-of-hospital succinylcholine-assisted endotracheal intubation by paramedics. Ann Emerg Med 35:568-572
45. Ochs M, Davis D, Hoyt D et al (2002) Paramedic-performed rapid sequence intubation of patients with severe head injuries. Ann Emerg Med 40:159-167
46. Stout J, Pepe PE, Mosesso VN Jr (2000) All-advanced life support vs tiered-response ambulance systems. Prehosp Emerg Care 4:1-6
47. Pepe PE (2001) Current issues in resuscitative trauma management: an overview. Curr Opin Crit Care 7:409-412
48. Omert L, Yeaney W, Mizikowski S et al (2001) Role of the emergency medicine physician in airway management of the trauma patient. J Trauma 51:1065-1068
49. Mackay CA, Terris J, Coats TJ (2001) Prehospital rapid sequence induction by emergency physicians: is it safe? Emerg Med J 18:20-24
50. Genzwuerker HV, Hilker T, Hohner E et al (2000) The laryngeal tube: a new adjunct for airway management. Prehosp Emerg Care 4:168-172.
51. Doerges V, Ocker H, Wenzel V et al (2000) The laryngeal tube: a new simple airway device. Anesth Analg 90:1220-1222
52. Katz SH, Falk JL (2001) Misplaced endotracheal tubes by paramedics in an urban emergency medical services system. Ann Emerg Med 37:32-37
53. Lossius HM, Soreide E, Hotvedt R et al (2002) Prehospital advanced life support provided by specially trained physicians: is there a benefit in terms of life years gained? Acta Anaesthesiol Scand 46:771-778
54. Regel G, Stalp M, Lehmann U et al (1997) Prehospital care, importance of early intervention on outcome. Acta Anaesthesiol Scand Suppl 110:71-76
55. Miller TR (1994) Costs of head and neck injury and a cost-benefit analysis of bicycle helmets. In: Levine RS (ed) Head and neck injury. Society of Automotive Engineering, New York
56. Kwan I, Bunn F, Roberts I (2002) Spinal immobilisation for trauma patients. (The Cochrane Library, issue 2) WHO Pre-Hospital Trauma Care Steering Committee, Oxford (update software)
57. Burney RE, Maio RF, Maynard F et al (1993) Incidence, characteristics, and outcome of spinal cord injury at trauma centers in North America. Arch Surg 128:596-599
58. De Lorenzo R, Olson J, Boska M et al (1996) Optimal positioning for cervical immobilisation. Ann Emerg Med 28:301-308

59. Davis JW, Phreaner DL, Hoyt DB et al (1993) The etiology of missed cervical spine injuries. J Trauma 34:342-346
60. Lampl L, Helm M, Winter M (1992) Zum Problem der präklinisch nicht erkannten Wirbelsäulenverletzung. Notarzt 8:99-103
61. Hauswald M, Ong G, Tandberg D et al (1998) Out-of-hospital spinal immobilization: its effect on neurologic injury. Acad Emerg Med 5:214-219
62. Muckart D, Bhagwanjee S, Van der Merwe R (1997) Spinal cord injury as a result of endotracheal intubation in patients with undiagnosed cervical spine fractures. Anesthesiology 87:418-420
63. National Spinal Cord Injury Statistical Center (1998) Spinal cord injury: facts and figures at a glance. University of Alabama, Birmingham, Ala
64. Orledge JD, Pepe PE (1998) Out-of-hospital spinal immobilization: is it really necessary? Acad Emerg Med 5:203-204
65. Davies G, Deakin C, Wilson A (1996) The effect of a rigid collar on intracranial pressure. Injury 27:647-649
66. Butman AM, Schelble DT, Vomacka RW (1996) The relevance of the occult cervical spine controversy and mechanism of injury to prehospital protocols: a review of the issues and literature. Prehosp Disast Med 11:228-233
67. Totten VY, Sugarman DB (1999) Respiratory effects of spinal immobilization. Prehosp Emerg Care 3:347-352
68. Houghton DJ, Curley JW (1996) Dysphagia caused by a hard cervical collar. Br J Neurosurg 10:501-502
69. Hewitt S (1994) Skin necrosis caused by a semi-rigid cervical collar in a ventilated patient with multiple injuries. Injury 25:323-324
70. Kim SH, Stezoski SW, Safar P et al (1997) Hypothermia and minimal fluid resuscitation increase survival after uncontrolled hemorrhagic shock in rats. J Trauma 42:213-222
71. Stern SA, Dronen SC, Birrer P et al (1993) Effect of blood pressure on hemorrhage volume and survival in a near- fatal hemorrhage model incorporating a vascular injury. Ann Emerg Med 22:155-163
72. Capone AC, Safar P, Stezoski W et al (1995) Improved outcome with fluid restriction in treatment of uncontrolled hemorrhagic shock. J Am Coll Surg 180:49-56
73. Bickell WH, Bruttig SP, Millnamow GA et al (1991) The detrimental effects of intravenous crystalloid after aortotomy in swine. Surgery 110:529-536
74. Bickell W, Wall M, Pepe P et al (1994) Immediate versus delayed resuscitation for hypotensive patients with penetrating torso injuries. N Engl J Med 331:1105-1109
75. Tisherman SA (2003) Trauma fluid resuscitation in 2010. J Trauma 54:S231-234
76. Rizoli SB (2003) Crystalloids and colloids in trauma resuscitation: a brief overview of the current debate. J Trauma 54:S82-88
77. Kwan I, Bunn F, Roberts I (2002) Timing and volume of fluid administration for patients with bleeding following trauma. (The Cochrane Library, issue 2) WHO Pre-Hospital Trauma Care Steering Committee, Oxford (update software)
78. Roberts I, Evans P, Bunn F et al (2001) Is the normalisation of blood pressure in bleeding trauma patients harmful? Lancet 357:385-387
79. Pepe P, Stewart R (1986) Role of the physician in the prehospital setting. Ann Emerg Med 15:1480-1483
80. Marcin JP, Pollack MM (2002) Triage scoring systems, severity of illness measures, and mortality prediction models in pediatric trauma. Crit Care Med 30:S457-467
81. Ornato J, Mlinek EJ Jr, Craren EJ et al (1985) Ineffectiveness of the trauma score and the CRAMS scale for accurately triaging patients to trauma centers. Ann Emerg Med 14:1061-1064
82. van Wijngaarden M, Kortbeek J, Lafreniere R et al (1996) Air ambulance trauma transport: a quality review. J Trauma 41:26-31
83. Baxt WG, Berry CC, Epperson MD et al (1989) The failure of prehospital trauma prediction rules to classify trauma patients accurately. Ann Emerg Med 18:1-8

84. Norwood SH, McAuley CE, Berne JD et al (2002) A prehospital Glasgow Coma Scale score < or = 14 accurately predicts the need for full trauma team activation and patient hospitalization after motor vehicle collisions. J Trauma 53:503-507
85. Coats TJ, Wilson AW, Cross FW (1993) On-scene medical decision making and overtriage. Br J Surg 80:1291-1293
86. Anderson I, Woodford M, De Dombal F et al (1988) Retrospective study of 1000 deaths from injury in England and Wales. BMJ 296:1305-1308
87. Longnecker D (1997) Navigation in uncharted waters: Is anesthesiology on course for the 21st century? Anesthesiology 86:736-742
88. Sampalis J, Lavoie A, Williams J et al (1993) Impact of on-site care, prehospital time, and level of in-hospital care on survival in severely injured patients. J Trauma 34:252-261
89. Ivatury R, Nallathambi M, Roberge J et al (1987) Penetrating thoracic injuries: in-field stabilization vs. prompt transport. J Trauma 27:1066-1073
90. Sampalis J, Lavoie A, Williams J et al (1992) Standardized mortality ratio analysis on a sample of severely injured patients from a large Canadian city without regionalized trauma care. J Trauma 33:205-211
91. Spaite D, Criss E, Valenzuela T et al (1998) Prehospital Advanced Life Support for major trauma: critical need for clinical trials. Ann Emerg Med 32:480-489
92. Pepe P, Wyatt C, Bickell W et al (1987) The relationship between total prehospital time and outcome in hypotensive victims of penetrating injuries. Ann Emerg Med 16:293-297
93. Bulinski P, Bachulis B, Naylor DF Jr et al (2003) The changing face of trauma management and its impact on surgical resident training. J Trauma 54:161-163
94. Gisvold SE (2002) Helicopter emergency medical service with specially trained physicians - does it make a difference? Acta Anaesthesiol Scand 46:757-758
95. Scope A, Lynn M, Farkash U et al (2001) Military trauma life support: a comprehensive training program for military physicians. Mil Med 166:385-388
96. Spaite D, Criss E, Valenzuela T et al (1995) Emergency medical service systems research: problems of the past, challenges of the future. Ann Emerg Med 26:146-152

Severe thermal burn injury: assessment and early management

P. Y. GUEUGNIAUD, M. BERTIN-MAGHIT, P. PETIT

Despite rational progress in prevention, burns remain a major cause of traumatic injury in all age groups of the population worldwide. Nevertheless, survival after extensive burn injury has improved substantially during the past 30 years [1], thanks to various factors: immediate prehospital care, early care for the burn shock and of the potential post-burn pulmonary dysfunction, better understanding of pathophysiological mechanisms involved in burn shock and some progress in acute surgical approach [2].

Assessment and pathophysiological changes

Burn injury induces an immediate, acute, total or partial destruction of the skin and possibly the underlying tissues. When the surface area of the body involved and the depth of burn injury are significant, the burn shock secondary to hypovolaemia appears in the first several hours post-burn. The size of the burn (relative to that of total body surface area: TBSA), the depth of injury, the location of injury, the patient's age, and the presence of associated injuries determine morbidity and mortality [3].

Calculation of burn size

To calculate the extent of the burn, Wallace's "rule of nines" is a useful guide. The adult body configuration is such that anatomical regions represent 9% or a multiple of TBSA: head plus neck and each arm, 9%; anterior, posterior trunk, and each lower extremity, 18%. To be more precise and to adjust the calculation for children according to age, the Lund and Browder chart is indicated: in children, the relative body surface area of the head and the neck is larger and that of the lower extremities smaller than in adults (Table 1). A useful adjunct for calculating the size of partially burned areas of skin is the palm of the patient's

Table 1 Lund and Browder Chart

Years old	0-1	1-4	5-9	10-15	Adult
Head	19	17	13	10	7
Neck	2	2	2	2	2
Anterior trunk	13	13	13	13	13
Posterior trunk	13	13	13	13	13
Right buttock	2.5	2.5	2.5	2.5	2.5
Left buttock	2.5	2.5	2.5	2.5	2.5
Perineum	1	1	1	1	1
Right forearm	4	4	4	4	4
Left forearm	4	4	4	4	4
Right arm	3	3	3	3	3
Left arm	3	3	3	3	3
Right hand	2.5	2.5	2.5	2.5	2.5
Left hand	2.5	2.5	2.5	2.5	2.5
Right thigh	5.5	6.5	8.5	8.5	9.5
Left thigh	5.5	6.5	8.5	8.5	9.5
Right leg	5	5	5.5	6	7
Left leg	5	5	5.5	6	7
Right foot	3.5	3.5	3.5	3.5	3.5
Left foot	3.5	3.5	3.5	3.5	3.5

hand, which represents 0.5% of TBSA. The palm area plus the palmar surface of the five digits represents 0.8% of TBSA in males and 0.7% in females [4].

The initial assessment of surface area involved in a burn injury remains a general approximation, even in adults. Whatever formula is used, the initial calculation of %TBSA affected only predicts initial fluid resuscitation requirements.

Criteria to define a "major" burn

Major burns in adult patients have been defined as thermal injury-induced lesions which justify intensive care treatment for at least 3 days post-injury. Table 2 (adapted from [5]) lists criteria that can be used to define a "major" burn. Major burn was classically defined as burn greater than 15 to 20% of TBSA in adults and 5 to 10% in infants and small children. Indeed such burns justify admission to a specialised centre. But today, critically burned patients are defined as victims who have sustained a size of deep burn over 50% of TBSA, which is usually considered to cause a mortality rate of about 50% in healthy young adults [6].

Table 2 Criteria for different major burns. Adapted from [5]

Total body surface area burned 25% in adults or 20% at extremes of age
Full thickness burns 10%
Burns involving face and/or neck
Inhalation burns
Associated trauma
Burns in patients with serious pre-existing medical disorders (ASA Status II)

This paper provides a short update focused on the initial resuscitation of these critically burned patients.

Depth of burn injury

Traditionally, burn depth has been classified into three degrees of injury. Nevertheless, for an initial emergency evaluation, classification of burn degrees must only distinguish between superficial burn and deep burn: each burn injury which induces more than a cutaneous erythema must be considered a deep burn. All patients with deep burns greater than 20 per cent of TBSA require fluid resuscitation and referral to a burn center [7].

Severity index

The prediction of burn mortality is not easy. The indices of severity usually applied in intensive care units, e.g. Apache II, are not relevant for burn patients.

Only clinical parameters can be used to prospectively assess a prognosis. The "Baux index" is calculated by adding patient's age and TBSA: an index level at 95 is associated with a 50% mortality rate [8]. The "unit of burn skin"

(UBS) of Sach and Watson takes into account TBSA and the third-degree area: UBS is only applicable retrospectively. Probably the most valuable index is the "abbreviated burn severity index" (ABSI) from Tobiasen: it is suitable from admission onward [9] (Table 3).

Table 3 Abbreviated burn severity index. From [9]

		Score
Sex	Male Female	1 0
Age (years)	0-20 21-40 41-60 61-80 81-100	1 2 3 4 5
Inhalation injury		1
Third-degree burn lesions		1
TBSA (%)	1-10 11-20 21-30 31-40 41-50 51-60 61-70 71-80 81-90 91-100	1 2 3 4 5 6 7 8 9 10

-Score < 4, probability of survival rate = 0.99
-Score = 4-5, probability of survival rate = 0.98
-Score = 6-7, probability of survival rate = 0.8 – 0.9
-Score = 8-9, probability of survival rate = 0.5 – 0.7
-Score = 10-11, probability of survival rate = 0.2 – 0.4
-Score >11, probability of survival rate ≤ 0.1.

Pathophysiological changes after extensive cutaneous burns

Systemic inflammatory response

A zone of ischaemia is present below the dead tissue in the early post-burn period. This zone has been heat-injured but not destroyed, and its vasculature is compromised [6]. This marginally viable tissue can be readily converted to nonviable tissue by a further insult, such as hypoperfusion, hypoxia or infection. Prevention of wound conversion from viable to nonviable tissue is of major importance in the resuscitation period for the final prognosis of the most severely burned patients. In its turn, this zone of ischaemia is surrounded with inflammatory tissue. Various chemical mediators of inflammation (kinins, histamine, thromboxane, free radicals, and also multiple cytokines), which are produced and released at the burn site, cause increased capillary permeability locally and, when burns are extensive, in distant injured organs [1]. During the post-burn first 5 days' resuscitation, interleukin-1 [10, 11], and interleukin-8 [12, 13], and especially interleukin-6 [10, 11, 14] reach abnormal plasma levels, suggesting that interleukin-6 could be involved in cell membrane permeability and therefore in fluid shifts and haemodynamic instability [15]. On the other hand, recent studies suggest that burn trauma activates cardiomyocyte secretion of TNF-alpha [16] and that apoptosis may be an important pathway for cardiac injury through decreased nitric oxide levels [17]. Anyhow, whatever the precise pathophysiological mechanisms involved, burn injury is consistent with the general pattern of the systemic inflammatory response syndrome [2, 18].

Fluid shifts and haemodynamic disturbances

Hypovolaemia is the initial mandatory consequence of the fluid shifts after an extensive burn injury. The problem of hypovolaemia, when aggressively corrected, is replaced by a generalised burn oedema formation, that can result in serious morbidity [6]. Massive tissue oedema results in an increase in tissue pressure and a decrease in tissue oxygen tension, leading to a further ischaemic insult to already damaged cells. Oedema in the upper airway after severe burns and airway oedema after inhalation injury are well described. Hypoproteinaemia characteristically occurs due to the loss of protein from leaky capillaries in burn tissue, which can further accentuate oedema formation in non-burned tissues and distant organs: life-threatening cerebral oedema has also been reported in the early period after injury [19].

In the haemodynamic field, all patients with serious burns suffer burn shock. From the injury until 12 - 24 hours post-burn, burn shock is linked with hypovolaemia: increased systemic vascular resistances and depressed cardiac output occur because of this hypovolaemia. The decrease in myocardial contractility could also be accentuated by a myocardial depressant factor, which remains controversial [16, 17, 20, 21]. Then, from day 2 to day 5 after injury, a hyperdynamic shock arises with an increase in cardiac output and a significant decrease in systemic vascular resistance [22]. This specific haemodynamic profile, initially described 20 years ago by Shoemaker et al. [23], has been corroborated [15, 24, 25]. The reversal of the haemodynamic trends occurs simultaneously with the highest level of tissue oedema and circulating interleukin-6 [15] (Fig. 1).

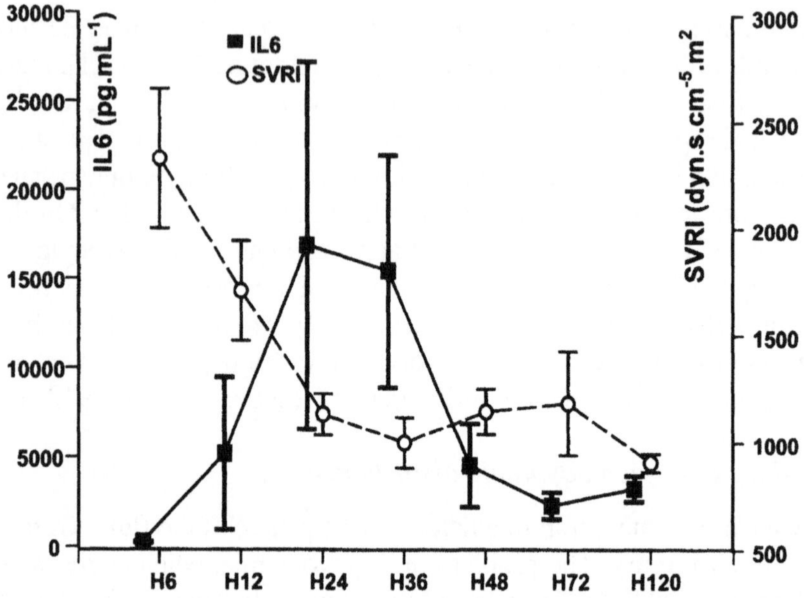

Fig. 1 Trends of systemic vascular resistances (SVRI) and circulating interleukin-6 (IL6) during the first 5 days after injury in a group of 13 severely burned patients (TBSA = 72 ± 4 %) [15]

Prehospital care

The quality of prehospital care is probably of prime importance to reduce the local and general after-effects of a burn injury. At the scene of the injury, burn is only considered as a wound which must be protected from superinfection whereas the burned patient is a critical patient potentially suffering from hypovolaemic shock, hypoxia, hypothermia and severe pain [7].

First aid

First aid must be provided quickly at the site of the accident. The first priority is to stop the burning process and to alert the Emergency Medical System immediately [26].

As a thermal burning process can continue long after the exposure, it is usually recommended to use cool fresh water (15°C) as quickly as possible for at least 10-15 minutes [27]. However, the danger of hypothermia contraindicates the cooling of large thermal burns, especially in paediatric or elderly populations. Similarly, the gel-impregnated blankets which aim to transfer heat from the wound to the dressing should be avoided in very extensive burns [3, 7].

Finally, the rescuers must promptly remove smouldering clothing and clothing, soaked with chemicals only, and otherwise must not remove burned clothing especially when it is sticking to the wound. Patients sustaining chemical burns need early copious irrigation of the affected area with cool water (20°C) for at least 30 min [28]. Otherwise the burn should be covered only with clean dry dressings; any topical agents should be avoided at the scene of the accident [26].

Prehospital (medical) care

This permits a (medical) assessment of lesions (burn and associated injuries) [29]; an early initiation of fluid resuscitation and airway management should be achieved before a safe transportation to a general hospital and then to a burn centre.

Initial fluid resuscitation

One of the first priorities at the scene of the injury is to commence adequate fluid resuscitation as soon as possible for all major burns. Recent data suggest that fluid resuscitation, given within 2 h of a thermal injury, may be one of the most important steps in the prevention of multi-organ failure and mortality [30]. Two large peripheral vein catheters (if possible through nonburn tissue) is the preferable route of administration of fluids. A central IV line is needed only if large peripheral access is impossible: femoral venous puncture is the easiest central route at the scene of the injury.

Blood samples are taken to measure carboxy haemoglobin levels before patients are treated with oxygen. Fluid resuscitation should be initiated only with the administration of crystalloids, such as lactated Ringer's solution or isotonic salt solution. Following a modified Parkland Formula, the initial rate of fluid administration should be 2 ml/kg/% TBSA during the first 6-8 h post-injury [7, 26]. This initial fluid loading must be sufficient, and the loading rate must be as constant as possible: each decrease in fluid rate induces collapse, and increases extend the burn oedema [7]. Because of the capillary permeability impairment, colloids are not indicated in the first 8 h post-burn: if the burn shock is worsening in spite of adequate crystalloid infusion, nonprotein colloids could be proposed such as hetastarch (up to 20 ml/kg).

In electrical injuries, initial rate of fluid resuscitation must be increased to 4 - 6 ml/kg/% TBSA during the first 8 h [31, 32]. Acute renal failure due to rhabdomyolysis could be prevented by this large fluid loading associated with sodium bicarbonate and early diuretics [33].

Airway management

The second priority at the scene of the injury is the establishment of an adequate airway. Oxygen should be systematically administered by face mask. Endotracheal intubation and mechanical ventilation are indicated when there is clinical evidence of respiratory failure, major inhalation injury or massive facial swelling, and finally when the burn size exceeds 60 to 70% of TBSA of deep burn [22]. Intubation must be achieved in patients with usual crash induction (with etomidate and succinylcholine). Mechanical ventilation is maintained by continuous hypnosis and narcotic analgesia (e.g., midazolam and fentanyl) and reduces hypoxia [3] and compensates the increased oxygen consumption secondary to an increase in the work of breathing after smoke inhalation [34].

Analgesia and anaesthesia

Prehospital general anaesthesia is rarely indicated except to intubate conscious critical patients. In contrast, the extreme pain of second-degree burn requires analgesia. In conscious patients with spontaneous breathing, morphine is generally necessary to maintain adequate initial pain control [7]. The anxiety caused by an extensive burn often justifies resorting to addition of low doses of benzodiazepines to analgesia [35].

Transportation

The final priority at the scene for the medical team is to establish whether the patient should be treated in a general hospital (if there is no close burn centre) or referred to an appropriate centre for further treatment. All patients with deep burns greater than 10 - 15% TBSA, electrical burns, inhalation burns and burns with a high risk of cosmetic or functional deformities, such as on face, hands or joint surfaces, should be referred to a specialised centre [3, 26].

The initial management of the patient at the scene determines the safety of the transportation. The ambulance frame must be heated to limit the hypothermia of the patient (thermal comfort for a burned patient is between 25 and 33°C). The maintenance of the fluid loading rate and of the analgesia is achieved simultaneously with careful monitoring (cardioscope, pulse oximetry, non-invasive arterial pressure and central temperature).

Resuscitation during the first 72 h

This initial post-burn period is marked by the cardiovascular instability which can lead to deleterious tissue hypoperfusion.

Acute management in ICU

Following admission to the ICU, a burned patient suffering an extensive and deep thermal injury requires:

- Oxygen: this should be administered either through a high-flow face mask, or by mechanical ventilation if previously described criteria are met.
- Intravenous access: if over 40% of TBSA is affected, the insertion of a double-lumen central catheter is the preferred route for fluid administration (distal lumen) and drug infusions (proximal lumen). If possible, this catheter should be sited through non-burn tissue, preferably subclavian or jugular.
- Continuous electrocardiographic monitoring.
- Arterial catheterisation (usually through femoral artery): this permits continuous monitoring of arterial blood pressure and frequent blood sampling.
- Pulse oximetry: for continuous monitoring of arterial oxygenation.
- Urinary catheter: to measure urine output at hourly intervals.
- Continuous electronic monitoring of core temperature.
- Double-lumen nasogastric tube.
- Fibre-optic pulmonary artery catheterisation: this could be considered in all patients suffering initial and prolonged burn shock in spite of theoretically optimal resuscitation, or when respiratory failure supervenes with a PaO_2/FiO_2 ratio below 300. This catheter permits improved fluid resuscitation and catecholamine administration, when necessary, to optimise cardiac output and oxygen delivery. An indirect calorimeter which continuously measures oxygen consumption completes the haemodynamic survey [22].

Initial fluid resuscitation

Numerous fluid resuscitation formulae have been developed to maintain arterial pressure and urine output. As proposed by Parkland, most formulae suggest a 3 - 4 ml/kg/%. TBSA crystalloids for the first 24 h [18, 22, 36]. Other groups favour colloidal fluid and/or hypertonic saline to limit the total volume of fluid infused [18, 37, 38]. The use of albumin solutions remains controversial [39]. Prolonged hypoalbuminaemia does not reduce survival though unwarranted albumin infusions could increase mortality [40]. Thus, albumin infusion only seems to appear necessary when serum albumin levels <20 g/l [41, 42]: this is the case for virtually all severely burned patients suffering more than 60% TBSA as early as the 1st day post-burn.

As with all fluid resuscitation formulae, the exact volume of crystalloid, or the amount and rate of colloid administration, cannot be appraised by urine output and vital signs alone [43]. If theoretically adequate fluid loading is not sufficient to control burn shock (MAP $\leq$70 mmHg and urine flow $\leq$0.5 ml/kg/h), catecholamines are indicated and pulmonary artery catheterisation is then necessary [15, 25, 44]. In our clinical practice, the patient's fluid resuscitation is commenced with crystalloid alone (2 ml/kg/% TBSA with lactated Ringer's solution) until the 6th hour. For the next 18 h, 1 ml/kg/% TBSA crystalloid and 1 ml/kg/% TBSA colloid volumes are given simultaneously. This formula is intended only as a guideline for planning fluid therapy which should not exceed 4 ml/kg/% TBSA for the first 24 h [22]. Hypertonic saline solutions have also been proposed as they reduce the volume of fluid infused [37, 45, 46] and the tissue oedema [47, 48] and may improve myocardial function [38, 49]. In contrast, others authors reported that this strategy could increase the rate of acute renal failure as well as mortality [50].

From 24 to 48 h half of these calculated volumes are used. From 48 to 72 h the requirement becomes maintenance plus considerations for increased insensible water losses and electrolyte imbalance. Nevertheless, the infusion rate, which needs to be as constant and regular as possible, appears more important than the daily infused volume [22, 36].

Some authors have suggested that basic vital signs (heart rate, arterial blood pressure and urine flow) provide insufficient data for prediction of adequate resuscitation [43]. For the most seriously burned patients, even those without previous cardiac disease, measurement of cardiac output could be a useful means of optimising tissue perfusion and oxygen delivery both to burned tissues and to healthy organs [51, 52]. Other general or regional cardiopulmonary monitoring could also be valuable [53, 54]. However, for most authors, a urine flow between 0.5 and 1 ml/kg/h reflects satisfactory fluid replacement.

Finally, if burn shock persists in spite of well-conducted treatment, inotropic drugs such as dobutamine are indicated, sometimes as early as the hypovolaemic period to improve unsatisfactory cardiac output (CI > 4 $l/min/m^2$) and during the hyperdynamic state, alpha adrenoceptor-stimulating drugs such as noradrenaline to maintain systemic vascular resistance at acceptable levels (SVRI 800 $dyn.s/cm^5$) [15, 51].

Some authors believe that hyperdynamic resuscitation with theoretically optimal therapeutic goals could improve survival and reduce the incidence of organ failure [44, 51]. These hyperdynamic end-points appear all the more important because some degree of post-burn cardiac injury could exist, as suggested by a usually elevated serum level of troponin-I [55]. Several days after the injury, the patients enter an anti-diuretic phase. Diuretics, sometimes combined with continuous haemofiltration, may be necessary to reduce the salt and water excess [56]. However, early fluid resuscitation remains the only treatment which obviously reduces the incidence of acute renal dysfunction [57].

Pulmonary support

Injuries to the airways and lungs include several mechanisms [22]:

- Direct thermal damage to the tracheobronchial tree due to flame, liquid or steam inhalation is rare because the humid airway gas transfers heat poorly.
- Smoke and toxic products are frequently inhaled. Inhalation injury induces mechanical complications such as airway oedema and mucosal hypersecretions, and toxic after-effects through two distinct mechanisms: smoke poisoning (e.g. hydrogen cyanide) and carbon monoxide intoxication [3, 58].
- Blast injury, which occurs only in the case of explosion in a closed place. The initial diagnosis of inhalation burn injury is achieved by of fibreoptic bronchoscopy. The incidence of inhalation injury increases with increasing extent of the burn, so that it is present in two thirds of patients with flame burns that exceed 70% of TBSA [18]. Nevertheless, for these extremely critical patients, early endotracheal intubation is preferable to avoid difficult late intubation or respiratory failure and to manage continuous and sufficient analgesia and sedation. The mechanical ventilation permits management up to the end of the oedema phase. Arterial blood gases twice a day and daily chest radiograph are necessary to adjust ventilatory parameters (e.g. PEEP). In case of inhalation injury, fibreoptic bronchoscopy is desirable once a week and before extubation [59].

The principal pulmonary complications (e.g. pneumonia or atelectasis) generally occur after the first 72 h post-burn [60]. For that reason, newer treatments such as high-frequency percussive jet ventilation, permissive hypercapnia or nitric oxide inhalation are not indicated in this initial period. On the other hand, carbon monoxide poisoning necessitates mechanical ventilation with a fractional concentration of oxygen in inspired gas of 1.0 for at least 6 h. Hyperbaric oxygen should be considered for comatose patients or for those with carboxyhaemoglobin levels 30% [5]. High levels of carboxyhaemoglobin associated with prolonged and elevated lactic acidosis must be considered due to cyanide poisoning, necessitating infusion of hydroxocobalamin [61].

Complementary therapy

Some others components of ICU management are important. For patients requiring mechanical ventilation adequate pain control and sedation must be achieved by a continuous infusion of midazolam-sufentanil, for example [62]. No antibiotics should be utilised prophylactically: antibiotics are initially used only in the perioperative period. In contrast, guidelines for tetanus prophylaxis are the same as for any wounds.

Diuretics can be considered after the first 24 h to accelerate the decrease in oedema. Nutritional support to keep up with early hypermetabolic demand can be managed as early as the 2nd day post-injury by both parenteral and enteral routes if the gastrointestinal tract is still functioning adequately. This has been shown to be the best stress ulcer prophylaxis [63], as well as maintaining gut mucosal integrity and modulating the inflammatory response [64].

Wound management

Finally, in an extensive burn wound management is not an initial priority. The only emergency is represented by the escharotomies indicated in all full-thickness circumferential and constricting burns of trunk and extremities, including the digits, regardless of the pulse status [3]. Burns should ideally be dressed twice a day (after washing with iodine polyvidone or chlorhexidine gluconate and water) with topical antiseptics: silver sulphadiazine is the mostly widely used for routine prophylaxis [3, 7, 36]. Aggressive surgical excision and skin grafting are the treatment of choice for full-thickness burns, if possible begun after 48-72 hours post-burn [65]. On the day of admission, a small skin biopsy (5 to 10 cm^2) can be taken to start autologus cultured keratocytes for the most extensively burned patients (more than 60-70% of TBSA) [20].

Conclusions

The major improvement in burn therapy in the near future is likely to focus on the early management of haemodynamic problems and respiratory failure, achieved in part through a better understanding of the inflammatory syndrome's pathophysiology and through early optimised resuscitation. Nevertheless, because of the cost of extensive burn care and the unavoidable major sequelae, efforts focused on the prevention must first be reinforced [66].

References

1. Muller MJ, Herndon DN (1994) The challenge of burns. Lancet 343:216-220
2. Gueugniaud PY, Bertin-Maghit M (1995) Burn therapy. Curr Opin Anaesthesiol 8:187-192
3. Briggs SE (1990) First aid, transportation and immediate acute care of thermal injuries. In: Martin JAJ (ed) Acute management of the burned patient, Saunders, Philadelphia, pp 1-11
4. Rossiter ND, Chapman P, Haywood IA (1996) How big is a hand? Burns 22: 230-231
5. MacLennan N, Heimbach DM, Cullen BF (1998) Anesthesia for major thermal injury. Anesthesiology 89:749-770
6. Demling R (1990) Pathophysiological changes after cutaneous burns and approach to initial resuscitation. In: Martyn JAJ (ed) Acute management of the burned patient. Saunders, Philadelphia, pp 12-24
7. Gueugniaud PY, Bertin-Maghit M, Bouchard C, Petit P (1995) Prise en charge pré-hospitalière des brûlés graves. In: SFAR (ed) Médecine d'Urgence, 37th Congrès national. Masson, Paris, pp 19-28
8. Saffle JR (1998) Predicting outcomes of burns. N Engl J Med 338:387-388
9. Tobiasen J, Hiebert JH, Edlich RF (1982) Prediction of burn mortality. Surg Gynecol Obstet 154:711-714
10. De Bandt JP, Chollet-Martin S, Hernvann A et al (1994) Cytokine response to burn injury: relationship with protein metabolism. J Trauma 36:624-628
11. Drost AC, Burleson DG, Cioffi WG et al (1993) Plasma cytokines following thermal injury and their relationship with patient mortality, burn size, and time postburn. J Trauma 35:335-339
12. Mc Millen MA, Huribal M, Cunningham ME et al (1996) Endothelin-1, interleukine-6, and interleukine-8 levels increase in patients with burns. J Burn Care Rehabil 17:384-389
13. Struzyna J, Pojda Z, Braun B et al (1995) Serum cytokines levels (IL-4, IL-6, IL-8, G-CSF, GM-CSF) in burned patients. Burns 21:437-440
14. Gueugniaud PY, Bertin-Maghit M, Joly MO et al (1993) Rôle de l'interleukine-6 dans la phase oedèmateuse du brûlé grave. Presse Med 22:735
15. Gueugniaud PY, Vilasco B, Pham E et al (1996) Brûlés graves: état hémodynamique, transport et consommation d'oxygène, cytokines plasmatiques. Ann Fr Anesth Réanim 15:27-35
16. Mass DL, Hybki DP, White J, Horton JW (2002) The time course of cardiac NF-kappaβ activation and TNF-alpha secretion by cardiac myocytes after burn injury: contribution to burn-related cardiac contractile dysfunction. Shock 17:293-299
17. Wang CG, Xia ZF, Yu BJ et al (2001) Cardiac apoptosis in burned rats with delayed fluid resuscitation. Burns 27:250-253
18. Monafo WW (1996) Initial management of burns. N Engl J Med 335:1581-1586
19. Gueugniaud PY, Jauffray M, Bertin-Maghit M et al (1997) Cerebral oedema after extensive burn injury: prognostic significance of early intracranial and cerebral perfusion pressure. Ann Burns Fire Disast 10:72-77
20. Carleton SC (1995) Cardiac problems associated with burns. Cardiol Clin 13:257-262
21. Cioffi WG, De Meules JE, Gamelli RL (1986) The effects of burn injury and fluid resuscitation on cardiac function in vitro. J Trauma 26:638-642
22. Bertin-Maghit M, Petit P, Gueugniaud PY (2003) Réanimation du brûlé. In: Pourriat JL, Martin C (eds) Principes de réanimation chirurgicale. Blackwell, Arnette, Paris, pp 1289-1302
23. Shoemaker WC, Vladech BC, Bassin R et al (1973) Burn physiopathology in man. J Surg Res 14:64-73
24. Bernard F, Gueugniaud PY, Bertin-Maghit M et al (1994) Prognostic significance of early cardiac index measurements in severely burned patients. Burns 20:529-531
25. Miller JG, Bunting P, Burd DAR, Edwards JD (1994) Early cardiopulmonary patterns in patients with major burns and pulmonary insufficiency. Burns 20:542-546
26. Gueugniaud PY, Bouchard C, Bertin-Maghit M, Petit P (1992) Prise en charge pré-hospitalière d'un brûlé grave. Revue des SAMU 5:218-221

27. Raine TS, Heggers JR, Robson M (1981) Cooling the burned wound to maintain microcirculation. J Trauma 21:394-397
28. Sykes RA, Mani MM, Hiebert JM (1986) Chemical burns: retrospective review. J Burn Care Rehabil 7:343-347
29. Carsin H, Ainaud P, Le Bever H (1995) Le brûlé polytraumatisé. In SFAR (ed) Médecine d'Urgence, 37th Congrès national. Masson, Paris, pp 29-39
30. Barrow RE, Jeschke MG, Herndon DN (2000) Early fluid resuscitation improves outcomes in severely burned children. Resuscitation 45:91-96
31. Demling R, Lalonde C (1989) Electrical Burns. In: Blaisdell FW, Trunkey DD (eds) Burn trauma, trauma management vol. IV. Thieme, New York, pp 221-224
32. Remensnyder JP (1990) Acute electrical injuries. In: Martyn JAJ (eds) Acute management of the burned patient. Saunders, Philadelphia, pp 66-86
33. Dubien PY, Bertin-Maghit M, Gueugniaud PY et al (1996) Brûlures par électrisation: aspects épidémiologiques et thérapeutiques. Presse Med 25:1781-1785
34. Demling R, Lalonde C, Heron P (1994) Initial effect of smoke inhalation injury on oxygen consumption (response to positive pressure ventilation). Surgery 115:563-570
35. Ashburn MA (1995) Burn pain: the management of procedure-related pain. J Burn Care Rehabil; 16:365-371
36. Carsin H, Le Bever H (1995) Brûlures graves. In: Samii K, (ed) Anesthésie-réanimation chirurgicale. Flammarion, Paris, pp 1657-1665
37. Kreimeir U, Messmer K (2002) Small-volume resuscitation: from experimental evidence to clinical routine. Advantages and disadvantages of hypertonic solutions. Acta Anaesthesiol Scand 6:625-638
38. Suzuki K, Ogino R, Nishina M, Kohama A (1995) Effects of hypertonic saline and dextran 70 on cardiac functions after burns. Am J Physiol 268:H856-H864
39. Cochrane injury group albumin reviewers (1998) Human albumin administration in critically ill patients: systematic review of randomised controlled trials. BMJ 317:235-240
40. Greenhalgh DG, Housinger TA, Kagan RJ et al (1995) Maintenance of serum albumin levels in pediatric burn patients: a prospective randomized trial. J Trauma 39:67-73
41. Conférence de Consensus (1996) Utilisation des solutions d'albumine humaine en anesthésie-réanimation chirurgicale de l'adulte. Ann Fr Anesth Réanim 15:411-570
42. Sanchez R (1996) Rôle de l'albumine chez les brûlés: son efficacité au cours de leur réanimation. Ann Fr Anesth Réanim 15:1124-1129
43. Dries DJ, Waxman K (1991) Adequate resuscitation of burn patients may not be measured by urine output and vital signs. Crit Care Med 19:327-329
44. Schiller WR, Bay RC, Garren RL et al (1997) Hyperdynamic resuscitation improves survival in patients with life-threatening burns. J Burn Care Rehabil 18:10-16
45. Guha SC, Kinski MP, Button B et al (1996) Burn resuscitation: crystalloid versus colloid versus hypertonic saline hyperoncotic colloid in sheep. Crit Care Med 24:1849-1857
46. Milner SM, Kinsky MP, Guha SC et al (1997) A comparison of two different 2400 mOsm solutions for resuscitation of major burns. J Burn Care Rehabil 18:109-115
47. Kinsky MP, Milner SM, Button B et al (2000) Resuscitation of severe thermal injury with hypertonic saline dextran: effects on peripheral and visceral edema in sheep. J Trauma 49:844-853
48. Elgjo GI, Poli de Figueiredo LF, Schenarts PJ et al (2000) Hypertonic saline dextran produces early (8-12 hrs) fluid sparing in burn resuscitation: a 24-hr prospective, double-blind study in sheep. Crit Care Med 28:277-278
49. Elgjo GI, Mathew BP, Poli de Figueriedo LF et al (1998) Resuscitation with hypertonic saline dextran improves cardiac function in vivo and ex vivo after burn injury in sheep. Shock 9:375-383
50. Huang PP, Stucky FS, Dimick AR (1995) Hypertonic sodium resuscitation is associated with renal failure and death. Ann Surg 221:543-557

51. Gueugniaud PY, Bertin-Maghit M, Hirschauer C et al (1997) In the early stage of major burns, is there a correlation between survival, interleukin-6 levels and oxygen delivery and consumption? Burns 23:426-431
52. Holm C, Melcer B, Horbrand F et al (2000) Haemodynamic and oxygen transport: responses in survivors and non-survivors following thermal injury. Burns 26:25-33
53. Lorente JA, Ezpeleta A, Esteban A et al (2000) Systemic hemodynamics, gastric intramucosal PCO_2 changes, and outcome in critically ill burn patients. Crit Care Med 28:1728-1735
54. Second Conference on Supportive Therapy in Burn Care (1981) J Trauma 21:664-668
55. Murphy JT, Horton JW, Purdure GF, Hunt JL (1998) Evaluation of troponin-I as an indicator of cardiac dysfunction after thermal injury. J Trauma 45: 700-704
56. Leblanc M, Thibeault Y, Querin S (1997) Continuous haemofiltration and haemodiafiltration for acute renal failure in severely burned patients. Burns 23:160-165
57. Chrysopoulo MT, Jeschke MG, Dziewulski P et al (1999) Acute renal dysfunction in severely burned adults. J Trauma 46:141-144
58. Kirk MA, Gerace R, Kulig KW (1993) Cyanide and methemoglobin kinetics in smoke inhalation victims treated with the cyanide antidote kit. Ann Emerg Med 22:1413-1418
59. Micak R, Cortiella J, Desai M, Herndon D (1997) Lung compliance, airway resistance, and work of breathing in children after inhalation injury. J Burn Care Rehabil 18:531-534
60. Hollingsed TC, Saffle JR, Barton RG et al (1993) Etiology and consequences of respiratory failure in thermally injured patients. Am J Surg 166:592-597
61. Baud FD, Barriot P, Toffis V et al (1991) Elevated blood cyanid concentrations in victims of smoke inhalation. N Engl J Med 325:1761-1766
62. Bertin-Maghit M, Gueugniaud PY, Bouchard C, Petit P (1995) Problèmes posés par l'anesthésie du brûlé grave. Cah Anesthésiol 43:215-222
63. Raff T, Germann G, Hartmann B (1997) The value of early enteral nutrition in the prophylaxis of stress ulceration in the severely burned patient. Burns 23:313-318
64. O'Leary MJ, Coakley JH (1996) Nutrition and immunonutrition. Br J Anaesth 77:118-127
65. Giro Z, Sheng Z, Diao L et al (1995) Extensive wound excision in shock stage in patients with major burns. Burns 21:139-142
66. Gueugniaud PY, Carsin H, Bertin-Maghit M, Petit P (2000) Current advances in the initial management of major thermal burns. Intensive Care Med 26:848-856

OBSTETRICS

Perioperative obstetric anaesthesia - haemorrhage and coagulation

G. Lyons

In the United Kingdom a national hospital service is freely available to all citizens. Apart from a small number who deliver at home, virtually all the 700,000 women who deliver each year do so in public hospitals. Private maternity units are unknown outside London. Blood banks, coagulation laboratories and intensive care facilities are often available on site. This may have some significance for the way that haemorrhage is managed in the UK.

Maternal deaths from haemorrhage

A unique feature of practice in the UK is that data collection is well developed. Mortality statistics are available from the early part of the last century, and have been collected without a break since the last world war [1]. Maternal mortality has declined steadily over the last 50 years (Fig. 1).

The introduction of routine ultrasound scans and elective caesarean section has reduced deaths from placenta praevia, but deaths from abruptio placentae and uterine atony have also declined. This suggests that the factors responsible for the improvement in mortality are general in nature and common to all causes of obstetric haemorrhage. Consequently, haemorrhage is now the eighth most important cause of maternal death in the UK, accounting for a smaller proportion than cardiac disease or suicide (Fig. 2).

Pathophysiology of haemorrhage

Haemorrhage is accompanied by an increasing sympathetic response, diverting circulation away from the periphery and the gut. Rising systemic vascular resistance and failing perfusion generate acid metabolites in the tissue groups deprived of circulation. A falling pH has a negative impact on myocardial

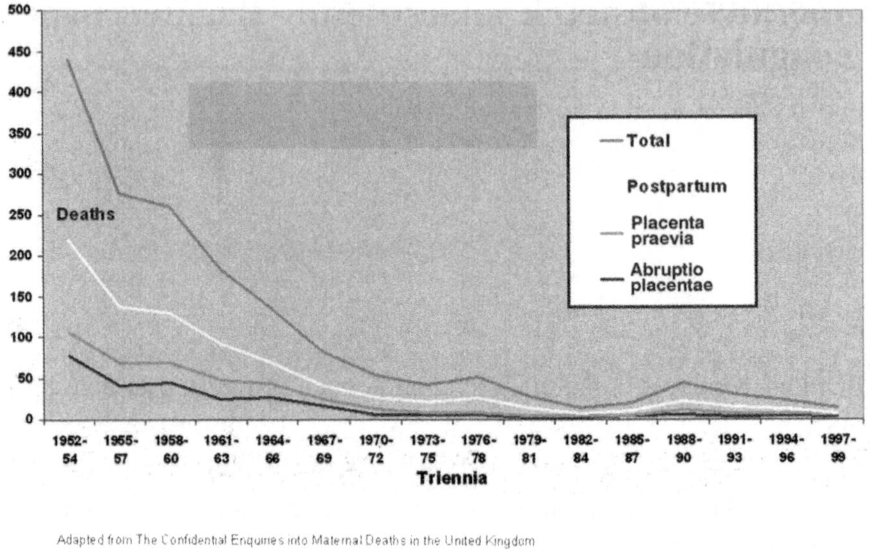

Fig. 1 Maternal mortality from haemorrhage in the United Kingdom 1952-1999. Adapted from Department of Health (2001) Confidential enquiries into maternal deaths in the United Kingdom

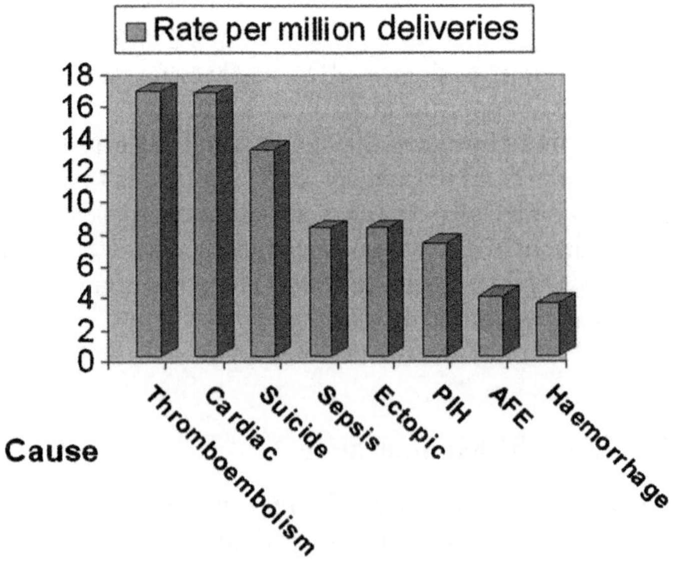

Fig. 2 Causes of maternal death in the UK 1997-1999. Haemorrhage is seen to be the eighth most common

function, which only serves to generate further acidosis. This will be offset, initially, by the increase in catecholamine production. Volume replacement on the appropriate scale is required to reverse the trend of acidosis and failing myocardium. Because obstetric losses can be brisk, a particularly efficient administration system is required. Monitoring pH can be a useful measure of success where replacement is concerned. Short-term adrenaline administration can help to overcome the negative effects of acidosis [2].

Risk factors for haemorrhage

Age, parity and caesarean delivery are associated with increased risk of bleeding. In the UK, the mean maternal age is now 29, with 27 being the mean age for a first baby [3]. The risk associated with caesarean delivery increases with advancing age. An elective operation involves three times the mortality of a vaginal delivery, and an emergency operation has six times the risk [4]. Parity, though, is declining as women choose to have fewer babies.

Placenta praevia, abruptio placentae and uterine atony are responsible for most instances of significant bleeding. Coagulation failure complicates a small number of cases.

Placenta praevia

The traditional grading for placenta praevia reflects the risk attached to vaginal delivery. An alternative grading based on the position of the placenta relative to a uterine incision and the presence of a uterine scar, has been suggested. A low anterior placenta attached to a uterine scar can cause torrential bleeding. Blood loss may be reduced with regional anaesthesia, and increasingly this is being used.

Placental abruption

Even a small central abruption can cause fetal demise. Bleeding may be concealed or revealed. A consumptive coagulopathy can complicate the condition. Because abruption can be a feature of pre-eclampsia and HELLP syndrome, associated renal and hepatic dysfunction contribute to a syndrome of multiorgan failure. Management of haemorrhage in these circumstances can cause further complications, and organ support may be required.

Uterine atony

Long, obstructed labours predispose to failure of uterine contraction. Medical management includes oxytocics, ergot derivatives, prostaglandin analogues and manual compression. Examination should first exclude undetected tears and lacerations.

Surgical management

Temporary control of bleeding might be achieved by direct compression of the aorta. Ligation of the internal iliacs is the next step, with progression to hysterectomy if control is not obtained. Interventional radiologists can offer embolisation if temporary control allows transfer to an imaging suite.

Coagulation failure

Intravascular volume replacement may give rise to a dilutional coagulopathy, as factors V and VIII, together with platelets, are washed out. Massive haemorrhage can trigger a consumptive coagulopathy and also create the circumstances required for dilutional coagulopathy. Conditions such as abruption and amniotic fluid embolism are associated with a coagulopathy that might contribute to the haemorrhage. For all these reasons, a practical approach does not seek to distinguish between dilutional and consumptive causes of coagulopathy.

Coagulation monitoring

The traditional coagulation screen is useful provided the response time is short enough for the results to have some meaning. An alternative is to use a point-of-care coagulation monitor, and most experience has been obtained with the thromboelastograph, which will give a response in 10-20 minutes [5]. Use in cardiac surgery has allowed a reduction in the use of expensive blood components. Each system has its strengths and weaknesses.

Practical approach

Haemorrhage is a potential problem in every obstetric unit, and all units should have a protocol for its management. More recent recommendations suggest that the protocol is tested regularly by practices in the same way as a fire drill. The basis for a protocol will be discussed.

Success requires mobilisation of the necessary resources, additional staff, the transfusion service and the coagulation laboratory.

Short large-bore cannulae, which give the greatest flow, attached to a rapid infusion system are necessary to keep up with loss. Simple alternatives to expensive infusion devices are available. Blood warmers and pressure channels for arterial and central venous monitoring should also be available.

Target values are an important way of directing activity. When the mean arterial pressure is below 80 mmHg infusion should be brisk. The central venous pressure is not the best guide to replacement when there is hypotension, but when hypotension has been corrected, it is useful for the fine-tuning of fluid replacement. For this reason, an arterial cannula should be preferred over cannulation of a great vein.

Infusion should be managed in such a way as to keep the pH above 7.2. A falling pH suggests that losses are not being adequately replaced. The target haematocrit might be set at 30%, this being the threshold that triggers blood replacement.

Serial measurement of blood count, blood gases, and coagulation screen are needed. Serum calcium can also be useful.

Finally, continuing support should be available in a high-dependency or intensive care unit.

Lessons from successive maternal mortality reports suggest that the commonest error is underestimating the severity of blood loss. Setting clinical targets to guide management and monitoring intensively are one way to avoid this mistake.

References

1. Department of Health (2001) Confidential enquiries into maternal deaths in the United Kingdom, 1997-1999. RCOG Press, London
2. Pargger M, Schneider M (1997) Major haemorrhage. In: Russell I F, Lyons G (eds) Clinical problems in obstetric anaesthesia. Chapman and Hall, London, pp 33-46
3. Thomas J, Paranjothy S, Royal College of Obstetricians and Gynaecologists: Clinical Effectiveness Support Unit (2001) The National Sentinel Caesarean Section Audit Report. RCOG Press, London, pp 24-32
4. Hall M, Bewley S (1999) Maternal mortality and mode of delivery. Lancet 354:776
5. Gorton H, Lyons G (1999) Is it time to invest in a thromboelastograph? Int J Obstet Anesth 8: 171-178

Caesarean section in an emergency

R. ALEXANDER

The last two decades have seen a steep rise in the rates of caesarean sections for both elective and emergency cases [1]. The World Health Organisation has concluded that no extra health benefits are associated with a caesarean section rate above 10-15% [2]. However, recent statistics for England showed a rise in the caesarean section rate from 9% in 1980 to 18.8% in 1997-1998 [3]. This led to the collection of data for the National Sentinel Caesarean Section Audit (NSCSA) report, which reported an incidence of 21.3% [4]. The urgency of the operation was classed into four categories listed in Table 1 [5].

Table 1 Classification of urgency of caesarean section

Category 1	"Immediate threat to the life of the woman or fetus" e.g., severe fetal bradycardia, severe APH, cord prolapse, uterine rupture, pH.2.
Category 2	Maternal or fetal compromise which is not immediately life threatening.
Category 3	Needing early delivery but no maternal or fetal compromise.
Category 4	At a time to suite the woman and maternity team.

Sixteen percent of all sections (4% of all births) were classified as category 1, but only 8% 'should have been' and 32% as category 2. Only 33% of women who had a caesarean section went on to have a normal delivery after the next pregnancy. The relative risk of mortality following caesarean section was 12 times as high for category 1, falling to 6 times for category 2, as for vaginal delivery.

The 'ideal' decision to delivery time for category 1 caesarean section is currently regarded as less than 30 min [6]. There is little clinical or theoretical evidence to support this timing, but its widespread adoption has major medicolegal implications [7]. However, Tufnell et al. listed 33 steps that had to be performed before caesarean section, indicating the difficulty in achieving the target time [6]. Despite these obstacles, 25% of all emergency caesarean sections were reported to be followed by delivery in 30 min and 50% within 60 min. The odds ratio was examined for both grades of urgency and time to delivery, and baby outcome. Those parturients classified in category 1 had a higher chance of stillbirth or severe baby compromise (Table 2). When the authors examined the time from decision to delivery they found that mothers for whom the interval was over 30 min had healthier babies than those for whom the interval was less then 30 min (Table 3).

Table 2 Odds ratio for grade of urgency and baby outcome

	5 min Apgar		Stillbirth
	<7	<4	
Category 1 Life threatening	9.8 (2.5, 10.1)	8.6 (4.3, 17.0)	11.5 (3.6, 36.8)
Category 2 Maternal or fetal compromise, not life threatening	2.5 (1.7, 3.6)	1.7 (0.8, 3.7)	0.8 (0.2, 3.3)
Category 3 Needs early delivery	1.00	1.00	1.00

Unadjusted OR (995 CI) National Collaborating Centre for Women's and Children's Health

Table 3 Odds ratio for time to delivery and baby outcome.

Minutes from decision to delivery (min)	5 min Apgar <7	<4	Stillbirth
<30	1.00	1.00	1.00
31-75	0.4 (0.3, 0.5)	0.3 (0.2, 0.5)	0.2 (0.1, 0.4)
>75	0.5 (0.4, 0.6)	0.4 (0.3, 0.6)	0.4 (0.2, 0.9)

Unadjusted OR (995 CI) National Collaborating Centre for Women's and Children's Health

There was very little outcome difference between babies born after an interval of ≤30 min and after 31-75 min when the odds ratio was adjusted for indication, urgency, anaesthesia and CTG trace.

Anticipating the emergency section

The role of the anaesthetist starts with participation in the multidisciplinary group approach to the care of the mother. Morgan et al. anticipated 87% of 360 consecutive emergency caesarean sections in a unit where the duty obstetric anaesthetists accompanied the obstetric team on three ward rounds a day [8]. Though they are not so easy on smaller units without dedicated obstetric anaesthetists, such ward rounds allow early maternal review and improve communication. This is the single most effective method of reducing the decision to delivery interval without compromise. Consent should be obtained as much in advance as possible for any anticipated anaesthetic intervention and while the patient still has the capacity to consent.

The 'decision to anaesthetic' interval

Once the decision has been made to perform a caesarean section, a team approach should be adopted. There should be clear communication between team members about the urgency as this may have a direct effect on the anaesthetic morbidity, as discussed above. No parturient should be transferred to theatre without the institution of intra-uterine resuscitation (IUR) of the fetus. Many episodes of acute fetal distress are associated with a transient reduction of oxygen delivery to the fetus. Occasionally there may be a major event during labour, which is associated with disruption of the placental or fetal oxygen delivery (placental abruption, fetal haemorrhage, umbilical cord prolapse with vasospasm). Every obstetric department should incorporate an intra-uterine resuscitation guideline as part of the protocol for emergency section. This guideline should include:

- Turning off the oxytocin infusion to reduce the strength of the contraction.
- Turning the parturient into the full lateral position, which should be maintained until the patient is transferred to the operating table and is ready to be operated on.
- Oxygen should be administered at high flow as effective oxygen delivery to the mother improves fetal oxygenation.
- Intravenous fluid (normal saline 1000 ml) stat unless fluid intake is restricted.
- Low blood pressure should be treated as appropriate.
- Tocolysis should be given if there is no evidence of abruption or bleeding (terbutaline 0.25 mg administered subcutaneously or 2 puffs of glyceral trinitrate sublingual spray).

All the above manoeuvres may transform a category 1 caesarean section to category 2 or less by the time the woman arrives in theatre [9]. Some women may even be returned to their rooms because the cardiotachograph (CTG) has improved, and they may not need any further intervention for the immediate future.

Anaesthesia for emergency section

The choice of anaesthetic technique will depend upon the urgency of the section, the presence of a working epidural, the availability of a fully staffed operating room and the skill of the anaesthetist. The 7th Annual Report of the Confidential Enquiry into Stillbirths and Deaths in Infancy (June 2000) focused on 25 neonatal deaths related to anaesthetic problems [10]. Four related to serious anaesthetic complications, which all occurred under general anaesthesia. Ten neonatal deaths (all ten started as attempted regional block) were due to delay in provision of anaesthesia once the anaesthetist was present. The report concluded that although general anaesthesia is reliably quick, it increases the risk to the mother and should only be used when clear reasons exist. However, anaesthetists should avoid repeated attempts at spinals and should start epidural top ups in the room; on occasion, it may be appropriate for the obstetrician to interrupt an anaesthetist who is having difficulties.

General anaesthesia

General anaesthesia, especially for emergency caesarean sections, has always been a significant cause of maternal mortality. Although the actual number of deaths attributable to general anaesthesia was small, anaesthesia was at one time the third commonest cause of death reported in obstetric patients in the UK (Fig. 1).

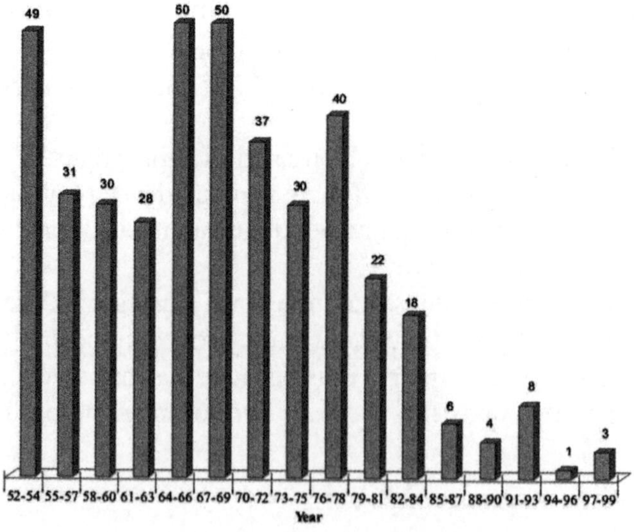

Fig. 1 Maternal deaths reported due to anaesthesia in Confidential Enquiry of Maternal Deaths

However, at one time it was the only choice for emergency caesarean section on account of the speed of induction and patient preparation for skin incision. Two of the major advantages of general anaesthesia in obstetric practice are the lack of contraindications to the technique and the speed of onset. The technique is reliable and controllable, especially in the presence of major haemorrhage. It also the most familiar anaesthetic technique for anaesthetists who do not undertake routine obstetric practice. Lack of a high sympathetic block makes the treatment of hypotension less problematic. The only absolute contraindication is patient refusal.

Anaesthesia for caesarean section requires minimising the risk of aspiration of gastric contents, minimising aorto-caval compression, ensuring anaesthesia and analgesia, maintaining oxygenation and minimising sedation and respiratory depression in the neonate. A standardised technique used in the author's institution is shown in Table 4.

Table 4 General anaesthesia for caesarean section

- 15° lateral tilt
- Preoxygenation and cricoid pressure
- Thiopentone 5 mg/kg
- Suxamethonium 1-1.5 mg/kg
- Tracheal intubation ± cricoid pressure
- O_2 48.5% N_2O 50% and Sevoflurane 1.5%
- Atracurium 0.3 mg/kg
- Opioid of choice after clamping of cord
- Reduction of inspired oxygen after delivery

There are several problems associated with the administration of general anaesthesia for caesarean section, which are discussed below:

Difficult airway and intubation

An assessment of the airway is vital, and there are several published methods of assessing a patient for the risk of encountering a difficult airway or laryngoscopy and intubation. The incidence of failed intubation is approximately 1:300. This is ten times that in the general surgical population, for a number of reasons, such as:

- Oedema around the pharynx and the glottis, especially in pre-eclampsia
- Application of cricoid pressure

- Large breasts
- Weight gain
- Patient tilted
- Protruding teeth

The introduction of new anaesthetic equipment has led to a modification of the algorithm of the American Society of Anesthesiologists for failed intubation. The most significant item has to be the laryngeal mask airway (and more recently the intubating model) [11]. Every anaesthetist should know their department's own protocol and always remember that it is hypoxia that kills patients and not the failure to intubate.

Aspiration of gastric contents

Aspiration of gastric contents is always a risk in the obstetric population. There is a very high prevalence of women with gastro-oesophageal reflux as a result of progesterone-mediated relaxation of the lower oesophageal sphincter and raised intra-abdominal pressure [12]. Also, the administration of opioids for pain relief during labour will delay gastric emptying, so increasing the risk of regurgitation.

The documentation of deaths following aspiration of regurgitated gastric contents by Mendelson [13] highlighted the dangers of the problem and the cricoid pressure manoeuvre was introduced as part of the routine for rapid sequence induction. It was not until the introduction of H_2 antagonists that the problem of acidity and volume of gastric contents could be seriously tackled. When the decision is made, ranitidine 50 mg and metoclopramide 10 mg iv (slowly) should be administered, and within 15 min of surgery 30 ml sodium citrate 0.3 M po. The use of proton pump inhibitors is less clear with conflicting published evidence [14-16]. This is all very well for elective sections, where time is available for the medication to work, but in the case of the emergency section the drugs should be administered im. The only medication that works almost immediately is sodium citrate, and this should never be omitted because of the urgency of the case.

Inadequate anaesthesia

In the attempt to protect the fetus from the sedative effects of opioids and anaesthesia and reduce the relaxing effects on the uterus contractility, anaesthetists run the risk of providing inadequate anaesthesia. The common practice in the 1970s of avoiding volatile agents and using a 50:50 mixture of nitrous oxide and oxygen led to an incidence of 12-26% of cases. The addition of halothane in low concentrations reduced the incidence of inadequate anaesthesia to less than 1% [17]. However, in a more recent review on this topic the widespread availability of expired volatile agent concentration monitoring and the greater use of opioids has led to a reduction in the incidence of awareness from 1.8% to less then 0.4% over the next 3 years [18]. Bispectral index monitoring is a new method of measuring EEG waves to assess depth on anaesthesia that is easy to set up and interpret. It may have a place in obstetric practice in the future [19].

Regional anaesthesia

Epidural anaesthesia

The use of epidural anaesthesia will depend on the category of section. In category 2 or less, epidural analgesia during labour can be extended to provide surgical anaesthesia for emergency caesarean section very effectively. The commonly used solutions for converting a low-dose labour epidural into a block adequate for emergency caesarean section are bupivacaine 0.5%, a 50: 50 mixture of bupivacaine 0.5% and lignocaine 2% with 1: 200 000 adrenaline (final concentration); and lignocaine 2% with 1: 200 000 adrenaline. In a recent publication the authors demonstrated no difference in the time taken to achieve the required block [20].

The volume of anaesthetic used (up to 20 ml approx.) can lead to complications secondary to intravascular injection and intrathecal injection. The comorbidity is less, however, following an epidural than a general anaesthetic for caesarean section. Epidural anaesthesia is associated with less pain and discomfort in the immediate postoperative period than general anaesthesia following elective caesarean section. Fewer patients have gastrointestinal stasis, pyrexia and coughing [21]. Other advantages to using epidural anaesthesia compared with spinal anaesthesia include:

- Good extended postoperative analgesia
- Extension of block if required
- No dural puncture
- Slow onset of block for cardiovascular stability

However, the incidence of patchy and less profound block makes many anaesthetists opt for spinal anaesthesia. There is also a greater need for intravenous opioid supplementation in the recovery period than after spinal anaesthesia [22].

Spinal anaesthesia

There has been a major shift in obstetric anaesthesia practice from general to regional anaesthesia. The use of spinal anaesthesia will depend on the category of the section and the skill and experience of the operator. Most anaesthetists would make at least one attempt while preoxygenating the patient so not losing any time. The left lateral position is probably the most appropriate for an emergency section to prevent aorta-caval compression and so maximise placental perfusion. Head-down tilt after the spinal will result in a speedy block but this may be higher than anticipated. The dose administered should be reduced.

Absolute contraindications to the procedure include:

- Patient refusal
- Sepsis, local or systemic
- Coagulopathy or anticoagulation

Relative contraindications may include:

- Anticipated major blood loss
- Neurological disease
- Fixed output states
- Cardiovascular disease

Some of the more controversial contraindications, such as placenta praevia and aortic stenosis, have been the subject of fierce debate [23, 24].

Hypotension

The block of the sympathetic outflow from the thoracic and lumbar roots leads to vasodilatation and hypotension. There have been many publications on the subject of prevention of hypotension, and the debate rages between preloading and vasopressors. There is then debate as to the optimal vasopressor. The use of metaraminol, an alpha agonist, has been shown to be more beneficial than ephedrine for both the mother and baby when administered as an infusion [25]. Care must be taken to avoid the reflex bradycardia commonly seen with metaraminol.

Post-dural puncture headache (PDPH)

The incidence of PDPH following the use of 25–27 G pencil point spinal needles is approximately 2-4% [26]. The incidence following dural puncture with a 16 G Tuohy needle is in the order of 70-90%. The flow of cerebral spinal fluid (CSF) through the Tuohy needle can be distinguished from saline by the temperature of the fluid and the presence of glucose.

Combined spinal epidural (CSE)

There is little place for a combined spinal epidural technique for category 1 emergency section, but it may be considered for categories 2 and 3.

Postoperative analgesia

Analgesia can be provided in many ways. If there is an epidural catheter in situ then the patient may receive an infusion of opioid, local anaesthetic or both. One of the mainstays of treatment is the rectal administration of diclofenac sodium 100 mg [27, 28]. Morphine 15 mg im is usually prescribed to follow a regional technique or for patient-controlled analgesia.

Conclusions

The choice of anaesthesia for emergency section will depend on the presence of a working epidural and the urgency of the section. General anaesthesia, although not considered the first choice, is now a safer technique due to advances in equipment and monitoring.

References

1. Caesarean section on the rise [editorial] (2000). Lancet 356:1697
2. World Health Organisation (1985) Appropriate technology for birth. Lancet 2:436-437
3. NHS Maternity Statistics, England: 1995–6 to 1997 – 8. Bulletin 2001/14. ISBN 1 84182 373 3
4. The National Sentinel Caesarean Section Audit Report. RCOG Clinical Effectiveness Unit, Royal College of Obstetricians and Gynaecologists. 2001
5. Lucas DN (2000) Journal of the RSM 93:346-350
6. Tuffnell DJ, Wilkinson K, Beresford N (2001) Interval between decision and delivery by caesarean section – are current standards achievable? BMJ 322:1330-1333
7. James D (2001) Caesarean Section for foetal distress. BMJ 322:1316-1317
8. Morgan BM, Magni V, Goroszenuik T (1990) Anaesthesia for emergency caesarean section. Br J Obstet Gynaecol 97:420-424
9. Thurlow JA, Kinsella SM (2002) Intrauterine resuscitation: active management of foetal distress. Int J Obstet Anesth 11:105-116
10. Confidential Enquiry into Stillbirths and Deaths in Infancy (2000): 7th Annual Report. London, HMSO
11. Benumof JL (1996) Laryngeal mask airway and the ASA difficult airway algorithm. Anesthesiology 84:686-699
12. Hart DM (1978) Heartburn in pregnancy. J Int Med Res 6: Suppl 1:1-5
13. Mendleson CL (1946) The aspiration of stomach contents into the lungs during obstetric anesthesia. Am J Obstet Anesth 52:191-205
14. Lin CJ, Huang CL, Hsu HW, Chen TL (1996) Prophylaxis against acid aspiration in regional

anesthesia for elective cesarean section: a comparison between oral single-dose ranitidine, famotidine and omeprazole assessed with fiberoptic gastric aspiration. Acta Anaesthesiol 34:179-184
15. Yau G, Kan AF, Gin T, Oh TE (1992) A comparison of omeprazole and ranitidine for prophylaxis against aspiration pneumonitis in emergency caesarean section. Anaesthesia 47:101-104
16. Ewart MC, Yau G, Gin T et al (1990) A comparison of the effects of omeprazole and ranitidine on gastric secretion in women undergoing elective caesarean section. Anaesthesia 45:527-530
17. Moir DD (1970) Anaesthesia for Caesarean section. An evaluation of a method using low concentrations of halothane and 50 per cent of oxygen. Br J Anaesth 42:136-142
18. Lyons G, Macdonald R (1991) Awareness during Caesarean section. Anaesthesia 46:62-64
19. Yeo SN, Lo WK (2002) Bispectral index in assessment of adequacy of general anaesthesia for lower segment caesarean section. Anaesth Intensive Care 30:36-40
20. Lucas DN, Ciccone GK, Yentis SM (1999) Extending low-dose epidural analgesia for emergency Caesarean section. A comparison of three solutions. Anaesthesia 54:1173-1177
21. Morgan BM, Aulakh JM, Barker JP et al (1984) Anaesthetic morbidity following caesarean section under epidural or general anaesthesia. Lancet 1(8372):328-330
22. Riley ET, Cohen SE, Macario A et al (1995) Spinal versus epidural anesthesia for cesarean section: a comparison of time efficiency, costs, charges, and complications. Anesth Analg 80:709-712
23. Parekh N, Husaini SW, Russell IF (2000) Caesarean section for placenta praevia: a retrospective study of anaesthetic management. Br J Anaesth 84:725-730
24. Brighouse D (1998) Anaesthesia for caesarean section in patients with aortic stenosis: the case for regional anaesthesia. Anaesthesia 53:107-109
25. Ngan Kee WD, Lau TK, Khaw KS, Lee BB (2001) Comparison of metaraminol and ephedrine infusions for maintaining arterial pressure during spinal anesthesia for elective cesarean section. Anesthesiology 95:307-313
26. Vallejo MC, Mandell GL, Sabo DP, Ramanathan S (2000) Postdural puncture headache: a randomized comparison of five spinal needles in obstetric patients. Anesth Analg 91:916-920
27. Dennis AR, Leeson-Payne CG, Hobbs GJ (1995) Analgesia after caesarean section. The use of rectal diclofenac as an adjunct to spinal morphine. Anaesthesia 50:297-299
28. Lim NL, Lo WK, Chong JL, Pan AX (2001) Single dose diclofenac suppository reduces post-Cesarean PCEA requirements. Can J Anaesth 48:383-386

Obstetric emergencies and anaesthesia

H. SINGH, R. ALEXANDER

In the generally accepted sense of the term, life-threatening conditions imply illnesses that will inevitably lead to death without immediate medical intervention. Many anaesthetists fear obstetric emergencies, because these are some of the most extreme challenges of their professional lives. Obstetric emergencies can be life-threatening to the mother-to-be, the fetus or both. Worldwide, the commonest causes of the maternal mortality are pre-eclampsia, haemorrhage, cardiac disease and sepsis. While critical illness requiring admission to intensive care units (ICUs) are uncommon in pregnancy, accounting for between 1 and 9 per 1,000 deliveries [1-5], mortality can be as high as 20%, depending upon the severity of illness and entry requirement to ICU. The majority of admissions to general, surgical, or obstetric ICUs are due to obstetric complications rather than intercurrent medical disease. Of obstetric complications, hypertensive diseases of pregnancy and obstetric haemorrhage make up the majority of problems [4]. Anaesthetic complications can account for 13% of admissions [1].

A few life-threatening conditions are discussed.

Pre-eclampsia and eclampsia

These conditions complicate about 10% of pregnancies, being severe in about 5-10% of these (systolic blood pressure ≥160 mmHg, diastolic pressure ≥110 mmHg, proteinuria ≥5 g/24 hours, oliguria ≤400 ml/24 hours, growth restriction, HELLP syndrome, or symptoms of headache, epigastric pain, or visual disturbance).

Prevention

To date, no treatment instituted after recognition of clinical disease has reduced the major prenatal morbidity, since many of the pathophysiological changes antedate clinical disease. Antiplatelet agents, largely low-dose aspirin, have small or moderate benefits when used for prevention of pre-eclampsia [6]. Magnesium sulphate could prevent progression to eclampsia [7].

Management

Early diagnosis, close medical supervision and timely delivery are the requisites for management. The goal of antihypertensive therapies is to prevent maternal stroke. Antihypertensive medication does not prevent eclampsia or change the pathology in pre-eclamptic patients. However, the fetus may remain in utero for a sufficient number of days to allow pharmacological induction of lung maturity with corticosteroids. There is no clear benefit of drug treatment. Guidelines for management for severe pre-eclampsia must be available in all obstetric units. Senior obstetricians should lead the discussion on timing and mode of delivery, but the plan should be implemented by team management. Monitoring a stable patient will include: hourly blood pressure record, fluid balance chart, daily urine analysis, daily or more frequent review of the symptoms and signs, twice-weekly blood count, especially platelets, uric acid, urea and electrolytes, creatinine and liver function test, 24-hourly urinary protein estimation and weekly weighing. If platelets are less than 100×10^9, further clotting studies need to be investigated. If these are abnormal, the haematology department needs to be alerted and blood should be sent for fibrinogen and fibrin degradation product assessment. All women should have these recorded on the pre-eclampsia chart. Monitoring should continue for 72 hours post partum for the severe form of the disease, and the decision to transfer to the ward should be made in conjunction with the anaesthetist. Treatment should be given if blood pressure is more than 160/110 mmHg on three consecutive readings. Until better evidence is available, the choice of antihypertensive should depend on the experience and familiarity of an individual clinician with a particular drug and what is known about adverse maternal and fetal side effects. Parenteral hydralazine is given as 5 mg i.v, with similar boluses every 20 minutes until the BP is reduced or the heart rate is more than 120 beats/minute or 20 mg hydralazine is given. Alternatively, after the initial bolus, an infusion can be commenced at 5-20 mg/h, with the infusion rate titrated. Hydralazine is associated with several side effects, such as headache, vomiting mimicking severe eclampsia and maternal tachycardia. The dose range of labetalol is variable and starts at 20 mg followed at 10 minutes interval the incremental doses of 40, 60 and 80 mg until the cumulative dose of 300 mg. Nitroglycerin is used only if other agents have failed and would necessitate invasive BP monitoring. Diuretics are usually contraindicated unless fluid overload has occurred. Accurate fluid input control is required. If urine output is less than 25 ml/h, CVP should be instituted and the fluid and diuretic administration guided with the help of CVP. Eclampsia is an emergency situation and resuscitation team is called to assess the ABC of basic resuscitation. Magnesium is a first-line drug now. The dose is 4 g over 10-15 min followed by infusion of 2 g/h, and infusion is continued for 24-48 h after delivery. Magnesium is kept in different strengths and it should not cause confusion. An ampoule of calcium gluconate should be available as an antidote. Magnesium infusion is used if there is adequate clinical monitoring. The patellar-reflex cannot be relied on in the presence of epidural analgesia. The infusion should be stopped if saturation drops below 90%. ECG is mandatory during and for 1 h after the loading dose. Dose alteration is required if oliguria develops, if plasma urea is over 10 mmol/l or liver function deteriorates. A subtherapeutic or toxic concentration also requires dose adjustment. Consider diazepam for recurrent fits and then infusion of thiopentone with an input from intensive care. Epidural analgesia is advantageous in women with severe pre-eclampsia, because it increases the utero-placental blood flow and improves maternal blood pressure control [8]. Spinal anaesthesia is not contraindicated, but meticulous attention must be paid to blood pressure. Ephedrine is still the best vasopressor, but small increments are advised to avoid rebound hypertension. Pre-hydration is initially limited to 1 L. In some patients neuraxial block is contraindicated due to fetal distress or concurrent coagulopathy. The main goal of general anaesthesia is to prevent haemodynamic instability during intubation and extubation. The use of antihypertensives alone or in combination with short-acting opiates is indicated.

Thromboembolism

Thromboembolism is the leading cause of death, as shown in the Confidential Enquiry into Maternal Deaths in the UK. The current rate of 16.5 per million deliveries has fallen from the all time high of 21.8 per million deliveries in the last report. There were two key findings in this report. The number of deaths from thromboembolism following caesarean section has fallen since the introduction of the Royal College of Obstetrics and Gynaecology guidelines published in 1995. There also was a significant rise in deaths due to missing the diagnosis or not offering thromboprophylaxis to women who had known risk factors. The use of antipsychotic drugs has recently been described as independent factor for first-time idiopathic venous thromboembolism [9]. The risk factors and thromboprophylaxis are shown in Table 1.

Table 1 Risk factors and approach to prophylaxis in vaginal and caesarean delivery

Thromboprophylaxis in vaginal deliveries	Thromboprophylaxis in caesarean section
Low risk: early mobilisation and hydration Assessment: uncomplicated pregnancy	**Low risk:** early mobilisation and hydration Assessment: uncomplicated pregnancy and elective section
Moderate risk: subcutaneous enoxaparin 40 mg once daily, elasticated compression stockings if heparin contraindicated	**Moderate risk:** consider one of the variety of prophylactic measures
Assessment: Any of two factors: • Age over 35 years • Obesity (> 80 kg at booking) • Parity 4 or more • Labour 12 hours or more • Gross varicose veins • Current infection • Pre-eclampsia • Immobility for 4 or more days prior to labour • Mid cavity or rotational forceps delivery • Major current medical illness	Assessment: Any two factors • Age over 35 years • Obesity (> 80 kg at booking) • Parity four or more • Labour 12 hours or more • Gross varicose veins • Current infection • Pre-eclampsia • Immobility prior to surgery four or more days • Major current medical illness • Emergency section in labour
High risk: subcutaneous enoxaparin 40 mg plus graduated elastic compression stockings	**High risk:** heparin prophylaxis with or without leg stockings
• Assessment: any vaginal delivery with one of these factors: • Four or more moderate risk factors • Extended major pelvic or abdominal surgery • Patient with family history of DVT/ PE/ thrombophilia • Paralysis of lower limbs • APL antibody or lupus anticoagulant	• Assessment: • Patient with three or more moderate risk factors • Extended major pelvic or abdominal surgery • Patient with family history of DVT/ PE/ thrombophilia • Patient with APL antibody or lupus anticoagulant

Prevention and management

The recent RCOG guidelines make five key recommendations, as follows [10]:

- Any woman with signs and symptoms suggestive of VTE should have objective testing performed to avoid the risks, inconvenience and cost of inappropriate anticoagulation. Individual hospitals should each have an agreed protocol for this.
- In clinically suspected DVT or pulmonary thromboembolism, treatment with unfractioned heparin or low-molecular-weight heparin should be given until the diagnosis is excluded, unless it is strongly contraindicated.

- Subcutaneous unfractioned heparin is an effective alternative to intravenous unfractioned heparin for the initial management of DVT.
- Low-molecular-weight (LMW) heparins are more effective with low mortality and fewer bleeding complications in the initial management of DVT in nonpregnant patients. LMW heparins are as effective as unfractionated heparin in treatment of pulmonary thromboembolism
- During pregnancy, adjusted-dose subcutaneous, unfractioned heparin and LMW heparins are effective alternatives to oral anticoagulants in maintenance treatment of VTE.

All the above recommendations except first are grade A evidence based (requiring at least one RCT), and the first one is grade B (requiring well-controlled studies). Table 2 shows the recommended therapeutic dosage of LMW heparin.

Table 2 Therapeutic dosage for low-molecular-weight heparin

Early pregnancy weight	Initial dose of enoxaparin
< 50 kg	40 mg twice daily
50-69 kg	60 mg twice daily
70-89 kg	80 mg twice daily
> 90 kg	100 mg twice daily

Haemorrhage

There was a fall from 5.3 to 3.3 per million deliveries in the rate of death due directly to haemorrhage according to the last Confidential Enquiry into Maternal Deaths. Haemorrhage can occur before, during or after delivery. The situations are premature placental detachment, placenta praevia, uterine rupture, retained placenta, uterine atony, placenta accreta and uterine inversion. A recent survey suggests that life-threatening haemorrhage may occur in 6.7 per 1,000 deliveries [11].

Prevention

Where a delivery is known to involve an elevated risk of major haemorrhage, for example when placenta praevia, especially with a previous caesarean section, myomectomy scars, uterine fibroids, premature placental detachment or previous third-stage complications are known of, the following steps are important:

- Possible prenatal anaemia should be checked and corrected in the antenatal period if possible.
- All elective or emergency surgery should be performed by a consultant.
- Any anaesthetics should be given by consultant.
- Adequate intravenous access (two large-bore cannulae) should be in place before the start of surgery.
- A central venous access should be in place, either preoperatively or whenever it is apparent that bleeding is excessive.
- Women at known risk should be delivered in a consultant unit with an on-site blood bank.
- A multidisciplinary massive haemorrhage protocol should be available and rehearsed regularly in conjunction with the blood bank. It should also be included in life support training.

Management

Maternal fluid resuscitation should be optimised. Close liaison with blood bank services is required. The option of using cell salvage has now become viable [12]. The pregnant patient is more prone to disseminated intravascular coagulation (DIC), so that input from a haematologist is invaluable. The blood and its component therapy are ideally based on laboratory results, but clinical judgement may be the only tool available in a rapidly changing emergency situation. The use of other utero-tonic drugs, such as methylergonovine (two doses of 0.4 mg intravenous) and carboprost (0.2 mg intramuscular or intramyometrial, total not exceeding 0.6 mg) may be necessary. Prostaglandins are more promising in treatment of haemorrhage than in routine attempts at prevention of blood loss in the third stage of labour. Uterine packing is staging a comeback as an interim measure for bleeding patients or for stabilising a patient with DIC. Embolisation of uterine arteries by an interventional radiologist or further surgical procedures, such as internal artery ligation, hysterectomy, B-Lynch suture or Billings suture, may be considered. Help should be sought from surgical colleagues or, if necessary, a vascular surgeon. In the case of a retained but separated placenta, tocolysis can be obtained using general anaesthesia and halogenated agents. Under regional anaesthesia nitroglycerin, 50 to 250 μg i.v. or two puffs (800 μg) inhalation can be used, depending upon the haemodynamics of the mother. Beta-adrenergic agents can also be used. If placenta increta or percreta is diagnosed preoperatively, preoperative placement of balloon catheters in the hypogastric arteries under light sedation may prove helpful to control bleeding before proceeding to hysterectomy. In all cases of significant haemorrhage before delivery, intensive resuscitation of the newborn in the presence of a neonatologist is essential.

Cardiac disease

The joint most common cause of maternal death in the UK is cardiac disease and women with pulmonary vascular disease have a very high mortality risk. The most frequent disorders include rheumatic mitral valve stenosis, treated or untreated CHD, cardiomyopathies and ischaemic heart diseases.

Prevention

The risks should be transmitted to the patient and her partner as clearly and as humanely as possible. The cultural pressure of continuing the pregnancy could be high, so that they should not be alienated in prepregnancy counselling to such an extent that they do not come for antenatal checkups. Women may deny or minimise the symptoms

- The delivery must be planned. At the very least, this will involve discussion with the consultant anaesthetist. The centre accepting the care should be staffed at consultant level by physicians with specialised medical experience.
- Correction of the problem before pregnancy whenever possible and monitoring throughout by the experts is the cornerstone of successful outcome.

Management

The detailed description of management is beyond the scope of this text, but readers are referred to a paper of outstanding interest in this field [13].The anaesthetic management of the pregnant cardiac patient is a challenge to the anaesthetist, whether the patient is delivering vaginally or by caesarean section, or undergoing cardiac or minor noncardiac surgery. Generally, during vaginal delivery local anaesthetic/narcotic infusion or the CSE technique can be used safely. In the later technique, an intrathecal narcotic initially, followed by a dilute local anaesthetic/opioid infusion provides adequate analgesia with minimal haemodynamic effects. During caesarean section single-shot spinal or epidural anaesthesia may be used, except in patients with severe aortic stenosis, mitral valve stenosis or aortic coarctation. General anaesthesia can be safely administered provided adequate monitoring is undertaken.

Special considerations

Occasionally an explosive combination of risk factors can easily make a situation life threatening.

Difficult airway

The frequency of difficult airway is estimated to be as high as 1 in 250 [14]. Fortunately, failed ventilation by mask is rarer than failed intubation. Precise airway assessment is important, although no single test is 100% accurate. Every obstetric theatre should have a difficult-intubation trolley with equipment including a full range of oral airways and intubating laryngeal mask airways, McCoy laryngoscope blades, a cricothyroidotomy kit and a means of ventilation. The optimal maternal position should be achieved before induction, and administration of a second dose of suxamethonium will depend on the experience of the clinician. The anaesthetic assistant should be appropriately experienced and trained, and failed intubation protocols should be rehearsed on a regular basis. Help should be sought at the earliest opportunity. Our department's algorithm is shown in Fig. 1.

Morbid obesity

Maternal obesity increases the chances of delivery by caesarean section, and could also be a contributing factor in life-threatening situations. A 'stat' section could be unrealistic and dangerous. Evaluation of the airway is most important. The problem with difficult venous access should be addressed in good time. Labour pain relief should be encouraged and the opportunity for timely correction of a failed epidural should not be missed. Appropriate antacid prophylaxis is given if delivery is to be done by operation. If the airway is not favourable, an alternate airway strategy should be planned. Meticulous attention to all detail could prevent serious mishaps.

Maternal cardiac arrest

Fortunately, the need for cardiac resuscitation of a parturient is infrequent (1 in 30,000) [15]. Standard resuscitative measures should be used, and the need to maintain left uterine displacement during resuscitation must be borne in mind. After 20 weeks of gestation, aortocaval compression may prevent effective

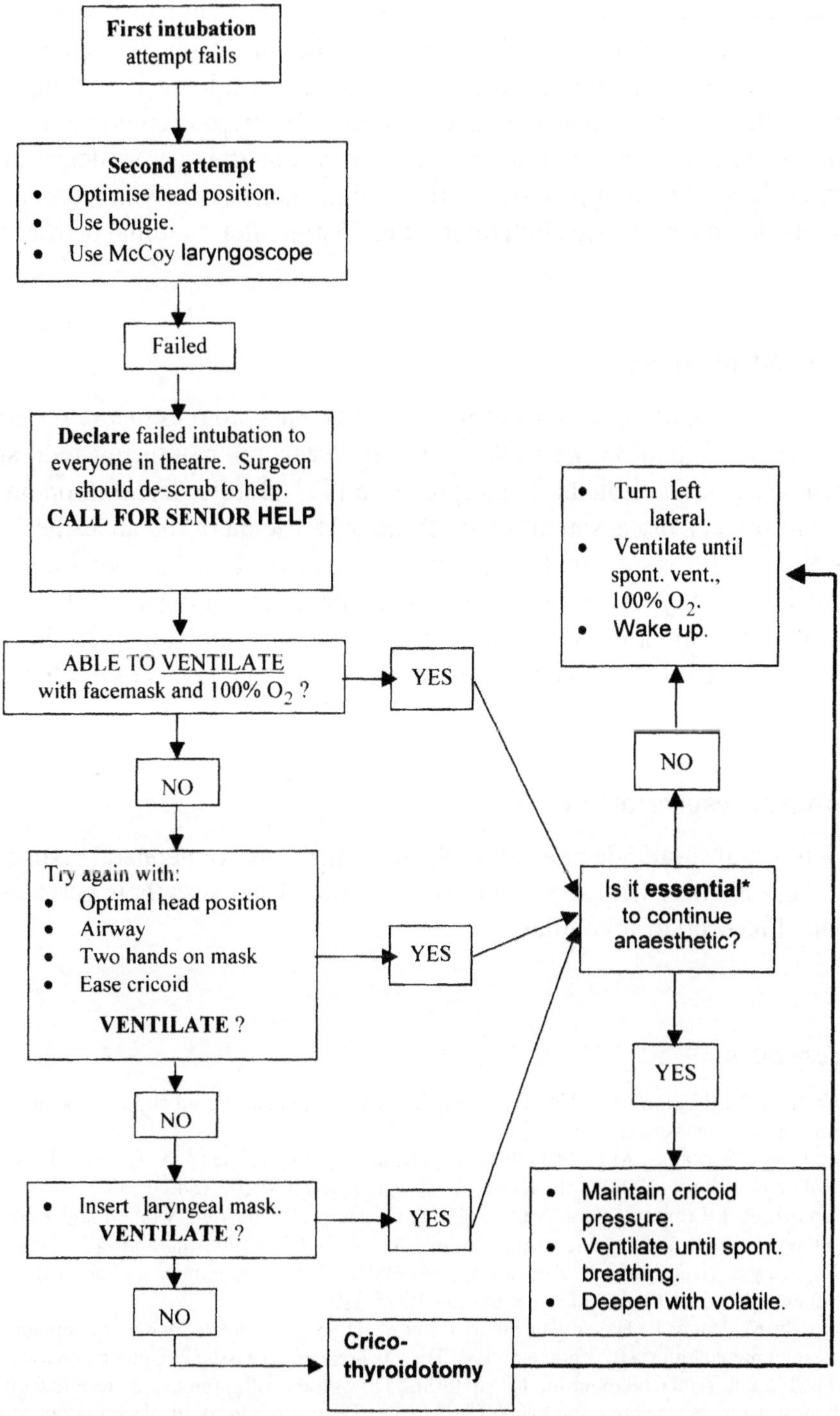

Fig. 1 Failed intubation drill

resuscitation; hence, section should be initiated with in 5 min of arrest to achieve most favourable outcome for the mother and her newborn [16]. Open cardiac massage by an experienced surgeon should be considered if section fails to improve the maternal condition. Cardiopulmonary bypass could be life saving in few situations, such as massive embolism, but is not a standard of care. Section should be attempted even after 5 min, because many newborns with a normal outcome have been delivered 11 to 15 min after maternal cardiac arrest.

Fetal compromise

The American College of Obstetricians and Gynaecologists has suggested that the term 'fetal distress' be replaced by the term 'nonreassuring fetal status', which describes a clinician's interpretation [17]. Before deciding on an intervention (forceps or caesarean section) the obstetrician or the anaesthesiologist or both should ensure that in utero fetal resuscitation has been attempted. Supplemental oxygen to the mother, adequate maternal position, discontinuation of oxytocin, normalisation of blood pressure and tocolysis in uterine hypertonus are all effective manoeuvres with variable levels of evidence.

Neonatal resuscitation

Each hospital should decide where the responsibility for neonatal resuscitation lies. Anaesthetists who work in obstetrics should reassess their knowledge of neonatal resuscitation regularly.

References

1. Graham SG, Luxton MC (1989) The requirement for intensive care support for the pregnant population. Anaesthesia 44:581-584
2. Kilpatrick S, Mathey M (1990) Obstetric patients requiring critical care. Chest 101: 1407-1412
3. Collop N, Sahn S (1993) Critical illness in pregnancy. Chest 103:1548-1552
4. Umo-Etuk J, Lumley J, Holdcraft A (1996) Critically ill parturient women and admission to intensive care: a 5 year review. International Journal of Obstetric Anaesthesia 5:79-84
5. Lapinsky S, Kruczynski K, Seaward G et al (1997) Critical care management of the obstetric patient. Canadian Journal of Anaesthesia 44:325-329
6. Knight M, Duley L, Henderson-Smart DJ et al (2003) Antiplatelet agents for preventing and treating pre-eclampsia (Cochrane review: The Cochrane library issue 2) Update Software, Oxford
7. The Magpie Trial Collaboration Group (2002) Do women with pre-eclampsia, and their babies, benefit from magnesium sulphate? The Magpie Trial: a randomised placebo-controlled trial. Lancet 359: (9321)1877-1890

8. Jouppila P, Jouppila R, Holimen A et al (1982) Lumbar epidural analgesia to improve intervillous blood flow during labour in severe pre-eclampsia. Obstet Gynecol 59:158-161
9. Zornberg GL, Jick H (2000) Antipsychotic drug use and risk of first time idiopathic venous thromboembolism: a case control study. Lancet 356:1219-1223
10. Royal College of Obstetricians and Gynaecologists (2001) Thromboembolic disease in pregnancy and the puerperium: acute management (guideline no. 28). RCOG, London
11. Waterstone M, Bewley S, Wolfe C (2001) Incidence and predictors of severe obstetric morbidity: case control study. BMJ 322: 1089-1093
12. Rainaldi MP, Tazzari PL, Scagliarini G et al (1998) Blood salvage during caesarean section. BJA 80:195-198
13. Gei A, Hankins GDV (2001) Cardiac disease and pregnancy. Obstet Gynecol Clin North Am 28:465-512
14. Barnardo PD, Jenkins JG (2000) Failed tracheal intubation in obstetrics: a 6 year review in a UK region. Anaesthesia 55:685-694
15. Rees GA, Willis BA (1988) Resuscitation in late pregnancy. Anaesthesia 43:347-349
16. Katz VL, Dotters DJ, Droegemueller W (1986) Perimortem caesarean delivery. Obstet Gynecol 68:571-576
17. American College of Obstetrician and Gynecologists (1998) Inappropriate use of the terms fetal distress and birth asphyxia. ACOG Committee Opinion, ACOG, Washington DC

Pre-eclampsia and anaesthesia

A. BHUVANAGIRI, R. ALEXANDER

Pre-eclampsia (PE) and eclampsia are the most common pregnancy-related conditions leading to admission to critical care unit [1]. Although the death rate has fallen over the last four decades, there is still a small but significant mortality rate [2]. Epidemiological studies suggest the true incidences of PE and eclampsia are approximately 3% and 0.05% of all deliveries, respectively [3]. Hypertensive disease of the pregnancy is also the second leading cause of direct deaths according to the statistics of the Confidential Enquiry of Maternal Deaths, 1977 – 1999 [4]. The rates, however, have fallen from 9.1 to 7.1 cases per million maternities compared with the previous report. Recommendations for treatment have been published in the CEMD 1997-1999 report, Appendix 1.

Pre-eclampsia is the term used to describe a disorder of pregnancy characterised by hypertension, proteinuria and often oedema and usually manifesting after the 20th week of gestation [5]. Proteinuria is defined as a 24-h urine collection with total protein excretion of equal to or greater than 300 mg 24 h^{-1} or two specimens of urine collected more than 4 h apart with ≥2+ on the protein reagent strip [6]. Severe PE is diagnosed if the patient suffers from any one of a number of symptoms [7] (Table 1). Eclampsia is defined if the parturient convulses.

Table 1 Clinical signs defining severe eclampsia

•	Severe hypertension (systolic blood pressure > 160 mmHg or diastolic blood pressure > 110 mmHg)
•	Proteinuria > 5.0 g / 24 h
•	Oliguria < 400 ml / 24 h
•	Cerebral irritability
•	Epigastric or right upper quadrant pain (liver capsule distension)
•	Pulmonary oedema

A diagnosis of eclampsia is made when a patient demonstrates seizure activity or coma in addition to the signs and symptoms of PE. The precise aetiology remains unknown. Epidemiological studies have suggested that genetic and immunological factors are involved. PE is twice as common in primiparas as in multiparas. However, with a change of partner, the risk in multiparous woman increases, suggesting that primipaternity is important. Particular men seem to have an increased risk of fathering a pre-eclamptic pregnancy [8]

Hypertension in pregnancy may be defined as pre-existing or pregnancy associated [9].

Pre-existing hypertension (3-5% of pregnancies)

Hypertension before pregnancy or found earlier than at 20 weeks of gestation or persisting after the pregnancy ends. Most such patients have essential hypertension, but some have renal disease and other medical disorders.

Pregnancy-associated hypertension (12% of pregnancies)

Hypertension occurring de novo after the 20th week of gestation and settling within 6 weeks postpartum. This category is divided into two groups :

a) *Gestational hypertension (6 – 7%).* Hypertension alone with no associated features.

b) *Pre-eclampsia (5 – 6%).* Hypertension with proteinuria of at least 0.3 g / 24 h (24-h urine collection or protein/creatinine ratio).

Pathophysiology of pre-eclampsia

PE is the result of (a) an initial placental trigger that has no adverse effect on the mother and (b) a maternal systemic reaction that produces the clinical signs and symptoms of the disorder [10].

Placental trigger

PE only occurs in the presence of a placenta [11]. It is associated with a failure of the normal invasion of trophoblast cells, leading to maladaptation of maternal spiral arterioles that are the source of the blood supply to the fetus. Maladaptation of these vessels can interfere with normal villous development, which may lead to placental insufficiency. Secondary damage such as fibrin deposition and thrombosis can then occur within the placenta. Not all women with the potential placental trigger develop PE; therefore the maternal response is the decisive factor in the development of the disease.

Maternal response

Although PE is said to be a vascular endothelial disorder it is a multisystem disorder with various forms [12]. Triglyceride-rich remnants are known to cause endothelial dysfunction and are positively correlated with elevations in BP. These proteins may contribute to the pathophysiology of PE [13]. Nitric oxide dysfunction, strong maternal inflammatory and immunological responses are all postulated to be significant factors [14].

HELLP syndrome

*H*aemolysis, *e*levated *l*iver enzymes and a *l*ow *p*latelet count constitute HELLP syndrome. It involves the combination of microangiopathic haemolytic anaemia, thrombocytopenia and hepatic ischaemia with periportal haemorrhage and necrosis, which can occur with severe pre-eclampsia. Some studies suggest that HELLP occurs in up to 50% of such cases [15]. Partial HELLP may be diagnosed if only one or two of the signs are present. Occasionally it may occur when hypertension or proteinuria is minimal [16]. Twenty per cent of the patients may present post partum with epigastric or right hypochondrial pain, malaise, nausea and vomiting.

Differential diagnoses include acute fatty liver of pregnancy, cholethiasis, viral hepatitis and thrombocytopenia from other causes. HELLP is associated with an increased risk of developing other serious complications, e.g. seizures. Maternal and fetal mortality are both increased.

Diagnosis

Hypertension is the most common diagnostic sign, although some women present with convulsions, abdominal pain or general malaise. Because there are no specific diagnostic investigations, the initial diagnosis of PE remains clinical. However, plasma uric acid concentrations are elevated in women with PE and may be used as a marker of the disease. Measurement of uric acid may aid in the diagnosis, particularly in those with pre-existing hypertension. Concentrations of 360 μg/L (6.0 mg / dl) are associated with PE, and there is often further rise in those who develop eclampsia. The range of clinical signs is listed in Table 2.

Table 2 Systemic effects of pre-eclampsia

RS	Pulmonary oedema, facial & laryngeal oedema, ARDS
CVS	Widespread vasoconstriction, normal or increased systemic vascular resistance, left ventricular failure, increased vascular permeability and oedema, decreased circulating blood volume
CNS	Headaches, visual disturbances, convulsions hyperreflexia, cerebral haemorrhage
Renal	Reduced glomerular filtration rate, reduced urea clearance and increased uric acid concentrations proteinuria and hypoproteinaemia, oliguria, acute renal failure
Liver	Abnormal LFT's (increased AST & ALT) subcapsular haemorrhage & epigastric pain liver rupture
Coagulation	Increased turnover of fibrinogen, fibrin & platelets thrombocytopenia, impaired platelet function, DIC
Fetal	Decreased placental perfusion, placental ischaemia & infarction, IUGR, placental abruption, preterm labour

Treatment

The goals of treatment are; (1) prevention of convulsions, (2) control of hypertension, (3) optimisation of intravascular volume and (4) treatment of coagulopathy.

Prevention of convulsions

Magnesium sulphate is considered the drug of choice for the prevention of convulsions [17]. The mechanism of action of Mg^{2+} involves a generalised depression of the CNS activity as well as cerebral arterial dilatation, relieving cerebral ischaemia. Other beneficial effects include mild antihypertensive effect, a tocolytic activity and lowering of plasma endothelin^{-1} levels. The results of a recent study indicated that Mg^{2+} does not affect overall coagulation [18]. Magnesium sulphate reduces the risk of eclampsia, and it is likely that it also reduces the risk of maternal death. It does not have any substantial harmful effects on the mother or the fetus in clinical doses, although a quarter of women may have side effects [19].

Control of hypertension

The aim should be to maintain MAP between 100 – 140 mmHg [20]. A sudden drop in BP or reductions below these pressures should be avoided, as this will further compromise placental perfusion. Careful volume expansion should be achieved prior to the use of vasodilators or epidural analgesia to maintain perfusion.

Fluid therapy

Intravenous fluid therapy is often necessary, as there is usually volume depletion. However, there is also a propensity to develop pulmonary oedema. There is an inverse relationship between intravascular volume and severity of hypertension. With plasma volume 30 - 40% below normal in severe PE, a significant decrease in plasma volume may precede the clinical appearance of the disease [21]. Volume expansion alone has been shown to reduce SVR and systolic BP. Optimum fluid therapy is difficult to achieve, since the combination of low colloid oncotic pressure and LV dysfunction in severe PE makes the risk of pulmonary oedema very high. Crystalloid alone causes a further decrease in colloid oncotic pressures, whereas colloids will increase the CVP and thus the risk of pulmonary oedema. The most usual regimens involve crystalloid at 1-2 ml kg^{-1} h^{-1} with colloid used if the CVP and serum albumin are low. Blood and blood products should be given as necessary. Oliguria should be treated with a fluid challenge of 250 ml of crystalloid, and if there is no response CVP monitoring should be instituted before any further fluid is given.

Treatment of coagulopathy

The regular monitoring of clotting factors and platelets will help identify the onset of thrombocytopenia or disseminated intravascular coagulopathy. Platelets should be given to maintain a count greater than 80×10^9 L^{-1} if regional anaesthesia is indicated, to prevent the possibility of epidural or subdural haematoma formation.

Anaesthetic management

A joint plan has to be developed with obstetricians and physicians for resuscitation, monitoring, anaesthesia, delivery and postpartum care. Resuscitation of the parturient should include the prevention and treatment of seizures and fluid resuscitation. Aorto-caval compression should be avoided at all times by placing the patient in the left lateral position and restoring the circulating blood volume. Antihypertensive treatment (according to local protocols) should be started to lower the blood pressure. Oxygen therapy should be started, as there is mounting evidence that there is an oxygen extraction defect at tissue level [22]. Even at high oxygen delivery levels, oxygen consumption is still low for pregnancy. Investigations should include full blood count, electrolyte function, liver enzyme tests including uric acid, coagulation studies and arterial blood gases. Adequacy of resuscitation should then be assessed (with repeat investigations if required) and a plan for delivery be drawn up with the rest of the multidisciplinary team.

For patients with severe PE, it is vital to have a flexible anaesthetic plan with more than one option, as the situation may change suddenly without prior warning.

Analgesia for labour

Epidural analgesia is suitable for providing pain relief for labour and delivery. There are numerous benefits of an epidural block, including the reduction of blood pressure to more manageable levels requiring less hypotensive medication. With pain relief, the serum concentration of catecholamines decreases, resulting in an increase in uteroplacental and intervillous blood flow, which is highly beneficial in patients with severe PE, who already have vasospasm of the uteroplacental circulation [23]. In addition, the neuroendocrine stress response to surgery is significantly weaker with epidural than with general anaesthesia [24]. Prolonged epidural infusions have been reported to improve the pre-eclamptic condition [25]. With judicious hydration and slow induction of the block, hypotension can be minimised with little change in central venous pressure, cardiac index and pulmonary artery wedge pressure, though recent reports state that the magnitudes of maternal BP declines were similar after spinal and epidural analgesia [26]. Vasoconstrictors should be used sparingly. The choice of epidural versus combined spinal-epidural blockade is an individual one, as there are advantages and disadvantages with each technique. A low-dose local anaesthetic and opioid solution should be administered intrathecally when a combined spinal/epidural (CSE) technique is used to initiate the block and then topped up with epidural boluses. There are good arguments for using an infusion as opposed to boluses of solutions to reduce the risk of hypotension as a result of vasodilatation in a venoconstricted, hypovalaemic patient. Small boluses delivered more frequently by patient controlled epidural analgesia may be preferable to infusions, as there is less accumulation of drug and less motor block [27].

Anaesthesia for caesarean section

Regional analgesia is the method of choice for caesarean deliveries owing to its proven records of maternal and fetal safety. It is however absolutely contraindicated when (a) the patient refuses permission, (b) there is evidence of coagulopathy and/or (c) there is evidence of sepsis. All other contraindications are relative. There are no significant changes in central venous pressure, cardiac index, and pulmonary artery wedge pressure (PAWP) from baseline during epidural analgesia for caesarean section [28]. There is also less risk of severe hypotension as the block may be increased in incremental doses. The drawbacks, however, are that the block will take longer to initiate than with a spinal anaesthetic and there may be a higher incidence of failed block for caesarean section [29].

The use of a single-shot spinal is controversial. Pre-eclamptic women have a depleted intravascular volume and decreased uteroplacental perfusion. Rapid and profound hypotension may occur with spinal anaesthesia, and prophylactic hydration does not reliably prevent spinal hypotension. Despite these concerns, recent evidence indicates that spinal analgesia may be safely used without adverse maternal or fetal outcome [26]. Continuous spinal anaesthetic may be a viable alternative for operative delivery in PE when epidural anaesthesia cannot be established [30]. An alternative plan is to apply a CSE technique, as mentioned for labour analgesia.

A suggested technique for regional analgesia for caesarean section is as follows:

1) Administer aspiration prophylaxis.
2) Ensure blood products are available as needed.
3) Start a second peripheral IV line and initiate CVP or PAWP monitoring as indicated.
4) Apply all the monitors.
5) Hydrate with 1000 ml of crystalloid or infuse enough fluids to increase CVP to no more than 4 mmHg or PCWP of 5 – 8 mmHg [31].
6) Monitor the FHR until the beginning of surgery.
7) Insert epidural catheter and administer either 2% lidocaine or 0.5% bupivacaine in incremental doses to extend the sensory level of block to the fourth thoracic dermatome. Administer 50-100 μg fentanyl.
8) For CSE administer 7.5 mg of hyperbaric bupivacaine with 25 μg fentanyl intrathecally.
9) Maintain left uterine displacement and treat hypotension with vasoconstrictors, fluid volume or both.
10) At the end of surgery, start epidural fentanyl infusion or give preservative-free morphine for postoperative pain relief.

General anaesthesia

If regional anaesthesia is contraindicated then one has to consider the potential problems associated with general anaesthesia and pre-eclampsia. These include:
1) Airway oedema and the possibility of difficult airway management
2) An exaggerated sympathetic, hypertensive response to laryngoscopy and tracheal intubation.
3) Drug interaction between Mg^{2+} and muscle relaxants.

Recommended technique for general anaesthesia.
1. Steps 1-3 as above.
2. Place an arterial line. Start haemodynamic monitoring with CVP or PCWP if required.
3. Ensure smaller endotracheal tubes and different sizes and types of laryngoscopic blades are available in the theatre. Make sure all the necessary equipment for the management of a difficult airway is readily available.
4. Begin preoxygenation and apply all the monitors.
5. Monitor FHR and gradually lower MAP as tolerated by the fetus, with labetolol 0.5-1.0 mg kg^{-1}, or use intravenous vasodilators guided by CVP or PCWP.
6. Induce anaesthesia according to your skill and personal preference for anaesthesia agents. Give labetolol 5-10 mg iv before extubation to prevent emergence hypertension.
7. Ensure adequate postoperative analgesia has been administered. Consider using patient-controlled analgesia.

Postoperative care

The patient should be monitored in the recovery room or a high dependency bed for the next 12–24 h. Magnesium infusion should be continued once started to prevent the risk of further fits. The risk of pulmonary oedema is very high, and careful monitoring of pulmonary congestion is required.

Intensive care management

Severe cases of pre-eclampsia and eclampsia should be managed in the intensive care unit (ICU) especially if there is prolonged fitting, marked coagulopathy or substantial renal impairment. Most admissions to the ICU are post partum. However, if delivery has not occurred, management should be directed at obtaining a safe MAP of 105–125 mmHg, controlling any convulsions, protecting the airway and delivering the fetus.

Hypertension

Invasive monitoring of the arterial pressures should occur. The use of hydralazine would now be regarded as the first-line therapy [32]. For immediate control of BP not responding to Mg^{2+}, the use of sodium nitroprusside is indicated [33]. It should be limited prior to delivery or in renal failure owing to potential thiocyanate toxicity. For long-term BP control, clonidine, hydralazine, calcium channel antagonists, beta-blockers and prazosin can be used [34].

Most patients with pre-eclampsia are volume-depleted. In some cases, fluid loading may result in lowering of BP, but usually the BP is preserved with a resultant increase in cardiac output. In severe cases the left ventricular compliance is markedly reduced and even small volumes (500 ml) may cause large increases in left-sided filling pressures with the development of pulmonary oedema. These changes will occur with little or no change in CVP.

Seizures

Management of the initial fit must be directed at its termination, usually with a benzodiazepine, and protection of the airway. An infusion of magnesium sulphate should be started. Management of recurrent fitting is directed again at terminating the seizures either with a benzodiazepine or, in refractory cases, thiopentone and intubation to protect the airway.

Renal failure

Oliguria is a common finding in PE patients and usually responds to fluid loading, delivery of the fetus and control of any hypertension. However, there is a small group of patients who develop acute tubular necrosis, requiring dialysis [35]. Initial management should be directed at adequate volume loading and vasodilatation using PAWP to optimise left ventricle pre- and afterload. Severe PE can also cause haemolytic uraemic syndrome. This should be kept in mind in patients with acute renal failure, especially when there is complete anuria. These patients will have to undergo plasma exchange.

The anaesthetic management of the pre-eclamptic parturient can be complex and difficult, requiring a multi-disciplinary approach. It should start in the antenatal period and finish well after delivery, with particular attention being given to pain and blood pressure control.

Appendix

Recommendations of the Confidential Enquiry into Maternal Deaths, 1997--1999

- Pregnant women with headache of sufficient severity to seek medical advice or with new epigastric pain should have their BP measured and urine tested for protein, as minimum investigation.
- Clear, written, management protocols for severe PE should guide initial and continuing treatment in the hospital.
- Automated blood pressure recording systems can systematically underestimate BP in PE, to a serious degree. BP values should be compared at the beginning of treatment with those obtained by conventional mercury sphygmomanometers.
- Severe life-threatening hypertension must be treated effectively.
- Magnesium sulphate is the anticonvulsant drug of choice in the treatment of eclampsia.
- There should be early engagement of intensive care specialists in the care of women with severe PE.
- Women with moderate to severe PE require a level of clinical observation that may be incompatible with location in a single side room in hospital.
- Women with multiple pregnancies are at increased risk of PE, and their antenatal care should reflect that awareness.

References

1. Department of Health (1999) Report on confidential enquiries into maternal deaths in the United Kingdom,1994-1996. HMSO, London
2. Leitch CR, Cameron AD, Walker JJ (1997) The changing pattern of eclampsia over 60 year period. Br J Obstet Gynecol 104:917-922
3. Saftlas AF, Olson DR, Franks AL et al (1990) Epidemiology of pre-eclampsia and eclampsia in the United States 1979-1986. Am J Obstet Gynecol 163:460-465
4. Department of Health (2001) Report on confidential enquiries into maternal deaths in the United Kingdom, 1997-1999. HMSO, London
5. Higgins JR, de Swiet M (2001) Blood pressure measurement and classification in pregnancy. Lancet 357:131-135
6. Brown MA, Buddle ML (1996) Hypertension in pregnancy. Maternal and fetal outcomes according to laboratory and clinical features. Med J Aust 165:360-365
7. Fadigan AB, Sealy DP, Schneider EF (1994) Preeclampsia: progress and puzzle. Am Fam Physician 49:849-856
8. Lie RT, Rasmussen S, Brunborg H et al (1998) Fetal and Maternal contributions to risk of pre-eclampsia: population based study. BMJ 316:1343-1347

9. Magee LA, Ornstein MP, vonDadelszen P (1999) Fortnightly review: management of hypertension in pregnancy. BMJ 318:1332-1336
10. Redman CW, Sacks GP, Sargent IL (1999) Preeclampsia: an excessive maternal inflammatory response to pregnancy. Am J Obstet Gynecol 180:499-506
11. Myatt L (2002) Role of placenta in Preeclampsia. Endocrine19:103–111
12. Roberts JM, Lain KY (2002) Recent insights into the pathogenesis of pre-eclampsia. Placenta 23:359-372
13. Winker K, Wetza B, Hoffmann MM et al (2003) Triglyceride rich lipo proteins are associated with hypertension in preeclampsia: Clin Endocrinol.Metab 88:1162–1166
14. Lowe DT (2000) Nitric oxide dysfunction in the pathophysiology of preeclampsia. Nitric Oxide 4:441-458
15. Saphier CJ, Repke JT (1998) Hemolysis, elevated liver enzymes and low platelets (HELLP) syndrome. A review of diagnosis and management. Semin Perinatol 22:118-133
16. Sibai BM,Taslimi MM, el-Nazer A et al (1986) Maternal perinatal outcome associated with the syndrome of hemolysis, elevated liver enzymes and low platelet in severe preeclampsia-eclampsia. Am J Obstet Gynecol 155:501-509
17. Sibai B, Ramanathan J (1992) The case for magnesium sulphate in preeclampsia-eclampsia. Int J Obstet Anaesth 1:167-171
18. Harnett MJ, Data S, Bhavani-Shankar K (2001) The effect of magnesium on coagulation in parturients with preeclampsia. Anaesth Analg 92 :1257-1260
19. Do women with pre-eclampsia, and their babies, benefit from magnesium sulphate? The Magpie Trial: a randomized placebo controlled trial. Lancet 2002:359:1877-1890
20. Mushambi MC, Halligan AW, Williamson K (1996) Recent developments in the pathophysiology and management of preeclampsia.Br J Anaesth 76:133-148
21. Bosio PM, McKenna PJ, Conroy R (1999) Maternal central hemodynamics in hypertensive disorders of pregnancy. Obstet Gynecol 94: 978-984
22. Belfort MA, Anthony J, Saade GR et al (1993) The oxygen consumption/oxygen delivery curve in severe preeclampsia: evidence for a fixed oxygen extraction state. Am J Obstet Gynecol 169:1448-1455
23. Jouppila P, Jouppila R, Holeman A et al (1982) Lumbar epidural analgesia to improve intervillous blood flow during labour in severe preeclampsia. Obstet Gynecol 59:158-161
24. Ramanathan J, Coleman P, Sibai B. (1991) Anaesthetic modification of haemodynamic and neuroendocrine stress responses to caesarean delivery in women with severe preeclampsia: Anaesth Analg 73:772-779
25. Kanayama N, Belayet HM, Khatun S et al (1999) A new treatment of preeclampsia by long-term epidural anaesthesia. J. Hum Hypertens 13:167-171
26. Hood DD, Curry R (1999) Spinal versus epidural anaesthesia for caesarean section in severely preeclamptic patients: a retrospective survey. Anaesthesiology 90:1276–1282
27. Ramanathan J, Vaddadi AK, Arheart KL (2001) Combined spinal and epidural with low doses of intrathecal bupivacaine in women with severe pre eclampsia: preliminary report. Reg Anaesth Pain Med 26:46–51
28. Hodgkinson R, Hussain FJ, Hayashi RH (1980) Systemic and pulmonary blood pressure during caesarean section in parturients with gestational hypertension Can Anaesth Soc J 27:389-394
29. Beilin Y, Bernstein HH, Zuncker-Pinchoff B (1995) The optimal distance that a multi orifice epidural catheter should be threaded into epidural space. Anaesth Analg 81:301-304
30. Overdyk KF, Harvery SC (1998) Continuous spinal anaesthesia for caesarean section in a parturient with severe pre eclampsia. J Clin Anaesth 10:510–513
31. Young P, Johanson R (2001) Hemodynamic, invasive and echocardiographic monitoring in the hypertensive parturient. Best Pract Res Clin Obstet and Gynaecol 15:605-622
32. Cotton DB, Gonik B, Dorman KF (1985) Cardiovascular alterations in severe pregnancy-induced hypertension seen with intravenously given hydralazine bolus. Surg Gynecol Obstet 161:240-244
33. Ellis SC, Wheeler AS, James FM 3rd et al (1982) Fetal and maternal effects of sodium

nitroprusside used to counteract hypertension in gravis ewes. AM J Obstet Gynecol 143:766-770
34. Mabie W, Gonzales A, Sibai B et al (1987) Comparative trial of labetolol and hydrallazine in the acute management of severe hypertension complicating pregnancy. Obstet Gynecol 70 328-333
35. Stratta P, Besso L, Canavse C et al (1996) Is pregnancy- related acute renal failure disappearing clinical entity? Ren Fail 18: 575-584

Prevention and management of eclampsia

F. PARUK, S. BHAGWANJEE

Eclampsia is a pregnancy-specific multisystem disorder associated with substantial fetomaternal morbidity and mortality [1-6]. The incidence of eclampsia is variable, but is generally low in well-resourced regions compared with resource-deficient countries. However, once eclampsia ensues the potential for both morbidity (immediate and long term) and mortality is cause for equal concern. In the context of its elusive aetiology, the prevention and management of this multiorgan disease challenge even the most experienced of clinicians. This paper focuses on the definition of pre-eclampsia/eclampsia, the suggested pathophysiology of the disease, current potential preventative strategies and specific issues of concern in the management of the critically ill eclamptic patient.

Definitions

Pre-eclampsia was traditionally defined as the occurrence of new-onset hypertension in combination with proteinuria (=0.3 g/24 h) after 20 weeks of gestation. It is now accepted that proteinuria is not an absolute prerequisite for the diagnosis of pre eclampsia. Therefore, hypertension together with other features, such as headache, thrombocytopenia, hyperuricaemia, deranged liver function or fetal compromise *in the absence of proteinuria* is likely to represent pre-eclampsia [7].

Eclampsia is defined as the occurrence of generalised seizures associated with the signs of pre-eclampsia during pregnancy or labour or within 7 days after delivery and not caused by epilepsy or other known causes of convulsions.

Pathophysiology

Pre-eclampsia

The aetiology of pre-eclampsia has yet to be adequately delineated. In fact it is often referred to as the "disease of theories". Certainly the accompanying pathological features are not characteristic of hypertension. The recurring findings of necrosis and haemorrhage in the brain, liver and adrenal glands are best explained by reduced perfusion [8]. The pathophysiological changes of pre-eclampsia support the theory of reduced maternal systemic organ perfusion. The most recently accepted model is that proposed by Roberts (Fig. 1) [9]. It is postulated that an interplay of immunological factors, environmental factors and genetic predisposition in a susceptible individual results in defective placental implantation, which is characterised by a failure of spiral artery modification into a low-resistance vascular circuit. This results in placental ischaemia. This in turn causes the release of various circulating factors (including VWF, fibronectin, thrombomodulin, endothelin and thromboxane) and the generation of oxidative stress, which leads to endothelial dysfunction. The resultant multiorgan hypoperfusion culminates in the widespread multiorgan dysfunction characteristic of pre-eclampsia. This two-stage model proposes maternal predisposition to the disease, hence increasing the possibility of preventative strategies targeted to susceptible women. The model also implies that by virtue of the multifactorial origin of the disease, there is no single "magic bullet' to prevent or treat the disorder.

Recent reviews by Redman et al. and Sargent et al. allude to the role of the maternal systemic inflammatory response (MSIR) in the pathogenesis of pre-eclampsia [10, 11]. In a nutshell, they propose that the normal inflammatory response of pregnancy (which is most probably stimulated by the placenta and characterised by apoptotic or necrotic debris shed into the maternal circulation from the syncytial surface of the placenta) is markedly exaggerated in pre-eclamptic patients. Thus, the MSIR associated with pre-eclampsia represents the extreme end of a spectrum of response to all pregnancies. There is therefore no clear distinction between normal and abnormal responses. The clinical implication of this is that the prediction and diagnosis of the disease is neither simple nor absolute.

Eclampsia

The pathophysiology of cerebral lesions is controversial. The two main theories that have emerged are those of vasospasm (resulting in cytotoxic oedema) and hypertensive encephalopathy (resulting in vasogenic oedema).

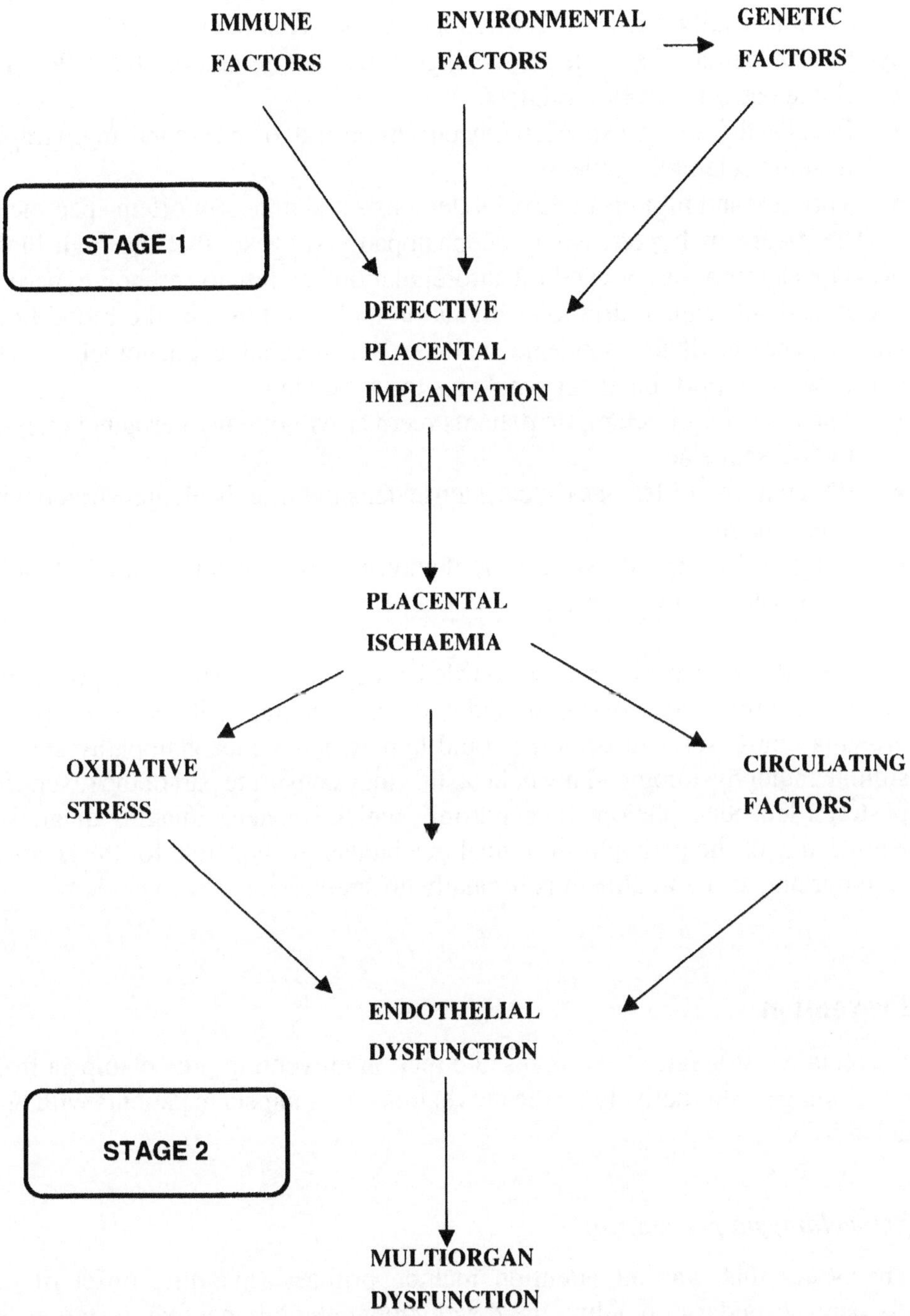

Fig. 1 Pathophysiology of pre-eclampsia

The vasospasm theory proposes that high blood pressure leads to cerebral vasospasm, resulting in cerebral hypoperfusion. This leads to ischaemia and cytotoxic oedema. The evidence to support this theory includes the following:

- Some patients develop infarcts.
- Focal or diffuse vasospasm has been demonstrated on cerebral angiography in some eclamptic patients.
- Thrombi and infarcts have been demonstrated in post-mortem specimens.

The theory of hypertensive encephalopathy suggests that the high blood pressure causes a loss of cerebral autoregulation, leading to cerebral hyperperfusion and subsequent arteriolar dilatation and disruption of the blood-brain barrier. The resultant vasogenic oedema is a reversible phenomenon. The evidence to support this theory includes the following:

- The majority of eclamptic patients recover without any permanent neurological sequelae.
- Reversibility of lesions (hyperintense densities) can be demonstrated with neuroimaging.
- Cerebral hyperperfusion can be demonstrated with transcranial Doppler studies and SPECT scans.

This latter theory is currently regarded as the more plausible. It is postulated that if it is untreated, vasospasm and cytotoxic oedema will ensue. There is a growing consensus that eclampsia and hypertensive encephalopathy share a similar pathophysiology. Many believe that they constitute part of the reversible posterior leucoencephalopathy syndrome, which is a neuroimaging diagnosis. Knowledge of the pathophysiological mechanism responsible for the seizures is important, as the treatment is basically different.

Prevention

Preventative strategies have focused either on preventing pre-eclampsia from developing or alternatively on the prevention of eclampsia in patients with pre-eclampsia.

Pre-eclampsia prevention

The issues that warrant attention include primary (avoiding onset of the disease), secondary (avoiding the development and clinical manifestations of the disease) and tertiary (avoiding the emergence of complications of the disease) prevention. Avoiding pregnancy is the absolute preventative measure.

However, certain risk factors for the development of pre-eclampsia have been identified (Table 1), and the manipulation of some of these factors may prevent the occurrence of the disease.

Table 1 Risk factors for pre-eclampsia

- Family history
- Primipaternity
- Nulliparity
- Minimal sperm exposure
- Male partner – history of pre-eclampsia in a previous relationship
- Female- previous history of pre-eclampsia
- Advanced maternal age
- Assisted reproduction
- Chronic hypertension
- Chronic renal disease
- Insulin resistance
- Antiphospholipid antibody syndrome
- Hyperhomocysteinaemia
- Activated protein C resistance
- Protein S deficiency
- Gestational diabetes
- Type I diabetes mellitus
- Multiple gestation
- Fetal hydrops
- Gestational trophoblastic disease
- Trisomy 13

Many clinical (e.g. maternal weight gain, second trimester blood pressure evaluation and Doppler velocimetry) and laboratory tests have been investigated as potential tools for the prediction of pre-eclampsia. To date no accurate predictor of pre-eclampsia has been identified.

Various methods have been explored to address the issue of secondary prevention of the disease. The following strategies are currently under investigation

Antiplatelet drugs

Antiplatelet drugs (and aspirin in particular), by virtue of their ability to alter the prostacyclin-thromboxane A_2 ratio (in favour of the vasodilatory prostacyclin), constitute an attractive option for the prevention of pre-eclampsia [12]. A recent systematic review by Duley et al. includes 39 trials (30 563 women), with most of them (28 802) comparing aspirin with placebo [13]. In essence, the authors conclude that antiplatelet drugs are associated with a moderate reduction (15%) in the risk of pre-eclampsia. There is a suggestion that an aspirin dose of >75 mg may be more beneficial. However, the subgroup was small and furthermore current pregnancy safety data suggest a dose of 60 mg.

The authors further suggest that apart from the drug dosage, both the time of treatment initiation and the individual risk of the disease are important considerations that might have influenced the overall (pooled) data.

Calcium supplementation

A recent systematic review concluded that calcium supplementation appears to benefit women at high risk of gestational hypertension even in communities characterised by a low calcium diet. The authors rightly suggest that further research is necessary in this field: while several small trials suggested a benefit, this was not demonstrated in the largest trial to date [14].

Fish oil supplementation

The omega-3 fatty acids are considered important by virtue of their protective effect on prostacyclin-thromboxane A_2 balance. The findings of the European Multicentre Fish Oil Supplementation trial do not support its use for the prevention of pre-eclampsia [15].

Antenatal

Appropriate antenatal care is a salient factor in the tertiary prevention of pre-eclampsia. In the United Kingdom, over the past 60 years the incidence of eclampsia has declined by more than 90% [16]. This is probably attributable to improvements in socioeconomic status as well as the provision of accessible and appropriate antenatal care.

Eclampsia

The international multicentre Magpie study, a double-blind randomised controlled trial involving 10 123 patients from 33 counties and designed to assess the role of magnesium sulphate ($MgSO_4$) in preventing eclampsia in women with pre-eclampsia demonstrated a significantly lower incidence of eclampsia in the $MgSO_4$ group than in the placebo group (1.1% versus 1.9%) [17]. There was also a 48% lower maternal mortality, although this was not shown to be statistically significant. Interestingly only 2.6% and 3.3% of the maternal deaths in the control and placebo groups, respectively, suffered an eclamptic seizure. There were no substantive side effects. It was noted that adverse effects were more frequent in the $MgSO_4$ group than in the placebo group; however, intravenous administration of $MgSO_4$produced significantly fewer adverse effects than the intramuscular mode of drug administration. The results of the follow-up study of the babies born in the trial are awaited. The

Magpie study has generated debate on the following issues:

- The specific indications for $MgSO_4$ in the scenario of pre-eclampsia.
- The questionable value of $MgSO_4$ prophylaxis in developed regions, where the incidence of eclampsia is very low.
- The practicality, safety and cost of $MgSO_4$ administration in under-resourced regions, where the incidence of eclampsia is generally high.
- In developing countries, where the incidence of eclampsia is high, many patients present following the onset of seizures. It has been suggested that in such situations the strategy of $MgSO_4$ prophylaxis will obviously not be the sole factor in reducing the incidence of eclampsia.

The South African Magpie Trial Collaborators Group suggest that in poor countries $MgSO_4$ be considered for moderate to severe pre-eclampsia at the time of delivery and during transport of the patient to a more appropriate level of care and also for the expectant management of pre-eclampsia at tertiary institutions [18]. The group also highlights the fact that current data provide safety data for 24-h use of $MgSO_4$ and therefore longer treatment should be undertaken with caution. The authors concede that the value of $MgSO_4$ prophylaxis depends on the ability to administer the drug safely and that site-specific costs and benefits must also be considered.

Recently, Belforte et al. compared $MgSO_4$ and nimodipine (a calcium channel blocker with specific cerebral vasodilatory properties) for the prevention of eclampsia [19]. The results showed significant benefit of parenteral $MgSO_4$ over oral nimodipine in the prevention of eclampsia in severely pre-eclamptic patients. The lack of efficacy of a specific cerebral vasodilator has led the authors to question the hypothesis that cerebral vasospasm with resultant ischaemia is the predominant cause of eclampsia. Belforte et al. had previously reported on a cohort of 192 patients with either mild or severe pre-eclampsia [20]. Cerebral perfusion pressure (CPP) of the middle cerebral artery was almost always (87%) normal in mild pre-eclampsia but increased in a significant proportion (52%) of severe pre-eclampsia patients. The majority of patients (mild and severe cases) had a normal cerebral flow index. The authors therefore hypothesise that raised CPP results in barotrauma and vessel damage, leading to hypertensive encephalopathy and overperfusion injury. Nimodipine has been shown to increase CPP, and $MgSO_4$ to decrease it [21]. This may explain the poor performance of the drug as a preventative agent for eclampsia. It also favours the hypertensive encephalopathy theory of the pathogenesis of the eclamptic seizure.

Management

The management of pre-eclampsia has been extensively reviewed [22, 23].

The important issues in the management of the critically ill eclamptic patient include the following:

- Assessment of the severity of illness.
- Principles of management.
- Non-specific interventions.
- Specific interventions.

Assessment of the severity of illness

There is a paucity of data on critically ill eclamptic patients. In most series the eclamptic patients constitute a subset of a larger critically ill obstetric population [24-37].

Traditionally, severity of illness has been quantified in accordance with the degree of physiological derangement at the time of ICU admission; this has formed the basis for scores such as the APACHE Sytems [38, 39]. The introduction of organ dysfunction assessment and organ failure scores suggests that organ dysfunction constitutes an *important* marker of illness severity. More recently, consensus conference definitions of SIRS have caused this to emerge as an important marker of severity of illness [40]. With SIRS the spectrum of severity ranges from sepsis to severe sepsis and ultimately septic shock. The non-septic correlates to this have been suggested as SIRS, severe SIRS and sterile shock [41].

Our observation of 105 critically ill eclamptic patients managed in an ICU over a period of 3 ½ years has been as follows [6]:

- The Glasgow Coma Score (GCS) alone was as effective as the APACHE II in identifying non-survivors.
- No fatalities were observed among the patients who were admitted to the ICU with a GCS>10.
- The presence of >2 organ failures for a period exceeding 48 h was invariably associated with a fatal outcome.

Currently there is no scoring system that accurately assesses severity of illness in patients with hypertensive disorders of pregnancy (or obstetric patients for that matter). Existing systems have yielded variable results when tested in obstetric populations [24, 26, 30, 35, 37]. This is not unexpected, as pregnant patients are a unique population whose members have a markedly different physiological behaviour than do their non-pregnant counterparts.

Principles of management

Although delivery of the fetus and the placenta is the cornerstone of the management of the disease, it is of paramount import to ensure that organ perfusion and tissue oxygen delivery is optimised and maintained. Table 2 outlines the general principles of management; nonetheless, it is imperative that an individually tailored approach be adopted. In addition, one should be cognisant of the point that the post-delivery period in eclampsia is extremely volatile (largely attributable to major fluid shifts) and renders the patient susceptible to cardiovascular complications in particular.

Table 2 Principles of management of eclampsia

- ABC/left lateral position
- Abort seizure
- Prevent further seizures (magnesium sulphate)
- Blood pressure control (MAP of 95-105 mmHg)
- Maternal-fetal assessment
- Patient stabilisation
- Expedite delivery (within 8-12 h of onset of initial seizure)
- Post delivery monitoring (intensive surveillance for first 24 h at least)

Indications for ventilation:

- Upper airway obstruction (oedema, tongue biting)
- Seizures without recovery of consciousness
- Multiple seizures
- Persistently low GCS
- Cardiorespiratory complications

It is important to note that pre-ICU care and stabilisation is a crucial determinant of maternal outcome. Antenatal care is better in developed countries (available, accessible and appropriate). Patients reach health care facilities promptly should they develop eclampsia. Thus, their GCS is usually not markedly depressed and they are physiologically less deranged than their counterparts in developing countries. This probably explains the lower mortality associated with eclampsia in developed countries.

Non-specific interventions

Benzodiazepines

These are ideal sedative and anticonvulsant agents and should be routinely administered. A very low seizure recurrence rate (0.9%) was reported in a cohort of 105 ventilated eclampsia patients receiving a midazolam infusion as part of their ICU care [6].

Analgesia

This is mandatory in order to prevent restlessness and agitation in the post-surgical patient.

IPPV

The aim is to achieve normocarbia, normoxia and a normal pH. Control of these factors is essential to ensure optimal cerebral perfusion.

Magnesium sulphate

The Collaborative Eclampsia Trial has provided clear evidence to support the use of $MgSO_4$ as the drug of choice in eclampsia, to prevent further seizures [42]. An accepted regimen is a loading dose of 6 g over 20 min, followed by an infusion of 2 g/h for 24 h post delivery. Serum magnesium levels are checked in selected situations, viz. oliguria, development of symptom or signs of magnesium toxicity, renal dysfunction or in the scenario of recurrent seizures. The intravenous regimen is preferred (despite the need for meticulous maternal surveillance) in view of the following:

~ Painful repeated injections are avoided.
~ The risk of abscess development at the injection site is obviated.

Blood pressure control

This is essential. A diastolic blood pressure of 110 mmHg should be targeted. The blood pressure should not be dropped too rapidly, nor should the drop be excessive: the MAP should not be reduced by >25% or the diastolic blood pressure should not be reduced by >30 mmHg. This is to prevent a sudden or marked drop in the cerebral perfusion pressure. Marked fluctuations in the blood pressure should also be avoided, particularly in the context of raised intracranial pressure. In our experience, dihydrallazine infusions produce good blood pressure control without producing marked fluctuations. A more detailed description of rapid-acting antihypertensive agents is given elsewhere [23].

Specific interventions

Neurological

This entails a 15° head tilt, maintenance of a neutral head position, attainment of normocarbia, normoxia and normal pH, blood pressure control and seizure prophylaxis.

Haemodynamic

The goal is to obtain cardiovascular stability with minimal variation in the blood pressure. Invasive blood pressure monitoring and serial CVP assessments are fundamental. The trend in CVP is an important tool to assess adequacy of fluid resuscitation and prevent circulatory overload. Echocardiography is indicated in selected patients to detect cardiac lesions or in the presence of ARDS (to assist with haemodynamic manipulations). A recent systematic review suggests that there is no data from randomised clinical controlled trials illustrating the clinical utility of pulmonary artery catheters or echocardiographic techniques in hypertensive disorders of pregnancy [43].

Respiratory

PEEP should be utilised judiciously as it may increase intracranial pressure. Pressure-limited ventilation with permissive hypercarbia is absolutely contraindicated as a ventilatory strategy in patients who develop ARDS whenever there is proven or suspected intracranial pathology.

Renal

The incidence of renal dysfunction has declined from 21% (1990) to 2.7% in our most recent series of patients (2000) [5], and this has been achieved without a rise in the incidence of pulmonary oedema in our unit. This is probably attributable to our policy of careful fluid titration, serial central venous pressure monitoring and meticulous surveillance of fluid balance status. We have observed reasonable success with low- or high-dose Lasix in the scenario of acute renal failure. Lack of an appropriate response to Lasix should lead to the consideration of haemodialysis (indications for dialysis are as for any patient with renal failure).

Haematological

Haematological disturbances are not uncommon and may range from mild thrombocytopenia to full-blown DIC: 25% of patients exhibit a thrombocytopenia of 100×10^5, while HELLP syndrome occurs in 10% [5]. Therapy should be guided by conventional laboratory investigations or the thromboelastogram.

Hepatic

Whilst liver dysfunction is common (approximately 10% in the general eclamptic population, and probably higher in complicated cases), there is no specific treatment. Management is supportive.

In summary, the prevention and management of eclampsia necessitate strategies to prevent global ischaemic and hypoxic events. Whilst delivery of the fetus is the cornerstone of management, general supportive measures should be instituted once eclampsia ensues, as there are no specific organ-supporting measures that will profoundly influence outcome. The critical care outcome is influenced by the severity of neurological insult as well as the presence of organ dysfunction. Meticulous maternal surveillance and general supportive measures are of paramount importance. The lack of knowledge regarding the aetiology of the disease represents a fertile area for research.

References

1. Moodley J, Naicker RS, Mankowitz E (1983) Eclampsia – a method of management. S Afr Med J 63:530
2. Lewis G (ed) (2001) Why mothers die 1997-1999. The fifth report on the confidential enquiries into maternal deaths in the United Kingdom. RCOG Press, London
3. Buga GA, Lumu SB (1999) Hypertensive disorders of pregnancy at Umtata General Hospital: perinatal and maternal outcomes. East Afr Med J 76:217-222
4. Mwinyoglee J, Amoko DH, Simelela N, Marivate M (1996) Eclampsia at Garankuwa Hospital. S Afr Med J 86:1536-1539
5. Paruk F, Moodley J (2003) Eclampsia: a prospective audit of 112 patients admitted to King Edward VIII Hospital Obstetric High Care Unit (in press)
6. Bhagwanjee S, Paruk F, Muckart DJJ, Moodley J (2000) Morbidity and mortality in critically ill eclamptic patients and the efficacy of APACHE II, the organ failure score and GCS in outcome prediction. Crit Care Med 8:120-124
7. Higgins JR, de Swiet M (2002) Blood pressure measurement and classification in pregnancy. Lancet 357:131-135
8. Friedman SA, Taylor RN, Roberts JM (1991) Pathophysiology of pre eclampsia. Clin Perinat 18:661-682
9. Roberts JM (2000) Pre eclampsia: what we know and what we do not know. Semin Perinat 24:24-28
10. Redman CW, Sargent IL (2003) Pre-eclampsia, the placenta and the maternal systemic inflammatory response – a review. Placenta 24:S21-27
11. Sargent IL, Germain SJ, Sacks GP et al (2003) Trophoblast deportation and the naternal inflammatory response in pre-eclampsia. J Reprod Immunol 59:153-160
12. Norwitz ER, Robinson JN, Repke JT (1999) Prevention of pre-eclampsia: is it possible? Clin Obstet Gynaecol 42:436-454
13. Duley l, Henderson-Smart D, Knight M et al (2001) Antiplatelet drugs for prevention of pre eclampsia: systematic review. BMJ 322:329-333
14. Hofmeyr JG, Roodt A, Atallah AN, Duley L (2003) Calcium supplementation to prevent pre eclampsia – a systematic review. S Afr Med J 93:224-228
15. Olsen S, Secher NJ, Tabor A et al (2000) randomised clinical trials of fish oil supplementation in high risk pregnancies. Br J Obstet Gynaecol 107:382-395
16. Leitch CR, Cameron AD, Walker JJ (1998) The changing pattern of eclampsia over a 60 year period. Br J Obstet Gynaecol 104:917-922
17. The Magpie Trial Collaborative Group (2002) Do women with pre eclampsia, and their babies, benefit from magnesium sulphate? The Magpie Trial: a randomised placebo-controlled trial. Lancet 359:1877-1890

18. South African Magpie Trial Collaborative Group (2003) The Magpie study-clinical implications for poor countries. S Afr Med J 93:264-265
19. Belforte MA, Anthony J, Saade GR et al (2003) A comparison of magnesium sulphate and nimodipine for the prevention of eclampsia. NEJM 348:304-311
20. Belforte MA, Varne MW, Dizon–Townson DS et al (2002) Cerebral perfusion pressure and not cerebral blood flow, may be the critical determinant of intracranial injury in pre eclampsia: a new hypothesis. Am J Obstet Gynecol 187:626-634
21. Belforte MA, Saade GR, Yared M et al (1999) change in estimated cerebral perfusion pressure after treatment with nimodipine or magnesium sulphate in patients with pre eclampsia. Am J Obstet Gynecol 181:402-407
22. Paruk F, Moodley J (2000) Treatment of severe pre eclampsia/eclampsia syndrome. In: Studd J (ed) Progress in Obstetrics and Gynecology. 14:103-119
23. Paruk F, Moodley J (2001) Untoward effects of rapid acting antihypertensive hypertensive agents. Best Prac Research Clin Obstet Gynecol 15:491-506
24. Hazelgrove JF, Price C, Pappachan J, Smith GB (2001) Multicenter study of obstetric admissions to 14 intensive care units in southern England. Crit Care Med 29:770-775
25. Platteau P, Engelhardt T, Moodley J, Muckart DJJ (1997) Obstetric and gynaecological patients in an intensive care unit: a 1year review. Tropical Doctor 27:202-206
26. El-Sohl AA, Grant BJB (1996) A comparison of severity of illness scoring systems for critically ill obstetric patients. Chest 110:1299-1304
27. Mabie WC, Sibai BM (1990) Treatment in an obstetric intensive care unit. Am J Obstet Gynecol 162:1-4
28. Johanson R, Anthony J, Domisse J (1995) Obstetric intensive care at Groote Schuur Hospital, Cape Town. J Obstet Gynecol 15:174-177
29. Heinonen S, Tyrväinen E, Saarikoski S, Ruokonen R (2002) Need for maternal critical care in obstetrics: a population-based analysis. Int J Obstet Anesth 11:260-264
30. Lewinsohn G, Herman A, Leonov Y, Klinowski E (1994) Critically ill obstetrical patients: Outcome and predictability. Crit Care Med 22:1412-1414
31. Lapinsky SE, Kruczynski K, Seaward GR et al (1997) Critical care management of the obstetric patient. Can J Anesth 44(3):325-329
32. Harris CM, Foley M (2002) Critical care obstetrics; 13 years of experience in a community practice setting. Obstet Gynecol 99 Suppl 1:S79
33. Kilpatrick SJ, Matthay MA (1992) Obstetric patients requiring critical care. Chest 101:1407-1412
34. Cohen J, Singer P, Kogan A et al (2000) Course and outcome of obstetric patients in a general intensive care unit. Acta Obstet Gynecol Scand 79:846-850
35. Taylor R, Richards GA (2000) Critically ill obstetric and gynaecology patients in the intensive care unit. S Afr Med J 90:1140-1144
36. Umo-Etuk JI, Lumley J, Holdcroft A (1996) Critically ill parturient women and admission to intensive care: a 5 year review. Int J Obstet Anesth 5:79-84
37. Afessa B, Green B, Delke I, Koch K (2001) Systemic inflammatory response syndrome, organ failure and outcome in critically ill obstetric patients treated in an ICU. Chest 120:1271-1277
38. Knaus WA, Zimmerman JE, Wagner DP et al (1981) APACHE –acute physiological and chronic health evaluation: a physiologically based classification system. Crit Care Med 9:591-597
39. Knaus WA, Draper EA, Wagner DP, Zimmerman JE (1985) APACHE II: a severity of disease classification syndrome. Crit Care Med 13:818-829
40. Members of the American College of Chest Physicians/Society of Critical Care Medicine Consensus Conference Committee (1992) Definitions for sepsis and organ failure and guidelines for the use the use of innovative therapies in sepsis. Crit Care Med 20:864-874
41. Muckart DJJ, Bhagwanjee S (1997) The ACCP/SCCM Consensus Conference definitions of the systemic inflammatory response syndrome (SIRS) and allied disorders in critically injured patients. Crit Care Med 25:1789-1895

42. The Eclampsia Trial Collaborative Group (1995) Which anticonvulsant for women with eclampsia? Evidence from the Eclampsia Collaborative Trial. Lancet 345:1455-1563
43. Young P, Johanson R (2001) Haemodynamic, invasive and echoecardiographic monitoring in the hypertensive patient. Best Prac Res Clin Obstet Gynaecol 15:605-622

PALLIATIVE CARE

The organisation of palliative care

G. LINKLATER

What is palliative care?

History

The modern hospice movement was founded in the 1960s as a reaction to an increasingly biomedical model of health care. The focus of medical management, spurred on by rapid advances in diagnostic and therapeutic options, was on treatment and cure. Symptomatic treatments were seen as less important, and death was seen as failure by doctors and a taboo by society as a whole [1].

Experience with terminally ill cancer patients showed a very high symptom load and unmet information and psychological needs [2, 3]. From this developed an 'approach' which returned to a patient-centred model of care. This holistic approach is exemplified by the concept of 'total pain'. This emphasises that pain is not just a physical phenomenon but has significant social, spiritual and psychological components (Fig. 1). It naturally follows that for effective assessment and treatment of pain a multidisciplinary approach is needed to explore all the possible facets of the individual's experience [4].

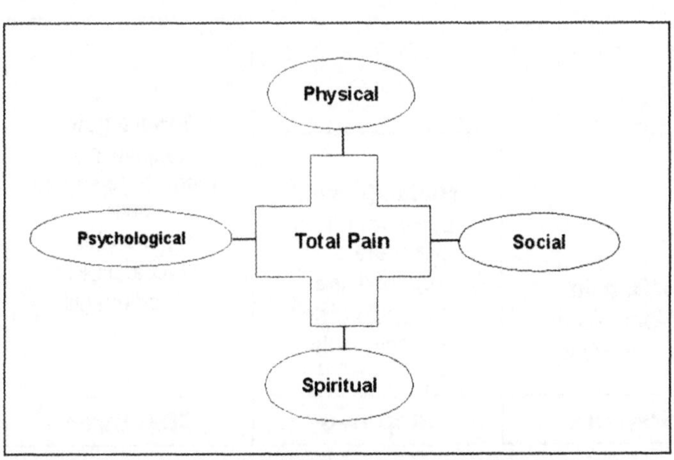

Fig. 1 Factors influencing the perception of pain

Accompanying this was the development by a working group of the World Health Organisation of the WHO pain control guidelines incorporating the ladder approach (Table 1, Fig. 2) [5]. Much work has been done to validate the ladder in different clinical settings, and its basis has been reaffirmed in several recent evidence-based guidelines [6-11].

Table 1 Basic principles of pain management

·	Thorough (multidisciplinary) assessment
·	Individualised approach
·	Analgesic 'ladder' according to pain severity
·	Concurrent use of adjuvant therapies according to pain type
·	Regular (by the clock) administration
·	Oral delivery unless contraindicated, e.g. by bowel obstruction
·	Regular review

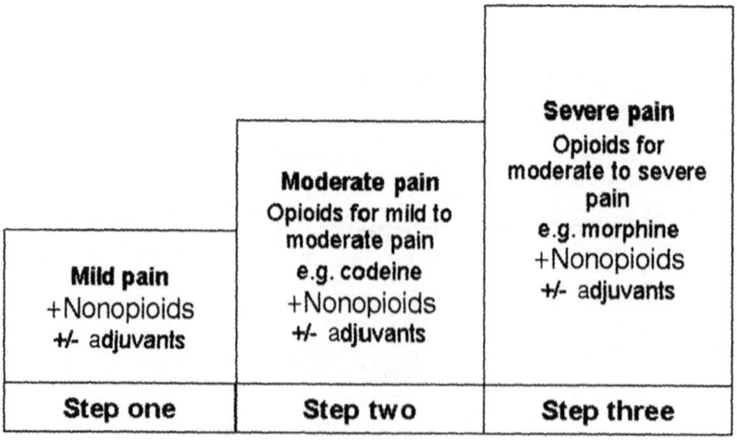

Fig. 2 The ladder approach to pain management

Definitions

Over the years, and in different countries, a number of different terms have been coined to represent this patient-centred holistic approach. The principal role of the early hospices was end-of-life care. With the recognition that the 'palliative approach' was appropriate much earlier in the disease process, the term palliative care (or supportive care in the US) was considered to be more appropriate and to be free of the potentially negative connotations of 'terminal' or 'end-of--life' care. This evolution can even be seen within the last 15 years. In 1987, when palliative medicine was recognised by the Royal College of Physicians in the UK as a medical specialty, the definition used spoke of patients with 'active, progressive, far-advanced disease' [12]. The original WHO definition of palliative care, although alluding to the provision of palliative care earlier in the disease process, still specifically focused on cancer [5]. This contrasts with the new WHO definition of palliative care (Table 2) [13].

Table 2. The WHO definition of palliative care

Palliative care is an approach that improves the quality of life of patients and their families facing the problems associated with life-threatening illness, through the prevention and relief of suffering by means of early identification and assessment and treatment of pain and other problems, physical, psychosocial and spiritual. Palliative care:

- Provides relief from pain and other distressing symptoms
- Affirms life and regards death as a normal process
- Intends neither to hasten nor postpone death
- Integrates the psychological and spiritual aspects of patient care
- Offers a support system to help patients live as actively as possible until death
- Offers a support system to help the family to cope
- Uses a team approach to address these needs
- Is applicable early in the course of illness, in conjunction with other therapies intended to prolong life

Specialists, generalists and the 'palliative approach'

Given the relatively recent genesis of palliative care and the ongoing evolution of relevant terms and definitions, it is perhaps unsurprising that there is confusion about what palliative care has to offer [14, 15]. When considering this and the provision of services for patients it is useful to look at the palliative care 'approach', generic palliative care and specialist palliative care separately.

Palliative care approach

It can be argued that the palliative care approach, i.e. patient centred and holistic care with an emphasis on promoting quality of life through multidisciplinary working, is really synonymous with the good basic care that we would all recognise is appropriate for all our patients, irrespective of diagnosis or indeed prognosis.

Generic palliative care

This relates to the skills that all health professionals should have when dealing with patients who have life-limiting conditions. These skills would include communication skills (particularly breaking bad news), multidisciplinary working, basic symptom relief (e.g. WHO ladder) and terminal care.

Specialist palliative care

This is obviously provided by professionals with additional knowledge and training and is aimed at those patients who have complex, difficult needs. Taking pain as an example, 10-15% of patients do not get good pain control with the WHO ladder [6, 7, 11]. These patients often need more complex interventions [16, 17]. Perhaps even more important than the intensive management of such patients is the educational and supportive role specialists in palliative care have in facilitating the provision of generic palliative care to the majority of patients by nonspecialist health professionals.

What about terminal care?

Despite what I have said above, end-of-life care remains a large and important part of specialist palliative care. Experience in this area has highlighted a number of important issues that need to be addressed to ensure that terminal care is done well [18]. To achieve this it can be argued that good terminal care requires an intensive critical care approach. By this I do not mean the rapid introduction of invasive technical procedures, but more the emphasis on rapid accurate diagnosis of the terminal phase, accompanied by speedy and effective multidisciplinary assessment and treatment of distressing symptoms. Unnecessary or futile monitoring and interventions should also be withdrawn. After all, we only have one chance to improve each patients terminal care, and the positive effects of a 'good death' are starkly contrasted with the distress and anguish of a 'bad death'.

The need for palliative care

Cancer

According to the WHO the worldwide annual incidence of cancer is 10 million. Six million people die of cancer per year, with 22 million living with the disease. These figures are expected to increase by 50% by the year 2020 [19].

Cancer patients often suffer multiple symptoms, usually worsening as the disease progresses. The prevalence of moderate to severe cancer pain is 30-60% during active treatment and up to 80% in advanced disease [20]. In another study, patients with advanced cancer had a median of three pains [21]. The common symptoms reported to affect more than 50% of cancer patients are reduced appetite, constipation, dry mouth, nausea, dyspnoea, low mood and insomnia [3].

Noncancer

A large retrospective study showed that 16.8% of noncancer patients who had died had a symptom load equivalent to or worse than the average experienced by cancer patients admitted to a specialist palliative care unit. Around half these patients died of cardiac disease, and 20% had respiratory pathology. Extrapolation of these data suggested that the caseload of patients requiring specialist palliative care would double if it were to be made equally available to symptomatic patients with and without cancer [22].

Another study in the US demonstrated that in the acute hospital setting 50% of conscious patients who died had uncontrolled pain in the last 24 hours of life. This was accompanied by the demonstration that only a minority of patients had the opportunity to discuss their wishes about end-of-life care with their doctors [23].

Barriers to effective palliative care

It would be easy to point to deficiencies in the education of health professionals and the financing of health services as potential reasons for the lack of palliative care provision in many countries round the world. It is perhaps more illuminating to look more specifically at issues surrounding the use and availability of opioids for symptom control. There has been considerable research into these issues, and they have been the subject of several WHO publications [24-30]. Opioids are the mainstay of the WHO cancer pain management guidelines and have potential benefits in the management of other symptoms, including dyspnoea and cough [31]. Barriers to the use of opioids appear to exist at both individual health professional and institutional/ governmental levels.

Individual

The term 'opioidphobia' has been used to describe the unwillingness of physicians to prescribe opioids for fear of intolerable side-effects, addiction or even concerns about hastening death [24].

Intolerable side-effects

The most serious opioid side-effect often feared by clinicians is respiratory depression. This can certainly happen with high-dose parenteral administration to opioid-naïve patients, but when opioids are used regularly to control cancer pain respiratory depression is extremely rare [31]. It can occasionally be seen when a patient who has had chronic pain suddenly becomes pain free, e.g. after a successful nerve block [32]. This suggests that chronic pain 'antagonises' any potential respiratory depressant effects of opioids [33].

Other commonly encountered side-effects either usually improve within a few days of initiating therapy, e.g. sedation and nausea, or are easily prevented, e.g. constipation [31].

Addiction

There is evidence that the prolonged use of opioids can cause physical tolerance [34]. This must, however, be distinguished from addiction. Addiction is characterised by psychological changes including craving and drug-seeking behaviour and is generally not seen when opioids are used for pain control [31, 32]. This is confirmed by clinical experience indicating that patients with stable pain can have stable opioid requirements over considerable periods of time and that patients whose pain improves can be weaned off opioids. Increasing opioid requirements often simply indicate disease progression rather than drug-seeking behaviour [35].

Hastening death

The doctrine of double effect is an ethical principle that allows a physician to act in a way that may be harmful to a patient if the primary aim of the act was intended to benefit the patient. It is unfortunate that the most commonly quoted clinical example involves the use of opioids to control pain. It is stated that when an opioid is used with the intended aim of benefiting the patient by controlling their pain, the inevitable consequence of shortening their life is justified. Following this argument suggests that to control pain physicians have to participate in a form of active euthanasia [27]. However, there is no evidence that opioids used at reasonable therapeutic doses cause premature death. Indeed there is even a suggestion that adequate pain control may prolong life by relieving distress and allowing patients to recover from exhaustion [36].

Institutional/ governmental

The most important barriers to the appropriate use of opioids at a national level fall into two categories: first the desire to ensure that drug misuse and abuse are controlled by limiting access to opioids, and second the relatively low profile that palliative care and such 'soft' subjects as communication skills have been given in medical curricula [27].

Opioid misuse and abuse

Opioid analgesics are essential for the adequate management of moderate to severe pain. Governments therefore have an obligation to ensure that opioids are readily available in appropriate formulations and doses to all patients who need them [25]. Global opioid consumption increased from two tonnes in 1972 to over 20 tonnes in 2000. This increase can mostly be accounted for by increases in a small number of countries (notably US, Canada, UK, France, Germany and Japan) in which opioids have been made freely available for use according to the WHO approach [27].

However, opioid analgesics do have the potential for abuse. They are considered controlled drugs, and governments are obliged to ensure there are statutory controls over their manufacture, distribution and use [25]. In the drive to prevent the diversion of opioids from medical uses to the illicit drug trade many countries have resorted to the strengthening of these statutory controls to the point where opioids are practically unavailable for medicinal use. In 1995 an International Narcotics Control Board report highlighted that under half the countries of the world have morphine available in all their cancer hospitals. Almost a third did not have morphine in their list of essential drugs [27].

The fears that increased volumes of opioid analgesics in the community will automatically lead to increases in the abuses of these drugs have been shown to be unfounded. A 6-year (1990-1996) study in the US showed that despite rapid increases in the medicinal use of opioids (59% for morphine, 27% for oxycodone and 20% for hydromorphone) there was no corresponding increase in the abuse of these drugs. Morphine abuse only rose by 3%, and there were actually reductions in oxycodone and hydromorphone abuse (reduced by 30% and 15% respectively). In 1996 only 3.8% of all episodes of drug abuse involved opioid analgesics [29]. These facts highlight the need to lessen restrictions on the medical use of opioids in most countries of the world.

Education

When countries with prohibitive restrictions on opioid prescribing and limited knowledge of the WHO pain management approach, and the obvious educational needs in these countries, are considered, it is sobering to reflect on the persistent failures in pain control in countries without these limitations. An audit in the US showed that 44% of cancer patients had uncontrolled pain, and yet 66% of these patients were not receiving a strong opioid and 39% were receiving no analgesics at all [30]. Even in Scotland, with a well-developed specialist palliative care service, free access to opioids in a variety of formulations and broad awareness of the WHO approach, a recent national audit showed 50% of cancer pain to be poorly controlled. Simple prescribing errors and omissions were found to contribute in large measure to the poor pain control demonstrated [37].

These findings can only emphasise the need for palliative care and symptom control to be given increasing importance in both undergraduate and postgraduate medical teaching.

Conclusions

There is a massive, and growing, need for palliative care throughout the world. The interventions used in palliative care are simple and effective, yet in many instances neglected. We have a responsibility both individually and collectively to improve our education about palliative care, to ensure that the facilities, drugs and knowledge are available to all patients who need them.

References

1. Doyle D, Hanks GW, MacDonald N (eds) (1998) Oxford textbook of palliative medicine, 2nd edition. Oxford University Press, Oxford, pp 4-8
2. Jenkins V, Fallowfield L, Saul J (2001) Information needs of patients with cancer: results from a large study in UK cancer centres. Br J Cancer 84:48-51
3. Addington-Hall J, McCarthy M (1995) Dying from cancer: results of a national population-based investigation. Palliat Med 9:295-305
4. Doyle D (1998) The provision of palliative care. In: Doyle D, Hanks GW, MacDonald N (eds) Oxford textbook of palliative medicine, 2nd edition. Oxford University Press, Oxford, pp 41-53
5. World Health Organisation (1990) Cancer pain relief and palliative care. (Technical report series 804). WHO, Geneva

6. Ventafridda V, Tamburini M, Caraceni A et al (1987) A validation study of the WHO method for cancer pain relief. Cancer 59:850-856
7. Zech DFJ, Grond S, Lynch J et al (1995) Validation of World Health Organisation guidelines for cancer pain relief: a 10-year prospective study. Pain 63:65-76
8. The Expert Working Group of the European Association of Palliative Care (1996) Morphine in cancer pain: methods of administration. BMJ 312:823-826
9. Scottish Intercollegiate Guidelines Network and Scottish Cancer Therapy Network (2000) Control of pain in patients with cancer. (SIGN publication number 44) Royal College of Physicians, Edinburgh
10. Hanks GW, de Conno F, Cherny N et al (2001) Morphine and alternative opioids in cancer pain: the EAPC recommendations. Br J Cancer 84:587-593
11. Meuser T, Pietruck C, Radbruch L et al (2001) Symptoms during cancer pain treatment following WHO-guidelines: a longitudinal follow-up study of symptom prevalence, severity and aetiology. Pain 93:247-257
12. Hillier R (1988) Palliative medicine. BMJ 297: 874-875
13. World Health Organisation (2002) National cancer control programmes, policies and managerial guidelines, 2nd edition. WHO, Geneva pp 83-91
14. Payne S, Sheldon F, Jarrett N et al (2002) Differences in understanding of specialist palliative care amongst service providers and commissioners in South London. Palliat Med 16:395-402
15. Gott CM, Ahmedzai SH, Wood C (2001) How many inpatients at an acute hospital have palliative care needs? Comparing the perspectives of medical and nursing staff. Palliat Med 15:451-460
16. Linklater GT, Leng MEF, Tiernan EJJ et al (2002) Pain management services in palliative care: a national survey. Palliat Med 16:435-439
17. Linklater GT, Leng MEF (2001) Recent advances in pain management in palliative care. Curr Anaesth Crit Care 12:296-301
18. Ellershaw J, Ward C (2003) Care of the dying patient: the last hours of life. BMJ 326:30-34
19. World Health Organisation (2003) Global action against cancer. World Health Organisation, Geneva
20. Cherny NI, Portenoy RK (1999) Cancer pain: principles of assessment and syndromes. In: Wall PD, Melzack R (eds) Textbook of pain, 4th edition. Churchill Livingstone, Edinburgh, pp 1017-1064
21. Twycross R, Harcourt J, Bergl S (1996) A survey of pain in patients with advanced cancer. J Pain Symptom Manage 12:273-282
22. Addington-Hall J, Fakhoury W, McCarthy M (1998) Specialist palliative care in nonmalignant disease. Palliat Med 12:417-427
23. The SUPPORT principal investigators (1995) A controlled trial to improve care for seriously ill hospitalized patients: The Study to Understand Prognoses and Preferences for Outcomes and Risks of Treatments. JAMA 274:1591-1598
24. Zenz M, Willweber-Strumpf A (1993) Opioidphobia and cancer pain in Europe. Lancet 341:1075-1076
25. World Health Organisation (2000) Narcotics and psychotropic drugs. Achieving balance in national opioids control policy. Guidelines for assessment. WHO, Geneva
26. Reidenberg MM (1996) Barriers to controlling pain in patients with cancer. Lancet 347:1278
27. UN International Narcotics Control Board (1995) Report: Availability of opiates for medical needs. International Narcotics Control Board, United Nations, Vienna
28. Wall PD (1997) The generation of yet another myth on the use of narcotics. Pain 73:121-122
29. Joranson DE, Ryan KM, Gilson AM et al (2000) Trends in medical use and abuse of opioid analgesics. JAMA 283:1710-1714
30. Zhukovsky DS, Gorowski E, Hausdorff J et al (1995) Unmet analgesic needs in cancer patients. J Pain Symptom Manage 10:113-119
31. Twycross R, Willcock A, Charlesworth S et al (2002) Palliative care formulary, 2nd edition. Radcliffe Medical Press, Oxon, pp168-175

32. Hanks GW, Twycross RG, Lloyd JW (1981) Unexpected complication of successful nerve block. Anaesthesia 36:37-39
33. Borgbjerg FM, Nielsen K, Franks J (1996) Experimental pain stimulates respiration and attenuates morphine-induced respiratory depression: a controlled study in human volunteers. Pain 64:123-128
34. McQuay H (1999) Opioids in pain management. Lancet 353:2229-2232
35. Collin E, Poulain P, Gauvain-Piquard A et al (1993) Is disease progression the major factor in morphine 'tolerance' in cancer pain treatment? Pain 55:319-326
36. Twycross R (1997) Symptom management in advanced cancer, 2nd edition. Radcliffe Medical Press, Oxford, pp 86-91
37. Welsh J, Brewster D, Cornbleet M et al (2001) A Scottish national audit of prevalence of pain in patients with active cancer. Poster presented the Seventh Congress of the European Association of Palliative Care

Death in the ICU: why integrate palliative care?

L. Scott Wilner, M.A. DeVita

As society increasingly demands better end-of-life care, it is incumbent upon critical care practitioners in particular to learn to manage death and dying with the same expertise they bring to other complex problems encountered in the care of critically ill patients. Patients dying – and surviving – in a critical care unit should be cared for by providers with expertise in palliative care and critical care. It is possible, but not necessary, that a single provider may be able to have both skill sets. The proposition that there is a place for palliative care in the critical care unit is not unchallenged, and is ambitious. Nevertheless, it is not unrealistic and demands further exploration. There is significant data indicating that many intensive care unit (ICU) patients' needs are unmet by current practice patterns. There is also preliminary data indicating that integrating palliative care practice into the ICU environment is not only feasible, but results in improved outcome (though not survival). Incorporating palliative care into critical care practice will require considerable attitude change and education. The ideal methodology for educating critical care professionals and trainees in end-of-life care continues to evolve as a work in progress. We believe that there is no longer any doubt that competence in these matters – such as conducting a resuscitation, managing a ventilator, or placing vascular access – will be a requisite fundamental skill for intensivists in the future.

In this paper we will focus on two major issues: the rationale for delivering palliative care in the critical care setting, and the need for improving educational initiatives for teaching palliative care goals and techniques to critical care practitioners.

Since its inception, the critical care unit has been the place in the hospital where the most invasive therapies have been delivered to patients. Indeed, the critical care unit grew from the need for operating room and recovery room patients to continue to receive prolonged respiratory and/or circulatory support. Since the Karen Ann Quinlan case in the United States in 1976 and other similar cases in Europe, there has been a trend toward identifying patients who refuse this intensive care, or who will not benefit from it, and then removing the support. Today, the vast majority of patients who die in the critical care unit do so after a decision to limit or withdraw support. (In this paper we will use the term "forgo" to encompass both withdrawal and withholding of medical treatments.) The transition from "full go" to "no go" is often problematic in the critical care unit, resulting in delays, emotional or psychological upset for patients, families and medical caregivers alike, and even perhaps harm to patients. Without established consensus, the care of dying patients in the intensive care unit (ICU) varies considerably [1, 2].

Caring for terminally ill ICU patients is becoming an increasingly common reality for intensivists. Already, nearly one in four Americans dies in an acute care setting [3], and the number of critically ill patients is likely to increase in the years ahead as evolving medical technology is brought to bear on an ageing population [4]. Familiarity with death does not, by itself, confer any particular expertise in the management of dying patients [5].

For all these reasons, the Society of Critical Care Medicine has identified end-of-life care as a priority [6] and issued recommendations to guide practitioners [7]. The challenge intensivists now face is to treat dying patients in the critical care unit with the same degree of skill, finesse, and scientific rationale as are utilised in the management of other clinical situations from respiratory failure to sepsis [8]. Pursuit of that goal begs the question of whether the historical division between intensive care and palliative care is really in the best interest of any ICU patient [9-12].

The case for palliative care in the ICU

What's wrong with the status quo?

A growing body of evidence demonstrates that current end-of-life practices in the critical care unit are not meeting the needs of patients, families, nurses or physicians. Studies suggest that "...the prevalence of distressing symptoms among critically ill patients is substantial... and... underestimated by caregivers [13]," and seem to lend credence to the fear among some patients that they will die with unrelieved pain or other symptoms [14].

The landmark Study to Understand Prognoses and Preferences for Outcomes and Risks of Treatment, commonly known as "SUPPORT" [15], was a four-year, multi-centre, analysis of 9,105 adult patients with advanced illness. In phase I, decision-making was described, hospital outcomes were observed, and perceived shortcomings of care were identified. In phase II, a randomised controlled intervention was instituted to provide improved prognostic information to physicians, and to facilitate communication among patients, families, and caregivers about treatment preferences, pain control and advanced care planning. While the intervention was ineffective, the study findings are notable – and have been widely cited - because of the unflattering view of end-of-life care they portray. For example, almost one-third of the phase I patients preferred not to receive resuscitation, but this preference was correctly identified by fewer than half of their physicians. Also, nearly half of these same patients never had a "do not resuscitate" order written during the hospitalisation, and almost 30% of them died without that order. Additionally, more than half of the patients who died in the hospital spent at least 8 days in an "undesirable state" before death: nearly half had been in the ICU within 72 hours prior to death, with many of them receiving mechanical ventilation; more than one-third had spent at least 10 days in the ICU; and as many as half were felt by their surrogates to have experienced moderate or severe pain in their last days of life. More than half of the patients who would have preferred to die at home were unable to realise that goal [16]. Finally, consequences for families were substantial as well – a relative reported having to quit work in 20% of cases, and one-third of families reported the loss of most or all of their savings [16].

The Hospitalized Elderly Longitudinal Project ("HELP"), concerned with the subset of SUPPORT patients over 80 years of age, has revealed shortcomings in the terminal care of older patients specifically [17]. Surrogate decision makers for the more than 400 patients who died within one year of enrolment reported that, in the course of dying, 40% of patients had severe pain, more than 50% had severe shortness of breath, 20% felt alone or isolated, and 25% were moderately depressed or anxious. More objectively, the data demonstrate that in the last 72 hours of life, 11% underwent resuscitation, 25% were mechanically ventilated and 40% were receiving tube feeding. Overall, 56% of the patients had at least one of these three interventions. A majority of the patients reportedly would have preferred care focused on their comfort, even if this meant dying sooner. Overall, the surrogates reported that patient care was inconsistent with this preference about 10% of the time.

Nelson and colleagues have recently provided the first description of ICU patients' real-time, self-reported, symptoms [18]. Between 55% and 75% of the patients reported experiencing pain, discomfort, anxiety, sleep disturbances, thirst and hunger that were "moderate" or "severe." Additionally, 33% of the patients reported dyspnoea and 40% identified their own depressed mood. Procedures they rated as the *most* painful included not only invasive measures, such as endotracheal intubation and arterial blood gas sampling, as might be expected, but also less aggressive manoeuvres, such as turning and tracheal suctioning, which many practitioners might consider more benign. Importantly, these results were found among patients who received automatic palliative care consultation and who were treated with what the authors described as "liberal" doses of analgesics and sedatives in advance of interventions thought to be potentially painful.

Studies of critical care nurses' experiences are similarly concerning. For more than 25 years, ICU nurses have recognised care of the dying as an important component of their practice, proclaimed their central role in the care of terminally ill patients and voiced frustration at seeing these patients therapeutically "bombarded" by their physicians [19]. This sentiment persists today, leading some ICU nurses to conclude that patients are not dying in comfort as they deserve [20], and motivating others to "work" the medical system by soliciting certain orders from specific physicians whom they consider particularly receptive to their concerns [21]. Some nurses may take things farther, as suggested by Asch in a controversial recent study that anonymously surveyed 852 randomly selected ICU nurses [22]: 17% reported being asked by a patient or family to perform euthanasia or assisted suicide; 16% acknowledged having actively done so at least once, typically by giving extra narcotics; and 4% described having complied more passively by secretly failing to provide some physician-ordered therapy such as vasopressors. While this study was criticised on methodological grounds, the finding that ICU nurses are likely to encounter these situations has been confirmed by a more recent study. Puntillo et al. [23] surveyed 906 critical care nurses and found that 37% had been asked by a patient or family member to hasten death, 5% had been asked to participate in such an act by another nurse, and 6% had been asked to do so by a physician. No data on compliance with these requests was reported. Taken together, these studies raise serious concerns about the way we care – or fail to care – for ICU patients in their final hours.

More evidence of the shortcomings of our current practices can be found in the professional and personal experiences of physicians. Facilitating good end-of-life care, particularly in a critical care unit, is not easy. Deciding to forgo life-sustaining treatment is unlike any other medical judgment: though sometimes shrouded in the ill-defined concept of "futility", it always seems to require the sometimes difficult concession that a patient is dying [24].

Another possibility is described by Levy [25, 26], who posits that the difficulty for many physicians lies not in recognising a duty to identify the point at which intensive treatment is no longer beneficial, but rather with the emotionally difficult task of *discussing these issues* with patients and families. Thus, in his view, it is this very discomfort, rather than recognition of terminal illness, that may be the major obstacle to quality end-of-life care. The literature offers little direction on how to choose which treatment(s) to stop and what kinds(s) of therapy to provide [27]. As a result, attitudes and practices with regard to withholding and withdrawing life-sustaining therapies vary greatly among practitioners, often without obvious rationale [13]. For example, Faber-Langendoen [28] has described such variability - and numerous misconceptions – among physician members of the Society of Critical Care Medicine. Kollef [29, 30] has shown that access to a private attending physician can strongly influence the nature of end-of-life care in the ICU. Christakis [31, 32] has described physician biases across specialties and forms of therapy. These details matter because "…the manner in which critically ill patients die is usually entrusted to physicians… (and)…the choices made…influence the speed, comfort, and dignity with which patients die" [31]. Notably, the literature also contains anecdotal reports by physicians who describe their inability to secure optimum end-of-life ICU care even for their own family members [33, 34]. Such accounts offer some indication of how overwhelming this same experience surely must be for the lay public, and a poignant reminder of the universal importance of these issues.

Potential advantages of palliative care in the ICU

Routine integration of palliative care principles and practices into ICU care (and culture) seems to make intuitive sense as a response to the concerns described above. On reflection, there are a number of reasons to expect this course to be successful. Some relate directly to patients and families, others to ICU staff members, and a few to the larger contexts of the ICU as a practice environment and the viability of our healthcare system.

First, and most importantly, *the fundamental precepts of palliative medicine can be applied to almost every critically ill patient and family* [13]. Care designed to (1) ensure the control of pain and other symptoms, (2) clarify and pursue specific therapeutic goals (as opposed to treatment modalities), and (3) recognise and integrate the patient's and physician's personal belief systems, as well as informing and encouraging participation of loved ones, is appropriate for all ICU patients. Symptom management rarely – if ever – interferes with curative therapies or efforts to sustain life [5]. Waiting until patients appear to be dying to incorporate these objectives is naïve and destines patients to fail to receive palliative care for days (if not weeks) after symptoms appear. While scoring systems exist to predict outcomes for groups of critically ill patients, it is difficult to prognosticate for a given individual [8], and no one has yet created a critical care scoring system that identifies which patient needs *palliative* therapies. *Optimum critical care, therefore, should incorporate proactive and aggressive palliative strategies throughout the ICU stay of every patient* [14], whether the ultimate goal is cure or comfort [35]. When palliation is thus "built in" to the ICU plan of care, the necessary shift in goals for patients who are not expected to survive can evolve as a process, rather than being condensed into a discrete event [36].

Second, there are logistical characteristics of the critical care unit that make it a desirable setting for the provision of palliative care. Most importantly, some patients will have such intense or variable symptoms that staff need to be at the bedside in order to titrate comfort therapies and manage symptom burden [8, 13, 37]. In many institutions, this degree of staffing – whether of nurses, respiratory therapists, or physicians – is possible only in the critical care unit, or in a designated hospice unit. Specific expertise is required to manage typical end-of-life symptoms in critically ill patients, and it is optimal if the transition from curative therapy to so-called comfort measures does not cause any added stress for the patient [38]. Additionally, the continual reassessment of patients that typifies the critical care unit sends an important psychological message: that the withdrawal of life-sustaining *therapy* is decidedly not a withdrawal of *care*. Patients will not be abandoned in dying – as many of them fear [39]. Perhaps not coincidentally, the structure of the care teams in both critical and palliative care emphasises the value of the input from many disciplines [14, 37, 38]. Finally, there are simple – but often overlooked – environmental features of good palliative care that can be well accommodated by most critical care units. These include such considerations as liberalised (if not unrestricted) visitation hours, reasonably private patient accommodations, and thoughtfully equipped waiting areas so that families can remain close by while having space and facilities to attend to their own needs [7, 39].

Third, adopting palliative care practices has the potential to "humanise" the critical care unit, benefiting not only terminal patients, but all ICU patients (and providers as well) [40]. Offsetting the psychological impact of the highly technological ICU environment can reduce patient and family stress and improve the work environment.

Candid discussion of unfavourable prognoses or deteriorating patient status is perhaps the most difficult task expected of critical care clinicians [41], who are generally not as comfortable providing psychosocial and emotional support to families as they are with providing physiological support to patients [42]. Additionally, the appropriate management of specific symptoms, sometimes requiring substantial doses of narcotics or sedatives, can be troubling, even for experienced clinicians [43]. An apparent lack of "logical" consistency in patients' wishes regarding resuscitation (for example, chest compressions without intubation, or vice versa), and the inability to predict patients' wishes based upon perceived quality of life, can cause additional frustration for medical caregivers who view technological interventions according to an "aggressiveness scale" that may be different from the patient's or family's perspective [44]. By focusing on patient and family goals, and evaluating treatments individually in terms of both their ability to achieve those goals and their potential to increase burden [14], palliative care makes it possible to redefine the meaning of a good outcome [41, 45]. That is, a "good death" can be as important as a "cure". This emphasis can help minimise any sense of failure when a patient does not survive. This approach to the care of patients and families need not necessarily be complicated or time consuming [14, 41]. Like other critical care procedures that can be anxiety-provoking in their unfamiliarity, competence in end-of-life care can be learned and practised to the point of becoming second nature (discussed in detail later in this paper).

Fourth, there is practical experience at one progressive centre to suggest that providing palliative services to critically ill patients can potentially benefit both patients and the healthcare system, by limiting unwanted aggressive care and achieving some conservation of scarce ICU resources in the process. Campbell has described the impact of the Comprehensive Supportive Care Team, established at Detroit Receiving Hospital in 1985 [46, 47]. This programme, which is staffed in part by ICU practitioners but typically transfers patients to other areas of the hospital to provide interdisciplinary end-of-life care, has reduced ICU lengths of stay, hospital costs, and non-beneficial interventions (as measured by the Therapeutic Interventions Scoring System). There were presumed to be other, unmeasured, "savings" in terms of improved ICU bed availability, family satisfaction and staff morale. More recently, Campbell has described a proactive palliative care consultative approach to ICU patients with the specific diagnoses of cerebral ischaemia following cardiac arrest and multi-system organ failure [1]. This programme limited the amount of time that terminally ill patients spent receiving invasive care prior to a transition to comfort measures. This patient-centred benefit may be the most important aspect of these studies, since questions of monetary cost – in addition to being somewhat unpalatable – might also be premature: to date, we have no way to put a price on a "good" or a "bad" death [48], no measure of the tremendous costs in pain, suffering, and indignity that accompany dying in the hospital [49], and no proof that the use of ICU beds for noncurative care accounts for a significant amount of the overall costs of care in this country [50].

Potential challenges to palliative care in the ICU

There are a number of factors that pose challenges to the ready integration of palliative care into ICU practice. None of these obstacles is likely to be insurmountable – but they must be identified and managed in a structured way.

First, the successful incorporation of palliative care into the ICU will require cultural adjustment for many. The typical ICU staff is accustomed to a high--technology, aggressive approach to saving lives and restoring function. Patients and families may share this so-called rescue mentality [51]. Palliative care, with its emphasis on holistic treatment including symptom management as well as a commitment to end-of-life planning, can address and resolve difficult ethical, social and medical issues. This approach may be difficult for some to embrace – even when the relevant issue is symptom management and the patient is expected to survive. Indeed, some have dismissed the very idea of palliation within the critical care unit [52, 53, 54], and others have cited the potential difficulty of charging one unit with such seemingly different missions [37, 55].

Second, the expansion of palliative care into the critical care unit requires firm backing at the institutional level. Though effective communication with patients and families about prognosis and treatment preferences is increasingly recognised as a valued "process of care" outcome [56], there may be a similar cultural resistance to the idea of palliative care in the ICU among hospital administrators. Palliative care services are unlikely to flourish without "top-down" support to assure necessary financial and personnel resources, to foster an environment supportive of innovation, research, and education and to assist with the development and implementation of policies and protocols.

Third, concerns have been raised that some palliative goals may not be compatible with best critical care practice for patients still receiving aggressive therapy. Attention seems to be focused on the potential untoward side effects of sedatives and narcotics. For example, Nelson posits that maximising comfort therapies may contribute to cardiovascular instability, ventilatory impairment, slowed gastrointestinal function, and an inability to perform adequate neurological or abdominal examinations [13]. Nelson and Mosenthal note that patients with respiratory failure are likely to spend less time on the ventilator and in the ICU if they are awakened and stimulated on a regular basis [13, 14]. The competing interests of curative and palliative goals highlight the importance of carefully addressing those goals and of balancing therapies so as to best benefit the patient.

Fourth, in order to provide good end-of-life care in the intensive care unit, it is inevitable that there need to be adequately trained providers. In the best circumstances, patients destined to die in the ICU could be cared for by physicians with a mastery of both critical care skills *and* palliative care sensibilities [38]. That goal is ambitious, but realistic. This important proposition is the focus of the remainder of this paper.

Teaching palliative care to critical care practitioners

As described above, there is now a growing consensus that palliative care does indeed have a place in the critical care unit. That begs the question of what strategy should be undertaken to implement palliative care when the vast majority of critical care practitioners are not specifically trained for this duty. The two favoured interventions include training attending physicians in end-of-life care (undertaken by the American Medical Association in their Education for Physicians on End-of-life Care {EPEC} programme [57]) and educating Critical Care Medicine (CCM) trainees, as advocated by Danis and others.

Danis and colleagues have outlined the content areas that need to be developed and taught in order to improve the capability of critical care physicians to meet the needs of patients dying in the intensive care unit [38]. They list the following content components:

a) *Goals* of care should guide technology use;
b) Understanding of the science of critical care prognostication;
c) Medical and ethical understanding of withholding and withdrawing technological support;
d) Recognition that effective communication and trusting relationships are crucial to good care, whether palliative in nature or not;
e) Need for cultural differences to be acknowledged and respected;
f) Acknowledgement of the delivery of excellent palliative care as appropriate in the ICU.

In addition to these core competencies, our group at the University of Pittsburgh would add the following additional skill set (described more fully by DeVita et al. [58]):

a) The ability to conduct a family meeting.
b) The ability to deliver "bad news" sensitively and effectively.
c) The ability to "manage" emotions that accompany dying in the ICU. This includes the emotions that occur in patients, families and other loved ones, and the health care providers.
d) The ability to foster decision-making when outcome is uncertain.
e) The ability to medically manage the pain, as well as the emotional and psychological discomfort that accompany dying.

The model of care that should be taught includes the above elements and is preferably delivered by a critical care physician who is adept at the above palliative skill set. There are two broad categories of "things" that need to be taught: cognitive (or knowledge based) and skills (or behaviourally based). The former set described by Danis et al. are possible via the more routine forms of education: reading, lectures, and observation. Practice will solidify the knowledge acquired by other means, but will not replace it. The latter set is skillsbased. That is, because they are skills, they require both knowledge *and* practice/experience for staff to master the material (because demonstration to a trainee, and possession of knowledge by a trainee are insufficient to create a skilled practitioner).

There are barriers to teaching effective palliative care. The first is attitude. There is a historical preference to avoid admitting "hopeless" patients to an ICU, and to favour moving patients for whom care is being "limited" out of the ICU for others to manage. In fact this was taught to, and by, many of our critical care predecessors until relatively recently. It is essential that the critical care practitioner have an attitude of "ownership" of managing the dying process and a feeling that end-of-life care is important in order to foster an educational opportunity.

The second barrier is that the workload and stress of "keeping people alive" can compete with the ability to teach anything, let alone how to allow a patient to die. Effective palliative education programmes will "free up" trainees so that they can have time to learn.

Third, important ICU management skills such as speedy decision-making, rapid interventions, and moving from bedside to bedside are often counterproductive to good palliative care. Indeed, the notion that the caregiver is no longer trying to "keep the patient alive" can cause a sense of relaxation toward medical concerns that can result in palliative care concerns being left unaddressed. These behaviours and the attitude that these behaviours are most important must be overcome before or as part of palliative care education in order for the trainee to learn the core materials.

Fourth, there is not a clear-cut curriculum or ideal model (or a residency review committee (RRC) requirement for this) for palliative care for critical care professionals, though it is now emerging. Danis, DeVita, Levy [41] and others have published their opinions on the required elements of palliative care education for CCM trainees. In our opinion, there will soon be clearer training requirements for palliative care for critical care trainees and a consensus on content.

Fifth, there are a limited number of critical care professionals trained in or expert in palliative care. According to the American Board of Hospice and Palliative Medicine, there are only two critical care physicians who have been certified by them. Hopefully, in the future cross-training and -certification will become more common and overcome this barrier. Placing some emphasis upon this education may foster the notion among trainees that this is an important patient care area and perhaps a career opportunity.

Sixth, communication skills per se have not been emphasised in medical education even though one might think that this would be a core competency for all physicians. It is especially important in the ICU, where stress levels are high, time is short, and life and death hang in the balance. Azoulay and colleagues recently reported that 50% of families of ICU patients reported inadequate communication with physicians [59]. While many might quibble over whether the family assessment of physician communication is fact or perception, the point remains: families' needs are not met. DeVita and Sirio reported that most patients who were likely to die in the ICU did not have any discussion of prognosis and goals of care [60]. Lilly and colleagues have published their experience on "mandatory" family meetings and have shown that frequent meetings are feasible, and are effective in overcoming this problem [61].

Finally, the methodology for palliative care training is largely unexplored, and will be discussed in detail below. There are several major questions to be answered. Ought palliative care training for physicians be performed in a setting filled with terminally ill patients, where 100% of the patients need palliation, but are rarely critically ill, or should it occur in a critical care setting, where any patient might die, but only 8% do so? Who should lead the training, palliative care physicians, or CCM physicians? How should the many disciplines involved in, and resources available to, the care of terminally ill patients be introduced to the trainee? Which is the most effective way of teaching communication skills in the ICU: role play, supervised experience, or observation of experts?

DeVita et al. have now reported their preliminary findings from implementing an end-of-life curriculum for two consecutive years for first-year CCM trainees [58]. They utilised several strategies with varying success. The components of the training were:

a) Knowledge based:
   i. required readings from palliative care and critical care literature
   ii. lecture series
b) Skills based:
   i. Expert-facilitated skills sessions (including role-play to enhance skill acquisition) for communication skills and emotional management
   ii. Participation in the palliative care service providing care to terminally ill patients throughout the hospital

Content included symptom management during dying (including pain, anxiety, itching, nausea, bleeding, delirium, dyspnoea, and excessive secretions). In addition, such patient concerns as isolation, loss of control, fear of death or pain, grief and depression were introduced. Skills sessions included delivering "bad news", managing emotions, requesting organ donation and decision making in the face of uncertain outcome. The last session is important. Most trainees felt it was impossible or impermissible to make a decision about end-of-life care unless outcome (in this case, death) was assured. Of course this "certainty" standard would preclude end-of-life planning and management for many critically ill patients. It is a fact that all individuals make decisions in spite of uncertainty (for example, marriage, changing jobs or schools, and even gambling). While recognition of uncertainty is important, uncertainty should not preclude a decision to forgo therapy in patients when the therapies are unwanted by the patient or are unlikely to produce benefit.

After two years, the authors reported improvement in the trainees' palliative care knowledge base, as well as their attitudes towards – and confidence in – caring for dying patients. They rated the skills sessions highly in terms of relevance and impact on their learning. However, the trainees saw the clinical time spent on the palliative care rotation as being irrelevant to their critical care training or practice. Future attempts at providing supervised clinical experience in palliative care should probably be conducted in the ICU. While the appropriate methodology for palliative care training is in evolution, the content appears to be supported by a consensus of palliative care and critical care authors on the topic. It is our opinion that this should be a core competency for all critical care training programmes.

Conclusions

The need to clarify the aims of medical therapy to avoid providing nonbeneficial treatment is not a new concept [62]. We are now past the issue of *whether* it is ethical to limit aggressive care; now the question is *how* to go about doing so in the best way [63]. Most Americans now die in hospital – frequently in the ICU, and typically after some form of limitation of therapy. The results of SUPPORT and other studies suggest that in these circumstances, our current end-of-life care practices are not meeting the needs of our patients, their families or our colleagues. Once taboo, these issues have now become a focus of public attention and there is growing acceptance of the fact that, despite all of our technological innovations and therapeutic advances, sometimes we cannot change the inevitability of death [64].

Our society and the increasing acuity of our in-patient population render it impractical to manage decisions about treatment limitation with such simple strategies as the "do-not-resuscitate" order [55]. Rather, it is time for end-of-life care for critically ill patients to be addressed comprehensively [23], and there is an emerging school of thought suggesting that integrating palliative care into intensive care is one way to accomplish that goal [51]. This approach has both advantages and disadvantages, and is as yet unproven on a large scale. Success may ultimately depend on our ability to impart the necessary skills and knowledge to future generations of critical care practitioners. For it now seems clear that communicating effectively with critically ill patients and families about end-of-life decisions, and skilfully managing both physical and psychological symptoms of dying patients, will rank with resuscitation, mechanical ventilation, and central line placement as core competencies for intensivists in the new millennium [5, 14].

References

1. Campbell ML, Guzman JA (2003) Impact of a proactive approach to improve end-of-life care in a medical ICU. Chest 123:266-271
2. Danis M (1998) Improving end-of-life care in the intensive care unit: what's to be learned from outcomes research? New Horiz 6:110-118
3. Truog RD, Burns JP (2002) Excellence in end-of-life care: a goal for intensivists. Intensive Care Med 28:1197-1199
4. Curtis RJ, Rubenfeld GD (2001) Introducing the Concept of Managing Death in the ICU. In: Curtis JR, Rubenfeld GD (eds) Managing death in the ICU. Oxford University Press, New York, pp 3-6
5. Prendergast TJ, Puntillo KA (2002) Withdrawal of life support: intensive caring at the end of life. JAMA 288:2732-2740
6. Parks L (1996) Society of Critical Care Medicine initiative to address care at the end of life. Crit Care Med 24:1106
7. Truog RD, Cist AF, Brackett SE et al (2001) Recommendations for end-of-life care in the intensive care unit: The Ethics Committee of the Society of Critical Care Medicine. Crit Care Med 29:2332-2348
8. Faber-Langendoen K, Lanken PN (2000) Dying patients in the intensive care unit: forgoing treatment, maintaining care. Ann Intern Med 133:886-893
9. Faber-Langendoen K (2000) Forgoing treatment, maintaining care. J Palliat Care 16 Suppl:S7-8
10. Rocker GM, Shemie SD, Lacroix J (2000) End-of-life issues in the ICU: a need for acute palliative care? J Palliat Care 16 Suppl:S5-6
11. Miller FG, Fins JJ (1996) A proposal to restructure hospital care for dying patients. N Engl J Med 334:1740-1742
12. Jastremski CA (2001) Caring for those who need critical care: understanding the patient experience. Crit Care Med 29:449-450
13. Nelson JE, Danis M (2001) End-of-life care in the intensive care unit: where are we now? Crit Care Med 29(2 Suppl):N2-9
14. Mosenthal AC, Lee KF, Huffman J (2002) Palliative care in the surgical intensive care unit. J Am Coll Surg 194:75-83
15. The SUPPORT Principal Investigators (1995) A controlled trial to improve care for terminally ill hospitalized adults. JAMA 274:1591-1598
16. Freeborne N, Lynn J, Desbiens NA (2000) Insights about dying from the SUPPORT Project. J Amer Geri Soc 48(5 Suppl):S199-205
17. Lynn J, Teno JM, Phillips RS, et al (1997) Perceptions by family members of the dying experience of older and seriously ill patients. Ann Intern Med 126:97-106
18. Nelson JE, Meier DE, Oei EJ, et al (2001) Self-reported symptom experience of critically ill cancer patients receiving intensive care. Crit Care Med 29(2):277-282
19. Boland M (1977) Care of the dying patient in intensive care areas. Nurs Mirror 145:20-21

20. Davidson P, Introna K, Daly J, et al (2003) Cardiorespiratory nurses' perceptions of palliative care in nonmalignant disease: data for the development of clinical practice. Am J Crit Care 12:47-53
21. McClement SE, Degner LF (1995) Expert nursing behaviors in care of the dying adult in the intensive care unit. Heart Lung 24:408-419
22. Asch DA (1996) The role of critical care nurses in euthanasia and assisted suicide. N Engl J Med 334:1374-1379
23. Puntillo KA, Benner P, Drought T, et al (2001) End-of-life issues in intensive care units: a national random survey of nurses' knowledge and beliefs. Am J Crit Care 10:216-229
24. Karlawish JH, Hall JB (1997) Managing death and dying in the intensive care unit. Am J Respir Crit Care Med 155:1-2
25. Levy MM (2001) Evaluating our end-of-life practice. Crit Care (London) 5:182-183
26. Levy, MM (2001) Making a personal relationship with death. In: Curtis JR, Rubenfeld GD (eds) Managing death in the ICU. Oxford University Press, New York, pp 31-35
27. Holzapfel L, Demingeon G, Piralla B, et al (2002) A four-step protocol for limitation of treatment in terminal care. An observational study in 475 intensive care unit patients. Intensive Care Med 28:1309-1315
28. Faber-Langendoen K (1994) The clinical management of dying patients receiving mechanical ventilation. A survey of physician practice. Chest 106:880-888
29. Kollef MH (1996) Private attending physician status and the withdrawal of life-sustaining interventions in a medical intensive care unit population. Crit Care Med 24:968-975
30. Kollef MH, Ward S (1999) The influence of access to a private attending physician on the withdrawal of life-sustaining therapies in the intensive care unit. Crit Care Med 27:2125-2132
31. Christakis NA, Asch DA (1993) Biases in how physicians choose to withdraw life support. Lancet 342:642-646
32. Christakis NA, Asch DA (1995) Medical specialists prefer to withdraw familiar technologies when discontinuing life support. J Gen Int Med 10:491-494
33. Nash I (1984) An ICU death: a Gordian knot in search of Alexander. N Engl J Med 311(26):1705
34. Moeller RA (1993) If doctors can't die with dignity, who can? Med Econ 70(17):30,33-34,36
35. Levetown M (1998) Palliative care in the intensive care unit. New Horiz 6:383-397
36. Cook DJ (2001) Transdisciplinary research to understand the role of bias and heuristics. In: Curtis JR, Rubenfeld GD (eds) Managing death in the ICU. Oxford University Press, New York, pp 59-67
37. Mularski RA, Bascom P, Osborne ML (2001) Educational agendas for interdisciplinary end-of-life curricula. Crit Care Med 29 (2 Suppl):N16-N23
38. Danis M, Federman D, Fins JJ, et al (1999) Incorporating palliative care into critical care education: principles, challenges, and opportunities. Crit Care Med 27:2005-2013
39. Brody H, Campbell ML, Faber-Langendoen K et al (1997) Withdrawing intensive life-sustaining treatment – recommendations for compassionate clinical management. N Engl J Med 336:652 -657
40. Fisher M (2002) ICU Cornerstone: a lecture that changed my practice. Crit Care (London) 6:403-404
41. Levy MM (2001) End-of-life care in the intensive care unit: can we do better? Crit Care Med 29 Suppl.:N56-N61
42. Jastremski CA (1998) Caring for the families of those who die in the critical care unit. Crit Care Med 26:1150-1151
43. Coyle N, Truog RD (1994) HealthCare Ethics Forum '94: pain management and sedation in the terminally ill. AACN Clin Issues Crit Care Nurs 5:360-365
44. Phillips RS, Wenger NS, Teno J, et al (1996) Choices of seriously ill patients about cardiopulmonary resuscitation: correlates and outcomes. SUPPORT Investigators. Am J Med 100:128-137
45. Dunn GP, Milch RA, Mosenthal AC, et al (2002) Palliative care by the surgeon: how to do it. J Am Coll Surg 194:509-537
46. Campbell ML, Field BE (1991) Management of the patient with do not resuscitate status: compassion and cost containment. Heart Lung 20:345-348

47. Campbell ML (1996) Program assessment through outcomes analysis: efficacy of a comprehensive supportive care team for end-of-life care. AACN Clin Issues Crit Care Nurs 7:159-167
48. Pronovost P, Angus DC (2001) Economics of end-of-life care in the intensive care unit. Crit Care Med 29(2 Suppl):N46-51
49. Marik PE (1995) The cost of dying. Am J Crit Care 4:56-58
50. Crippen DW (2003) End of life care in the ICU: toward a newer concept of futility. In: Vincent JL (ed) 2003 Yearbook of intensive care and emergency medicine. Springer, Heidelberg
51. Rushton CH, Williams MA, Sabatier KH (2002) The integration of palliative care and critical care: one vision, one voice. Crit Care Nurs Clin North Am 14:133-140
52. Wanzer SH, Federman DD (1989) The physician's responsibility toward hopelessly ill patients: a second look. N Engl J Med 320:844-849
53. Cassel CK (1996) Hospital care for dying patients (letter). N Engl J Med 335:1765-1767
54. Hill L (1996) Hospital care for dying patients (letter). N Engl J Med 335:1765-1767
55. Daly BJ (2000) Organizational change and delivery of multidisciplinary palliative care. Respir Care 45:1501-1510
56. Curtis JR (1998) The "patient-centered" outcomes of critical care: what are they and how should they be used? New Horiz 6:26-32
57. Emanuel LL, von Gunten CF, Ferris FD (1999) The Education for Physicians on End-of-life Care (EPEC) curriculum. American Medical Association, Chicago
58. DeVita MA, Arnold RM, Barnard D (2003) Teaching palliative care to critical care medicine trainees. Crit Care Med 31:1257-1262
59. Azoulay E, Chevret S, Leleu G, et al (2000) Half the families of intensive care unit patients experience inadequate communication with physicians. Crit Care Med 28: 3044-3049
60. DeVita M, Sirio CA, Paronish R, et al (1999) ICU Patients Are Unlikely to Receive Council Regarding Levels of Support. Chest 116:239S
61. Lilly CM, De Meo DL, Sonna LA, et al (2000) An intensive communication intervention for the critically ill. Am J Med 109:469-475
62. Anonymous (1976) Optimum care for hopelessly ill patients. A report of the Clinical Care Committee of the Massachusetts General Hospital. N Engl J Med 295:362-364
63. Rubenfeld GD, Randall Curtis J (2001) The End-of-Life Care in the ICU Working Group. End-of-life care in the intensive care unit: a research agenda. Crit Care Med 29: 2001-2006
64. Levy MM (2001) Paying attention to death. Crit Care Med 29:2037-2038

Nursing the dying in intensive care

J. SEYMOUR

While at first sight being at opposite ends of a spectrum, closer inspection of intensive care and palliative care reveals many similarities. Both specialities developed during a similar time period and care for patients and their families at moments of extreme vulnerability and need. Staff in both must face death frequently and repeatedly manage its consequences for patients, families and themselves. In so doing, both specialities rely on models of specialist nursing care in which the 'total' care of patients and their families is paramount and in which recognition of the interdependence of medicine and nursing and the importance of team work is highly developed.

The key goals of palliative care nursing in intensive care are to relieve suffering during end-of-life care and to support dying patients and their families as it becomes clear that the focus of care is moving from 'rescue' to 'palliation'[1]. Intensive care nurses have been shown to engage in a range of behaviours directed at achieving these goals [2], most of which are difficult to articulate and which, until recently, have been little emphasised in the 'technical' literature that has predominated in the intensive care field. A key difficulty for nurses working in intensive care is that there may seem to be little room to create space for a philosophy of palliative care in which dying people and their families can 'draw meaning and solace from their personal lives and culture in the face of death' [3], not least because one of the central tenets of palliative care, patients' awareness of dying, is usually absent [4]. Moreover, the process of reaching nontreatment decisions is marked frequently by extreme ethical and diagnostic complexity, with nursing and medical staff at the 'sharp end' of resolving potentially irreconcilable interests [4-5]. During this time, intensive care nurses and their medical colleagues are caught between two goals of caring: *hippocratic*, in which the controlling the disease from an objective standpoint is paramount; and *askelepian*, in which the caregiver tries to enter the experience of suffering for the patient and his family and focuses on preparing a space of safety and security for them [6-7].

This paper explores these issues by drawing on interview data from an ethnography[1] of death and dying conducted in two general adult intensive care units in the UK [4]. The paper concludes by making some recommendations for nursing dying people in the challenging environment of intensive care.

Caring and coping with death in intensive care

The analysis of the data on which this paper is based suggests that, when caring for dying people and their families, nurses strive to create a sense of 'occupational integrity', both personally and in a team context, in which the following key elements stand out:

- Attempts to separate the 'professional' and 'personal' self.
- An emphasis on the comfort of the dying person and the presentation of their body.
- The compassionate disclosure of appropriate information to family.
- Protection of the 'team' by balancing the different orientations of medicine and nursing.

Separation of the personal and professional self

Intensive care staff consciously deploy certain strategies or 'rules' to ensure the distressing emotions and feelings are controlled. This is particularly the case for nursing staff, for whom close intimacy with patients and their family is a defining feature of their work. A key theme in nurses' accounts is that of 'involvement' and of emotional investment. They describe incidents that might be interpreted as formative 'rites of passage', in which they overstepped the invisible line between self and professional. Such experiences had led to subsequent efforts to ensure that their emotions were 'managed' and separation achieved between personal and professional selves. This process of separation is, however, complex and difficult to sustain because such involvement and

[1] Fourteen case studies were completed in two intensive care units in the UK. Each 'case' consisted of the health care staff and families of selected critically ill patients (see Seymour 2001 for methodological details). This paper is largely based on seventeen interviews completed with staff: four were with consultant medical staff and three with junior medical staff. Ten interviews were conducted with nurses, seven of whom were experienced in the area and three of whom were relatively inexperienced. Respondents were asked to describe their work and those aspects that they found either difficult or rewarding. They were then asked to describe intensive incidents of particularly 'difficult' deaths in which they could remember being involved. The issues that emerged from these incidents and from their recollections about the particular case in which they had been involved were explored during each interview.

expression of emotion is integral to their professional identity. One junior nurse tries to explain the basis of this:

> I think it's because we are all human, you do get close ... I try to think of my patients as family, like when you're a student nurse and you're taught to think 'that's my granny there', so you try to look after them as well as you would your granny ... (Staff nurse)

A more experienced nurse describes how she had once become 'over-involved' with a young patient who had eventually died from severe injuries. She likens this experience to:

> ... Getting my fingers burnt ... it was so painful, I decided I wasn't ever going to do that again ... (Staff nurse)

Another nurse recalls the feelings of extreme anxiety and stress experienced during the delivery of care to a young man, who did eventually survive. She describes a high level of personal involvement which was personally exhausting and which constituted a threat to her 'professional self':

> ... He was only 28 and I was determined that he wasn't going to die ... I was so wound up, if he had died I would have probably just not wanted to come back to work again. I'd put so much of myself into making him better ... it just drained me. (Staff nurse)

In their emphasis on the precarious nature of the separation between 'personal' and 'professional' selves, nurses appear to be acutely aware that it is the nature of nursing as a caring occupation that is the root of such difficulties. Intensive care nursing, in particular, perhaps in contrast to the lay perception of intensive care nurses as 'technical experts', is perceived as demanding intimate exchange in interpersonal relationships with patients and their family. Although the opportunity to become emotionally involved is welcomed, nurses are conscious of the personal tensions that emerged from *work* that is essentially constituted by *care*. The more experienced nurses describe strategies of de-personalisation employed to cope with these tensions. However, it was clear that these were only partially successful and required high levels of energy to execute them:

> Nurse: I can still do it [caring] on a partially impersonal [level] ... I hope they never get the impression of this, but because you're dealing

> with so many people all of the time you can't get totally involved all of the time ... you put a bit of a mask on ... you've got to say, this is a nurse doing her job. I think that the reason you're successful is in the sign of the family thinking that you are wonderful [laughter] that's the impression they get, when really it's ... just acting a part, being a nice person who cares.
>
> I: How do you feel at the end of a few days or a shift looking after a patient and there family where it is, as you describe, quite draining and you have to put on a mask?
>
> Nurse: I feel quite exhausted. Not even after a few days, after each shift ... I try to use the time from leaving work to coming home and then back again to get rid of it. I try not to think about it too much. It makes one sound very automated, I suppose, but you have to cut off ... as it is now, it's very busy and people die. And they die young. It can all get too much sometimes. (Staff nurse)

In certain circumstances, this type of coping strategy became untenable. These occurred in situations in which a particular sense of identity developed between the nurse and the patient or the patient's family. Nurses experienced this as puzzling, and described how some patients evoke such strong feelings within them that they cannot 'let go' of those individuals. A common pattern was described in which care can be delivered across the course of many weeks or months without undue distress being experienced, but then close contact with one patient, or with a particular family suddenly engenders powerful feelings of almost familial identification that are extremely hard to contain. This does not occur in a predictable way: it is not only the classically 'tragic' deaths of previously fit, young and attractive patients that elicit such a response.

'Little things': giving comfort to the dying person

Nursing staff report high levels of satisfaction from giving what they termed 'basic nursing care' to their patients. Such care is referred to frequently, but in terms which appear to marginalise its role vis à vis the overall management of patients: the terms 'little things' or 'just basic care' are used in many instances when nurses describe their daily work:

> I care for one patient per shift ... I provide all their care for them, just basic care, mouth care, pressure area care, washing ... things like that. (Staff nurse)

> I get satisfied when ... somebody says 'oh, they look really comfortable' or 'they look well looked after' and it might have been that you've just shaved somebody that you've not managed to shave before ... the little things we do like that matter ... (Staff nurse)

The status of such care is heightened when a patient is known to be approaching death: in such instances physical care and careful presentation of the body apparently become the means of affirming the individuality of the dying person. Such bodily attention appears to be central to nurses' attempts to portray to family the social worth of dying people: individuals whom nurses often never 'known' as conscious beings. Further, it becomes the means by which nurses themselves *relate to* their patients as subjective individuals and the way in which their relationships with patients' family are sustained. The nurses below are all referring to their care of unconscious patients:

> I looked after him the previous week on nights and came back onto days and looked after him again. That was my choice. I wanted to do it because I felt like he knew me, because now and again he would open his eyes. I just wanted to be there for him, I wanted him to know I was there. (Staff nurse)

> You don't know the patients at all. You don't know what sort of person you have on the unit, what sort of people they are, what they've done in their life or anything like that ... it's just looking after their body until they die and looking after their relatives. It's only by talking to their relatives that you piece together a picture of what this person might be like ... you have to go on photographs and then you can see what the person might be like. (Staff nurse)

> ... [Relatives] sometimes watch you do things and that's enough, that you're doing something whether it's to help [the patient] get better or to help them die. Just that in a way is enough. (Staff nurse)

Nurses try to discover details of patients' lives, family relationships, personality and usual appearance. This serves two purposes: it strengthens the sense of 'person' within the body of each dying individual and it creates a bond with each person's family, since they are the providers of such information. Bodily attention given in this way is both an expression of respect for personhood and a means of portraying 'doing' in a situation where hope of recovery has gone. In some circumstances, however, such bodily care becomes problematic for nurses. This is especially the case in those situations where death is sudden and traumatic, or when the process of dying is prolonged.

Disclosure of information to patients' families

A major issue for all staff in intensive care is that of achieving a balance between the delivery of nursing care to their patients and the preparation of family for the possibility of the patient's death by the gradual disclosure of information:

> You had to watch what you said to her because she sort of clung to every piece of hope and she wanted to know exactly everything, which was fine, but it took up a lot of your time. [It meant] you had to be with her and not with [patient] ... I think with [her] you had to go into every tiny thing and if one nurse said a slightly different thing she would ask you to make sure [but] then she couldn't take it in because she was really upset ... she had so much faith that he was going to pull through ... I couldn't not encourage her faith, because without that she would have had nothing, so you couldn't be too pessimistic and you couldn't be too optimistic, but then he was very ill. (Staff nurse)

As this illustrates, nurses are acutely aware of tensions in their relationship with family and struggle to ensure that they achieve a balance between the delivery of patient care and the disclosure of information. The informal way in which nurses give information sometimes creates difficulties in achieving consistency with the disclosures of other team members. Further, while it is accepted that the nurse's role in disclosing information is to prepare family members for the likelihood of death, this causes anxieties about the extent and form that such disclosure should take. Of particular concern among nurses is the possibility of encroachment on the 'formal' disclosure of bad news or of intensive decisions concerning treatment withdrawal that were seen to be the province of medical staff:

> Nurse: I'll always remember my first death on intensive care, I think more so than on the general wards – I hadn't been on the unit long and they'd decided to withdraw [treatment] on a chap ... the doctors decided to withdraw but felt that they couldn't speak to his wife who was sitting out in the waiting room on her own. They thought they had to wait for her family to come in. ... [but] she knew what was going on, she knew that he had deteriorated and that we would be discussing it, [that] it was inevitable. I remember going out to see her and I was just going to say 'he's not doing well and the doctors will probably have a talk with you later on', knowing at the back of my mind that they were going to see her when the son came in and that they were going to withdraw ... but when she came in beside the bed ... and she

> was asking questions, I couldn't lie ... [but] I didn't know where to stop or how far to go. (Staff nurse)

Sometimes, in those circumstances where no 'formal decision' has been agreed upon regarding the continuation of treatment, nurses find themselves having to forestall the enquiries of patient's family. This can lead to extreme feelings of discomfort and can create a barrier between the nurse and the patient's family at a time when the latter are very vulnerable.

Medical staff assume a more formal relationship with patients' families and have a more clearly delineated view of their responsibilities regarding both the disclosure of information and regarding their remit in patient care. Their concerns are to consolidate in a clear way the preparatory 'groundwork' that nurses had undertaken with family. They want to ensure that they had been seen to have done 'all' that was possible with regard to treatment. These concerns are associated with a belief that responsibility for intensive treatment decisions should not be assumed by family:

> Doctor: ... We did what we could and there [was] nothing more that could be done – you can only do your best ... it was pushing our knowledge and expertise forward and that's what we are here for ... [with family] you can only reassure them that what you are doing is right, that you are doing everything that you possibly can ... I'm very keen for relatives to be informed of decisions but ... not to actually put the burden on them of making the decision ... it's *not* their decision, there must be a lightening of that load ... [they should be told] we've done our best and do you agree with what's happening? (Consultant)

These extracts reveal clearly the division of labour that exists between doctors and nursing staff in intensive care with regard to the care of dying patients and the support of patients' families. The roles that each assume during the process of patient care are interdependent, but enacted according to clearly defined boundaries. Of key importance was the notion of 'teamwork'.

Promoting teamwork

Both medical and nursing staff emphasise the importance of 'teamwork' in their management of dying people. The 'team' is seen to offer informal staff support as well as a means of 'getting through the work' of caring for dying people. It is seen, for example, as a means of defusing some of the more extreme pressures associated with such care:

> Nurse: I think that it's teamwork that we have here, you know a good rapport with everybody and we're all able to help one another. We have dinner time when we laugh about stupid things ... you can laugh about things even though they're not laughable, even though they're deadly serious – you have to laugh at them because otherwise you'd just go silly, you'd go mad. (Staff nurse)

In possible contrast to other areas of the hospital, nurses and doctors within intensive care work closely together in the delivery of care to intensively ill and dying people. This prompted some nurse respondents to describe the more 'respectful' attitudes of intensive care doctors to nurses as the basis for team work in intensive care. Such opinions were reinforced by the doctors who were interviewed. They tend to emphasise their co-operation and consultation with nurses during the care of intensively ill patients. However, two issues emerged from the interview data that threw doubt on the extent to which 'teamwork' actually operated in the intensive care environment. The first of these concerns the extent to which nurses are able to influence the management of particular patients; the second issue concerns the organisation of medical work both within intensive care and within the wider hospital. This operates to reinforce doctor-to-doctor, collegial consultation rather than multidisciplinary teamwork. This style of working adds an element of unpredictability to patient management and ensures that many aspects of the care of dying patients are outside the sphere of influence of nursing staff.

Nurses frequently voice concerns about the extent to which they can participate in, or question, 'medical' decisions about patients. Their anxieties seem to centre upon their rather ambiguous relationship with doctors. Indeed, much of the medical work involved in caring for patients is shared between nurses and doctors: for example, nurses assume a great deal of responsibility for the assessment and analysis of blood results and for the adjustment of analgesia and sedation given to patients. One nurse describes how she spends part of her time: 'prompting doctors without telling them' and how she is aware that many medical decisions concerning patients were based on observations reported by nurses. Nurses are also expected to play a central role in ward rounds, which are a central feature of intensive care work. However, nurses report a lack of confidence and a lack of ability to question doctors. Commonly it is felt that doctors are always in the position of being able to 'veto' the opinion of nurses by setting the agenda for acceptable, 'sensible' knowledge:

> Nurse: ... If you think one thing and the doctors think another ... although they'll listen to you they'll then tear what you've got to shreds if they don't agree with it. I think it can be quite frustrating. ... (Staff nurse)

> Nurse: I do find it difficult when they're pulling all the stops out on somebody and then say within half an hour they will have said: 'Let's just stop everything' ... I find it difficult to take in sometimes ... I think its up to me to stand up and get a bit more confidence and ask questions [but] the other thing is, I don't want to appear stupid – you don't want to be seen as being silly ... (Staff nurse)

The more experienced nurses report a greater role in treatment decisions but are still aware that the extent to which they can influence decision making is determined in part by the willingness of each particular doctor and by the personality of the nurse:

> Nurse: ... For the nurses, I think they would welcome a bit more notice of what they feel [but] really to be honest, I think it depends very much on which particular consultant it is and I think it also depends on how assertive the nurse is, what sort of personality she has and how she makes her general feelings known ... (Staff nurse)

Nurses of all levels of experience are aware that much medical decision making takes place 'behind the scenes' and operates to effectively exclude the influence of other disciplines. Further, nurses feel constrained by the need for them to remain at the bedside of the patient. This means that they cannot participate fully in behind the scenes negotiations that crucially affect the process of medical decision making. Doctors acknowledge that their relationships with other doctors determine, in large part, the outcome of deliberations about the treatment of patients and that a crucial factor in this process is the issue of patient 'ownership':

> Doctor: ... Basically the decision ... with most people is that the intensive care doctors come to an opinion ... once we come to that opinion and before we talk to the relatives we ask the nurses and they usually unanimously agree ... and then depending on which admitting team it is we inform them or discuss it with them: it very much depends on the admitting surgeon [if] we have a good rapport with him, if he's used to dealing with ITU. (Consultant)

Summary and recommendations

This paper has highlighted some of the special difficulties that intensive care nurses face when caring for dying patients and their families. The delicate balance between personal and professional 'selves' has been revealed as of critical importance in coping with work that demands high levels of intimacy across a series of relatively short-term, intense exchanges. We have seen how nurses learn to manage the demands of caring for dying people by exposure to painful experiences of dying and death that might be likened to formative 'rites of passage'. The nature of 'teamwork' in intensive care has been briefly explored, with reference to the varying influence of medical and nursing staff on aspects of the management of potentially dying patients. Teamwork is highly valued in intensive care and is essential to high quality palliative care. However, as we have seen, a lack of attention to team dynamics means that nurses and doctors will tend to work in parallel and from their own somewhat insular and well-defended disciplinary perspectives, rather than jointly and from a position of shared understanding about the objectives of care [8]. In discussing this problem, Corner [8] draws on the work of Rosenfield [9], who developed a taxonomy of cross-disciplinary working in which 'transdisciplinary working' is the ultimate goal. This model of teamwork involves developing a shared conceptual framework and working out together how to address common problems of patient care. In many intensive care units, and other types of health care settings, this may seem almost unattainable. Problems which need to be addressed in order to achieve this model of team working are: inadequate organisational support; lack of training in teamwork; lack of interprofessional trust; lack of clear goals; lack of continuity among team members; the dominance of particular discourses and the exclusion of others [10].

What can be concluded from this by way of recommendations that may be helpful for staff working in intensive care? Most notably, as Puntillo [11] notes, care for the caregivers must be afforded a high priority. Opportunities to reflect on the experiences of caring for dying people in intensive care arise infrequently, and often the dying process is telescoped into a few days and hours: these are critical moments [4] in which staff risk emotional exhaustion as they strive to provide good care to their patients while putting their own fears and feelings 'on hold'. Creating time and space for reflection and case discussion can be done, but it requires a commitment from management and from all team members. Such discussion is best when it involves both doctors and nurses, perhaps by way of a regular 'separation review' in which the circumstances of the illness, care and death of a patient can be discussed [12]. Structured opportunities such as these can provide a much needed opportunity for doctors and nurses to share their 'narratives of care' [13] in such a way that they develop a sense of shared understanding about the goals and particular constraints that fashion their work and influence their differing perspectives on clinical decision making [14]. This can provide an opportunity for intensive care staff to explore together how patients' dignity can be maximised, and may allow a greater focus on the 'just little things' that are so important to nurses, patients and families. Block [15] suggests that developing models of bereavement care and family support, by drawing on the expertise of colleagues in specialties such as palliative care and psychiatry, can enable staff to broaden their definitions of success to include both rescue and an appropriate, dignified death. In turn, this can lead to a change in culture so that intensive care is better suited to give care to those who die and those who are bereaved within its confines.

References

1. Seymour JE (2003) What's in a name? A concept analysis of key terms in palliative care nursing. In: Payne S, Seymour JE, Ingleton C (eds) (in preparation) Palliative care nursing: principles and evidence for practice. Open University Press, Buckingham (in press)
2. McClement SE, Degner LF (1995) Expert nursing behaviours in care of the dying adult in the intensive care unit. Heart Lung 24:408-419
3. Miles SH (2001) The role of the physician in sacred end of life rituals in the ICU. In: Randall-Curtis J, Rubenfeld GD (eds) Managing death in the intensive care unit. The transition from cure to comfort. Oxford University Press, Oxford, pp 207-214
4. Seymour JE (2001) Critical moments: death and dying in intensive care. Open University Press, Buckingham
5. Seymour JE (2000) Negotiating natural death in intensive care. Soc Sci Med 51:1241-1252
6. Kearney M (2000) A place of healing: working with suffering in living and dying. Oxford University Press, Oxford
7. Mount BM (2003) Existential suffering and the determinants of healing. Eur J Palliat Care, 10 (Suppl):40-42
8. Corner J (2003) The multidisciplinary team-fact or fiction? Eur J Palliat Care, 10 (Suppl):10-12
9. Rosenfield PL (1992) The potential of transdisciplinary research for sustaining and extending linkages between the health and social services. Soc Sci Med 35:1343-1357
10. Opie A, Bernhofen DM (1997) Thinking teams and thinking clients: issues of discourse and representation in the work of health care teams. Sociol Health Illness 19:259-280
11. Puntillo KA (2001) The role of critical care nurses in providing and managing end of life care. In: Randall-Curtis J, Rubenfeld GD (eds) Managing death in the intensive care unit. The transition from cure to comfort. Oxford University Press, Oxford
12. McNamara B (2001) Fragile lives. Death, dying and care. Open University Press, Buckingham
13. Johnson N, Cook D, Giacomini M et al (2000) Towards a "good" death: end of life narratives constructed in an intensive care unit. Culture, Med Psychiatry 24:275-295
14. Hall K (2002) Medical decision-making: an argument for narrative and metaphor. Theoret Med Bioethics 23:55-73
15. Block SD (2001) Helping the clinician cope with death in the ICU. In: Randall-Curtis J, Rubenfeld GD (eds) Managing death in the intensive care unit. The transition from cure to comfort. Oxford University Press, Oxford

APPENDIX

Planning, designing and writing up scientific research

S. Martins, A. Zin, W. Zin

What is the meaning of research?

In a broad sense the word *research* can be used to mean finding out about unfamiliar matters, generally by retrieving bits of information here and there. In fact, research is the systematic process of collecting and analysing data in order to increase the knowledge available to those working in a specific field of interest. The whole process presents seven distinct characteristics:

1. Question or problem
2. Aim
3. Specific plan or procedure
4. Division of the main problem into subproblems
5. Acceptance of critical assumptions
6. Collection and interpretation of data
7. Cyclical nature

Question or problem

A question, problem or hypothesis should start off any research. There are so many unanswered questions in every field that it is just a matter of asking: "Why?" "What is the meaning of this?" or "What has caused that?" Accidents can happen, of course, but an experienced researcher will never start collecting data in the expectation that these data will show him/her which path to follow. The problem dictates the origin of formal research.

Most sections of this chapter have already appeared in the volume:
Planning and Designing Clinical Research: the Basics (S.B. Martins, W.A. Zin). Series Teaching and Training in Anaesthesiology and Critical Care. 2001, Springer-Verlag Italia

Aim

A clear and unambiguous statement of the aim of the research is imperative. Researchers must start up their projects in full knowledge of exactly what is intended. "What is the goal?" is the question to be answered at this stage of the project.

Specific plan for procedure

Research requires discipline: the plan for the procedure must be carefully and explicitly decided in advance. In other words, planning and designing are basic and essential steps. Clearly, depending on the specific project different designs and methods will be chosen to generate data of importance to the research problem. The question to be answered is: "How to reach the goal?"

Division of the main problem into subproblems

Sometimes it is wise to reduce the main problem to a logical series of subproblems. The independent solutions to these subproblems will lead to unravelling of the overall question. When applicable, this technique can change a cumbersome and unwieldy research project into a series of easily handled smaller studies.

Acceptance of critical assumptions

Assumptions are self-evident truths, which must be valid for the research to proceed. In other words, an assumption is a condition that is taken for granted, without which the research could not be carried on. It is essential that prospective readers know what assumptions underlie a research project. If any assumption is not self-evident the author should point it out explicitly.

Collection and interpretation of data

Data must be collected very carefully. If data are collected in a sloppy way, the meaning of the results may be distorted. Usually a series of experiments is carried out to train the members of the research team, in the same way as surgeons train their colleagues, until the group knows exactly what needs to be done. Notes must be taken as frequently as possible, so that later on any member of the group can understand the meaning of a sudden drop in arterial blood pressure during the experiment, for instance. Moreover, another researcher may want to repeat the experiment, and such precise notes taken at the time will help in this task.

Interpretation of the results allows recognition of the meaning of the data. Without this there can be no research. It must be stressed that data can be differently interpreted by different researchers. A magnificent analogy to this was given by Luigi Pirandello, an Italian dramatist, novelist and Nobel prize winner, in his play "*Così è si vi pare*" (1918), in which the same facts are presented to different characters, who then report back quite dissimilar views of them. The interpretation of the same set of data can also change with time; while the realities of time and space have not changed, the way we interpret them has.

Cyclical nature

The research process follows a cycle. It begins with the initial questioning; then comes the identification of a problem; data are collected and interpreted; a conclusion is reached; and the initial hypothesis is either supported or not supported (the initial question is partially/completely answered or not).

Although the circle seems to be neatly closed, this impression is deceptive. Research is never conclusive, because exploration of an area draws attention to further problems that need solving. Thus, research begets research, and the circle becomes a spiral.

Introduction to the general tools of research

Every professional needs specific tools to carry out his/her work. Without scalpel and scissors it would be difficult indeed for surgeons to do their job safely. Naturally, researchers have their own toolkits designed to achieve their aims. The specific tools required by a physiologist, for instance, will be quite different from those needed by an astronomer. Nonetheless, the great majority of researchers will share a general set of general research tools.

Four general research tools are frequently identified:

1. The library and its resources
2. The computer and its software
3. Statistics
4. Facility with language

The library and its resources

The library has evolved from a repository of writings, books, manuscripts, and so on into a very dynamic space that can even be visited electronically. As in the past, ease and speed of access to information are the priorities, but with the avalanche of new knowledge produced daily researchers have become more demanding.

In order to keep up with researchers' present needs and desires, the ambience of modern libraries has been changing in recent years. In addition to the card catalogue and the shelf after shelf of books and periodicals, banks of computer terminals and keyboards will now be found there. The ultimate goal is to access the whole realm of global knowledge rapidly and comprehensively.

The university library offers both printed material and electronically accessed information. Thus, it will provide readers with: (a) periodicals and books, with a card catalogue to help readers to find the ones they need; (b) databases stored on CD-ROM (Compact Disk – Read Only Memory); (c) databases stored on local computer(s); (d) remotely accessed databases; and (d) commuting facilities.

Typically, the card catalogue indicates whether the desired periodical/book is part of the library collection, in which case it just needs to be retrieved from its shelf for consultation. CD-ROMs contain a great deal of information (650 megabytes) and are still frequently used in libraries. Many databases are stored on CD-ROMs. Depending on the computer network available at the particular university, they can be browsed in the library or from users' own offices. In many universities information is stored on local computers or networks. These replace the card catalogue and also provide a way of searching by terms, authors, and keywords. Remotely accessed databases are physically located somewhere else, sometimes even in another country. The users purchase the right to access them electronically from specified computers.

CD-ROMs and locally and remotely located databases have characteristics that must be specified by the users when purchasing them. Users of this medium may be given only the complete reference to a paper or its abstract or the full paper. Some databases allow searching of the literature by author's name and/or terms, providing a fast and comprehensive way of finding the relevant papers in a specific field of knowledge. Finally, if any reader desires to have a copy of a certain paper that cannot be found in the library, it can be forwarded in a matter of hours by the library's commuting system. Basically, the librarian places an order with another library that does hold the required periodical. The librarian there scans the paper and sends it electronically to the requesting library, where it will be printed out on a high-quality machine.

In summary, it is astonishing how much shorter the modern library has made the process that begins with consulting the literature and ends with availability of the information for immediate reading.

The computer and its software

The computer is perhaps the workhorse among general research tools. It can perform myriad tasks at an incredible speed. However, it must be borne in mind that it is not a human brain but in fact a very limited machine that is dependent on a human at the keyboard to direct its actions. As a research assistant, the computer can play a part in: (a) planning of a study; (b) literature review; (c) reference management; (d) data collection; (e) data analysis; (f) statistical analysis; (g) production of graphics; and (h) reporting.

During the planning phase of the study, software can be used to help generate and organise ideas for the research, as well as to assist in budget planning. Computers can be used to review the literature by taking advantage of such technology as CD-ROM and online databases for information acquisition. They are also able to provide telecommunication assistance (e-mail, electronic bulletin boards, list servers, access to the Internet, World Wide Web, and so on). Software can easily assist with electronic storage and retrieval, so that valuable bibliographic citations and comments can be readily sorted and accessed by title, author, keywords, etc.

Analogue-to-digital (A-D) converters make it possible for computers to sample and store experimentally generated data. This is a fundamental step in setting the stage for data analysis. Paper records of information have long been a thing of the past, thanks to A-D boards. Data points can be sampled at very high frequencies, increasing the accuracy and precision of the results. Data analysis can be performed offline by means of general-purpose and/or dedicated software. Dedicated software usually suits novices better, whereas general-purpose software allows a more elastic and comprehensive analysis. Data analysis can also be performed online by dedicated programs that run in computer-controlled machines, such as ventilators, spirometers or capnographs. Different statistical and spreadsheet software packages can be used on a personal computer, thus allowing quick analysis of various types of data sets. Some of these programs even give the user guidance on the right statistical test to be used.

In the late 1980s plotting a curve or drawing a graph meant sharpening one's pencils and later calling in a graphic artist. Nowadays a fairly sophisticated figure can be prepared in no time by means of powerful software.

The preparation of the text is facilitated by the use of word processing to write and edit any number of versions and updates of the final report. Desktop publishing software can help to produce professional-looking documents that can be presented at conferences and elsewhere. Similarly, figures and text can be combined for a slide presentation by other software.

In summary, the computer and its software together are an extremely powerful research tool that is involved at practically every stage of a research project. Last but not least, laptops add the mobility factor to the "old" desktop personal computer, while maintaining the same degree of precision and usefulness.

Statistics

Statistical analysis is a powerful tool when used correctly. However, its limitations should be considered. Statistical values are never the final answer to any research problem. It must always be borne in mind that statistics are underlaid by the data reported in the tests. Statistics provide information about the data, but an experienced researcher will never be satisfied until the meaning of the data is unveiled. Statistics has two principal functions: descriptive and inferential. Descriptive statistics provide information, such as mean, standard deviation, median, etc. of the values recorded, and in the case of two or more groups of data, how they relate to each other. Inferential statistics seeks to fit data to the ideal form of a statistical model.

The fundamental problem in statistical analysis lies in the choice of the right test to be applied in order to reveal the meaning of the data. To start with, the experimented researcher finds out which major set of tests could be applied to his/her data: parametric or nonparametric. A great many scientific reports erroneously put forward conclusions based on parametric statistical analyses when the distribution of the data points is clearly not normal. Powerful software (that runs on personal computers) is now available that can guide novice researchers in the search for the most suitable test to answer their questions. In summary, statistics is a powerful research tool that can help researchers to understand the meaning of data, but it must be applied with caution to avoid misleading conclusions.

Facility with language

A successful research project culminates in a published document. To generate such a paper, the author must be able to use language with a degree of clarity that will make it easy for others to read the document in all its aspects. As a rule of thumb, after several drafts it is a good idea for the author to hand the manuscript to a colleague who has not been involved in the project, with the request that he/she check it for clarity. Many papers reporting on good work are not accepted for publication simply because the reviewers cannot understand them. An experienced writer will always make good use of a well-thumbed dictionary. The spelling of every single word must be checked. In summary, facility with language paves the way to a well-written document, and expert help is always needed in its preparation.

Literature search

When developing a protocol for a research project you require information relevant to the research question and study design. A review of current research evidence will yield detailed knowledge on the topic of interest and arguments that can be used to underline the need for the study in applications to funding agencies. The review does not have to be extensive, but it does need to highlight the current issues that are relevant to the specific research question.

The research question will guide the literature search. This will expand researchers' comprehension of the topic and make it possible to develop and focus the research question and underlying hypothesis further. Review papers are a good starting point to expand comprehension of a given subject; it is necessary to be aware of the potential for bias in narrative reviews.

In traditional reviews there is often no clear statement of the question that prompted the review, how the selection of primary studies was achieved, or how the author went about including and excluding studies. This makes it difficult for readers to evaluate how comprehensive the author's search for primary studies was and what the quality of the studies included and excluded was, and consequently, how valid the conclusions reached are. Such reviews have been criticised as unsystematic and biased, as they express the subjective impressions of the individual reviewer [1].

Systematic reviews, in contrast, are explicit about the question they aim to answer and the methodology used. The author of a systematic review describes the process used to select primary studies, the evaluation of quality markers and the statistical methods used to combine results. The quantitative combination of the results of different studies addressing the same question is called meta-analysis. The unique advantages of quantitative systematic reviews or meta-analyses are increased power and precision in the estimation of effects and risks. Qualitative and quantitative systematic reviews, with their explicit methods, may limit bias and improve the reliability and accuracy of recommendations [1]. "Researchers use the systematic review to identify, justify, and refine hypotheses; recognise and avoid pitfalls of previous work; estimate sample sizes; and delineate important ancillary or adverse effects and covariates that warrant consideration in future studies" [2].

The search for papers has become an easier task in recent years because of the Internet. Electronic access to databases and journals on the Internet is increasing every year. Access to much of this information, e.g. that saved in the PubMed database and published in the journals *BMJ* and *The Canadian Medical Journal*, is free. Some information is available through university connections, and some only by subscription. Computer skills are required, but the development of user-friendly software is making the procedures less "technical" and more accessible.

The decision on which databases to search for papers depends on the topic of interest. Studies on search strategies for various topics have shown that there is much to be gained from searching more than one database. Databases extract data from different journals, and the indexing terms used and the quality vary [3–8]. Talking to librarians and to other researchers in the field is a good way of finding out about the available databases. Language can be a constraint, so that the benefit of looking for primary studies in other languages, for example by searching LILACS (Latin American and Caribbean Health Science Information Database), must be evaluated.

The quality of indexing of bibliographic databases will have a bearing on how successful a search strategy is. The National Library of Medicine together with the Cochrane Collaboration is updating the indexing of clinical trials with the aim of improving researchers' access to them. The Cochrane Collaboration's database of clinical trials is regularly updated and aims to contain all clinical trials published. The content is not limited by journal of publication.

Efficient literature searching is a skill acquired through both experience and learning about the use of effective search strategies. Information is published in a range of sources, including journals, books, and research reports. Medline holds over 12 million references, and in 2002 alone 502,000 citations were added (http://www.ns.nlm.nih.gov/). The quantity of material may seem overwhelming, but there are four sources of evidence that can help make searching for clinical information more efficient:

1. Specialist organisations that are dedicated to summarising research findings and creating databases to aid dissemination:

A. The Cochrane Collaboration—An international organisation that aims to help people make well-informed decisions about healthcare by preparing, maintaining and ensuring the accessibility of systematic reviews of the effects of healthcare interventions. Italian Cochrane Center: http://www.areas.it/index.asp?IDL=ITA; http://www.areas.it/index.htmUK Cochrane Center http://www.cochrane.co.uk.

B. NHS Centre for Reviews and Disseminations (University of York)—Established in January 1994 to provide the National Health Service (United Kingdom) with important information on the effectiveness of treatments and the delivery and organisation of health care. It is a good resource for systematic reviews: http://www.york.ac.uk/inst/crd/.

2. Specialist journals which provide systematic reviews or review high-quality primary searches:

A. *ACP Journal Club*—A bimonthly publication containing structured abstracts of selected studies that have been published in over 50 journals concerned with internal medicine and have met explicit criteria for scientific merit and clinical importance. Commentaries from experts in the subject area are included. Published since 1991: http://www.acpjc.org/.

B. *Evidence-Based Medicine*—Articles on topics in the areas of internal medicine, general and family practice, surgery, psychiatry, paediatrics, and gynaecology and obstetrics are summarised in value-added abstracts and commented on by clinical experts if studies meet explicit criteria for scientific merit and clinical importance. Published since 1995: http://ebm.bmjjournals.com/.

C. *The Cochrane Library*—An electronic publication designed to supply high-quality evidence about healthcare-related issues and embracing the Cochrane Database of Systematic Reviews, the Database of Abstracts of Reviews of Effectiveness, and the Cochrane Controlled Trials Register: http://www.update-software.com/cochrane/.

3.General and specialised databases that can be searched by specific techniques to find relevant articles:

A. MEDLINE—National Library of Medicine (USA) bibliographic database of biomedical indexed journals. Free internet access through PubMed: http://www.ncbi.nlm.nih.gov/entrez/query.fcgi.

B. PubMed Central—A new service provided by the National Library of Medicine, this has as its objective the preservation and maintenance of open access to electronic literature. There is free access to full texts of articles from available journals. The list of journals available is growing rapidly: http://www.PubMedcentral.nih.gov/.

C. Embase—Published by Elsevier Science, this is a comprehensive pharmacological and biomedical database.

D. Cancer-CD—A compilation by Silver Platter of Cancerlit and Embase cancer-related records from 1984.

E. Psychlit—Produced by the American Psychological Association, this database covers the areas of psychology and psychiatry and related subjects. Journals from 1974 and books from 1987 are included.

F. LILACS—Latin American and Caribbean Health Science Information Database, published since 1982. The database indexes 670 journals in the region, with abstracts in English, Portuguese or Spanish. Only 41 journals overlap with MEDLINE or Embase.

4. The Internet offers direct links to organisations that may hold the information you need.

A. Medical associations.

B. Government organisations.

C. Pharmaceutical industry.

The search strategy

A structured question will help in focusing searches and deciding what sources and search strategies to use. When deciding on a search strategy it is advisable to start with a broader approach. While this may generate a lot of irrelevant material, limiting the search too early may cause some vital piece of information that is pertinent to answering the research question to be overlooked.

Deciding on the best words to use to start a search is critical in identifying key references. It is possible to start by using "ordinary" terms, such as *renal* or *renal disease*. These are known as "text words". These text words can be used to search the database directly or to identify keywords by which related articles are indexed. The search engine will search for the specific term in the title or the abstract.

However, most databases have their own indexing terms and are based on a controlled vocabulary. For example, PubMed uses Medical Subject Headings (MeSH), which is a controlled vocabulary. In MeSH, a deliberate choice of the terms to be used in describing the content of a study is made. Synonyms and spelling differences can be grouped under an indexing term to improve retrieval of relevant papers. The indexed vocabulary of the database that best describes the author's own keywords should be identified and included in the search strategy. For example, in Medline a search for "blood pressure" as a text word would retrieve only articles in which this exact term appears in the title or the abstract. If it were used as a MeSH term, articles for which "systolic blood pressure", "diastolic blood pressure" and "pulse pressure" are indexed would also be retrieved.

Search strategies have been developed to enhance users' ability to retrieve relevant articles in PubMed. The menu on the left in PubMed includes an option called "Clinical Queries". These enable the user to apply automated research methodology filters developed for different clinical queries, such as *therapy, diagnosis, aetiology* or *prognosis*. An option that will focus on specificity or sensitivity can also be selected. Choosing specificity will result in a more focused retrieval; if this option is used some relevant papers may be missed. If sensitivity is chosen retrieval will be broader and some irrelevant papers will be retrieved. The next step is to add a subject term to be searched by (Fig. 1).

Authors can also develop their own search strategies, rather than applying automatic queries. Specificity of the search can be improved by use of the "single term strategies" approach [8]. For example, in a search for studies on the aetiology of hypertension, use of the text word "risk" and the MeSH term "hypertension" improves retrieval. Table 1 describes the single-term strategies that provide the best specificity [8].

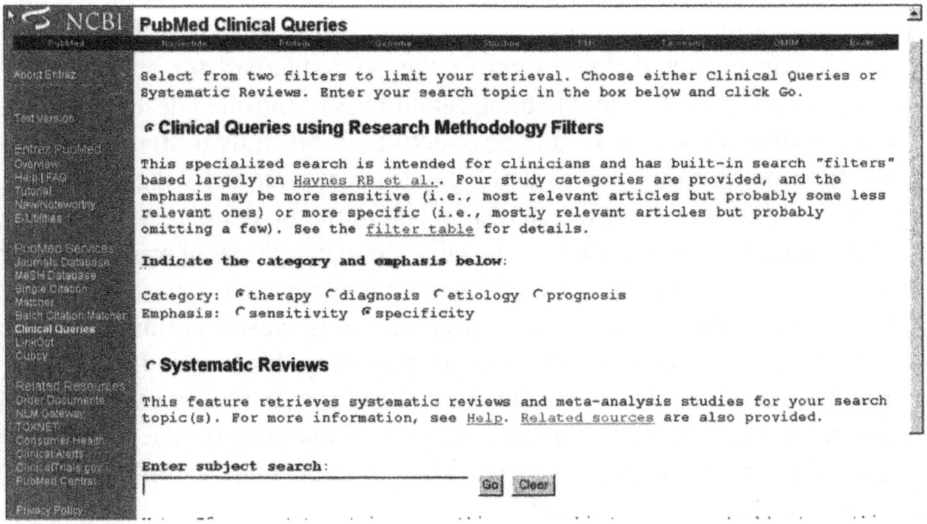

Fig. 1 Clinical Queries Web Page in PubMed

Table 1 Single term search strategies with highest specificity in Medline [8]

Area of interest	Best single-term search	Medline
Studies of therapy or prevention	Clinical trial	Field: publication type
Studies of aetiology	Risk	Textword
Studies of diagnosis	Sensitivity	Textword

Search strategies are constantly being improved and updated. Recently a search query has been added to PubMed specifically for systematic reviews [10]. Robinson & Dickersin report a highly sensitive search strategy for controlled trials [11].

No one strategy will pick up 100% of the articles relevant to the research question that has initiated the study. Checking the references of the papers, asking experts in the area, and using different databases are ways of expanding the bibliography and making sure no important pieces of work are missed.

Levels of evidence

The research question determines the type of study design in which the best evidence can be found. For example, the gold standard for evaluation of a therapy's efficacy is the double blind randomised controlled design, while that for evaluation of prognosis is the prospective cohort study design. The level of the evidence of a result in a research paper is determined by the fulfilment of quality indicators in the research design and implementation.

The highest level of evidence is usually found in reviews of primary research conducted in a scientific manner, i.e. in systematic reviews. A systematic review will give an explicit answer to a focused question, clearly defining the search criteria used in selection of the primary papers (published and unpublished) considered, evaluate these for quality markers, extract the data systematically and analyse the data by a validated method. Homogeneity (the direction and degree of the results of the primary studies) is evaluated for further reinforcement of the validity of the results.

Meta-analysis is the technique of pooling and re-analysing data from primary studies. The data can be abstracted from the primary research reports or from the original patient data requested from the authors. Unpublished data can also be collected for the meta-analysis. This technique allows for an increase in power by enlargement of the "sample size", i.e. adding together samples investigated in several different studies.

Level of evidence is used to define the grade of a recommendation for clinical practice. Clinical practice guidelines are increasingly defining the *grade of recommendation* for each recommendation developed [12–14]. Individual clinical practice guidelines generally state their definitions of level of evidence and grade of recommendation. Table 2 is a summary of the grades of recommendations for therapy issued by the Centre for Evidence Based Medicine [15].

Table 2 Levels of Grades of Recommendations and Evidence for Therapy and Prevention (taken from http://www.cebm.net/levels_of_evidence.asp [15])

Grade of Recommendation	Level of Evidence	Therapy/Prevention
A	1a	Systematic review (with homogeneity)
	1b	Individual RCT (with narrow confidence interval)
B	2a	Systematic review of cohort studies
	2b	Individual cohort study (including low-quality RCT; e.g., 80% follow-up)
	3a	Systematic review (with homogeneity) of case-control studies
	3b	Individual case-control study
C	4	Case series
D	5	Expert opinion without explicit critical appraisal, or based on physiology, bench research or "first principles"

Databases

Electronic databases are very important tools in the search for information on healthcare to be used for research or clinical purposes. Finding the best electronic databases for the area of interest requires some research; librarians and research colleagues should be consulted, and authors should also explore the Internet. We will describe "PubMed", "EMBASE" and "The Cochrane Library".

PubMed

PubMed is the National Library of Medicine (NLM) search service that provides access to over 12 million citations in MEDLINE, PreMEDLINE, and other related databases, with links to participating online journals, through the Internet - http://www.ncbi.nlm.nih.gov/PubMed (Fig. 2).

PubMed Central provides access to full texts of articles collected from a growing number of journals.

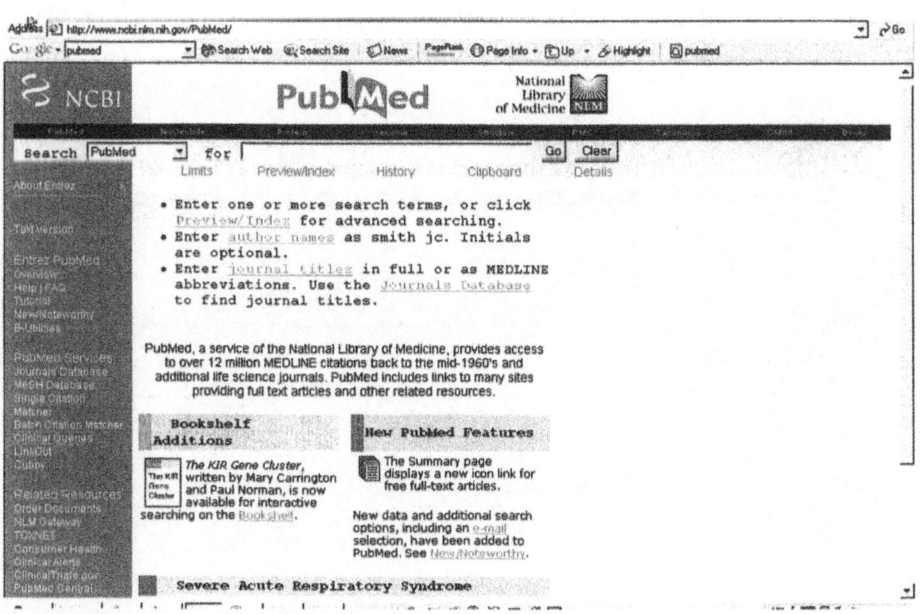

Fig. 2 PubMed Initial Screen

MEDLINE is the National Library of Medicine's premier bibliographic database, covering the fields of medicine, nursing, dentistry, veterinary medicine, healthcare systems and the preclinical sciences. MEDLINE contains bibliographic citations and author abstracts from more than 4,600 biomedical journals published in the United States and 70 other countries. The file contains over 12 million citations dating back to 1966. Coverage is worldwide, but most items are from English-language sources or have English abstracts.

Searching PubMed

The opening screen of PubMed is quite user friendly. The horizontal menu includes links that help in developing and focusing the search strategy. This menu includes "Limits", "Preview/index", "History", "Clipboard" and "Details"

- Limits

The "Limits" option can be activated by insertion of a check mark (Fig. 2). The "Limits" window displays field tags that are available to focus the search. There is an "All fields" option, where the choices to be selected from include: "Author Name", "Issue", "Journal Name", "Language", "MeSH Major Topic", "MeSH Term", Publication Type, "Text Word" and "Title Word".

Additional fields exist to give further support in focusing the search: "Publication Type", "Age Group", "Publication Date", "Languages", "Human

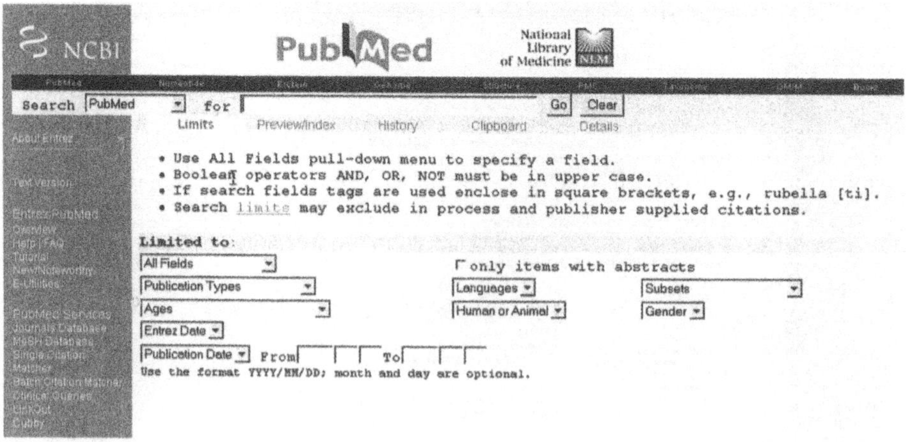

Fig. 3 PubMed "Limits" Screen
(http://www.ncbi.nlm.nih.gov/entrez/query.fcgi?CMD=Limits&DB=PubMed)

or Animal", "Database Subset" and "Gender". Examples of details of choices for different fields are described in Table 3.

Table 3 Description of Options Within "Field Tags" in the "Limits" Section of PubMed

Field: Publication type	Field: Ages	Field: Languages
Clinical Trial	Newborn: Birth to 1 month	English
Editorial	Infant: 1–23 months	French
Letter	Preschool child: 2–5 years	German
Meta-analysis	Child: 6–12 years	Italian
Randomised Controlled Trial	Adolescent: 13–18 years	Japanese
Practice Guideline	Adult: 19–44 years	Russian
Review	Middle Aged: 45–64 years Aged 65+: 65+ years Aged 80 and over: 80+ years	Spanish

- Preview/Index

In this window you can preview the number of articles retrieved during the search (Fig. 4). This feature helps you decide on the need to improve your search strategy before the abstracts are displayed.

Boolean logic operators allow you to combine search results. The most commonly used operators are "AND", "OR" and "NOT". If you use "AND"

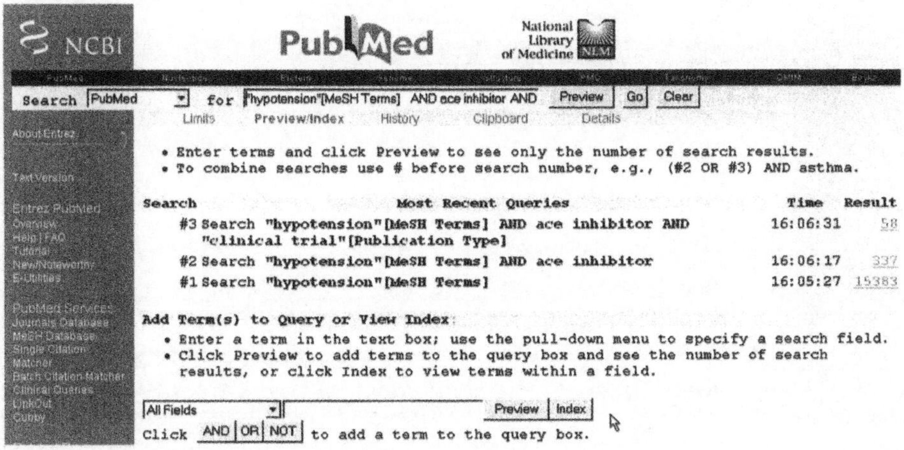

Fig. 4 Preview/Index Window in PubMed (http://www.ncbi.nlm.nih.gov/entrez/query.fcgi?CMD=Index&DB=PubMed)

this will narrow your results to articles that include search criteria of different search sets, while "OR" will combine all the articles found in different search sets, broadening the results. Use of "NOT" will exclude articles with a given characteristic from the search.

Using the index option you can search for terms indexed for a particular field (journal, MeSH) to see what is available. You can then choose to add the term to the search by clicking on Preview.

- History

A complete history of the search strategy is displayed. From this window search strategies can be incremented by using the numbers of previous searches rather than having to type out the whole strategy.

- Clipboard

The clipboard is a place where relevant citations can be saved during a search, by selecting Clipboard in the "Send to" box. The records that can be added are limited only in terms of a time interval (60 minutes of inactivity) or of total number, which cannot exceed 500. The records can be displayed in the available formats (citation, MEDLINE, etc.) at any time.

- Details

Details displays information about the search strategy being used. To save the search strategy for future use the text string can be copied and pasted into a Word document (Fig. 5).

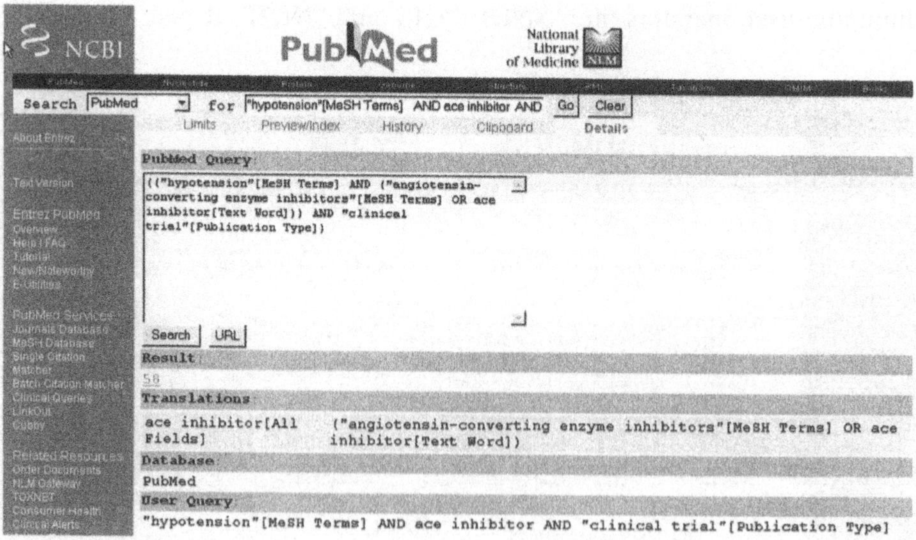

Fig. 5 Details screen in PubMed
(at http://www.ncbi.nlm.nih.gov/entrez/query.fcgi?CMD=Details&DB=PubMed)

- MeSH

MeSH is the controlled vocabulary used by the National Library of Medicine for indexing articles in PubMed. The MeSH terminology provides a consistent way of retrieving information in which different terms may be used for the same concepts.

The hyperlink MeSH Database (http://www.ncbi.nlm.nih.gov/entrez/query.fcgi?db=mesh) in the menu on the left of the PubMed screen can be used to find descriptors of interest and see how they relate to others. In MeSH the descriptors are organised in a hierarchical structure.

One useful feature is the "See related articles" tag that appears after any citation retrieved. If a search yields an article that meets an author's needs and more papers on the same topic are wished for, clicking on this link retrieves additional related articles.

EMBASE

EMBASE from Elsevier Science is a comprehensive biomedical and pharmacological database (biology, medicine, psychiatry and drugs), which is renowned for extensive indexing of drug information from 4,000 journals published in 70 countries. Embase is available only by subscription. Updates of the database appear less than a month after journal publication. The database contains over 9 million records from 1974 to the present. Around 450,000 new records are added annually. Each record contains the full bibliographic citation, indexing terms and codes. The database includes EMTREE, a hierarchically ordered controlled thesaurus, which contains 45,000 preferred terms and more than 190,000 synonyms.

The Cochrane Library

The Cochrane Library is an electronic publication designed to supply high-quality evidence about healthcare-related issues. It is published quarterly on CD-ROM and the Internet (http://www.update-software.com/cochrane/http://www.cochrane.org/cochrane/revabstr/ccsales.htm).

The Cochrane Library includes three databases plus other resources:

Cochrane Database of Systematic Reviews (CDSR): A rapidly growing collection of regularly updated, systematic reviews of the effects of healthcare. The systematic reviews are maintained by contributors to the Cochrane Collaboration, who are committed to 'preparing, maintaining and disseminating systematic reviews of the effects of healthcare.' New systematic reviews are added with each issue of *The Cochrane Library*. The Cochrane reviews deal mainly with randomised controlled trials.

Database of Abstracts of Reviews of Effectiveness (DARE): Includes structured abstracts of systematic reviews from around the world, which have been critically appraised by reviewers at the NHS Centre for Reviews and Dissemination at the University of York, England.

Cochrane Controlled Trials Register (CCTR): A bibliography of controlled trials identified by contributors to the Cochrane Collaboration and others. This is an international effort, with collaborators hand-searching the world's journals to create an unbiased source of data for systematic reviews. CCTR includes reports published in conference proceedings and in many other sources not currently listed in MEDLINE or other bibliographic databases.

Managing references

The development of software to manage references has greatly facilitated the organisation of references and the preparation of papers in general. Personal bibliographic software is designed to handle bibliographic information (journal articles, books, book chapters, conference proceedings, magazine articles, audiovisual material, patents, figures, images or even authors' own reference style) in a user-friendly way.

The software allows the organisation of references by subject area or by project. The software has a gateway to several databases on the Internet and allows direct downloads. References retrieved from a database can be saved in a specified format and then imported. Of course, there is still also the option of typing in the references individually.

When preparing a typescript, authors can insert citations automatically. To this end, the bibliography software is kept open, and on selection of any reference(s) insertion of it/them at the specific point in the text automatically follows. A powerful search capability helps in finding the references needed within the bibliography database. A personal reference database can be searched in the same way as online databases by using Boolean criteria. Once the reference(s) of interest are located they can be inserted in the text.

After insertion of the references the software will generate a bibliography and update citations in the manuscript to comply with the style defined. This can be done repeatedly, allowing changes to the text and addition or deletion of citations and any corresponding amendments to the body of the text and/or the bibliography to be made with a single mouse click. The software has predefined output formats for citations (e.g. Harvard or Vancouver style), but a personal style can also be defined. Some examples of personal bibliographic software are:

ENDNOTE- http://www.endnote.com/
PROCITE-http://www.procite.com/
REFERENCE MANAGER- http://www.refman.com/

Statistical analysis: data and distributions

Introduction

In order to read a scientific publication intelligently or to appreciate the results of a research project, it is essential to understand clearly how the data were collected and described. The lack of such information frequently results in a poor appraisal of a paper; more seriously, it can lead to erroneous conclusions.

Types of data

The information generated in a research project or published in a scientific paper usually falls in one of two broad categories of data: quantitative or qualitative.

Qualitative variables (also known as *categorical* or *nominal*) are not numerical, but denote different categories, rather than actual measurements of quantity (e.g., sex, marital status, presence/absence of diarrhoea). On the other hand, *quantitative* variables can take any numerical value along a continuous scale of measurement (*continuous* variables, e.g., temperature, arterial blood pressure, breathing frequency) or vary by finite specific steps (*discrete* variables).

Presentation of data

As a rule of thumb, for the presentation of qualitative data, the number of observations in each category of the variable should be counted and the absolute numbers and percentages displayed in a table. A very frequent problem faced by authors when preparing tables is the number of decimal places to be used in percentages. One decimal place is usually enough. It follows that the percentages may not add up to exactly 100%, and there is no universally accepted answer to this problem: one solution is to provide correct rounded values in the table so that the total does add up to 100%; alternatively, the correct total (99.9%, 100% or 100.1%) may be given or one of the percentages in the table is modified to give a total of 100%.

Qualitative data can also be presented as a *bar chart*, in which the categories of a variable (e.g. causes of death due to sepsis) are depicted on the horizontal axis and the frequencies (or relative frequencies, i.e. percentages), on the vertical axis. Another method of displaying categorical data is the *pie chart* or *pie diagram*, where the total area of a circle represents the total frequency, and each slice of the pie has an area proportional to the observed frequency in each category of the variable. Both presentations are depicted below.

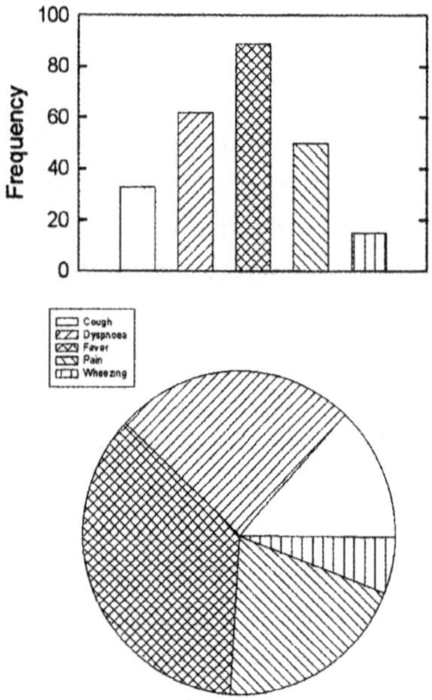

Fig. 1. The bar chart displays the number of individuals (population = 249) presenting with each of the five most prominent signs and symptoms associated with a certain respiratory disease. The pie chart shows the frequency of each as a percentage of the total count (or area)

Quantitative data can be also be presented in tables and in diagram form. The frequency with which the different possible values of a variable occur in a group of subjects is called the *frequency distribution* of the variable in the group. Both discrete and continuous variables can be expressed in the same way. Another point that must be stressed is that it is usually necessary to establish *class limits* for the data, e.g. body weight in *class intervals* of 5 kg: 50–55, 55–60, 65–70 etc. It is clear that the class intervals should not overlap and should cover the full range of the data. This concept of interval is also seen in *histograms*, which present the distribution of quantitative variables in a graphical way, usually with the data grouped into a number of intervals.

Reduction of the class interval (associated with larger and larger groups) makes it possible to transform the histogram (or frequency polygon) into a *frequency curve*. Frequency curves are often referred to in order to describe the shapes of distributions.

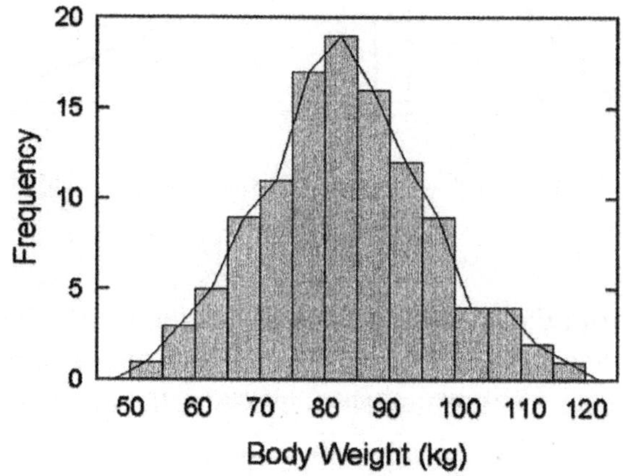

Fig. 2 The histogram shows the frequency distribution of the body weight of individuals admitted to an intensive care unit with a diagnosis of ARDS in a 6-month period. The *frequency polygon* is also shown superimposed on the histogram

Measures of central value

The most common measure of central value is the *arithmetic mean*. It is calculated by adding up all the observed values and dividing this total by the number of observations.

Although the (arithmetic) mean is the most commonly used measure of central value, there are other measures that are very useful. The *median* is the value that divides a distribution in half when the values are arranged in ascending or descending order. Generally, the mean and the median are not identical; in fact agreement between them depends on the shape and characteristics of the particular distribution concerned (see below).

The *mode,* another measure of central value, is defined as the most commonly occurring value. Data sets can have more than one mode (e.g. 3, 5, 5, 6, 7, 8, 8, 9, 10 has modes of 5 and 8) or no mode (e.g. 1, 2, 3, 4, 5). Thus, data with more than one mode are called *multimodal*, and a particular case, two modes, is that of the *bimodal* distribution.

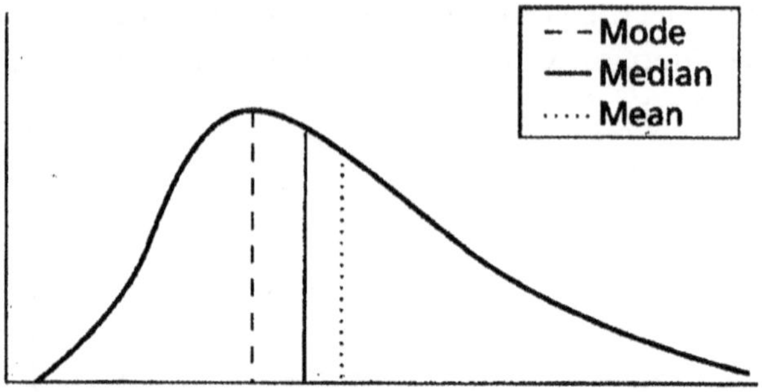

Fig. 3 Mean, median and mode in an asymmetrical distribution. Note that they do not coincide in this type of curve

It is obvious from the above definitions that the mean, the median and the mode are not identical except in the case of symmetrically distributed data. The mean is very sensitive to extreme values, whereas the median and the mode are not.

Quantiles

Mean, median and mode are measures of central value, meaning that they are intended to locate the centre of the distribution. It may be of interest to determine other points in the distribution. Thus, the total area under the frequency distribution curve can be divided into certain proportions, or *percentiles*. For instance, the value corresponding to 10% of the area under the curve is called the 10th percentile of the distribution. By definition, this means the median can also be called the 50th percentile. The 25th and 75th percentiles are sometimes given special names: the *lower quartile* and *upper quartile*, respectively.

Shapes of distributions

The *unimodal* distribution is a frequency distribution that rises to a maximum and then decreases. It is much more common than the *bimodal* distribution, where two "humps" can be seen.

Unimodal distributions can be divided into *symmetrical* and *skewed* distributions. In the former case a perpendicular drawn from the maximum point splits the area under the curve into two identical halves. In this case, mean, median and mode all have the same value. Skewed distributions are asymmetrical and tail off towards either the right (*positively skewed*) or the left (*negatively skewed*). Thus, for example, when a distribution is positively skewed most of the measurements are over to the left around the mode. *Normal distribution* is a very specific unimodal, symmetrical, bell-shaped distribution that will be described below.

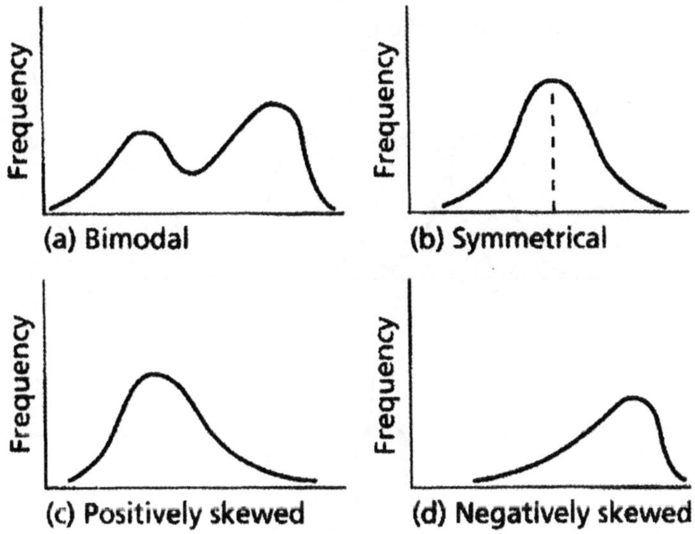

Fig. 4 Four examples of frequency distributions

There are some diverse transformations that can be applied to data to reduce skewness. In most cases it is necessary to proceed by trial and error, by representing the transformed distribution to look for the best result. However, some basic suggestions can be advanced: in the cases of low, medium and high positive skewness the square root, logarithmic and reciprocal transformations should be used, respectively, whilst in low and high negative skewness the square and cubic transformations, respectively, should be tried first. For instance, if the distribution presents a low positive skewness, each data point should be transformed by taking its square root, and the transformed frequency distribution should then be plotted to see whether the resulting profile is closer to being symmetrical.

Measures of dispersion

The *range* represents the interval between the largest and the smallest data values. It is based on only two observations and provides no idea whatsoever of how the observations are arranged between these two.

If the values of a variable do not vary much, observations will be dispersed closely around the mean, whereas if there is substantial variation observations will be scattered widely about the mean.

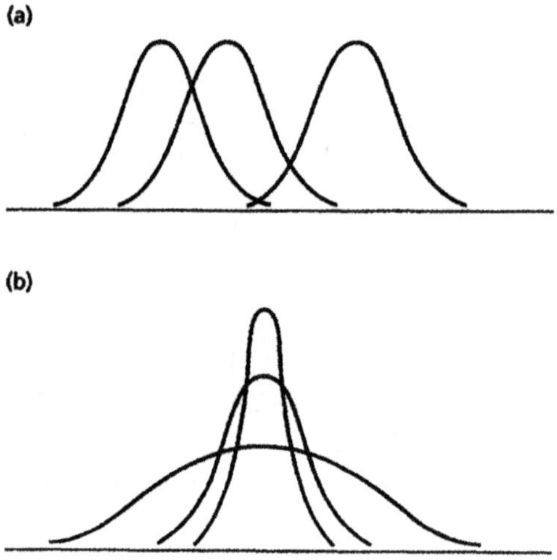

Fig. 5. Panels *a* and *b* show normal distributions. Note that in *a* the standard deviations are identical but the means do not coincide. In *b* the means coincide but the standard deviations diverge

This variability or *variance* (S^2) can be measured in terms of how far observations are, on average, from the mean or, in other words, by how far, on average, each observation deviates from the mean. Although the variance is a very useful mathematical measure of the average spread of the values around the mean, its interpretation is difficult because it is the square of the unit used for measurement, e.g. kilogram squared. Hence, it is more useful to take the square root of the variance to obtain the *standard deviation* (SD) (sometimes also called the *root mean square deviation*). The standard deviation is usually reported together with the mean.

If the variabilities of some measurements in two groups are to be compared, the standard deviation can be used. However, if the means of the two groups differ substantially, direct comparison of their standard deviations could be misleading. In such cases it might be useful to verify what the variation is relative to the mean. For this purpose the *coefficient of variation*, i.e. the SD expressed as a percentage of the mean, can be used.

Normal distribution

The *normal* or *Gaussian* distribution is unimodal, symmetrical and bell shaped and can be characterised entirely by its mean and standard deviation. Normal distributions can, naturally, have different means and diverse standard deviations. The term "normal" does not mean "common" or "typical"; nor is it used here to mean the opposite of "abnormal".

What distinguishes a normal distribution from other unimodal, symmetrical, bell-shaped distributions are its area properties, or, more precisely, some relationships between its percentile values and its mean and SD. First, 50% of the area lies above the mean and the remaining 50%, below the mean. In addition, 68.27% of the area under the normal distribution curve lies between mean±1 SD. Also, 95% of the area of a normal curve lies within mean±1.96 SD (mean+1.96·SD gives the 97.5th percentile, and mean–1.96·SD is the 2.5th percentile). These properties apply solely in the case of normal (or Gaussian) distributions.

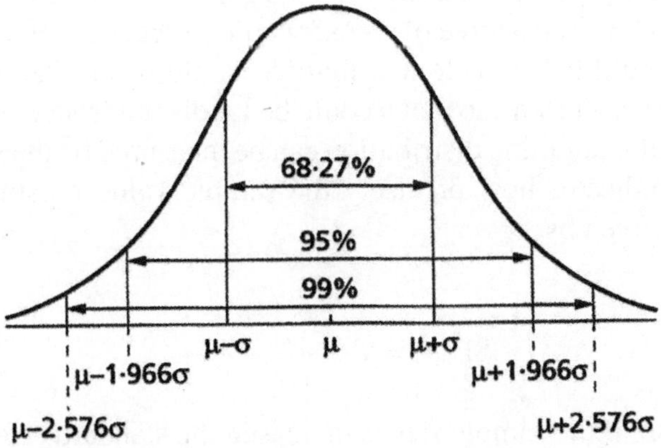

Fig. 6 Properties of the normal distribution. (μ population mean; σ standard deviation of the population mean)

Statistical inference

Populations and samples

Usually it is impossible to examine or study every single individual of a *population* of interest, and the researcher is left with the examination of a *sample of* n *individuals* drawn from this population, hoping that this sample is representative for the overall population. Without knowledge of the entire population it is impossible to know the true proportion of a population that carries a specific genetic trait or suffers from a certain disease. However, the proportion calculated from a random sample can be used as an estimate of the proportion in the entire population from which the sample was drawn.

In reality, different random samples will provide slightly different estimates of the true proportion of the population. It follows that any sample estimate is subject to *sampling error*. As an example, let us assume that a sample of 60 individuals resident in the same town revealed that 14 were smokers, so that the proportion of smokers was 23%. However, sampling error means it is unlikely that the proportion of smokers in the town is equal to exactly 23%. How far from 23% is it likely to be?

Suppose that all possible samples of 60 individuals in the town were studied, and the sample proportion p was computed. As mentioned above, the value of p will change from sample to sample. If all values of p were plotted, a *sampling distribution* of p would result. Most sample estimates would be located around the true (population) proportion π, whereas some would lie at some distance from this true value. The degree of spread would reflect how precise the sample proportion p would be. A wide distribution would mean that a great deal of sampling error was present, so that p could be far distant from π, and vice versa.

The spread of a sampling distribution can be measured by the *standard error* (SEp), which indicates how precisely the sample value π estimates the true value p, and is given by:

$$\mathrm{SE}(p) = \sqrt{\frac{p(1-p)}{n}}$$

In conclusion, if the sample size is increased the standard error will fall and the sampling distribution will become narrower. In addition, it is possible to demonstrate mathematically that 95% of all sample estimates will fall within two standard errors of π; 2.5% will fall more than two SEs below π and 2.5% will lie more than 2 SEs above π.

The initial sample of 60 individuals may have come from any part of the above distribution, but there is a 95% chance that the observed proportion p lies within 2 SEs of the true value π. In other words, it can be said with 95% confidence that the true proportion π is between:

$$p \pm [2 \cdot \mathrm{SE}(p)]$$

This interval is called a 95% confidence interval (or 95% confidence limits). The confidence interval is in fact a range of values that is likely to encompass the true population value, but there is no absolute certainty that it will. The confidence interval gives the precision of the sample estimate of a parameter. The size of the sample determines the precision of the estimate: the bigger the sample, the more precise the sample estimate is likely to be.

To be more confident that the interval includes the correct value, the 99% confidence interval can be computed. For this purpose 2.58 is substituted for 2 in the above formula, giving:

$$p \pm [2.58 \cdot \mathrm{SE}(p)]$$

It should be stressed that for all the above to apply the sample should be randomly selected from the population of interest, which has been thoroughly defined beforehand. In other words, every single individual in the population must have an equal chance of being in the observed sample.

When the degree of association between two variables is measured, the confidence interval can be used to determine whether the observed association might be due to chance. If it overlaps the null value (no association) it is equivalent to a nonsignificant result. If it excludes the null value the result is statistically significant.

Hypothesis testing

Statistical significance testing is a method used in attempts to quantify the chance of obtaining the observed results if there is no true difference between groups or association between factors in the whole population.

A researcher conducting a study should have a theory in mind. For example, low tidal volume is better than high tidal volume in the treatment of acute respiratory distress syndrome (ARDS). This theory is called the *study hypothesis*. The *null hypothesis* states that the treatments are equally effective. If the null hypothesis were true, then all ARDS patients with low and with high tidal volumes would have the same responses. The *alternative hypothesis* states that the results of the treatments are different.

Once the null hypothesis is defined, the main question is: If the null hypothesis is true, what are the chances of getting the observed difference? For instance, in the ARDS trial, what is the probability of getting a treatment difference as large as (or larger than) 45% versus 15%? This probability is determined by applying an appropriate statistical test.

Values of P in excess of 0.1 are generally considered large enough to accept the null hypothesis, i.e. to accept that there is insufficient evidence of a true difference. It is widely accepted that $P<0.05$ indicates that there is substantial evidence that the null hypothesis is untrue. This arbitrary cut-off value has been used to decide definitively between significant and nonsignificant. Rather, the true P-value should be reported and the results discussed accordingly.

In summary, when dealing with statistical significance testing investigators should always keep the following sequence in mind: (i) State the study hypothesis; (ii) formulate the null hypothesis; (iii) collect the data; (iv) apply the statistical significance test; and (v) reject or fail to reject the null hypothesis.

The significance test

The probability (P) that a result could have arisen if the null hypotheses were true must be calculated for every significance test. If the P-value is less than the significance level the hypothesis is rejected. It should be borne in mind that the significance level should be stated before the test is applied, i.e. the cut-off value for P determining whether a result is accepted as statistically significant or nonsignificant must be known beforehand ($P<0.05$ and $P<0.01$ are often used).

One-sided and two-sided tests. In patients with a particular disease the mean survival is 36 months. Investigators now wish to determine whether the use of a certain new drug improves the survival rate of the same population. The null hypothesis states that the new drug has no effect on survival, and can be written as:

$$H_0{:}\mu_D = 36 \text{ months}$$

where H_0 reads 'the null hypothesis is' and μ_D represents the mean survival in the population treated with the new drug. The alternative hypothesis:

$$H_A{:}\mu_D \neq 36 \text{ months}$$

does not distinguish between a significant positive or negative response. In this case, assuming that the cut-off point has been established as $P<0.05$, a *two-tailed* or *two-sided* significance test must be used. In other words, the significant result could lie at either extreme (or tail) of the normal distribution. Thus, the 5% value would be distributed as 2.5% at the lower extremity and 2.5% at the higher side.

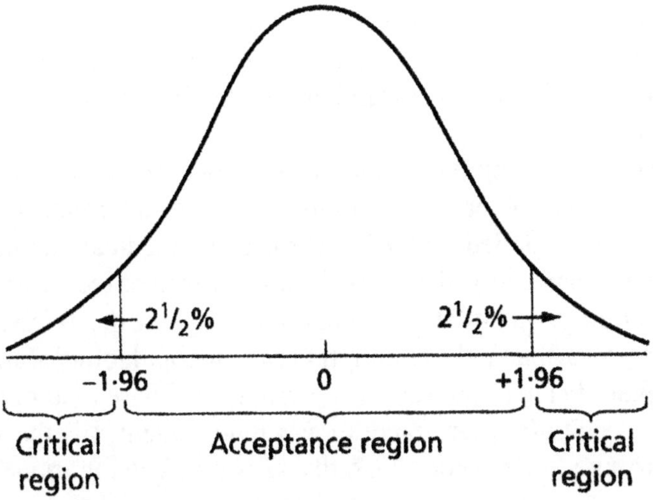

Fig. 7 The normal distribution. At each 'tail' there is a critical region for rejection of H_0 equal to 2.5%. The limits are the mean±1.966·SD for a 95% confidence interval

Naturally there will be situations in which the alternative hypothesis can only be either smaller or larger values than the control value, e.g. (H_A:μ_D < or H_A:μ_D >). In this case the *one-tailed* or *one-sided* test must be employed.

Independent and paired comparisons. *Independent samples* are taken from the independent populations under study. In other words, the selection of subjects for one sample group is not affected by the individuals already selected for the other groups. For instance, suppose that a cardiologist wishes to evaluate the effects of different hypotensive medicines. One group of patients will receive drug A, another will be treated with drug B and so on, up to the last drug of interest. Each of these groups can be considered to be a sample from one of the *n* populations defined by the hypotensive drug under consideration.

A *paired sample* occurs in two- or many-group comparisons when every individual in one of the groups has a unique match or pair in the other groups. Two or more treatments can be compared in a group of patients to whom different hypotensive medicines are administered one at a time. This particular situation is known as *self-pairing*. *Natural pairing* can be observed, for instance, when animal experiments use littermates: one group of rats is assigned to one treatment while the remaining littermates will receive another one. *Artificial pairing* commonly arises when controls can be chosen individually and matched to cases for potential confounding variables, such as age and weight.

Between the independent and paired data there are the *frequency-matched* data. These occur when the distribution of a variable, or variables, is required to be identical in the groups. For example, each group must display the same proportions of individuals in a number of weight categories, without any matching of individuals.

Parametric and nonparametric significance tests. The measurement scale of the variable under consideration can also determine the statistical hypothesis test to be applied. In the biomedical and medical literature, the vast majority of significance tests deal with the comparison of means or proportions with consideration of quantitative or qualitative data, respectively.

Significance tests that make assumptions about population parameters of the variable under study are known as *parametric tests*. These assumptions are: (i) the samples in each group are random and independent; (ii) the samples are normally distributed or not too markedly skewed (*Kolmogorov-Smirnov test with Lilliefors' correction* can be used to check the normality of the data distribution); and (iii) the variances of the groups are identical (*Levene's test of homogeneity of variance* may be used to test for this). Sometimes assumptions can be made valid with a suitable transformation of the data, as already discussed in this chapter. In summary, parametric tests are used for quantitative data, to test hypotheses about means and to make assumptions about parameters in the population.

In some situations, checking whether the aforementioned assumptions hold true is not feasible, especially when the sample size is relatively small and there is still doubt about the validity of a test in the face of a set of quantitative data. Most statistical tests of ordinal data are assumption free and are called *nonparametric, distribution-free* or *rank tests*. They are very useful, providing a fall-back since quantitative data can be analysed as ordinal data, but parametric tests are more powerful in detecting differences when the underlying assumptions hold. Nonparametric tests evaluate a null hypothesis relating to median values rather than mean values. It must also be said that many parametric tests do not have nonparametric counterparts. Briefly, it can be said that nonparametric tests are used for quantitative or ordinal data, and that they test hypotheses about medians, make few assumptions and are useful and easily applied to small sample sizes.

Type I and type II errors, sample size and power of the study

The table below depicts the main elements of the decision process. The columns correspond to reality: is the null hypothesis true or false? The rows represent the decision taken: is the null hypothesis (H_0) to be accepted or rejected?

If H_0 holds true and a nonsignificant result is obtained the correct decision has been reached. If the null hypothesis is true and a significant result is achieved the decision to reject H_0 is incorrect, yielding a *type I* or α (alpha) *error*, i.e. the probability of rejecting the null hypothesis when it is true. The significance level of the test must then be revised.

		Reality	
		Null hypothesis true	Null hypothesis false
	Do not reject H_0	Correct decision	β or type II error
Decision	Reject H_0 (significant result)	α or type I error	Correct decision

If the null hypothesis is false, and H_0 is not rejected, a *β* or *type II error* is made. The chances of type II errors depend on the true value of the population mean. The actual size of the ß probability depends on the overlap between the sampling distributions of the mean under: (i) the null hypothesis and (ii) a specific alternative hypothesis for which the type II error is to be calculated. Type II errors can be reduced by: (i) lowering the significance level to a value greater than 5% (this will increase α), and (ii) diminishing the spread of the sampling distribution of the mean, thus reducing the overlap between the null and alternative hypotheses distribution curves. In other words, type II error can be reduced by increasing the sample size (preferred method).

The *sample size* should be calculated by someone familiar with statistical methods rather than relying on clinical experience or judgment. When the sample size is too small it is impossible to distinguish between real and spurious results. The requirements needed to calculate a sample size are: (i) significance level; (ii) the accepted chance to make a type II error; (iii) the size of what would be considered an important result; and (iv) an estimate of the population variability.

The *power*, or *sensitivity*, of a test (1–ß) is the probability of detecting the difference that is looked for when it is present. The power depends on: (i) the significance level; (ii) the size of the effect or difference to be detected; (iii) the underlying population variability; and, (iv) the sample size. It is desirable to have a high power or probability of detecting a difference between treatments to justify the efforts and ethical issues involved in conducting an experiment. The power of a significance test increases as the true size of the effect augments. Both sample size and power computations are used to determine the parameters for an intended experiment before it is actually carried out. Power or sample sizes can be determined for: (i) paired and unpaired *t*-tests; (ii) one-way analysis of variance; (iii) z-test comparison of proportions; (iv) Chi-square analysis of contingency tables; and, (v) correlation coefficients, all of which are introduced below.

If the power to detect a true difference is established at 80%, then there is a 20% chance that this real difference could be missed. Generally, power levels of 80%, 90% or 95% are used, and it is accepted that the size of the type II error should be around four times that of the two-sided significance level chosen. It thus follows that 80% power and 5% significance is the most common combination in the determination of the sample size, whereas 95% power is linked with 1% significance.

Associations

An association occurs when the value of one variable in an individual yields some information about the possible value that another will have. If an association is found, it is necessary to ask whether there could be another explanation for the phenomenon before trying to conclude whether there is a causal effect relating the variables. It must be borne in mind that the finding may be due to chance, bias or a real (causal) effect.

One explanation for an observed association is *chance*. In fact, most statistical tests evaluate the possibility that chance alone could explain the result. Special care should be taken with small sample sizes.

A *bias* can be defined as any factor or process that leads to a conclusion that differs from the truth. In fact attention to the avoidance of bias is needed at every stage of a study, from the study design up to the inferences and conclusions drawn from the data. Last but not least, bias can also occur during the writing up of the resulting scientific paper. Many biases pertain to specific study designs and will be dealt with later in this book.

Perhaps the most important bias that can be pinpointed results from *confounding*. In broad terms, a *confounder* is any factor that is related to both variables under study. It can either thwart a true association or generate a spurious one. A confounder can be controlled by design (matching, restriction or randomisation) or analysis (stratification or regression). On the other hand, other causes of bias cannot be corrected.

There are criteria to evaluate whether an observed effect can be considered *causal*: consistency, strength, specificity, temporality, coherence and reversibility of the association. The *consistency* of an association is assured if different methods of study design and results from diverse populations all lead to similar conclusions. The *strength* of an association is related to the degree of association between the variables or, in other words, a strong association results when the effect of the risk factor is large. *Specificity* implies that there is an unequivocal relationship between the variables: a cause–effect relationship is present. *Temporality* means that the risk factor was present before the disease occurred, for instance. *Coherence* implies that the association fits in with known facts relative to the natural history and biology of a disease. *Reversibility* relates to a decrease in the risk of disease when exposure is removed.

Hypothesis testing: two-group comparisons

Comparison of two independent means

The parametric *t*-test is used for the comparison of two means. The null hypothesis naturally states that the two means are equal. This statistical test is associated with a known distribution originated from theoretical considerations, so that tables can be used to evaluate whether the calculated *t*-value lies in the tails of the *t* distribution. A cautionary note (not only for the *t* distribution): different texts can give rise to statistical tables in diverse formats. Hence, it is advisable to become familiar with one set of tables and the corresponding tests.

Comparison of paired means

The independent *t*-test cannot be used under paired-data conditions. Instead, the parametric paired *t* is applied to the data. By definition, the sample sizes in both groups must be the same.

Comparison of two independent proportions or risks (2 × 2 tables)

The *z* test for two independent proportions. This is a nonparametric test, because it makes no assumptions in relation to the distribution of the variables being examined (some authors would not include this sort of test in the 'nonparametric' category, arguing that the term should be reserved exclusively for 'rank tests'). As an example, let us imagine that a 5-year outcome (patients alive or dead) is being analysed in patients to whom two distinct drugs (A and B) have previously been administered. The 5-year outcome is the response variable and is entered as column headers in the 2 × 2 *contingency table*, while the drugs administered are aspects of the explanatory variable (exposure) and are shown as rows in the table. The null hypothesis states that the survival rates (outcome variable) are equal in both groups (taking drugs A or B).

The Chi-square test for two independent proportions. For this test the data are laid out in a 2 × 2 table, and the test is based on the observed and expected (null hypothesis) frequencies in each of the four cells of the table. Absolute numbers must be used, rather than percentages or proportions. It is noteworthy that when the expected values are added up across rows and down columns, the total number of cases must be identical to those resulting from the observed numbers. The calculated value for Chi-square is referred to tables of the Chi-square distribution, and the critical value given in the table must be exceeded for a result to be significant. For total sample sizes less than 20, *Fisher's exact* test (see below) should be used. Yates' correction is applied to the calculation of Chi-square for sample sizes between 20 and 40.

Fisher's exact test for two independent proportions. The Chi-square test is generally not recommended when the frequency in any of the cells in a 2 × 2 table is less than 5. In these conditions, *Fisher's exact* test is used instead. Fisher's exact test is based on fixed row and column totals and is therefore theoretically not applicable to all 2 × 2 tables. This test is quite complex to perform manually.

Comparison of paired proportions

McNemar's test for paired proportions. This is a test to be used with paired samples of a binary variable. Often the groups are cases and controls in a pair-matched case-control study and the binary variable is exposure/nonexposure to a risk factor (see below). Paired data are frequently incorrectly analysed by the Chi-square test, which does not take account of the fact that the groups are not independent.

Exact sign test. The *exact sign test* is used for small sample sizes; in fact, it may be regarded as one form of the McNemar test

Comparison of two independent medians

If the conditions are such that the assumptions inherent in the use of the parametric independent *t*-test do not hold, and especially with small sample sizes, the *Mann-Whitney U-test* for independent medians should be used instead. In this case two independent random samples from two populations (sizes may differ) with medians m_1 and m_2 are tested for the null hypothesis H_0: $m_1 = m_2$. The basic assumption is that the distribution of the variable is continuous and that it is skewed. In fact this test is valid for the comparison of both means and medians, but its power is lower than that of the *t*-test.

Comparison of paired medians

The sign test for paired medians. This nonparametric test examines the null hypothesis H_0: $m_1 = m_2$. The data may be quantitative or ordinal, but a continuous distribution of the data is assumed. It is extremely easy to perform. For instance, if the intention is to compare the reactions of a group of *n* patients to two different drugs, with the patients rating the effectiveness of each one on a scale of 0–10, two columns will result: one with the rating for the effect of drug A and another for that of drug B. A third column will result, in which the sign of the remainder when the score given by each patient to drug B is subtracted from that given by the same patient to drug A. Thus, a series of zeros (A=B), plus signs (A>B) and minus signs (A<B) will be written down. Tied pairs (A=B) will be disregarded, and the number of plus signs and untied pairs recorded, as seen in the table below. There are critical values for the sign test in specific tables.

Patient	Drug A	Drug B	Sign of A–B
1	5	3	+
2	7	3	+
3	5	5	0
4	4	5	-
5	4	2	+
6	8	6	+
7	8	8	0
8	8	9	-
9	3	2	+
10	6	4	+

n_+ = number of "+" signs = 6; n = number of untied pairs = 8.

The Wilcoxon signed rank test for paired medians. The sign test for paired medians does not take account of the magnitude of the difference between the effects of drugs A and B. The *Wilcoxon signed rank test for paired medians* can provide that missing magnitude and is hence more powerful than the former sign test. In this test two individually matched samples, each (*n* observations) of a quantitative or ordinal variable, are tested for H_0: $m_1 = m_2$. The differences between "before" and "after" for each pair are ranked and ordered irrespective of the sign (+ or –). Tables of critical values for the paired sign test are available.

Comparisons among more than two groups

When comparing more than two groups it is very tempting to use multiple *t*-tests (group A × group B, A × C, and B × C, for instance). This is not correct, because the significance level would be larger than the established one for a single *t*-test. The correct technique for comparing means or medians in three or more groups is known as *analysis of variance* (= ANOVA). A *one-way ANOVA* is used in the face of only one variable that defines the groups. When groups are defined by two variables, a *two-way ANOVA* is applicable, instead. There are parametric and nonparametric ANOVAs, and also ANOVAs for independent and repeated measures. Thus, ANOVA tests for differences among group means or medians and the result will allow acceptance or rejection of the null hypothesis (H_0: no difference among treatments; alternative hypothesis: at least one treatment differs from the others). In other words, the investigator will conclude that there are (or are not) differences among the groups. ANOVA does not determine which group(s) is(are) different, or the sizes of these differences. Multiple comparison tests isolate these differences by running comparisons between the experiment groups. Qualitative data relating to more than two groups can also be analysed.

Analysis of variance

To choose which ANOVA to apply to the data, first the normal distribution is tested in all groups, as is the similarity among the variances. If the data are deficient in any one of them, a nonparametric ANOVA is indicated; conversely, a parametric ANOVA should be used if both assumptions are accepted. Then the experimental design will indicate whether the groups are independent of each other or whether the same individual appears in all of them (repeated measures).

Under parametric conditions, therefore, the researcher will use an ANOVA or an ANOVA for repeated measures. Their nonparametric counterparts are, respectively, the *Kruskal-Wallis ANOVA on ranks* and the *Friedman repeated-measures ANOVA on ranks*. The result of an ANOVA is expressed as an *F* statistic, for which tables of critical values are available.

Multiple comparisons

There are two classes of multiple comparison procedures: all pairwise comparisons, where every pair of groups is compared, and multiple comparisons versus a control, where all treatments are compared with a single control group.

Tukey test. The *Tukey test* and the *Student-Newman-Keuls* test are conducted in a similar way to the Bonferroni *t*-test. The Tukey test is more conservative than the Student-Newman-Keuls (SNK) test and is therefore less likely to determine that a given difference is statistically significant. This test is used in the case of all pairwise comparisons (not recommended for multiple comparisons versus a control).

Student-Newman-Keuls test. The *SNK test* is less conservative than the Tukey test, which means it is more likely to determine that a given difference is statistically significant. The SNK test is usually more sensitive than the Bonferroni *t*-test and is only available for all pairwise comparisons.

Bonferroni *t*-test. The *Bonferroni t-test* performs pairwise comparisons with paired *t*-tests. It can perform both all pairwise comparisons and multiple comparisons versus a control and is the most conservative test for both conditions.

Fisher's least significance difference test. The *Fisher's least significance difference (LSD) test* is the least conservative of all pairwise comparison tests. Because it makes no attempt to control the error rate when detecting differences between groups, it is not recommended.

Dunnett's test. *Dunnett's test* is the analogue of the SNK test for multiple comparisons against a single control group. This test is less conservative than the Bonferroni *t*-test and is only available for multiple comparisons versus a control.

Duncan's multiple range test. *Duncan's test* is similar to the Tukey and SNK tests. Although it has greater power to detect differences than the other two tests, is has less control over the type I error rate and is therefore not recommended.

Dunn's test. *Dunn's test* must be used for ANOVA on ranks when the sample sizes in the different treatment groups are different. It can be used with both all pairwise comparisons and multiple comparisons versus a control. The all pairwise Dunn's test is the default for data with missing values.

Comparison of independent proportions in more than two groups

The usual Chi-square test is also appropriate for multigroup comparisons. In fact, the test is applicable to tables of any dimensions, providing the groups in the table are independent. If a Chi-square test comparing more than two groups gives a significant result it is not possible to determine which group(s) is(are) significantly different from which. Although more advanced tests are available to answer this question, visual inspection of the data may be sufficient to yield a conclusion.

The interesting aspect of the Chi-square test is that it also applies to quantitative data if quantitative variables are categorised, grouping them instead of using the exact data values. It must be borne in mind, however, that these categories must be picked before examination of the data to avoid any kind of bias.

Regression and correlation

Regression and *correlation* are methods of analysing relationships between quantitative variables. Before any regression or correlation analysis is started we strongly recommend plotting the data in a *scatter diagram* with the response (or 'dependent') variable plotted on the vertical (or y) axis, or ordinate, and the explanatory (or 'independent') variable on the horizontal (or x) axis, or abscissa.

Regression

Regression procedures use the values of one or more independent variables to predict the value of a dependent variable. The independent variables are the known, or predictor, variables. When the independent variables are varied they result in a corresponding value for the dependent, or response, variable.

Regression assumes an association between the independent and dependent variables, which, when plotted on a Cartesian coordinate system, produces a straight line, plane, or curve. Regression finds the equation that most closely describes the actual data.

Simple linear regression. The *linear regression* is used to predict a trend in data or predict the value of a variable from the value of another variable by fitting a straight line through the data. If the existence of more than one independent variable is suspected the multiple linear regression should be tested.

Linear regression assumes an association between the independent and dependent variables that can be adequately fitted by a straight line. Linear regression finds the straight line that most closely describes, or predicts, the value of the dependent variable, given the observed value of the independent variable.

The equation used for a simple linear regression is the equation that describes a straight line:

$$y = \mathrm{a} + \mathrm{b}x$$

where y is the dependent variable, x is the independent variable, a is the intercept (value of the dependent variable when $x = 0$, the point where the regression line intercepts the ordinate) and b is the slope (increase in the value of y per unit increase in x). As the values for x increase, the corresponding value for y either increases or decreases if b is positive or negative, respectively.

Linear regression is a parametric test, that is to say that for a given independent variable value the possible values for the dependent variable are assumed to be normally distributed with constant variance around the regression line.

Multiple linear regression. *Multiple linear regression* is used to predict the value of one variable from the values of two or more other variables by fitting a plane through the data.

When the independent variables are changed they produce a corresponding modification of the dependent variable.

If it is known that there is only one independent variable, the simple linear regression should be used. On the other hand, if it is not known for sure whether all independent variables should be used in the model (or take part in the description of the dependent variable), the stepwise or best subsets regressions are used to identify the relevant independent variables from the selected possible independent variables. If the relationship is not represented by a straight line or a plane, the polynomial or nonlinear regressions (or a variable transformation, see above) should be tried.

Multiple linear regression assumes an association between the dependent and n independent variables that fits the general equation for a multidimensional plane, where $a_1, a_2, \ldots, a_n$ are the n intercepts, and $b_1, b_2, \ldots, b_n$ are the n slopes.

Multiple linear regression is a parametric test: this means that for a given set of independent variable values, the possible values for the dependent variable are assumed to be normally distributed and have constant variance about the regression plane.

Polynomial regression. *Polynomial regression* is used to predict a trend in the data or predict the value of one variable from the value of another variable by fitting a curve through the data that does not follow a straight line when it is known that there is only one independent variable.

If the relationships between the independent variables and the dependent variable are straight lines, the multiple linear regression should be used instead. If the relationship is not a linear polynomial, the nonlinear regression should be tried.

Polynomial regression assumes an association between the independent and dependent variables that fits the general equation for a polynomial of order n:

$$y = a + bx + cx^2 + dx^3 + \ldots + zx^n$$

where y is the dependent variable, x is the independent variable, $a, b, \ldots, z$ are the regression coefficients.

The order of the polynomial n is the highest exponent of the independent variable. A first-order polynomial is a straight line, a second-order (quadratic) polynomial is a parabola, and so on.

Polynomial regression is a parametric test, meaning that for a given independent variable value the possible values for the dependent variable are assumed to be normally distributed and to have equal variance.

Stepwise linear regression. *Stepwise linear* regression is used to predict a trend in the data, or predict the value of one variable from the values of one or more other variables, by fitting a line or plane through the data. It is especially useful when it is not known which independent variables contribute to predicting the dependent variable and the intention is to find the model with suitable independent variables by adding or removing independent variables from the equation.

If the independent variables to be included are already known, multiple linear regression should be used instead. If the few best equations from all possible models are wanted, best subsets regression should be used. If the relationship is not a straight line or plane, polynomial or nonlinear regressions are recommended.

Stepwise regression is a technique for selecting independent variables for a multiple linear regression from a list of candidate variables. The use of stepwise regression instead of regular multiple linear regression avoids the inclusion of extraneous variables and under- or overspecification of the model.

Stepwise regression determines which independent variables to use by adding or removing selected independent variables from the equation:

$$y = \mathrm{a} + \mathrm{b}_1 x_1 + \mathrm{b}_2 x_2 + \mathrm{b}_3 x_3 + \ldots + \mathrm{b}_n x_n$$

where y is the dependent variable, $x_1, x_2, x_3, \ldots, x_n$ are the independent variables, and $a, b_1, b_2, \ldots, b_n$ are the regression coefficients. The independent variable is the known, or predicted, variable. As the values of x_i vary, the corresponding value for y either increases or decreases, depending on the sign of b_i.

There are two approaches to stepwise regression: (i) Forward and (ii) backward stepwise regression.

In *forward stepwise regression*, the independent variable that produces the best prediction of the dependent variable (and has an F value higher than a specified F-to-enter) is entered into the equation first, the independent variable that adds the next largest amount of information is entered second, and so on. Once each variable is entered, the F value of each variable already entered is checked and any variables with small F values (below a specified F-to-remove value) are removed. This process is repeated until adding or removing variables does not significantly improve the prediction of the dependent variable.

In *backward stepwise regression* all variables are entered into the equation. The independent variable that contributes the least to the prediction (and has an F value lower than a specified F-to-remove) is removed from the equation, the next least important independent variable is removed, and so on. Each time a variable has been removed, the F value of each variable removed from the equation is checked and any variables with large F values (above a specified F-to-enter value) are re-entered into the equation. This process is repeated until adding or removing variables does not significantly improve the prediction of the dependent variable.

Best subsets regression. *Best subsets regression* is used to predict a trend in the data, or predict the value of one variable from the values of one or more other variables, by fitting a line or plane through the data. It is needed when it is not known which independent variables contribute to the prediction of the dependent variable and the intention is to find the subsets of independent variables that best contribute to predicting the dependent variable.

If the independent variables to be used are already known, the multiple linear regression should be used. If the idea is to select the equation model by incrementally adding or deleting variables from the model, stepwise regression should be the method of choice. If the relationship is not a straight line or plane, polynomial or nonlinear regressions should be employed.

Best subsets regression is a technique for selecting variables in a multiple linear regression by systematically searching through the different combinations of the independent variables and selecting the subsets of variables that give the 'best' prediction of the dependent variable. There are three criteria for 'best', and the results depend on which criterion has been chosen. (i) r^2, The *coefficient of determination* for multiple regression, is a measure of how well the regression model describes the data. The higher the value of r^2, the better is the model. However, the number of variables used in the calculation is not taken into consideration, and, consequently, models with more variables will always perform better, i.e., have higher r^2 values, whether or not the additional variables do contribute to the prediction. (ii) *Adjusted* r^2 is a measure of how well the regression model describes the data based on r^2, but takes into account the number of independent variables. (iii) *Mallow's Cp*: *Cp* is a gauge of the size of the bias introduced into the estimate of the dependent variable when independent variables are omitted from the regression equation, as computed from the number of parameters plus a measure of the difference between the predicted and true population means of the dependent variable. The optimal value of Cp is equal to the number of parameters (the independent variables used in the subset) plus 1.

No predicted values, residuals, graphs, or other results are produced with a best subsets regression. To view results, it is necessary to note which independent variables were used for the desired model and then perform a multiple linear regression using only those independent variables.

Nonlinear regression. Nonlinear regression is used when the data follow a curve that is a nonlinear function. Nonlinear regression solves the regression problem directly without transforming the data and performing linear regression techniques.

The nonlinear regression algorithm (Marquardt-Levenberg) seeks the values of the parameters that minimise the sum of the squared differences between the observed and predicted values of the dependent variable. The process is iterative: it starts with a 'guess' at the parameters, checks to see how well the equation fits, then continues to make more accurate guesses until the differences between the residual sum of squares no longer decreases significantly. This condition is known as convergence.

Nonlinear regression can fit almost any equation.

Correlation

Correlation procedures measure the strength of association between two variables, which can be used as a gauge of the certainty of prediction. Unlike regression, it is not necessary to define one variable as the independent variable and one as the dependent variable.

The *correlation coefficient*, *r*, is a number that varies between –1 and +1. A correlation of –1 indicates that there is a perfect negative relationship between the two variables, with one always decreasing as the other increases. A correlation of +1 indicates that there is a perfect positive relationship between the two variables, with both always increasing together. A correlation of 0 indicates no relationship between the two variables.

There are two types of correlation coefficients: (i) the Pearson product moment correlation, a parametric statistic that assumes a normal distribution and constant variance of the residuals; and (ii) the Spearman rank-order correlation, a nonparametric association test that does not require the assumption of normality or constant variance of the residuals.

The *Pearson product–moment correlation* is used to measure the strength of the association between pairs of variables without regard to which variable is dependent or independent, to determine whether the relationship, if any, between the variables is a straight line. It is used when the residuals (distances of the data points from the regression line) are normally distributed with constant variance. To predict the value of one variable from another the simple or multiple linear regression should be used.

The *Spearman rank order correlation* is used to measure the strength of association between pairs of variables without specifying which variable is dependent or independent, and the residuals are not normally distributed with constant variance. The Spearman rank order correlation is computed by ranking all values of each variable, then computing the Pearson product moment correlation coefficient of the ranks. The Spearman rank order correlation is a nonparametric test that does not require the data points to be linearly related.

Finally, it can be shown that the *coefficient of determination*, r^2 (the square of the correlation coefficient), represents the proportion of the total variation in the dependent variable that is explained by the regression line. Assuming that the correlation coefficient of the linear regression between residual volume and age equals 0.52, r^2 amounts to 0.270. Hence, the variation in the age of the patients explains just 27% of the total variation in residual volume, and the other 73% of the variation remains unexplained and must result from other factors.

Study design

"The argument is not about the inherent value of different approaches and worthiness of investigators using them. The issue is which way of answering the specific question before us provides the most valid, useful answer."[16].

Medical research is usually divided into basic, epidemiological and clinical types. Basic research is often carried out in a laboratory, involving experimentation on animals or human beings. This kind of research can involve genetic, immunological, biochemical, physiological, pathophysiological and other types of investigations. Clinical and epidemiological research tends to be more patient centred. Epidemiology deals with the determinants and distribution of disease in populations, and clinical research deals directly with patients who have a disease.

Most clinical studies involve comparison of groups and can be broadly divided into two categories: observational and experimental.

Before considering the study designs, some concepts regarding what is being studied have to be established: the outcome, the primary exposure or risk factor of interest (the one which is included in the hypothesis) and other exposures that may influence the outcome (confounders).

An outcome can be a defined as a disease, death or a state of health.

A confounder is an alternative explanation for the outcome. In order to be a confounder, a factor has to be associated with the exposure being investigated and independently associated with the risk of developing the outcome of interest.

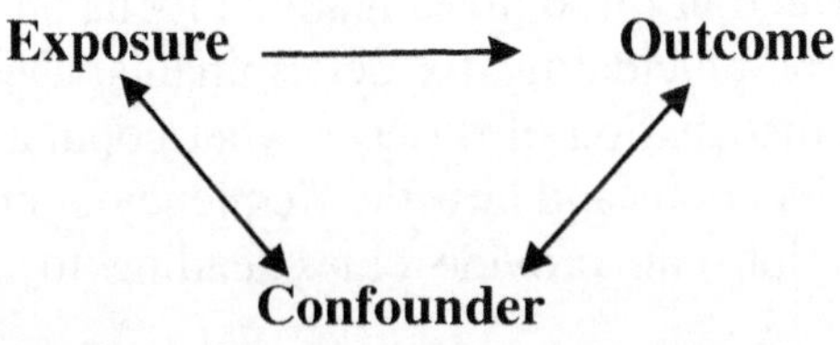

For example, the association of drinking coffee (exposure) and increased risk of myocardial infarction (outcome) could be due in part to the habit of cigarette smoking (confounder), since coffee consumption is associated with smoking and smoking is independently associated with the risk of myocardial infarction.

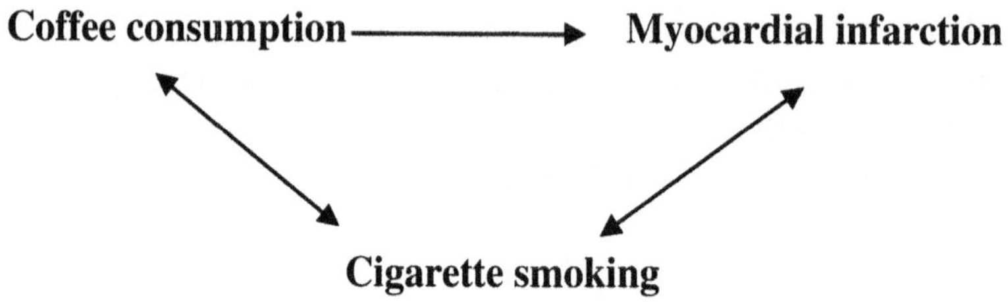

A factor can be an outcome in one study and an exposure in another.

The first step in a research study is to define the hypothesis that is to be tested. This should be done in a way that makes it clear what the primary outcome(s), exposure(s), and potential confounders are. Then, the most appropriate design will be chosen. In designing a study to determine whether there is an association between exposure (risk factor) and an outcome (a disease), the potential alternative explanations that might be responsible for such an association should be anticipated.

Awareness of the existence of a confounding factor is essential in clinical studies, and many study designs are built up around the control of confounding.

Observational studies

Observational studies collect information on events that are happening or have happened and over which we have no control. Data can be collected from populations or from individuals. In some observational studies the outcome of interest is described with no reference to exposure (descriptive studies), while others consider a possible association of outcome of interest and exposure (analytic studies).

The basic strategy designs used in clinical research can be broadly categorised according to whether these investigations focus on describing the distributions of disease or elucidating its determinants. Descriptive studies are concerned with the distribution of disease, what populations are affected and in what geographic locations and how the frequency of occurrence varies over time. Such information can provide clues leading to the formulation of a hypothesis that is consistent with existing knowledge of disease occurrence. Analytic studies focus on the determinants of a disease by testing the hypothesis formulated from descriptive studies.

Descriptive studies

A descriptive study describes the general characteristics of the distribution of a disease, mainly related to person, place and time. Information such as age, sex, race, marital status, occupation, medication use, consumption of foods, geographic distribution of a disease and seasonal patterns in disease onset are examples of the kind of data that can be collected. They can be done quickly and easily, as such information is usually freely available. Descriptive studies have usually provided reliable information about the possible determinants of a disease. However, owing to limitations of the design, this kind of study is mainly useful for the formulation of a hypothesis that can be tested later using an analytic design.

There are three main types of descriptive studies: correlational (ecological) studies, case reports or case series and cross-sectional studies.

Correlational or ecological studies. The correlational study uses data from entire populations to compare disease frequencies between groups during the same period of time or in the same population at different times. Since they refer to whole populations, it is not possible to draw conclusions about exposure in the individual and the risk of the outcome. Therefore, although correlational studies are useful for generating hypotheses, they have many limitations and can be very misleading at times.

In order to investigate the patterns of mortality from coronary heart disease in 1960, death rates from 44 states of the USA were correlated with per capita cigarette sales. Death rates were higher in states with the highest cigarette sales, and lower in states with lowest sales. The hypothesis that smoking cigarettes has a causal effect on coronary heart disease was then formulated. Various subsequent analytic studies have proved this hypothesis.

Correlational studies are frequently used as a first step in investigating a possible exposure–disease relationship. They are quick and cheap, and the information is readily available. The main limitation is the inability to link exposure with disease in individuals. A second limitation is the lack of any way of controlling for possible confounders. Thus, the presence of an association does not imply the presence of a statistically valid association.

Case reports and case series. The case report is the most basic type of descriptive study of individuals. Such reports are usually used to describe a new or unusual condition or circumstance and are often the first reported indications of a problem. Case series are collections of individual case reports in a short period of time; they usually indicate the beginning or presence of an epidemic. For example, acquired immunodeficiency syndrome, Crohn's disease and many other conditions were originally reported as case series. Case reports and case series are limited to careful description of single problems and suggestions for potential hypotheses to be tested in future studies.

Case reports are among the most common types of studies published in medical journals. Case reports document unusual medical occurrences and may be the first clues in the identification of a new disease or adverse effect of exposures.

Cross-sectional surveys. In cross-sectional studies the presence or absence of both the exposure and the disease are determined at the same time point. For example, a cross-sectional survey might determine whether subjects are current smokers (exposure) and whether they have evidence of emphysema (disease). Because both exposure and disease are determined at the same time, in most cases it is impossible to determine which came first. Therefore, cross-sectional studies can suggest associations between an exposure and a disease, but cannot prove causality. Cross-sectional studies are relatively cheap and simple to conduct and take only a short time. For these reasons, they are frequently used for planning purposes. In general, they are used to estimate the prevalence of common conditions of reasonably long duration or to determine the distribution of continuous variables within a population.

Hypothesis formulation from descriptive studies:

The first step in the search for the solution to a problem is to formulate a testable hypothesis. Descriptive data address such questions as:

1. Who is getting the disease?
2. Where are the rates of disease highest and lowest?
3. When does the disease occur commonly or rarely?
4. Is the frequency of this disease at present different from its frequency in the past?

Analytic studies

Analytic study designs are used for testing the hypotheses formulated by descriptive studies. These studies enable comparison among groups, determining whether or not the risk of disease is greater in individuals exposed or not exposed to a known risk factor.

Analytic studies can be divided into observational and experimental studies. In observational studies, the researcher does not interfere with the natural course of events. In experimental studies, the researcher allocates exposure at random in a sample of sufficiently large size, following up the groups to check for the development or not of the outcome of interest.

There are two main types of observational analytic studies: case-control and cohort.

Case-control study

A case-control study is designed to help determine whether an exposure is associated with the outcome of interest. The first step is to identify a group of cases, i.e. individuals with the outcome of interest (a disease) and a group of controls (individuals without the illness). The proportion exposed to a suspected risk factor is then measured in the two groups and compared. If the proportion of subjects exposed to the factor is higher in the case group than in controls, then the exposure might be a risk factor for the disease. If it is lower, it might be a protective factor.

A case-control study can be used to investigate the relationship between exposure and outcome. If there is a strong association and it meets temporal requirements, i.e. exposure occurs before the outcome, then the hypothesis that there is a causal connection can be set up. The relationship between lung cancer and smoking [17] is a historical example. Further research is required to support the theory of causation. Case-control studies are also useful to identify adverse effects of treatment.

Study question. The first step in designing a case-control study is to state clearly what the study question is.

Definition and selection of cases. The definition of a case is essential. Diagnostic criteria should be explicit and clear, to ensure the selection of cases that represent a homogeneous entity.

An important decision is whether to include both prevalent and incident cases. Prevalent cases include those in patients who may have had the disease for some time and may exclude those who died soon after the diagnosis was made. If the risk factor is related to early mortality then the effect will be diluted. These patients are still alive and still ill, and may have changed their habits because of the disease. Prevalent cases reflect determinants of duration as well as the development of the disease. The interpretation of such a study may be complicated. Incident cases include those of newly diagnosed patients. Whenever possible, it would be better to limit the cases to those newly diagnosed within a determined period.

Once the definitions of disease and diagnostic criteria have been clearly established, the individuals can be selected from different sources.

The study might be hospital based, which involves identifying patients with the disease who have been treated at a particular hospital during a specified period of time. This is the more common procedure, because it is relatively inexpensive and easy to conduct.

Alternatively, the study might be population based, which involves locating and obtaining data on all affected individuals in a defined population over a period of time. The advantage is that it avoids bias arising from selection factors. In general, these studies are easier to interpret, but much more difficult to conduct.

Selection of controls. Selection of the control group is a very difficult task within the design of a case-control study. The controls must be representative of the population that the the cases also come from; otherwise selection bias will be introduced. A member of the population is eligible to be a control if that person would have been selected for the study as a case if he/she had developed the disease or outcome of interest.

Source of controls: The question to keep in mind when selecting controls is "What is the population from which the cases originated?" When choosing hospital controls care should be taken to avoid selection bias. Hospitalised people usually tend to have a higher prevalence of adverse exposures than the general population. Also, patients with diseases known to be associated with the exposure of interest should be excluded from the control series. The best arguments for using hospital controls are cost and logistics. The use of general population controls ensures a high level of comparability. Identifying controls in the general population is usually more costly and time consuming than identifying controls from hospitals.

Matching: The effect of confounders can be adjusted for in the design of the study. Matching is the procedure for choosing controls for having the same distribution as cases in terms of confounders. Common matching variables are age, sex, place of residence or socio-economic status. Care should be taken not to match too many variables, which could lead to difficulties. There are other ways to control potential confounding in case-control studies: restriction, stratification, logistic regression, etc. Matching should not take place on variables related to the risk factor only, since this will result in equal distribution of risk factors in cases and controls and therefore no result. Cases could be individually matched to one or more controls or frequency-matched to controls (equal number of cases and controls at each level of matching variable). Matching design requires matched analysis.

Measurement of exposure. Data on exposure can be collected in many ways—by examining medical occupational records, by taking biological samples or by personal, postal or telephone interviews. It is important that the information is not influenced by whether anyone is a case or a control.

Case-control studies are vulnerable to information bias because the individuals are recruited on the basis of their disease status. If the information is based on recall, this is a particular problem. Response bias refers to the situation in which the information given by study subjects differs between controls and cases. Recall bias is an example: the fact of having a disease may influence the recall of exposure. Responder bias may be minimised by keeping the individuals who are interviewed blind to the study as well as ensuring that both cases and controls have similar incentives to remember the events. Information should be collected by means of the same questionnaires and forms for cases and controls. The interviewer should be blind to the hypothesis under study and to who is a case and who a control, in order to avoid observer bias.

Analysis. To calculate the relative risk it is necessary to know the population at risk, and this information is not available in a case-control study. The only measure of association that makes sense in a case-control study is the odds ratio. The odds of an event is defined as the number of occurrences divided by the number of nonoccurrences.

$$\text{Odds of disease} = \frac{\text{No of subjects who develop disease during follow-up}}{\text{No of subjects who do not develop disease during follow-up}}$$

The odds of disease and risk of disease are two different measures of the same process. If risk is low, both numbers are very similar. Odds tend to be expressed as a ratio.

Odds = Risk / (1–Risk)

The odds ratio is the comparison of two odds.

$$\text{OR} = \frac{\text{Odds of disease in exposed subjects}}{\text{Odds of disease in nonexposed subjects}}$$

or

$$\text{OR} = \frac{\text{Odds of exposure in those with disease}}{\text{Odds of exposure in those without disease}}$$

Case-control studies can estimate the ratio of the odds of exposure, which can be a valid estimate of the odds of disease. Since case-control studies deal with rare diseases, the odds ratio is an acceptable approximation of the relative risk.

Unmatched case-control studies: Data from exposed and unexposed cases and controls can be arranged in a 2×2 table as follows:

	Cases	Controls
Exposed subjects	a	b
Unexposed subjects	c	d
Total	a+c	b+d

The odds ratio is obtained by dividing the odds of exposure in cases (a/c) by the odds of exposure in controls (b/d):

$$OR = \frac{a/c}{b/d} = ad/bc$$

Confidence intervals can be calculated.

Individually matched case-control studies: If the study is matched, then a matched analysis is necessary. Matched pairs are analysed for whether they are concordant or discordant in relation to their exposure.

	Control exposed	Control unexposed
Case exposed	a	b
Case unexposed	c	d

The odds ratio is b/c. Confidence intervals can be calculated.

In case-control studies, restriction, stratification and logistic regression can be applied to unmatched and matched data to control for confounding. An adjusted odds ratio is used to control for confounders. Logistic regression and stratified analysis are used for unmatched data. Logistic regression is used for matched data. For frequency-matched data, stratified analysis should be employed.

Interpretation of results. Quality indicators should be sought in the analysis of case-control studies. In a major review of case-control studies 35 different sources of bias were identified [18]. The selection of subjects and measurement of outcomes of interest were the main problematic areas for introduction of bias. When a case-control study is to be appraised the quality indicators include:

1. Do the selection criteria for control subjects match those of the case subjects in every respect except for the presence of disease or risk factor under scrutiny?
2. Were the measurements in control subjects free of bias?

If an association is found, it is necessary to consider whether it was due to chance, selection bias in the choice of cases and controls, information bias in the gathering of exposure data or the presence of confounding factors not considered or controlled for in the design of the study.

Advantages of case-control studies

1. They are quick and cheap.
2. They are the only feasible method for studying very rare disorders or those with a long time gap between exposure and outcome.
3. They can be used to investigate a wide range of risk factors.
4. Fewer subjects are needed than in cross-sectional studies.
5. The consistency of measurement techniques is maintained.

Disadvantages of case-control studies.

1. There can be bias in determination of exposure (recall bias, interviewer bias, missing data, lack of standardisation of pre-recorded data, measures affected by disease onset, use of nonnewly diagnosed cases).
2. There can be bias in the selection of controls (inappropriate source, over-matching).
3. Sorting out the sequence of events can be problematic (because retrospective).
4. No estimate of the absolute risk is possible.
5. There is only one end-point (disease).
6. The method is not suitable for investigation of rare exposures (unless they are the only cause of disease).
7. They do not allow an estimate of disease incidence.

Cohort studies

In a cohort or follow-up study a group of individuals who are exposed and a group who are unexposed to a potential cause of disease are followed up over time and the incidence of disease in one group is compared with that in the other. When exposure status is defined, all subjects must be free of the disease under investigation. All participants are then followed up to assess the occurrence of the outcome.

The structure of a cohort study is shown schematically below.

	Disease present	Disease not present	Total
Exposed	a	b	a+b
Nonexposed	c	d	c+d

Cohort studies are useful to evaluate aetiology, prognosis (natural history) and incidence of a disease, as all subjects in both groups (exposed and nonexposed) are free of disease at the beginning of the study. Incidence can be calculated as follows:

$$\text{Incidence rate} = \frac{\text{No of new cases of disease (in a time period)}}{\text{Population size}}$$

A cohort study design can be used to investigate research issues in specific circumstances, such as when it is not ethical to carry out a randomised controlled trial to determine the outcome of a treatment. The findings from this type of study enable the elaboration of quality indicators, e.g. readmission rates, to be based on the evidence. Experiments in the organisation and delivery of health services are also ideal for the cohort design; for example, the relationship between the volumes of procedures carried out in a hospital and such outcomes as complication rates or mortality might be examined in such a study.

There are three study design features that are pivotal in the outcome of an appraisal of a cohort study. The first is the recruitment of subjects, which must be evaluated for completeness. It can be useful to ask about the subjects not recruited. The possibility of a selection bias before the entry point must also be assessed. For example, the more severe cases may be referred elsewhere. Secondly, the criteria for evaluating outcomes of care must be valid or validated; for example, hospital mortality may vary owing to variations in length of stay and therefore is not a valid measure. A validated measure would be 30-day mortality. Third, when the results are analysed it is essential to make sure that some measure of control for co-morbidities is taken into account, as this can systematically bias the results.

Types of Cohort. Cohort studies can be prospective or retrospective. These terms refer to the temporal relationship between the initiation of the study and the occurrence of the disease outcomes being studied.

Prospective: The groups of exposed and unexposed individuals have been assembled but there have not yet been any cases of the disease. The researcher must follow up the patients for a specific period to ascertain the outcome of interest.

Retrospective: The investigation begins after both exposure and outcome have already occurred.

A cohort study is bidirectional when data are collected both retrospectively and prospectively in the same cohort. This type is applicable for exposures that have both short-term and long-term effects.

Retrospective studies can be conducted more quickly and cheaply than prospective studies. Hence, retrospective studies are more suitable for investigation of diseases with long latency periods, which would require many years for significant results to be achieved in a prospective study. However, it depends on the availability of previously recorded data on exposure. Sometimes this can mean that data are not complete and comparable for all study subjects: for example, information on possible confounders (i.e. smoking, diet, coffee intake) is not recorded.

In prospective studies the investigator can assess information on exposure and potential confounders directly from study subjects.

Study hypothesis. A clear hypothesis is essential. Usually the hypothesis has already been tested (more cheaply and quickly) by means of other study designs (e.g. case-control studies).

Selection of the exposed population. The group of subjects selected to represent the exposed group can originate from different sources. The choice of a particular group will depend on the frequency of exposures under study, the need for accurate and complete information on exposure, follow-up of all participants, and the nature of the hypothesis of the study.

If the exposure of interest is a rare condition, or related to a particular occupation, it is more efficient to choose a specific exposure population (e.g. people working in uranium mining, shipbuilding), which would allow recruitment of a sufficient number of exposed individuals in a reasonable period of time.

If the exposure is a common condition, the exposure population can be chosen from members of certain groups (professions), such as doctors, nurses and labourers, in whom collection of the relevant information will be easier.

Selection of the control group. As in case-control studies, the selection of the control group is an important step in the design of a cohort study. Groups being compared should be as similar as possible with respect to all factors related to the disease except the exposure under investigation. In addition, it is fundamental that the data obtained from the unexposed group be comparable to that recorded in the exposed one.

In cohort studies, it is important to consider the potential confounders at the beginning of the study and measure them accurately later on, so they can be taken into account in the analysis.

Sources of data. Another crucial point in designing cohort studies is the availability of complete and reliable information on all cohort members concerning the exposure under investigation and/or development of any outcome of interest.

Information on exposure status can be obtained from existing records (hospital, employer). This source has the advantage of information availability for almost all participants of the cohort and to provide unbiased information on exposure. However, information recorded some time before is sometimes insufficient to address some specific questions of the research. Also, potential confounders may not have been considered at the earlier time. In this case information may be provided by the participants in questionnaires or interviews. Bias may be introduced when data is collected in this way, as patients may have preconceived ideas about the exposure under investigation.

A cohort study offers the possibility of examining a range of outcomes, which will depend on the chosen method of measurement. Whatever the procedure, it is crucial for the validity of the study that the method of ascertainment be identical for those exposed and those unexposed.

Follow-up. Failure to collect information on every subject is a source of potential bias in a cohort study and would have a drastic influence on the validity of the results. The longer the follow-up period the more difficult it will be to achieve complete follow-up, as more subjects are likely to move and change jobs. A drop out of 10–15% is usually considered acceptable.

Analysis. There are many ways of comparing the risks in exposed and nonexposed populations. A risk is the probability that an event will occur over a defined period of time. The rate is the amount of change per unit of time. Risks are defined with reference to persons alive at the start of the study. Rates are defined per person-year of follow-up (1 person-year means one person followed for 1 year). The absolute risk and the incidence rate of the end-point in cohort studies are defined as follows:

$$\text{Absolute risk} = \frac{\text{No of subjects with disease during follow-up}}{\text{No of subjects disease free at start}}$$

$$\text{Incidence rate} = \frac{\text{No of subjects with disease during follow-up}}{\text{Average population during the period}}$$

The most commonly used comparative measure of risk is the relative risk (RR), also called risk ratio. A relative risk greater than 1 means that the risk in the exposed population is greater than in the nonexposed one. Relative risk less than 1 means the exposure is protective. If the relative risk equals 1, there is no difference between groups. It is the best measure of strength of an association between exposure and outcome.

$$\text{Relative risk (RR)} = \frac{\text{Risk in exposed subjects}}{\text{Risk in unexposed subjects}}$$

Another comparative measurement is the risk difference (attributable risk or excess risk), which is the remainder when risk in nonexposed subjects is subtracted from risk in exposed subjects. If there is no difference there is no risk. This measure is a more direct and useful indicator of the impact of prevention.

$$\text{Risk difference} = \text{Risk in exposed subjects} - \text{Risk in nonexposed subjects}$$

For example: if the risk in exposed subjects is 7% and that in nonexposed subjects is 2%, there is an excess or attributable risk of 5% of developing the outcome under investigation in the exposed group compared with the unexposed group.

The attributable risk per cent (AR%) is defined as the percentage of the absolute risk in the group exposed to the risk factor.

$$\text{AR\%} = \frac{\text{Risk difference}}{\text{Risk in exposed subjects}}$$

Although OR is not very frequently used in the analysis of cohort studies, it is a good approximation to the relative risk in low-risk situations.

$$\text{OR} = \frac{\text{Odds of disease in exposed subjects}}{\text{Odds of disease in nonexposed subjects}}$$

or

$$\text{OR} = \frac{\text{Odds of exposure in those with disease}}{\text{Odds of exposure in those without disease}}$$

Interpretation. It is important to consider the possibility of bias, chance and confounding as alternative explanations for the results of a cohort study.

Misclassification of exposure and/or disease may increase the similarity between exposed and nonexposed groups. Hence, any possible association will be underestimated.

A major problem in cohort studies is the bias introduced by losses during follow-up. The only way of eliminating this effect is prevention to minimise losses.

Not all subjects who are eligible to participate on a study agree to do so. Nonparticipants may differ from participants in various ways, such as smoking habits, diet and health care. The results may be valid for the studied population but cannot be generalised.

Advantages of cohort studies

1. Such studies are ethically safe.
2. Subjects can be matched.
3. The timing and directionality of events can be established.
4. Rare exposures can be examined by appropriate selection of study cohorts.
5. Multiple outcomes can be studied for any one exposure.
6. The incidence of disease can be measured in both exposed and nonexposed groups.
7. If they are conducted as prospective studies they minimise bias in the ascertainment of exposure.
8. Eligibility criteria and outcome assessments can be standardised.
9. They are easier and cheaper to manage than a randomised controlled trial.

Disadvantages of cohort studies.

1. It may be difficult to identify controls.
2. Exposure may be linked to a hidden confounder.
3. Blinding is difficult.
4. Randomisation is not present.
5. In the case of rare diseases large sample size or long follow-up is necessary.
6. They are very expensive and time consuming, particularly if follow-up is long and outcome is rare.
7. If they are conducted in a retrospective manner the availability of adequate records is required.
8. Validity of the results can be affected by losses to follow-up.
9. Changes in exposure status and diagnostic criteria over time can affect the classification of individuals by exposure and disease status.

Experimental studies: clinical trials

In experimental research the researcher plans an intervention and observes the outcomes. For clinical trials the most representative design is the randomised controlled trial (RCT), which the scientific community considers the gold standard for determining causal effect.

The first description of a comparative clinical trial was issued in Britain in the mid-1700s. In 1834 Louis, in France, established a scientific approach to clinical trials and epidemiology by discussing the importance of accurate observations of patient outcome, knowledge of the natural progress of untreated controls, precise definition of disease prior to treatment and careful observation of deviations from intended treatment. Random allocation of subjects to treatment and blinding were concepts introduced in the early twentieth century. The first clinical trial in which a placebo control was used in a double blind manner was conducted in 1950 [19].

A clinical trial is a carefully and ethically planned experiment. The experiment involves a group of subjects, (an) intervention(s) and measurement of the outcome(s). The objective is to answer a focused research question on the most appropriate intervention for a specific condition in a given population. The measured outcomes of any clinical trial should be clinically relevant to the treatment of future patients [19]. There are many types of clinical trial designs; we will focus on the randomised controlled trial.

A well-conducted double blind randomised controlled trial produces the strongest evidence for a causal effect. *Double blind* means that both researchers and subjects are unaware of which intervention the subjects receive; *randomised* means the researchers have no influence on which subjects receive the experimental or control intervention; and *controlled* means there is a control group receiving either standard of care or placebo. This design is used to assess the efficacy of an intervention. This intervention can be a drug therapy/device (risk of myocardial infarction associated with antihypertensive drug therapy), a method of clinical/surgical management (management of patients with venous leg ulcers) or an evaluation of health service organisation (acute stroke intervention: special stroke unit vs. general medical ward). The double blind randomised controlled trial is the gold standard of scientific methodology for evaluating the efficacy of an intervention.

Advantages of the clinical trial design are that blinding and randomisation allow for the unbiased distribution of unknown confounders between study groups and this strengthens the validity of the results. The disadvantages of clinical trials include ethical constraints on the design of the study, the high cost both in financial terms and in time and a risk of *volunteer bias* in selection of subjects.

Clinical trials can have many different design characteristics. When a cross-over design is used subjects are exposed to both the experimental and the control intervention sequentially, usually with a washout period between [20, 21].

Drug development trials

Drug development trials within the pharmaceutical industry are classified into four sequential phases of experimentation:

Phase I trials: Evaluation of clinical pharmacology and toxicity. The first experiments in human volunteers are concerned primarily with drug safety and not efficacy. Drug metabolism and bioavailability studies are conducted, followed by studies of multiple doses to determine appropriate dose schedules for use in phase II. Cohort study designs are generally used.

Phase II trials: Initial clinical investigation for treatment effect. This is a small-scale investigation to determine the efficacy and safety of a drug. Close monitoring of each subject is required. Cohort study designs are most frequently used, although clinical trials can be implemented.

Phase III trials: Full-scale evaluation of treatment. Once a drug has been shown to be reasonably efficacious it is necessary to compare it with the current standard treatment(s) for the same condition in a larger study. The double blind randomised controlled trial is the design of choice.

Phase IV trials: Post-marketing surveillance. After a drug has been approved for marketing, substantial enquiry still needs to be undertaken. Monitoring for adverse effects and additional large-scale, long-term studies of morbidity and mortality are important. These studies can utilise case-control, cohort or clinical trial study designs.

The research protocol

The research protocol is a formal written document specifying the study design and the manner in which the study will be conducted. It is the blueprint for the study and serves as a guideline throughout the implementation and analysis phases. It details procedures to be followed so that valid results are achieved. The research protocol fulfils scientific, ethical and organisational requirements so that the study can be conducted efficiently and according to plan and standardises the procedures for research personnel to follow. The purpose of the study and the setting will determine which professionals will be consulted about the development of the research protocol. Subject area experts, epidemiologists and/or statisticians can be included.

If the research involves human subjects the Internal Review Board (IRB) must approve the study protocol before the study can begin. Even with careful planning and foresight, conditions in the field may require protocol adaptations to meet unexpected situations. The IRB must also approve any modifications made to the protocol before these can be implemented. Detailed documentation of any changes made to the protocol and dates of IRB approval must be kept.

The protocol document is the blueprint for all those working on the research project. It should be well organised to make it easy to find relevant information. The title page includes the study title, protocol number, study site, principal investigator's name/affiliation, study sponsor and final or draft date. A summary of the research protocol contains information on the study background, objectives, study design, subject eligibility criteria, intervention(s) and outcome measurements. The summary is followed by the introduction. The introduction describes the background information on the research topic, with a review of clinical studies relevant to the research question and to support for the study hypothesis.

All literature references used to support the background and methodology sections must be included. All documents and forms relevant to the implementation of the study are attached in the appendices, including schedules for assessments, informed consent form approved by the IRB and procedural requirements (source documentation, case report forms, data collection and storage methods, study monitoring, study medication accountability, conditions for modifying or terminating the study, disclosure of data/publication and conflict of interest) for the study and product information about drugs or devices (clinical trials) [24]. We will describe elements of a research protocol in more detail.

Objectives

The research study has as its main objective the answer to a research question. The main objective is also defined as the primary outcome of the study. There may be other questions (secondary objectives) to which answers are also sought. These are also called secondary outcomes and should be defined in the protocol. Adjustments can be made to the study protocol to guarantee the collection of the necessary data for secondary outcomes. All efforts, though, should be focused on collecting quality data to answer the primary question, since the secondary outcomes will generate hypotheses for future studies.

Hypothesis

The hypothesis is a statement of the expected outcome to the research question. Usually hypotheses are concerned with relationships between variables or with differences between groups. Clear definitions of the population, intervention and outcome of interest are important. For example, in a clinical trial the research question might be "Does high-frequency oscillatory ventilation (intervention) make for lower mortality (outcome) than conventional ventilation (comparison) in preterm infants with respiratory distress syndrome (population). The hypothesis would be "High-frequency oscillatory ventilation results in lower mortality than conventional ventilation in preterm infants with respiratory distress syndrome."

Study design

A statement summarising the main design elements should open the description of the study design. Standard terminology must be used for study designs, such as randomised, controlled, blinded, cohort, cross-over. The major elements of the study design, such as the subjects, intervention and outcome, must be specified, as must the temporal aspects relevant to the intervention and evaluation of outcomes. For example: "This protocol describes a randomised, double blind, placebo-controlled study of the safety and efficacy of drug A administered to HIV-infected subjects with HIV RNA levels<50,000 copies/ml with follow-up for 1 year." It is a good idea to look for examples of cohort and clinical trials.

Sample selection

One key objective of research studies is to be able to make inferences from the results of a study that are applicable to a more general population. The characteristics of patients included in the study will determine the extent to which the conclusions can be generalised to other patient populations. Such factors as age, sex, socio-economic status, education, and health consciousness can all affect subsequent morbidity and mortality. Results should be applicable to the reference population for which the research question is being posed, for example, "renal disease in patients with diabetes and hypertension".

The broader the inclusion criteria the easier it is to select study subjects and the more the results can be generalised. When exclusion criteria are designed an attempt must be made to exclude extraneous conditions that could distort the outcome; in some prospective subjects there might be contraindications for the intervention under scrutiny, for example, and these persons should be excluded, as should any who are judged unlikely to comply with the intervention.

Clear definition of the condition of interest is essential before subject selection. If the condition of interest is a disease then how accurately can a diagnosis be made? Are issues relating to staging of the severity of illness clearly described? When the clinical course of a disease is extremely variable, assessing treatment effects by clinical observation can be extremely unreliable. For example, patients with systemic lupus erythematosus have a variable clinical progression. The natural history of the condition of interest and the existence of validated prognostic markers must be taken into account to support the effect of the intervention on the outcome variables.

Patients who refuse to participate may be systematically different (in social class, severity of disease or other factors) from those who do agree to enter the study. Records must be kept of subject refusals, to allow a comparison between those who consented and those who did not.

Subject eligibility

Subject eligibility criteria are clearly defined by establishing inclusion and exclusion criteria. Characteristics frequently considered include: age, sex, function of major body systems, mental status, previous health conditions and/or previous drug treatment. The focus should be on criteria related to the condition of interest.

Sample size

Sample size is generally determined by a statistician rather than by subjective judgment. Important considerations in calculation of sample size include whether the outcome measures are continuous (e.g. height) or categorical (e.g. presence of diabetes) variables, and the size of effect and incidence of outcome in the control group. Data from previous studies or from a pilot study can support informed guesses in estimations of effect size, which is required for calculation of the sample size. If an outcome is rare a larger sample size will be needed to observe a difference between groups. The statistical power of the study will define how certain the researchers want to be of detecting a statistically significant result. Generally a power of 80--90% is regarded as adequate. This means the investigator accepts a 10–20% chance of not detecting a significant difference between interventions although such a difference may in reality exist (type II error).

Once the appropriate sample size is known, an extra percentage should be added to allow for dropouts or withdrawals. It is almost inevitable that some subjects will drop out, not comply with the study protocol or be lost to follow-up. As a general rule, a loss of up to 10–15% of subjects is acceptable and should not bias the result unless there is a strong confounder present.

Screening and recruitment

The recruitment procedure is selected with two goals in mind. The first is to recruit a sample that adequately represents the target population. If the source group is a hospital population this limits the generalisability of the results to a community population. The response rate of recruited subjects will also influence how far results can be generalised to a wider population.

The second is to recruit enough subjects to meet the sample size required.

The inability to enrol a sufficient number of subjects is a frequent problem in clinical research. The accessible population from which the study sample is recruited should have a greater number of probable subjects than is required for the study sample. There is always a tendency for investigators to overestimate the number of subjects meeting the study criteria who will agree to participate. Contingency plans must be developed if recruitment efforts fail initially [20]. The procedure for handling withdrawals and replacements and other foreseeable problems should be established in the protocol.

The procedure developed for screening subjects to see whether they meet inclusion criteria before being invited to participate in the study is detailed in the protocol. Where will the information about potential subject be obtained? Will there be any contact between researchers and potential subjects? What information will be collected? Ethical and privacy considerations are taken into account.

Screening and recruitment methods must be approved by the IRB. Subjects will be more highly motivated to participate by a design that avoids invasive and uncomfortable tests. Language barriers can be overcome by using bilingual staff [20].

Baseline evaluation

The purpose of measuring baseline variables is to define and describe the characteristics of the study population. In a clinical trial this allows the researcher to assess whether the characteristics in intervention and control groups are similar before the intervention. It is important to measure demographic characteristics, disease states, socio-economic aspects and/or predictors of outcome, such as risk factors or existing conditions that can influence the outcome. In the case of a chance misdistribution between study groups, the researcher can make statistical adjustments in the analysis phase. This adjustment reduces the impact of a sampling misdistribution, for example an age misdistribution, on the results.

Description of the intervention

A detailed description of the intervention includes the randomisation procedure, intervention assignment strategy, and schedule and duration of study intervention. If the intervention is a drug therapy, the description should include details of how the drug is dispensed, supplied (e.g. as capsules in bottles) and labelled. A clear account of the management of anticipated situations in drug therapy trials includes handling dose reduction, changes allowed in background therapy (e.g. use of other chemotherapeutic agents) and temporary study discontinuation.

Several types of control interventions can be used in clinical trials, including concurrent placebo, concurrent active drug, no treatment, different dose of the same drug and concurrent use of standard care. Historical controls can be either data collected from patients in the same cohort as used in trial before the intervention or from a similar cohort used in another study that received standard of care or no therapy.

Compliance bias occurs when compliance differs between the interventions being compared. These generate differences in patient adherence to treatment (e.g. one group receives a pill with a bitter taste and the other one with a sweet taste).

Randomisation procedure

The goal of randomisation is to maximise the probability that groups receiving differing interventions will be comparable. When an adequate randomisation procedure is used, the potential for bias in allocation to study groups is removed. With random selection, the assignment of subjects to the intervention is determined by chance alone. Study groups tend to be comparable with respect to all known confounding variables as well as to other, unsuspected, confounders. However, there is no guarantee that differences will not arise by chance between the two groups. The larger the sample size, the smaller the risk of differences between groups. The randomisation method should provide true random allocation. Computer-generated random numbers and tables of random numbers are the most commonly used methods. Alternate allocation and allocation by birth date are not true randomisation procedures. Central randomisation procedures are preferable to local randomisation; that is to say randomisation should be carried out by a statistician or a researcher not involved in the recruitment and follow-up of subjects.

Concealment of allocation means the researcher is unaware of which intervention group the next subject is allocated to. This removes any possibility of manipulation of subject allocation in the field. Concealment of allocation strengthens the randomisation process; it is achieved by using sequentially numbered, sealed, opaque envelopes.

A blocking procedure can be used when it is necessary to balance the number of subjects in different strata of subject characteristics. Subjects are first classified with respect to variables that will affect the outcome (e.g., age, sex, severity of disease) and then randomised.

People tend to modify their behaviour because they are receiving special care and attention; this is described as the *Hawthorne effect*. Also, the subjects can make changes in their life-style that are unrelated to the intervention, but nonetheless affect the outcome. The two most important elements in eliminating bias in clinical trials are randomisation and blinding.

Blinding

The study protocol must state clearly whether a blind or an open label design will be used. Open label means that the subjects, investigators, and outcome evaluators know the type of intervention given to each subject. Blinding means concealment of the identity of the intervention in clinical trials or of exposure status in cohort studies. The aim is to avoid bias in both study execution and interpretation of the results.

Investigators, clinicians and subjects are all prone to change their behaviour if they know who is receiving which treatment or who has been exposed to a condition of interest. Blinding avoids this. Blinding is especially important when the outcomes are subjective, e.g. pain, and may be influenced by the knowledge of the treatment received. Hard outcomes, such as death or recurrence, are not affected as much.

Ethical issues and practicability issues need to be taken into consideration when the level of blinding in a clinical trial is selected. A higher level of blindness involves higher costs, increased complexity and longer timelines for trials. Blinding can be described as single, double or triple, depending on who is unaware of the intervention given:

1. Single blind: Patients are unaware of the treatment they are receiving but the researcher evaluating the outcome is informed.
2. Double blind: Health professionals providing care and the subjects themselves are unaware of the intervention received. Health professionals assessing the outcome are also not aware of the intervention received. This is the most common type of blinding.
3. Triple blind: Health professionals, subjects and research personnel are all unaware of the intervention being given.

Data collection

Predictor variables are those that will be measured against the outcome variables to evaluate the presence of a relationship. In clinical trials the predictor variables are the experimental intervention and the control intervention. In cohort studies the predictor variable is the exposure of interest. Outcome variables are relevant clinical end-points to the condition of interest.

The measurement of the study variables should be clearly defined. For example, if stroke is the outcome of interest a clear definition of your measurement should include the signs, symptoms, results of diagnostic procedures and other reliable indicators. If the important parameters cannot be measured the trial may not be ethically justifiable.

Accuracy and precision are characteristics of measurements. Precision involves obtaining the same or very similar results after repeated measures. Precision is affected by observer variability (e.g. skill in using an instrument, measuring blood pressure), subject variability (e.g. mood when responding to a questionnaire) and instrument variability (e.g. screening tests of hearing can be affected by background noise). Action that can be taken to enhance precision includes standardising the measurement methods, training the observers, refining instruments, automating the instruments and repeating measurements [20].

Accuracy is defined by how close the measurement is to the "true" value. Systematic error is reflected by lower accuracy. An example is a manometer that is not calibrated. Its accuracy is assessed by using a "gold standard" or by comparing it with a technique of accepted accuracy. Strategies for enhancing accuracy include standardising the measurement methods, training the observers, refining the instruments, automating the instruments, developing measures that subjects are not aware of, blinding, and calibrating the instruments [20].

Measures that have been validated in the literature should be preferred. Continuous variables are those that can be ranked on a spectrum of quantifiable intervals, such as body weight and blood pressure. Categorical variables are those derived from characteristics that cannot be measured, such as sex and blood type. Continuous variables can provide more informative statistics (mean and standard deviation) than categorical variables (rates, counts and proportions), adding power to the study and reducing the sample size required [20].

The protocol must also set out the procedures for data collection and protection of subject confidentiality. Back-up methods, storage procedures and security measures to avoid access by nonresearch personnel to sensitive subject health information must all be detailed.

Follow-up evaluation

The follow-up period should be long enough to detect enough occurrences of the outcomes of interest. One common mistake investigators make is not allowing a follow-up period that is long enough, which means the investigator misses the effect of the intervention.

The frequency of follow-up contacts varies, depending on the requirement for data and the need to keep informed about the subject's status. In the protocol the strategies used to minimise the incidence of subject dropout and withdrawal must be described. Telephone calls and house visits are methods used in the follow-up of subjects who are not complying with the study procedures. The reasons for any subject's withdrawal from the study must be given.

Case report forms are created to permit accurate and systematic collection of individual subjects' data. The design of the case report forms is extremely important, because it facilitates data recording in such a way as to meet study objectives and promotes investigators' adherence to the protocol. The case report should allow for a rapid and effective review of subject data and facilitate generation of the database.

Subjects should always be actively asked about their use of other therapies. Subjects often use concurrent interventions inadvertently, and this can go unrecognised by study personnel. The protocol must contain information on what kind of concurrent therapy (medications, physiotherapy) will be accepted and which would be a reason for excluding a subject. This can happen either before or during the study, so that it is important to keep eliciting such information throughout the study period.

If loss of subjects in the follow-up period is related to the intervention it will affect the outcome. One illustration is when an intervention causes discomfort to the subjects and this leads to an increased dropout rate in the experimental group. This leads to under- or overestimation of the effects of the intervention. The potential bias resulting from dropouts or withdrawals should be carefully considered. If over 20% of subjects are lost to follow-up this causes serious concern about the validity of the trial data. *Intention-to-treat analysis* is a strategy used in analysis of clinical trial data to control for loss to follow-up.

Adverse events and safety

Thought should be given to how any complications arising from the disease or the intervention should be dealt with and how to respond to new problems. If adverse events arise will the intervention be discontinued temporarily or permanently? Will the dose be decreased? What other actions should be taken? For clinical trials studying new interventions, proactive safety procedures are determined in the protocol. Adverse event reporting defines the steps to be taken if an adverse event occurs.

Statistical specification

A statement about the analysis strategy to be used to evaluate primary and secondary outcome variables is included in the protocol. The types of variables to be collected for outcomes and the statistical tests planned must be documented. For clinical trials it must be made clear whether "intention-to-treat" or "as treated" analysis is to be performed. The handling of specific situations should be described in advance. For example, how will dropouts be dealt with? Will there be a subgroup analysis? Will data from ineligible subjects be included or excluded? [22].

An interim analysis is conducted at a predetermined time in the study. The strategy used for this analysis is defined in the protocol. In clinical trials an interim analysis is conducted to (a) assess trends in incidence of adverse events, and (b) assess efficacy results. If a new intervention is found to be particularly successful or obviously harmful at the interim analysis then early termination of the trial and publication of the results is mandatory. Ethical issues and cost are the main justifications for planning interim analyses. In drug development trials an independent monitoring group separate from the investigators conducts the interim analysis.

After data collection: analysing the results

Statistical analysis of the data collected provides information about the strength of the association between predictor variables and outcome variables. In the research protocol, the investigator defines the level of statistical significance (P-value) and the power of the study.

Descriptive statistical analyses

The data are summarised using noncomparative techniques such as frequency distributions (proportions), description of averages (mean, mode and/or median) and description of the spread of values (standard deviation and standard error). Assumptions for the statistical tests, e.g. whether the data have a normal distribution or not, must be assessed. Baseline characteristics are compared to search for differences that might impact on the outcome, such as demographic characteristics and prognostic factors.

Analytic statistical analyses

Primary hypotheses and secondary outcomes must be tested. Variables are compared to evaluate the pattern and strength of relationships. The adequate statistical test depends on a variety of factors (e.g. presence of normal distribution, variation between/within subjects) and circumstances (e.g. timeline) surrounding the data. A statistician should be consulted to plan the appropriate analysis methodology, including subgroup analysis, in advance. The analysis plan is dynamic, and additional analysis may be planned before the data are considered.

Hypotheses can be proved wrong, but they can never be proved correct, because the investigator cannot test all the potential subjects with the condition of interest. All the specific factors that may have influenced or biased the data and/or the interpretation reached must be considered [23].

- Analysis: Intention-to-treat

An intention-to-treat analysis is based on the inclusion of all randomised patients in the analysis, regardless of which intervention the subject has received in the study. The outcome is analysed by the intervention originally assigned to the subject and includes dropouts. It is the preferred approach for pragmatic studies. If one starts excluding patients from the analysis for a variety of apparently "justifiable" reasons (later realisation that they have not met criteria, noncompliance, missed study visits, house move, other illnesses or dropout of the trial before completion), a large percentage of patients may be excluded from the analysis and thus compromise the validity. Intention-to-treat analysis eliminates the risk of creating a bias through these exclusions. When an intention-to-treat analysis is planned differences between treatments can be obscured and sample size needs to be increased to compensate.

- Analysis As Treated

In the as-treated analysis strategy, an algorithm based on the degree to which the patient has "complied" with the protocol determines which subjects are included in the analysis. For example, subjects would be included only if they had taken all the study medications as defined in the protocol. The sample size used in this analysis is smaller, because not all subjects meet compliance criteria. The power of the study is thus compromised. Bias can be created, as the subjects who have not complied (e.g. because they have suffered adverse effects) may be different from subjects who have complied. The validity of the statistical testing is undercut, and an imbalance may result. It is advisable to perform an intention-to-treat analysis as well, so that both types of analysis support the results.

- Subgroup analysis

Data may be evaluated using subgroup analyses. The subgroups are decided in advance in the study protocol, with a hypothesis on how different subgroups might react differently. As sample size decreases there will probably not be enough power to answer many questions. If a decision to do subgroup analysis is made after the data is collected this is called post hoc analysis and can be helpful only in generating hypotheses for future studies [24].

Subject characteristics are frequently used for subgroup analyses such as: age, sex, race, severity of disease at baseline and duration of therapy. Within a subgroup, study data can be further divided into strata, for example: females <65 years of age versus 65 or older. The more strata are used the fewer the subjects in each stratum, resulting in less power to detect differences.

Drawing the conclusions: interpreting study results

Interpretation begins after the trial is completed: the data are collected, edited, and entered into a database, appropriate statistical tests are performed to analyse the data, and the statistical report providing a permanent and detailed record of the study is compiled. This report allows other investigators to repeat the study using the identical design and to audit the results in just the same way.

Analyses of data are primarily statistical exercises, whereas its interpretation is an exercise in discerning the clinical meaning of the data evaluated. The researcher is primarily concerned with drawing conclusions to report in publications. The goals of interpreting research data include establishing the meaning of the data collected, with an emphasis on clinical significance, reporting the results of the original objectives of the study while comparing them with the results from previous studies, developing hypotheses for future studies and gaining insight into interpretations of the condition of interest.

In the interpretation of the results of analyses factors that may bias the data or affect their interpretation should be sought. These include characteristics of the study design, subjects enrolled, condition being evaluated, study intervention, investigator and staff and trial environment. Other factors that can be responsible for bias are how the clinical trial is conducted, the characteristics of the tests and the measures used, statistical factors, characteristics of the data report and, possibly, errors of deceit committed accidentally or wilfully before, during or after the trial [23].

Statistical significance alone does not provide information about whether a result is clinically important. When clinical significance is considered the relevance of chosen outcomes, the size of the effect observed, the risk/benefit ratio and also the cost/benefit ratio should be evaluated [24].

Good clinical practice: conduct of a trial

In 1990, government agencies and pharmaceutical companies from the USA, Japan and Europe joined forces to create an international standard concerning both ethics and scientific quality to be observed in designing, conducting, recording and reporting clinical trials that involve human subjects. This group, known as the *International Conference on Harmonisation*, led to the Good Clinical Practice (GCP) guideline in 1996. Compliance with GCP ensures (a) protection of trial subjects' rights, safety and wellbeing and (b) credibility of the clinical trial data. This guidance facilitates mutual acceptance of clinical data by the regulatory authorities in the USA, Japan and Europe [25, 26].

The Medical Research Council describes the principles of the GCP guidelines [27]:

1. Clinical trials must be conducted in accordance with ethical principles originating from the Declaration of Helsinki and be consistent with current GCP and applicable regulatory requirements.

2. A clinical trial should be initiated and continued only if the anticipated benefits outweigh foreseeable risks for the individual participant.
3. Rights, safety, and the well-being of the individual participants should prevail over the interests of science or society.
4. The intervention proposed in the clinical trial should be supported by adequate information, clinical or nonclinical, justifying the trial design.
5. The design of the clinical trial should be scientifically sound and must be clearly described in the study protocol.
6. The clinical trial should be conducted in compliance with the protocol approved by the IRB.
7. Qualified health professionals should provide care to participants.
8. All individuals involved in conducting the clinical trial should be adequately qualified by training, education or experience to perform their roles.
9. Informed and freely given consent should be obtained from every participant prior to participation.
10. All clinical trial information should be recorded, handled and stored in a way that allows accurate reporting, interpretation and verification.
11. Confidentiality of records that could identify participants should be protected, with respect for privacy and confidentiality rules in accordance with the applicable regulatory requirements.
12. Investigational products should be manufactured, handled and stored in accordance with Good Manufacturing Practice and used in accordance with the protocol approved by the IRB.
13. Systems with procedures that ensure the quality of every aspect of the trial should be implemented.

Ethical considerations

The basic ethical principles of autonomy (respect for human subjects), nonmaleficence (do no harm), beneficence (do good) and justice (exclusion) underlie the ethical considerations in medical research [28]. Ethical considerations are important in all aspects of a study, from the development of the research question, through the decision on the study design and implementation of the study protocol through to analysis, interpretation and publication of the results. There are also concerns relating to individual study subjects and to scientific novelty and integrity. Ethical questions are not merely present or absent, but range from those which are obvious to those that can be strongly debated.

The ethical principle of autonomy incorporates two separate moral requirements: (a) acknowledgement of autonomy, and (b) treatment of individuals as autonomous agents and protection of those with reduced autonomy. In most cases of research involving autonomous human subjects, the principle of autonomy requires that subjects enter into the research voluntarily and are given adequate information about the study. In some cases, individuals are not capable of deciding in their own best interest, because of maturity (children), illness (coma), mental disability (Alzheimer's) or other circumstances (prison). Subjects that are not autonomous will require varying degrees of protection if they are to be included as human subjects in research.

The ethical principles of beneficence and maleficence involve an obligation to secure the well-being of human subjects, by maximising benefits and minimising or entirely avoiding harm. The critical decision is whether the risk of harm justifies the possible benefits. Ethical issues in research studies are concerned with *individuals* rather than society at large. The objective is for no individual to be exposed to an unreasonable risk for the sake of the community.

The third ethical principle, that of justice, refers to the selection of human subjects who derive the benefits of the research results. In the early twentieth century poor people were used as subjects for studies in hospitals, but they did not derive the benefits of the results; private patients were the ones who benefited. Another example of flagrant injustice was the use of unwilling concentration camp prisoners as study subjects during World War II. Selection of human subjects should be based on reasons directly related to the study question, not on easy access, convenience and/or availability.

Ethical concerns during development and implementation of a research protocol must also be taken into consideration with reference to scientific validity, recruitment procedure, participation procedures, potential harms and benefits and informed consent [29].

The ethical basis for the research question first needs to be established. Has the research question already been answered by good-quality studies? If this is the case, is it reasonable to deprive subjects of a therapy that has been proved to be effective? If your research question has not been answered and there are benefits that would justify the risk of harm, then the next step is to support this assertion in your protocol.

Once a research question has been established and a study protocol developed, the ethical considerations require that the research protocol be reviewed by an independent committee, the IRB, to assess whether any ethical principles have been violated. The IRB is a multidisciplinary committee whose objectives are to protect patients' rights and to ensure that the study protocol meets ethical standards. Its members review the protocol and any subsequent amendments, giving their approval and recommendations. They do not, however, check to see whether the study procedures described are being adequately followed. It is the responsibility of the sponsor and the researcher to ensure that the IRB is properly constituted and to conduct research in accordance with the guidelines recommended.

The IRBs are established in hospitals and educational institutions carrying out medical research, with the aim of protecting human subjects. National policy provides the guidelines for the IRB. For a multisite study, the study protocol has to be approved at each site. The IRB also serves as a resource for the investigator developing a protocol. The knowledge of the IRB requirements necessary to get the protocol approved helps the investigator to include all the necessary information for approval.

The IRB determines whether there is a need for an *Informed Consent Form* (ICF) and will approve the content. Informed consent should be obtained from all subjects entering the study and should be retained for future audit. The ICF is written in nontechnical language to facilitate subjects' understanding of the potential risks and benefits of entering the study. Some of the elements that should be included in the ICF [30] are listed below:

1. An explicit statement that the project involves research, a description of the purposes of the research, and the procedures for the selection of subjects.
2. A clear identification of the researchers and sponsors.
3. A description of the time and type of commitment required from the subjects.
4. An explanation of the concept of randomisation and blinding and the assignment of experimental and control intervention.
5. An explanation about the probability and magnitude of benefits and harm, with mention of procedures used to maximise benefits and minimise harms.
6. A description of alternative treatments if they are available outside the scope of the study.
7. Information about potential costs and the possibility of disclosure of the results.
8. A statement about procedures for maintaining confidentiality.
9. Reassurance that participation is voluntary and that declining to participate or withdrawing at any time during the study will not incur penalties.
10. An explicit offer to answer questions or provide further information.
11. Clear information about who can be contacted for further information, the rights of study subjects, and any adversities related to the study stated.

The ICF provides a procedure for certifying that the researcher has established each subject's autonomy, provided appropriate and adequate information on the study protocol, benefits and risk of harm, made it clear that the subject is able to withdraw from the study at any time without suffering any consequences and explained the protection of confidentiality so that the individual can decide whether or not to take part in the study.

Other issues that require clarification in the protocol are the protection of subject confidentiality and compensation. All study information about the subject's state of health must be confidential. If disclosure to a third party is required, specific consent must be obtained from the subjects beforehand. The staff involved in implementing the study procedure has to ensure subject confidentiality and comply strictly with protocol procedures. Study records should have an identifier, usually a subject number, which cannot be traced to the subject. Transmission of data over the Internet should meet strict standards to ensure that confidentiality is not broken.

Compensation of subjects requires IRB approval. Study subjects are usually not paid, unless it can be demonstrated that this is not an inducement. Only out-of-pocket expenses may be reimbursed. The sponsors, however, must provide compensation, regardless of legal liability, if the subject suffers deterioration in health or well-being as a result of participating in the study.

Once the IRB approves the study protocol and the ICF, the research study can be initiated, and not before. Ethical considerations are relevant to all individuals and groups connected with the study, the investigator research team and the sponsor.

In certain circumstances early discontinuation of the study is ethically required. For example, when a research staff fails to comply with study procedures or an interim analysis of a clinical trial may indicate an increase of harmful effects in the group receiving an experimental intervention. In the ALLHAT trial on hypertension management the study arm receiving an alpha blocker was discontinued because in the interim analysis the risk of congestive heart failure doubled [31]. If beneficial effects are determined in the interim analysis, ethical concerns are raised for patients not receiving this intervention.

Critical appraisal skills

Interpretation of scientific studies can be a daunting task, because professionals receive little training in this area. A common tendency is to read the conclusion of a research paper and then apply the information as presented. This is an inadequate approach, because the conclusion generally represents the author's subjective opinion. The professional needs to learn how to identify information that does, or does not, validate the results and conclusions of a research article. With this information to hand the reader is empowered to make a judgment of the limitations affecting the results and the stated conclusions of the research paper.

Some of the main areas of enquiry for critical appraisal of a medical research paper include the presence of a focused research question, the choice of the study design used to answer the research question, the adequacy of the study sample, the completeness of the study, the quality and adequacy of outcome measurements, the analysis procedures and the presence of distorting factors.

The Evidence-Based Medicine Working Group developed a manageable and user-friendly approach to critical appraisal. This approach greatly improves the ability to discuss and understand research papers and to apply the information consistently to clinical care and/or research [32-60]. The cited papers describe a systematic method of identifying components that support the interpretation of a variety of study designs from clinical trials to economic analysis extending to qualitative research. Worksheets with questions to guide researchers through the critical appraisal are available on the web (http://www.cche.net/usersguides/main.asp). Guyatt and Rennie's book, "*Users' Guides to the Medical Literature*" is an excellent resource to expand knowledge on interpretation of the medical literature and evidence-based clinical practice [61].

Based on the work developed by the Evidence-Based Medicine Working Group we will describe general questions used to elicit information about the validity and results of research papers. There are two basic categories of questions: screening for validity and interpretation and applicability of results. These are described in more detail below.

Screening for validity

Screening questions [36] can help in rapid assessment of whether it is worth investing more time in analysing a research paper. The answers to these questions help determine the validity of the results. If the validity is seriously compromised then it is best to devote the time to looking for research of a better quality.

As a general rule it should not be assumed that any aspect of research is sound, even if it is published in traditional journals. The initial search for quality markers helps in screening to select articles that are worth reading in detail. If the evaluation of these raises significant doubt about the quality markers used in the study, the validity of the study is compromised and the results can be rejected. The questions used in screening for validity vary according to the research study design used.

The first element to look for in a paper is the description of the study question. A research question contains three basic components: the population studied the intervention or exposure of interest and the outcomes considered.

For a controlled trial, a fourth component is the presence of a control group. The research question should be described in a clear and focused way. If the question the research report is addressing is not even clear how is it possible to evaluate the methodology used?

When a paper describing a controlled clinical trial is evaluated the methodology section should be reviewed for the presence of a randomisation procedure and concealment of allocation [62]. The randomisation procedure describes how subjects were allocated to control or experimental intervention. Some methods, e.g. allocation of the subjects alternately, or by record number or birth date, are not truly random. Lack of genuine randomisation seriously compromises the validity of the results. Concealment of allocation refers to the process used to prevent foreknowledge of the assignment group in a randomised control trial, the commonly used method is to use sealed envelopes containing each subject's assignment, which are only opened when the subject enters the study.

In all study designs completeness of follow-up should be sought. Completeness of follow-up means knowing what has happened to all subjects who entered the study. The subjects included in the study must be compared with the numbers used in the analysis. A dropout rate of up to 10–15% is usually acceptable unless there is something striking about those who dropped out. Some journals require authors to be explicit about dropouts or loss to follow-up and to use an algorithm for the purpose. If there is a large number of overall dropouts, or if patients are selectively excluded from analysis, this would seriously affect the validity of the results.

Blinding enhances the validity of the study results. In randomised trials procedures can be put in place so that subjects and caregivers and outcome evaluators can be made unaware of the intervention each individual subject has received. In cohort and case-control studies, researchers interviewing or following up the subjects can be made unaware of the study's real objective to avoid interview bias. Questionnaires can have questions on different topics to detract focus from the study objective.

Were outcomes measured in the same way? Researchers are interested in precision and accuracy of the measurements. If questions are asked about events in the past could there be a recall bias? For example, patients with leukaemia might be more aware of the fact that they lived near power plants than patients that do no have leukaemia. Another example of a strategy to improve accuracy of outcome measurement is to use prescription databases rather than depending on the patient's memory about use of a specific drug [63].

Appraisal questions

Once the research report has been screened and is considered worthy of further assessment, the next step is to examine the methodological details and the results. Appraisal questions in the Users' Guide [61] are specific to the type of research question and help you focus on key aspects of the research design that could possibly invalidate the results.

A first step in evaluating the methods is the assessment of the adequacy of the study sample, both in terms of being a representative sample and in terms of numbers required to answer the research question. A representative sample should include the section of the population of interest. Let us take the example of a study that is based on the following research question: Does use of thiazides as a first-line antihypertensive drug in patients with primary hypertension lower the incidence of stroke? The subjects for this study should be recruited from primary care clinics rather than from hypertension clinics, so that the results can be extended to patients in primary care. The hypertension clinic will have a selected sample of hypertensive patients that is different from the general population and would therefore answer a very different question.

The second element to be assessed from the aspect of sample adequacy is sample size. If the sample is too small to measure the effect expected a negative result is not meaningful. The scientific term used to express the probability of the study to achieve a true positive conclusion is *power*. Power is usually reported clearly in the Methods section. For example, a study that has 90% power means that there is a 90% chance of detecting a "true" difference between study groups and conversely a 10% chance of not finding such a result even if it is true (false negative) is accepted. As a standard cut-off, 80% is usually considered an acceptable power.

In studies that involve an intervention it is important to ascertain whether subjects, health personnel and study personnel were blind to the intervention. Sometimes this is not feasible, but the presence of blinding helps to strengthen the validity of the results. Subjects tend to change their behaviour in accordance with their beliefs of the effects of therapy if they know whether they are receiving placebo or active drug. A study investigating the effectiveness of arthroscopic surgery in reducing pain and improving function in patients with osteoarthritis of the knee used a sham procedure in the control group (three skin incisions under the effect of a short-acting tranquilliser). The conclusion was that there was no difference between arthroscopic surgery and the sham procedure in the outcomes measured [64]. Also, if the professional measuring the outcome knows which intervention the subject received he/she may evaluate the outcome differently.

The selection, definition and relevance of the outcome measurements are the next step in evaluating the methods and results. Do the outcomes adequately reflect the outcomes of interest for that patient group? For example, high-frequency oscillatory ventilation improves oxygenation levels in neonates with respiratory distress syndrome; the outcome measured, oxygenation level, is an important outcome in the initial development of new technology. In clinical care, though, relevant outcomes for the patient group would be mortality, morbidity and/or lung damage. The relevance of the outcomes depends upon the research question.

Studies usually are designed around one primary outcome measurement. Secondary outcomes are other outcomes of interest that the study was not designed to answer. The validity of secondary outcomes is limited, and they are used for generation of hypotheses. A new trial is necessary for specific evaluation of the secondary outcomes.

Accuracy of the primary outcome measurements requires close evaluation. A good example is measurement of blood pressure (BP), which is subject to great variability depending on the method of measurement. Some factors that affect BP measurement can be controlled, for example, by training the health professionals measuring BP, establishing a protocol for the measurement of BP to standardise the method, using high-quality instruments that are frequently calibrated, etc. A description of the effort invested to achieve proper BP measurement strengthens the validity of the results using BP as a primary outcome.

It is also important to assess the presence of confounding variables when reviewing a research paper. A confounding variable is a factor that is associated with the primary outcome and is also associated with the exposure studied. For example, in any study of the association between drinking and lung cancer, smoking is a confounder. People who drink frequently smoke, and smoking is associated with lung cancer, so that smoking is associated with both drinking and lung cancer. Unknown confounders are a challenge when a study is designed, which is why the randomised controlled trial is the gold standard in study design as it controls for unknown confounders [65].

When the results of a research report are evaluated, tables of baseline characteristics of subjects studied should be looked at to check for possible differences that could affect outcomes. In controlled trials and case-control studies it is necessary to compare the study groups to detect differences that may not validate the results. In cohort studies you want to check whether the study group is representative. For example, the incidence of recurrence of febrile seizures will vary depending on whether the subject pool is community based or hospital based. Another characteristic it is important to assess in the study sample is whether the subjects are at a similar point in the disease stage being studied. If you observe differences in factors relating to outcomes of interest validity may be seriously compromised.

Could study groups have been treated differently in a way that could affect the outcome of interest? To evaluate the way study groups were managed some factors that should be examined are time intervals for review of patients, general management for the disease being studied and types of healthcare support provided.

In evaluation of the primary outcome of a research report, we have assumed that the sample was representative, follow-up of subjects that entered the study was adequate and the data collection process was reliable and accurate. The next step is to look at the analysis and the results.

In a clinical trial, there are different ways to express the differences between the study groups. The simple subtraction of the experimental event rate (%) from the control event rate (%) is defined as Absolute Risk Reduction (ARR). Using ARR we can calculate the Number Needed to Treat (NNT) (NNT = 1/ARR), which gives us a more practical measure of how many people would have to undergo the intervention being studied to prevent one outcome event. For example, if a drug has an NNT of 10, it means 10 people will need to be treated to prevent one additional bad outcome. It is useful when comparing treatments, as it takes account of the baseline risk of having the bad outcome. Relative Risk Reduction is the ARR divided by the control event rate, denoting the percentage relative difference between the two groups. As an example we will use data from Schulman's clinical trial, "A comparison of six weeks with six months of oral anticoagulant therapy after a first episode of venous thromboembolism. Duration of Anticoagulation Trial Study Group". The outcome studied was recurrence of venous thromboembolism in patients that had a first episode of deep venous thrombosis or pulmonary embolism. Data are shown in Table 1; follow-up was for 2 years [66]. Other important issues in comparison of treatments are the rate and severity of adverse effects and cost.

Table 1 Results of the clinical trial "A comparison of six weeks with six months of oral anticoagulant therapy after a first episode of venous thromboembolism. Duration of Anticoagulation Trial Study Group" by Schulman et al. [66] and calculated reference data for interpretation

			Relative Risk Reduction (RRR) (95% confidence interval)	Absolute Risk Reduction (ARR)	Number Needed to Treat (NNT) (95% confidence interval)
Outcome	Control Event Rate (CER)	Experimental Event Rate (EER)	(CER – EER)/CER	CER – EER	1/ARR
Recurrence of venous thromboembolism	18.1%	9.5%	48% (23–63%)	8.6%	12 (8–24)

How precise was the estimation of the effect? Confidence intervals show the precision of the treatment effect. The width of the confidence interval determines precision of the results: the wider the confidence interval the less precise the results. In therapeutic trials, if the confidence interval straddles, e.g. 0.95-3.4, the interpretation is that it is possible that the treatment did not have the predicted effect.

Making a judgement

The perfect study is very hard to come by, and there are always issues to debate. The answers to most of the issues when the validity of the study results is checked are probably not clear (an unambiguous yes or no) but rather nuances of maybe/probably. The research report may not give enough information to make an evaluation, or the quality of the reporting may be poor. If this is the case, the reader has no other choice but to disregard the research report.

When results are accepted as valid, or as probably valid, other considerations then follow about the applicability of the results. In clinical care, it would be good to know whether the results could be applied locally. Is the study population sufficiently similar to the population the research is intended to benefit? Were all the relevant outcomes considered? Do the benefits outweigh any harm? What are the costs?

This method of systematically evaluating research reports increases understanding of limitations in studies and makes it possible to discuss the evidence with colleagues. It also helps researchers to be more selective in their reading and dismiss poor-quality papers. *ACP Journal Club* and *Evidence Based Medicine* are journals that produce one-page summaries of critically appraised research reports.

Writing up a scientific study

What is a scientific paper?

A scientific paper is a written and published report describing original research results. It should be stressed, though, that a scientific paper must be written in a certain way and be published under strict editorial practice and scientific ethics. An acceptable primary scientific publication must be the first disclosure of original research results containing sufficient information to enable peers:

1. To assess observations.
2. To repeat experiments.
3. To evaluate intellectual processes.

The key ingredient in science and scientific development is that an experiment cannot be considered to be completed until safely immortalised in a peer-reviewed publication. Hence, research is incomplete if it remains unpublished.

Writing a research paper

There is no single best way to write a research paper. There are some general rules that should be followed if the production of an acceptable publication is intended, but the overall sequence of events varies from paper to paper. In general, authors wait until data analysis is concluded and the results interpreted before they start writing, but not necessarily every time. Sometimes, the Methods section can be written up even before data analysis is completed. On the other hand, the activity of background reading should be continued. It should not be too extensive: some novice authors try to search all the literature and to read all the papers pertinent to the scope of their papers. They end up with a huge pile of documents and are not able to synthesise ideas: as a result there may be hundreds of references to be cited. When reading, researchers should make notes, make notes on the notes, and write down sentences or parts of them. There are different reasons for this: it may help to condense the major material necessary, and the act of making notes helps to ingrain the points in the memory. However, reading should not be undertaken during the time allocated for writing: there must be times for reading and times for writing, which should not be mixed.

Who is expected to read the paper?

Before the first version of the manuscript is actually written, the periodical for which the paper is destined must be chosen. In fact, the journal should be selected when the experiment is designed. Whether it should be sent to a general or to a subspecialty journal is a crucial question, and the pros and cons should be weighed up carefully by the author. A few helpful points for picking the most appropriate periodical follow:

1. Where were many of the recent papers to be cited in the new paper published?
2. Where do the scientists cited mostly publish their work?
3. Authors should read the advertising statements of society journals (and check society websites).
4. The "scope" paragraph in the "Instructions to Authors" is essential reading.
5. The Tables of contents of current issues of potential journals should be read to check whether any of the authors' names are familiar.

6. Several articles published in potential journals should be examined, for example to see how many figures and tables they have.

Most professional writers would say that when authors are writing they should please themselves, because the result will then also please its audience. This probably holds true in the case of a chapter in a novel. Unfortunately, such luxury does not apply to the writing of an original scientific paper: it is necessary to renounce personal gratification in favour of the technical aspects involved in the process of writing a scientific paper. The author should mentally pick out the toughest reviewer who might read the paper and pretend to be persuading him or her that the research reported is of the utmost importance.

Sequence

Once the journal has been selected, a realistic schedule for the work's progress must be fixed. A moderate approach is ideal, but the decision on how long it is going to take to write the paper must be sound and final. The schedule must be adhered to for a good outcome. Figures, tracings and tables come first, and form the basis for the writing of the Methods and Results sections. Discussion and Introduction follow, though not necessarily in this order. Not until the writing is well advanced should an author launch even a first attack on the Abstract and the Title.

Structure

A good article has a definite structure: it makes its point and does not waste space or time. This means that the most difficult element in writing a scientific paper is the planning of its structure. The reader must know where the authors began and where they are going to, and not get lost while reading the article. The biggest problems come first; when they have been dealt with the lesser ones are tackled.

Subheadings function as signposts to the reader. In early drafts of the manuscript subheadings in every paragraph are useful, but in the final version a subheading can never be used over a single paragraph. A scaffold of headings and subheadings obscures understanding of the paper; in fact three levels of subheadings are more than enough for typographical distinction.

Each section of the paper (Introduction, Methods, Results, Discussion, Abstract, and References) starts on a new sheet of paper. The first draft of the manuscript should be written in telegraphic style, ideas going onto the sheet of paper in random order for each of these sections. Any idea that might be even remotely related to the paper should be written down in no order whatsoever and not even in complete sentences. However, before the development of any part of the paper begins all these ideas must be numbered and put in order.

Writing tools

There are some books that are absolutely essential companions to a good writer: The first are a well-thumbed dictionary and a thesaurus, so that every word and its synonyms and shades of meaning can be checked out carefully. A waste paper bin easily accommodates unwanted bits of text, and good use of it is strongly recommended. Pencil, pen or computer? Whichever makes life easier is the best choice.

Methods section

Authors generally consider the "Methods" the easiest section to write because some of the material is usually contained in something they or one of the coauthors have already published. Obviously material cannot be taken from an earlier paper by anyone else. The Methods section must give enough information for an experienced investigator to be able repeat the work being reported. However, tiresome detail must be avoided at all costs. This is the first section of the paper in which subheadings should be used.

Results section

The Results section should be very concise. In order to accomplish this goal authors should always:
1. Refer to data (e.g. Fig. X, Table Y).
2. Refrain from repeating numeric data listed in tables in the text.
3. Replace a lot of numbers in the text by a table.
4. Repeat data from figures in the text only if particular precision is desired.

Introduction

This section defines the authors' credibility as investigators. A long boring Introduction will annoy reviewers, which increases the chances of the paper being rejected. Hence, a well-written Introduction will consist of no more than two or three paragraphs (restricted to a page and half of an average typescript, or about 450 words). The first paragraph introduces the broad area of interest, while the second presents the explicit rationale behind the work; the last one formulates the hypothesis.

In practice there are three rules of thumb that authors use when writing scientific manuscripts: first, they establish a territory by reviewing the previous work in the field, and begin to make generalisations; secondly, they create a niche by pointing out the gaps that exist in the field, by briefly discussing the findings in the literature, stressing the problems, giving the reasons for counterclaims and raising important scientific questions that need to be answered; finally, at the end of the Introduction the purpose of the study must be made clear: the niche is occupied.

Discussion

In the first paragraph of the Discussion the key findings are usually stated; if necessary the Abstract can be paraphrased, but a different sentence structure is strongly recommended. The last paragraph usually starts with "In summary, ..." or "In conclusion, ...": In the former case a brief summary follows, for which two or three sentences will suffice; speculation and "need more work" should be avoided; repetition of the key findings given in the first paragraph in the summary is inevitable, but different phrasing can persuade the reader that the paper is very important. Most authors recommend the use of a summary at both these points.

The last sentence is the most difficult, because it conveys the conclusion, the most important message of the paper, and the author generally revisits points raised in the Introduction. The way to finish up any argument is always to return to the questions presented at the beginning, because this gives the work a feeling of symmetry.

Each paragraph between the first and the last discusses a major result. The focus should always be on the author's own results, with no discussion of earlier work that does not involve reference to the current study. It must be borne in mind that the text is to be published as a scientific paper and not a review article, in which it would be correct for other investigators' results to be discussed separately. Almost every sentence will be linked to the current study; if any are not, it is necessary to take a long hard look at them. Tables and figures should be cited whenever necessary to clarify and shorten the text.

Abstract

A good abstract is written in précis format. It must be informative, not descriptive, and must be packed with information. Numbers can be used, but not to excess. At the same time the abstract must be easily read. The author must be aware that the abstract is one important determinant of whether the paper will be read and that abstracts are distributed freely in databases.

Title

The title should maximise information in the smallest possible number of words: fewer than 12 words or 100 characters will do. The title represents the label of the paper. It should almost never contain abbreviations, but results can be stated. A title in question form may have more impact on readers, because it will be easier for them to understand what issue(s) the paper intends to tackle.

Figures

On average the figures and tables make up one-third of the manuscript, and authors should therefore devote a great deal of attention to them. They represent the kernel of the report. Figures should be complete before writing begins. Experienced writers keep their eyes on the figures while preparing the text. Some simple rules of thumb must be borne in mind for good figures to be produced:

1. Redraw, redraw, prune clutter.
2. Reduce nondata ink as much as possible.
3. Do not use more than four lines, all solid; distinction through different symbols is recommended.
4. Minimise the number of tick marks and do not number each one.
5. Lettering should be uniform, lowercase, with bold fonts avoided; and after reduction to final size the lettering should be 2–3 mm high.
6. It is advisable not to have a caption as part of a figure.
7. Reduce the figure to one column width in the journal in which it is to be published (use a reduced photocopy to check it out).
8. The original figure should not be more than 3 times the size of the final one.

The legend itself should be sufficiently informative for figure+legend to be comprehensible as a "stand-alone" unit. The reader should be able to glean the information from each figure without going back to the text.

Tables

A table should also be a single unit that can be understood without referring to the text. Prune columns and rows, then reprune and reprune again: if the table occupies more than one sheet of paper it will be redrawn. If a line can be calculated from two other lines, it should be removed: authors should keep in mind that it is their primary data that count. Some novice authors believe that listing vast quantities of numbers will improve their credibility, but the true situation is rather the reverse. Very narrow and very wide tables should be avoided; some tables may look better if rotated through 90°. Vertical or horizontal lines should be avoided. If a table is too small the data will be moved to the text. Table titles should be concise.

About writing

This section is addressed directly to anyone proposing to write a scientific paper or papers for publication. Writing should be done at specific times; during these periods do not read (reading has its own predetermined times). Once writing is under way ideas will come to mind during or after the writing periods. Do not wait for inspiration from the muses: work hard, because writing is a craft rather than an art, and like any craft it must be practised again and again. Writing skills can be improved by reading good writers, especially good nonmedical writers. Reading and writing are related actions that provide inspiration for each other. Remember that any craft is learned by imitation.

Momentum

Experience has shown that a writing schedule must be fixed in advance, and monitoring progress may prove really important. Imagine writing one page a week: can there be a better means of torture? Skip trouble spots, leave them for later. Obey your biological clock: some people feel fresh in the early hours of the day, while others come alive in the evening. Write every day in your 'prime time', leaving less difficult activities for the rest of the day. Remember that there is no such thing thing as writer's block, and keep up your momentum.

Concentration

A good writing session requires a stretch of several hours. When time is short something else can be done instead: preparing, revising, etc. Avoid distractions: put away telephone, beeper, and everything else that can interrupt the session. Some people may feel inspired by the ocean or a field of corn, but a great many writers choose a dull corner as the place where they can reach and maintain the deepest concentration.

First draft

Write the first draft as quickly as possible, as if you were thinking out loud. You should get everything down, with no regard for spelling, grammar or style. Troublesome words are skipped over at this stage. No correction or rewriting should ever be done until the whole text is on paper, because this would hamper flow and rhythm. In addition, write the text with no help at all from the co-authors in this phase; in the worst-case scenario with preparation of the manuscript split among the co-authors the result would be a very patchy piece of nonsense.

Good writing

Good writing for a scientific paper depends mostly on the author's need to express his/her very important ideas, which is different from writing because the author wants to say something. There is a message underneath it all. A well-written paper should:

1. Convey accurate information (accuracy).
2. Be clear.
3. Be precise (with the right words used to convey your thoughts at all times–precision).
4. Have logic running through it and glueing it together.
5. Exhibit a logical order of presentation (maintained by logic).

Avoid ambiguity, inconsistency, and woolliness in the text and be concise (fewest possible words, short words). Always simplify the text, as in the following examples:

- In a considerable number of cases = often
- The majority of = most
- Small in size = small
- A greater number = more
- At the present time = now
- A considerable proportion = many
- Give rise to = cause
- In some cases = sometimes
- Is defined as = is
- On the basis of = by
- Pooled together = pooled
- Subsequent to = after
- With the result that = so that

Use and misuse of English

- Tense: Previously published work is an accepted piece of information and it is therefore described and discussed in the present tense. Your own work represents something that has been done but is not yet part of the universal "truth", so that it is referred to it in the past tense.
- Voice: The active voice is more precise and less wordy than the passive. Name the agent, even using "I" or "we".
- Singulars and plurals can be very tricky. Take special care with words in Latin.
- Punctuation: For young investigators it is better to use too many commas than too few. Do not forget the commas before "respectively" and "which".
- Hyphens: If the description comes before the noun the hyphen should be used, whereas the hyphen cannot be used if the description follows the noun.
- Pile-ups of nouns or phrases: These abound in scientific writing. English allows the use of nouns as adjectives. When more than two of these qualifying nouns are employed the sentence becomes hard to understand. Some prepositions should be added.
- Numbers: Spell out one to nine; use numerals for 10 and higher. Ordinals should be spelt out. If there is a number at the beginning of a sentence, rephrase it to avoid spelling out the number.

Bad writing

Bad writing must be suspected when words do not do justice to your ideas. It must be avoided, because multiple mistakes in spelling and syntax will lead reviewers to suspect that the study was characterised by similar sloppiness.

Style

Aim for a clear, orderly presentation that reads comfortably. Writing must be straightforward, linear and scientific. Science is not literature.

Writing

During the preparation of a paper a great deal of rewriting takes place. Reshape, refine and tighten up the text. Juggle words, change sentences around and keep on trying. Use the waste paper bin frequently. Strengthen transitions between sentences, so that no break in the narrative flow is apparent. After several drafts ask for a second opinion, if possible from an experienced researcher not active in your own field of interest. If the text is clear to him/her, it is probably fine.

Another important point is the avoidance of clutter. All first drafts have too many words. In successive drafts vigorous pruning is highly recommended; every sentence can probably be stripped. Excessive use of adverbs and adjectives contribute to clutter. In fact, writing improves in proportion to the deletion of unnecessary words.

Abbreviations and acronyms are popular with authors but anathema to readers. Reading should not require a glossary. Use of unwieldy words should be restricted.

Convey only one idea in a sentence that needs to be kept short (under 20 words. The length of the sentences must be varied throughout the text to keep it fluid. Remember that longer sentences involve a greater risk of grammatical error. Avoid excessive length.

There needs to be a connection from one paragraph to the next, but paragraphs differ from sentences in that the line of thinking is broken between them. The paragraph is the unit of thought and consists of a group of sentences. Normally it looks like a not-too-long solid block of printing containing not more than 125 words.

The paper should read like a story that the reader follows from start to end. Writing is sequential, and logic is the glue. If you use smooth transitions between sentences and paragraphs in your text the reader will later get the feeling that every step is inevitable.

Rewriting

The secret of writing is rewriting, and the secret of rewriting is rethinking. Stop when the new version is worse than the previous one: this means it is time to submit the paper for publication.

Typing

Clean typing on one side of the paper only reflects the profile of a careful professional. Margins should be wide (2.5 cm). There will be a check for adherence to the style of the journal. As a rule, to ensure that a clean document is submitted the experienced researcher proofreads, proofreads, and proofreads again.

Authorship

The authorship should be decided as early as possible in the process of writing a scientific paper, or preferably before the work to be reported starts. The key principle is that authorship should include only persons who can take public intellectual responsibility for the content, meaning that they

1. Can defend the intellectual content, including data and conclusions.
2. Must be willing to concede any errors publicly.
3. Must be willing, in the case of fraud, to make a public statement about its nature and extent, and account for its occurrence.

Criteria for authorship

All the following three criteria must be met:

1. Generation of at least part of the intellectual content (conception or design of the work, data analysis and interpretation).
2. Drafting, reviewing or critical revision with reference to important intellectual content.
3. Final approval of the version to be published.

Order of authorship

In some journals alphabetical order is used.

In most, however, it is assumed that the order in the paper as submitted is based on the individual authors' significance for the study. Thus, the first author is primarily responsible for collecting and analysing data and for writing the draft manuscript. The last will be an established investigator who assumes overall responsibility for the study. Any authors in between are listed in declining order of importance in the study.

Authorship responsibilities

With submission of a paper for publication, author(s) declare that:

1. The paper is not currently under consideration for publication elsewhere and that the research reported will not be submitted for publication elsewhere until a final decision has been made as to its acceptability for the journal it is submitted to.
2. The paper is a truthful report of original work, without fabrication, fraud, or plagiarism;
3. The authors named have each made an important scientific contribution to the study and are thoroughly familiar with the primary data.
4. All the authors have read the complete paper and take responsibility for its content and completeness, and they understand that if the paper, or any part of the paper, is found to be faulty or fraudulent, they share the responsibility.

Conflict of interest disclosure

All funding sources supporting the work and all institutional or corporate affiliations of the authors must be acknowledged. The authors must certify that they have no commercial association (e.g., consultancies, stock, ownership, equity interests, patent-licensing arrangements), except as disclosed in a separate attachment, that might represent a conflict of interest in connection with the article submitted (letter attached).

Benefits of writing

Last but not least, let us mention the benefits of writing. The benefits to the author are greater than any to the reader, because they enhance clear thinking and lead to invaluable mental discipline. Writing improves reading skills and satisfies a creative instinct.

Acknowledgement

The authors would like to thank Dr. Martin J. Tobin for contributing concepts included in the section "Writing up your scientific paper".

References

1. Mulrow CD (1987) The medical review article: state of the science. Ann Intern Med 106:485-488
2. Mulrow CD (1994) Systematic Reviews: rationale for systematic reviews. BMJ 309:597-599
3. Kleijnen J, Knipschild P (1992) The comprehensiveness of Medline and Embase computer searches. Searches for controlled trials of homoeopathy, ascorbic acid for common cold and *Ginkgo biloba* for cerebral insufficiency and intermittent claudication. Pharm Weekbl Sci 14:316-320
4. Woods D, Trewheellar K (1998) Medline and Embase complement each other in literature searches (letter; comment). BMJ 316:1166
5. Topfer LA, Parada A, Menon D et al (1999) Comparison of literature searches on quality and costs for health technology assessment using the MEDLINE and EMBASE databases. Int J Technol Assess Health Care 15:297-303
6. Watson RJ, Richardson PH (1999) Identifying randomized controlled trials of cognitive therapy for depression: comparing the efficiency of Embase, Medline and PsycINFO bibliographic databases. Br J Med Psychol 72:535-542
7. Minozzi S, Pistotti V, Forni M (2000) Searching for rehabilitation articles on MEDLINE and EMBASE. An example with cross-over design. Arch Phys Med Rehabil 81:720-722
8. Haynes RB, Wilczynski N, McKibbon KA et al (1994) Developing optimal search strategies for detecting clinically sound studies in MEDLINE. J Am Med Inform Assoc 1:447-458
9. McKibbon K, Walker-Dilks C (1994) Beyond ACP Journal Club: how to harness Medline for diagnostic problems. ACP J Club September/October:A10-A12

10. Shojania KG, Bero LA (2001) Taking advantage of the explosion of systematic reviews: an efficient MEDLINE search strategy. Eff Clin Pract 4:157-162
11. Robinson KA, Dickersin K (2002) Development of a highly sensitive search strategy for the retrieval of reports of controlled trials using PubMed. Int J Epidemiol 31:150-153
12. Jacobi J, Fraser GL, Coursin DB et al (2002) Clinical practice guidelines for the sustained use of sedatives and analgesics in the critically ill adult. Crit Care Med 30:119-141
13. MacIntyre NR, Cook DJ, Ely EW, Jr et al (2001) Evidence-based guidelines for weaning and discontinuing ventilatory support: a collective task force facilitated by the American College of Chest Physicians; the American Association for Respiratory Care; and the American College of Critical Care Medicine. Chest 120 (6 Suppl):375S-395S
14. Hirsh J, Warkentin TE, Shaughnessy SG et al (2001) Heparin and low-molecular-weight heparin: mechanisms of action, pharmacokinetics, dosing, monitoring, efficacy, and safety. Chest 119 (1 Suppl):64S-94S
15. Phillips B, Ball C, Sackett D et al. Oxford Centre for Evidence-based Medicine Levels of Evidence
16. Sackett DL, Wennberg JE (1997) Choosing the best research design for each question [editorial]. BMJ 315:1636
17. Doll R, Hill A (1952) The study of aetiology of carcinoma of the lung. BMJ II:1271-1986
18. Sackett D (1979) Bias in analytic research. J Chron Dis 32:51-63
19. Pocock S (1983) Clinical trials: a practical approach. Wiley, Chichester
20. Hulley S, Cummings S, Browner W et al (2001) Designing clinical research: an epidemiologic approach, 2nd edn. Lippincott / Williams & Wilkins, Philadelphia
21. Ebrahim G, Sullivan K (1995) Mother and child health research methods, 1st edn. Book-Aid, London
22. Chambers G, Fairbarn M (1998) Clinical trial design: an introduction to good clinical trial design and the protection of human subjects. Appl Clin Trials 7:60-66
23. Spilker B (1996) Fundamental principles, considerations, and techniques in the interpretation of clinical data. Guide to clinical trials. Lippincott-Raven, Philadelphia, pp 505-558
24. Detsky A, Naglie I (1995) Subgroup analyses: primary and secondary. ACP J Club May/June: A12-A14
25. Cook D, Sacket D (1992) On the clinically important difference. ACP J Club September/October: A16-A17
26. Federal Register (1997) 62(90):25691-25709
27. Medical Research Council (1998) MRC Guidelines for Good Clinical Practice. Clin Trials 1-49
28. The National Commission for the Protection of Human Subjects of Biomedical and Behavioral Research (1979) The Belmont Report. http://ohrp.osophs.dhhs.gov/humansubjects/guidance/belmont.htm
29. Hilsden R, Verhoef M (2000) Beginner's guide to the research proposal. Centre of Advancement of Health, University of Calgary, Calgary, Canada
30. Hulley S, Cummings S, Browner W et al (2001) Designing clinical research: an epidemiologic approach, 2nd edn. Lippincott / Williams & Wilkins, Philadelphia
31. ALLHAT Collaborative Research Group (2000) Major cardiovascular events in hypertensive patients randomized to doxazosin vs chlorthalidone: the antihypertensive and lipid-lowering treatment to prevent heart attack trial (ALLHAT). JAMA 283:1967-1975
32. Oxman AD, Sackett DL, Guyatt GH (1993) Users' guides to the medical literature. I. How to get started. The Evidence-Based Medicine Working Group. JAMA 270:2598-2601
33. Jaeschke R, Guyatt GH, Sackett DL (1994) Users' guides to the medical literature. III. How to use an article about a diagnostic test. B. What are the results and will they help me in caring for my patients? The Evidence-Based Medicine Working Group. JAMA 271:1615-1619
34. Jaeschke R, Guyatt G, Sackett DL (1994) Users' guides to the medical literature. III. How to use an article about a diagnostic test. A. Are the results of the study valid? Evidence-Based Medicine Working Group. JAMA 271:703-707

35. Levine M, Walter S, Lee H et al (1994) Users' guides to the medical literature. IV. How to use an article about harm. (Evidence-Based Medicine Working Group) JAMA 272:234-237
36. Guyatt GH, Sackett DL, Cook DJ (1994) Users' guides to the medical literature. II. How to use an article about therapy or prevention. A. Are the results of the study valid? (Evidence-Based Medicine Working Group) JAMA 271:59-63
37. Guyatt GH, Sackett DL, Cook DJ (1994) Users' guides to the medical literature. II. How to use an article about therapy or prevention. B. What were the results and will they help me in caring for my patients? (Evidence-Based Medicine Working Group) JAMA 271:389-391
38. Laupacis A, Wells G, Richardson WS, Tugwell P (1994) Users' guides to the medical literature. V. How to use an article about prognosis. (Evidence-Based Medicine Working Group) JAMA 272:234-237
39. Wilson MC, Hayward RS, Tunis SR et al (1995) Users' guides to the Medical Literature. VIII. How to use clinical practice guidelines. B. what are the recommendations and will they help you in caring for your patients? (The Evidence-Based Medicine Working Group) JAMA 274:1800-1804
40. Richardson WS, Detsky AS (1995) Users' guides to the medical literature. VII. How to use a clinical decision analysis. A. Are the results of the study valid? (Evidence-Based Medicine Working Group) JAMA 273:1610-1613
41. Hayward RS, Wilson MC, Tunis SR et al (1995) Users' guides to the medical literature. VIII. How to use clinical practice guidelines. A. Are the recommendations valid? (The Evidence-Based Medicine Working Group) JAMA 274:1630-1632
42. Oxman AD, Cook DJ, Guyatt GH (1995) Users' guides to the medical literature. VI. How to use an overview (see comments). (Evidence-Based Medicine Working Group) Can J Psychiatry 40:97-101
43. Naylor CD, Guyatt GH (1996) Users' guides to the medical literature. XI. How to use an article about a clinical utilization review. (Evidence-Based Medicine Working Group) CMAJ 155:1263-1268
44. Naylor CD, Guyatt GH (1996) Users' guides to the medical literature. X. How to use an article reporting variations in the outcomes of health services. (The Evidence-Based Medicine Working Group) JAMA 275:1435-1439
45. Guyatt GH, Sackett DL, Sinclair JC et al (1996) Users' guides to the medical literature. IX. A method for grading health care recommendations. (Evidence-Based Medicine Working Group) JAMA 275:554–558 (erratum in JAMA 275:1232)
46. Guyatt GH, Naylor CD, Juniper E et al (1997) Users' guides to the medical literature. XII. How to use articles about health-related quality of life. (Evidence-Based Medicine Working Group) Nurs Stand 11:32-33
47. Dans AL, Dans LF, Guyatt GH, Richardson S (1997) Users' guides to the medical literature: XIV. How to decide on the applicability of clinical trial results to your patient (see comments). (Evidence-Based Medicine Working Group) Ned Tijdschr Geneeskd 141:1804-1806
48. Drummond MF, Richardson WS, O'Brien BJ et al (1997) Users' guides to the medical literature. XIII. How to use an article on economic analysis of clinical practice. A. Are the results of the study valid? (Evidence-Based Medicine Working Group) JAMA 277:1802-1806
49. O'Brien BJ, Heyland D, Richardson WS et al (1997) Users' guides to the medical literature. XIII. How to use an article on economic analysis of clinical practice. B. What are the results and will they help me in caring for my patients? (Evidence-Based Medicine Working Group) JAMA 278:144-151 (erratum in JAMA 278:1064)
50. Bucher HC, Guyatt GH, Cook DJ (1999) Users' guides to the medical literature. XIX. Applying clinical trial results. A. How to use an article measuring the effect of an intervention on surrogate end points. (Evidence-Based Medicine Working Group) JAMA 282:771-778
51. Barratt A, Irwig L, Glasziou P et al (1999) Users' guides to the medical literature. XVII. How to use guidelines and recommendations about screening. (Evidence-Based Medicine Working Group) JAMA 281:2029-2034
52. Richardson WS, Wilson MC, Guyatt GH et al (1999) Users' guides to the medical literature. XV.

How to use an article about disease probability for differential diagnosis. (Evidence-Based Medicine Working Group) JAMA 281:1214-1219
53. Guyatt GH, Sinclair J, Cook DJ, Glasziou P (1999) Users' guides to the medical literature. XVI. How to use a treatment recommendation. (Evidence-Based Medicine Working Group and the Cochrane Applicability Methods Working Group) JAMA 281:1836-1843
54. Guyatt GH, Haynes RB, Jaeschke RZ et al (2000) Users' Guides to the Medical Literature. XXV. Evidence-based medicine: principles for applying the Users' Guides to patient care. (Evidence-Based Medicine Working Group) JAMA 284:1290-1296
55. McAlister FA, Straus SE, Guyatt GH, Haynes RB (2000) Users' guides to the medical literature. XX. Integrating research evidence with the care of the individual patient. (Evidence-Based Medicine Working Group) JAMA 283:2829-2836
56. McGinn TG, Guyatt GH, Wyer PC et al (2000) Users' guides to the medical literature. XXII. How to use articles about clinical decision rules. (Evidence-Based Medicine Working Group) JAMA 284:79-84
57. Hunt DL, Jaeschke R, McKibbon KA (2000) Users' guides to the medical literature. XXI. Using electronic health information resources in evidence-based practice. (Evidence-Based Medicine Working Group) JAMA 283:1875-1879
58. Giacomini MK, Cook DJ (2000) Users' guides to the medical literature. XXIII. Qualitative research in health care: A. Are the results of the study valid? (Evidence-Based Medicine Working Group) JAMA 284:357-362
59. Richardson WS, Wilson MC, Williams JW Jr et al (2000) Users' guides to the medical literature. XXIV. How to use an article on the clinical manifestations of disease. (Evidence-Based Medicine Working Group) JAMA 284:869-875
60. Giacomini MK, Cook DJ (2000) Users' guides to the medical literature. XXIII. Qualitative research in health care: B. What are the results and how do they help me care for my patients? (Evidence-Based Medicine Working Group) JAMA 284:478-482
61. Guyatt G, Rennie D (eds) (2002) Users' guide to the medical literature: American Medical Association, Chicago
62. Sackett DL, Straus SE, Richardson WS et al (2000) Evidence based medicine: how to practice and teach EBM. Churchill Livingstone, Edinburgh
63. Bennett CL, Connors JM, Carwile JM et al (2000) Thrombotic thrombocytopenic purpura associated with clopidogrel. N Engl J Med 342:1773-1777
64. Moseley JB, O'Malley K, Petersen NJ et al (2002) A controlled trial of arthroscopic surgery for osteoarthritis of the knee. N Engl J Med 347:81-88
65. Pocock S (1983) Clinical trials: a practical approach. Wiley, Chichester
66. Schulman S, Rhedin AS, Lindmarker P et al (1995) A comparison of six weeks with six months of oral anticoagulant therapy after a first episode of venous thromboembolism. Duration of Anticoagulation Trial Study Group. N Engl J Med 332:1661-1665

Suggested further reading

Alley M (1996) The craft of scientific writing, 3rd edn. Springer, New York
Booth WC, Colomb GG, Williams JM (1995) The craft of research. University of Chicago Press, Chicago
Christensen LB (1997) Experimental methodology, 7th edn. Allyn & Bacon, Needham Heights
Dixon WJ, Massey FJ Jr (1983) Introduction to statistical analysis, 4th edn. McGraw-Hill, New York
Fox J (1984) Linear statistical models and related methods: with applications to social research. Wiley, New York
Glantz SA (1992) Primer of biostatistics, 3rd edn. McGraw-Hill, New York

Glantz SA, Slinker BK (1990) Primer of applied regression and analysis of variance. McGraw-Hill, New York
Hennekens CH, Buring JE (1987) Epidemiology in medicine. Lippincott Williams & Wilkins, Philadelphia
International Conference on Harmonisation of Technical Requirements for Registration of Pharmaceuticals for Human Use - http://www.ich.org/ich1.html
Madansky A (1988) Prescriptions for working statisticians. Springer, New York
Matthews JR, Bowen JM, Matthews RW (2000) Successful scientific writing, 2nd edn. Cambridge University Press, Cambridge
Milliken GA, Johnson DE (1984) Analysis of messy data, vol I: Designed experiments. van Nostrand–Reinhold, New York
Mosteller F, Rourke REK (1973) Sturdy statistics: nonparametrics and order statistics. Addison-Wesley, Reading
Myers RH (1986) Classical and modern regression with applications. Duxbury Press, Boston
Ott L (1984) An introduction to statistical methods and data analysis, 3rd edn. PWS-Kent, Boston
Regulatory Framework for Clinical Trials with Medicines in Europe - http://www.efpia.org/ and http://www.efpia.org/6_publ/document/clinical.pdf
Rothman KJ, Greenland S (1998) Modern epidemiology, 2nd edn. Lippincott-Raven, Philadelphia
Snedecor WS, Cochran WG (1980) Statistical methods, 7th edn. The Iowa State University Press, Iowa City
Sprent P (1993) Applied nonparametric statistical methods. Chapman & Hall, London
Weisberg S (1985) Applied linear regression, 2nd edn. Wiley, New York
Winer BJ, Brown DR, Michels KM (1991) Statistical principles in experimental design, 3rd edn. McGraw-Hill, New York
Zar JH (1984) Biostatistical analysis, 2nd edn. Prentice-Hall, Englewood Cliffs

INDEX

GPSR Compliance

The European Union's (EU) General Product Safety Regulation (GPSR) is a set of rules that requires consumer products to be safe and our obligations to ensure this.

If you have any concerns about our products, you can contact us on ProductSafety@springernature.com

In case Publisher is established outside the EU, the EU authorized representative is:

Springer Nature Customer Service Center GmbH
Europaplatz 3
69115 Heidelberg, Germany

Batch number: 10704763

Printed by Printforce, the Netherlands